Antimicrobial Therapy in the Elderly Patient

INFECTIOUS DISEASE AND THERAPY

Series Editors

Brian E. Scully, M.B., B.Ch.
Harold C. Neu, M.D.

College of Physicians & Surgeons
Columbia University
New York, New York

1. Parasitic Infections in the Compromised Host, *edited by Peter D. Walzer and Robert M. Genta*
2. Nucleic Acid and Monoclonal Antibody Probes: Applications in Diagnostic Methodology, *edited by Bala Swaminathan and Gyan Prakash*
3. Opportunistic Infections in Patients with the Acquired Immunodeficiency Syndrome, *edited by Gifford Leoung and John Mills*
4. Acyclovir Therapy for Herpesvirus Infections, *edited by David A. Baker*
5. The New Generation of Quinolones, *edited by Clifford Siporin, Carl L. Heifetz, and John M. Domagala*
6. Methicillin-Resistant *Staphylococcus aureus*: Clinical Management and Laboratory Aspects, *edited by Mary T. Cafferkey*
7. Hepatitis B Vaccines in Clinical Practice, *edited by Ronald W. Ellis*
8. The New Macrolides, Azalides, and Streptogramins: Pharmacology and Clinical Applications, *edited by Harold C. Neu, Lowell S. Young, and Stephen H. Zinner*
9. Antimicrobial Therapy in the Elderly Patient, *edited by Thomas T. Yoshikawa and Dean C. Norman*
10. Viral Infections of the Gastrointestinal Tract: Second Edition, Revised and Expanded, *edited by Albert Z. Kapikian*

Additional Volumes in Production

Development and Clinical Uses of Haemophilus b Conjugate Vaccines, *edited by Ronald W. Ellis and Dan M. Granoff*

Herpesvirus Infections, *edited by Ronald Glaser and James F. Jones*

Immunotherapy of Infections, *edited by K. Noel Masihi*

Pseudomonas aeruginosa Infections and Treatment, *edited by Aldona L. Baltch and Raymond P. Smith*

Chronic Fatigue Syndrome, *edited by Stephen Straus*

Antimicrobial Therapy in the Elderly Patient

edited by

Thomas T. Yoshikawa
United States Department of Veterans Affairs and
George Washington University School of Medicine
Washington, D.C.

Dean C. Norman
West Los Angeles Veterans Affairs Medical Center and
University of California School of Medicine
Los Angeles, California

Marcel Dekker, Inc. New York • Basel • Hong Kong

Library of Congress Cataloging-in-Publication Data

Antimicrobial therapy in the elderly patient / edited by Thomas T. Yoshikawa, Dean C. Norman.
p. cm.—(Infectious disease and therapy; 9)
Includes bibliographical references and index.
ISBN 0-8247-9163-0 (alk. paper)
1. Geriatric pharmacology. 2. Anti-infective agents. I. Norman, Dean C. II. Series: Infectious disease and therapy; v.9.
[DNLM: 1. Anti-Infective Agents—therapeutic use. 2. Communicable Diseases—drug therapy. 3. Communicable Diseases—in old age. W1 IN406HMN v.9 1994 / QV 250 A6313 1994]
RC953.7.A56 1994
615'.329—dc20
DNLM/DLC
for Library of Congress 93-44026
CIP

The publisher offers discounts on this book when ordered in bulk quantities. For more information, write to Special Sales/Professional Marketing at the address below.

This book is printed on acid-free paper.

Marcel Dekker, Inc.
270 Madison Avenue, New York, New York 10016

Current printing (last digit):
10 9 8 7 6 5 4 3 2 1

PRINTED IN THE UNITED STATES OF AMERICA

To our wives, Catherine and Jane,
for their constant love and support

Series Introduction

Marcel Dekker, Inc., has for many years specialized in the publication of high-quality monographs in tightly focused areas in a variety of medical disciplines. These have been of great value to both the practicing physician and the research scientist as sources of detailed and up-to-date information presented in an attractive format. During the last decade, there has been a veritable explosion in knowledge in the various fields related to infectious diseases and clinical microbiology. Antimicrobial resistance, antibacterial and antiviral agents, AIDS, Lyme disease, infections in immunocompromised patients, and parasitic diseases are but a few of the areas in which an enormous amount of significant work has been published. The Infectious Disease and Therapy series covers carefully chosen topics that should be of interest and value to the practicing physician, the clinical microbiologist, and the research scientist.

Brian E. Scully, M.B., B.Ch.
Harold C. Neu, M.D.

Foreword

A decade ago, Tom Yoshikawa published an article highlighting the emerging importance of geriatric infectious disease (1). His article struck a particularly responsive chord in me at the time, because I was at a stage in my own career when I decided to address most of my remaining energy to geriatrics. Dr. Paul Beeson was then editing the *Journal of the American Geriatrics Society*, and I was honored to succeed him in this endeavor 3 years later. Initially, I was reluctant to do so because, aside from a passion for promoting primary, comprehensive, continuing, and preventive care for the elderly, I felt uncredentialed as a geriatrician. Not to be denied, however, was also a lifelong research obsession to enter the contest between host and parasite armed with this medical era's most precious gift of a spectacular antibiotic armamentarium. Dr. Beeson persuaded me that such credentials might be a good start for an editor of a geriatrics journal.

Now, as a grandfathered geriatrician and observant infectious disease-oriented internist, I have watched with much interest the emerging clinical art and science of the management of infections in the world's burgeoning old and old–old human population. Dr. Yoshikawa's prophetic article now has been superseded by a text that records the growing body of clinical experience concerning the use of antibiotics in the elderly. The challenge to apply these interventions skillfully deserves the earnest attention of the great majority of currently practicing physicians.

I take great pleasure in this text's organization and presentation. Drs. Yoshikawa and Norman present antibiotic therapy with a full understanding of the special problems that the knowledgeable use of these remarkable agents requires in aging hosts whose defenses are so commonly assailed by a variety of compromises. These compromises are clearly and concisely described. Comorbidity, organ failure, systemic disease, malnutrition, and senescence of some components of the immune system conspire to make the selection and administration of an antibiotic a paradigm of clinical acumen and judgment.

All of these factors are faithfully considered in the chapters on the use of each of the major classes of antibiotics as well as the particular pharmacodynamics of the agent in aging and compromised hosts who are particularly susceptible to drug side effects and vulnerable to drug interactions in settings of geriatric polypharmacy. Finally, the special use of antibiotics in the varying venues of geriatric treatment—the community, home, and nursing home rather than nosocomial settings alone—are addressed in specific chapters with which many physicians need to become increasingly expert.

Antibiotic therapy must be a basic clinical skill for all primary physicians for whom infectious diseases are "bread and butter" practice. With the graying of the population, geriatric care is consuming an increasing share of such practice. Drs. Yoshikawa and Norman have responded to a timely educational need in fine fashion by assembling this very practical and enjoyable text.

Gene H. Stollerman, M.D.
Co-Editor, *Hospital Practice*

REFERENCE

1. Yoshikawa TT. J Am Geriatr Soc 1983; 31:34–39.

Preface

Infections are among the top 10 causes of death in the geriatric population, and are often the most frequent cause of hospitalization for nursing home residents. Proper and timely treatment of infections in elderly patients requires a broad understanding of the special problems and unique aspects of managing these diseases. This book provides broad and in-depth analysis of the most up-to-date information on antimicrobial therapy in older adults.

Currently, there are many textbooks on infectious diseases, as well as a half-dozen books on infections in the elderly patient. However, they provide only a superficial description of antimicrobial biochemistry, pharmacology, clinical indications, dosage, and toxicity. Moreover, special issues and problems associated with treating older patients with antibiotics are not discussed. There is a need for detailed, current information on the proper approach to antimicrobial therapy in the elderly patient. In addition, special concerns such as therapy in nursing homes or at home—common problems facing practicing clinicians—are not dealt with in standard texts on infectious disease. *Antimicrobial Therapy in the Elderly Patient* is unique because it focuses on the geriatric patient and provides such needed information. Each chapter relates data and information in the context of the aging or elderly patient, and the special problems or needs of this age group are discussed in depth.

Chapters on appropriate antimicrobial therapy for seriously ill elderly patients and for ambulatory older adults, as well as antimicrobial prophylaxis and vaccinations, are also provided. Since no textbooks currently available in the field are similar to this one, infectious disease specialists and primary care physicians as well as geriatric specialists caring for elderly patients will find this book invaluable and of practical clinical use. In addition, pharmacists and pharmacologists can use it as a reference for information on antibiotic pharmacology in elderly persons.

Thomas T. Yoshikawa
Dean C. Norman

Contents

Contributors

Ariane An, Pharm. D. Resident, Geriatric Pharmacy, Geriatric Research, Education and Clinical Center, Veterans Affairs Medical Center–West Los Angeles, Los Angeles, California

Roger E. Bawdon, M.S., Ph.D. Associate Professor, Department of Obstetrics and Gynecology, The University of Texas Southwestern Medical Center, Dallas, Texas

Keith Beck, M.D. Associate Professor of Medicine, Division of Allergy and Clinical Immunology, Department of Medicine, Harbor-UCLA Medical Center, Torrance, and UCLA School of Medicine, Los Angeles, California

Bradley S. Bender, M.D. Chief, Division of Infectious Diseases, Geriatric Research, Education, and Clinical Center, Veterans Affairs Medical Center, Gainesville, Florida

Steven L. Berk, M.D. Professor and Chairman, Department of Internal Medicine, East Tennessee State University, Johnson City, Tennessee

Gloria Carandang Staff Research Associate, Division of Infectious Diseases, Department of Medicine, University of California–Irvine, Orange, California

Steven C. Castle, M.D. Assistant Professor of Medicine and Research Career Development Fellow, Multicampus Programs in Geriatrics and Gerontology, University of California, and Veterans Affairs Medical Center–West Los Angeles, Los Angeles, California

Mary Cesario, R.N. University of California–Irvine, Orange, California

Thomas C. Cesario, M.D. Professor and Chairman, Department of Medicine, University of California–Irvine, Orange, California

Chester Choi, M.D. Associate Clinical Professor, Department of Medicine, UCLA School of Medicine, Los Angeles, and St. Mary Medical Center, Long Beach, California

Anthony W. Chow, M.D. Chief, Division of Infectious Diseases, University of British Columbia, Vancouver, British Columbia, Canada

Burke A. Cunha, M.D. Chief, Infectious Disease Division, Winthrop-University Hospital, Mineola, and Professor, State University of New York School of Medicine, Stony Brook, New York

John S. Czachor, M.D. Associate Professor, Division of Infectious Diseases, Department of Medicine, Wright State University School of Medicine, and Miami Valley Hospital, Dayton, Ohio

Paul J. Drinka, M.D. Clinical Professor, Departments of Internal Medicine and Geriatrics, University of Wisconsin, Madison, and Wisconsin Veterans Home, King, Wisconsin

Asim K. Dutt, M.D. Chief, Medical Services, Department of Medicine, Alvin C. York Veterans Affairs Medical Center, Murfreesboro, and Meharry Medical College, Nashville, Tennessee

David M. Forrest, M.D., F.R.C.P.C. Senior Fellow, Department of Medicine, University of British Columbia, Vancouver, British Columbia, Canada

Richard A. Gleckman, M.D. Professor of Medicine, Boston University School of Medicine, and Director of Medicine, Carney Hospital, Boston, Massachusetts

Fred M. Gordin, M.D. Chief, Division of Infectious Diseases, Veterans Affairs Medical Center, Washington, D.C.

Stefan Gravenstein, M.D. Assistant Professor, Section on Geriatrics, Department of Medicine, University of Wisconsin, Madison, Wisconsin

David R. P. Guay, Pharm. D. Associate Professor, College of Pharmacy, University of Minnesota, Minneapolis, and Clinical Specialist, Geriatric Pharmacy Program, St. Paul-Ramsey Medical Center, St. Paul, Minnesota

Daniel Hancz, Pharm. D. Supervisor, Los Angeles County Regional Poison and Drug Information Center, Department of Poison and Drug Information, Los Angeles County–USC Medical Center, Los Angeles, California

Hearee Chung Julius, Pharm. D. Clinical Pharmacist, Department of Pharmacy, Harbor-UCLA Medical Center, Torrance, and Adjunct Assistant Professor of Pharmacy Practice, University of Southern California School of Pharmacy, Los Angeles, California

Carol A. Kauffman, M.D. Chief, Infectious Diseases Section, Department of Veterans Affairs Medical Center, and Professor, Department of Internal Medicine, University of Michigan Medical School, Ann Arbor, Michigan

Natalie C. Klein, M.D. Associate Director, Infectious Disease Division, Winthrop-University Hospital, Mineola, and State University of New York School of Medicine, Stony Brook, New York

Stephen A. Landis, Pharm. D. Ambulatory Care Pharmacist, Department of Pharmacy Services, Kaiser Permanente Hospital, Woodland Hills, California

Bengt Ljungberg, M.D., Ph.D. Associate Professor, Department of Infectious Diseases, University Hospital, Lund, Sweden

Mary Y. Ma, Pharm.D. Antimicrobial Clinical Specialist, Pharmacy Service, Veterans Affairs Medical Center–West Los Angeles, Los Angeles, California

Shookooh Yousefi Malekpour, Ph.D. Associate Professor, Department of Medicine, University of California–Irvine, Orange, California

Hope Marlow, M.A., Pharm.D. Clinical Pharmacist, Department of Pharmacy, Alvin C. York Veterans Affairs Medical Center, Murfreesboro, Tennessee

Glenn E. Mathisen, M.D. Associate Clinical Professor, Department of Medicine, Olive View-UCLA Medical Center, Sylmar, California

Jack D. McCue, M.D. Professor of Medicine and Vice-Chairman, Baystate Medical Center, Springfield, and Tufts University School of Medicine, Boston, Massachusetts

Barbara A. Miller, R.N. Senior Clinic Nurse Specialist, Institute on Aging, Madison, Wisconsin

Maury Ellis Mulligan, M.D. Staff Physician and Associate Clinical Professor of Medicine, Division of Infectious Diseases, Veterans Affairs Medical Center, Long Beach, and University of California–Irvine, Orange, California

Pamela H. Nagami, M.D. Clinical Associate Professor of Medicine, University of California School of Medicine, Los Angeles, and Infectious Diseases Section, Department of Internal Medicine, Kaiser Permanente Hospital, Woodland Hills, California

Ingrid Nilsson-Ehle, M.D., Ph.D. Associate Professor, Department of Infectious Diseases, University Hospital, Lund, Sweden

Dean C. Norman, M.D. Associate Professor of Medicine, University of California, and Chief of Staff, Veterans Affairs Medical Center–West Los Angeles, Los Angeles, California

Lynette H. Posorske, M.D. Division of Infectious Diseases, Veterans Affairs Medical Center, Washington, D.C.

William L. Quinn, M.D. Associate Chief of Staff, Division of Geriatrics and Extended Care, Department of Medicine, Department of Veterans Affairs Medical Center, Waco, and Associate Professor, Department of Medicine, Texas A&M School of Medicine, College Station, Texas

Jay P. Rho, Pharm.D. Associate Professor of Clinical Pharmacy, School of Pharmacy, University of Southern California School of Medicine, and Director, Department of Pharmacy, Shriners Hospital, Los Angeles, California

Ronald A. Sherman, M.D., M.Sc. (Lond.) Staff Physician and Director, Geriatric Evaluation and Management Program, Divisions of Geriatrics and Infectious Disease, Medical Service, Veterans Affairs Medical Center, Long Beach, and Assistant Clinical Professor, Department of Medicine, University of California–Irvine, Orange, California

Kimberly A. Shriner, M.D. Infectious Disease Specialist, Teaching Faculty, Huntington Memorial Hospital, Pasadena, California

Fawn C. S. Takemoto, Pharm.D. Resident in Geriatric Pharmacy, Geriatric Research, Education, and Clinical Center, Veterans Affairs Medical Center–West Los Angeles, Los Angeles, California

Edward G. Tessier, R.Ph., M.P.H. Clinical Pharmacist, Baystate Medical Center, Springfield, and Adjunct Assistant Professor of Clinical Pharmacy, Massachusetts College of Pharmacy and Allied Health Sciences, Boston, Massachusetts

Haragopal Thadepalli, M.D. Professor of Medicine, UCLA School of Medicine and Charles R. Drew University of Medicine and Science, and Chief, Geriatric Section, Department of Internal Medicine, King/Drew Medical Center, Los Angeles, California

Elizabeth Anne Williams, M.D., Ph.D. Assistant Professor, Department of Internal Medicine, East Tennessee State University, Johnson City, Tennessee

Leonard Williams, M.D. Clinical Pharmacology Fellow and Clinical Instructor, Department of Medicine, Geriatric Research, Education, and Clinical Center, Veterans Affairs Medical Center, and University of Florida College of Medicine, Gainesville, Florida

Thomas T. Yoshikawa, M.D. Adjunct Professor of Health Care Science, George Washington University School of Medicine, and Assistant Chief Medical Director, Office of Geriatric and Extended Care, United States Department of Veterans Affairs, Washington, D.C.

Darwin E. Zaske, Pharm.D. Professor, College of Pharmacy, University of Minnesota, Minneapolis, and Director of Pharmaceutical Services, St. Paul-Ramsey Medical Center, St. Paul, Minnesota

Antimicrobial Therapy in the Elderly Patient

1

Unique Aspects of Infection in Older Adults

Thomas T. Yoshikawa
George Washington University School of Medicine and United States Department of Veterans Affairs, Washington, D.C.

I. INTRODUCTION

A. Historical Perspective

Throughout the history of mankind, infectious diseases have been the major causes of death and morbidity (1). Until the mid–twentieth century, such diseases as typhoid fever, diphtheria, typhus, plague, smallpox, tuberculosis, scarlet fever, rheumatic fever, leprosy, syphilis, poliomyelitis, bacterial meningitis, measles, and pertussis accounted for the deaths, disabilities, deformities, functional limitations, and social rejection of hundreds of millions of people (1). Indeed, infectious disease was the major life-threatening and life-shortening process in modern civilization until in the early 1900s.

With the advent of antiseptics, asepsis, vaccination, antimicrobials, and public health measures, many of the life-threatening and disabling types of infectious diseases have been dramatically reduced in frequency or nearly eliminated during the past 50 years (2). The outcome of these advances in medicine was the reduction of infant and child mortality as well as deaths in younger adults. Hence, populations from modern civilization in recent times have experienced a dramatic increase in life expectancy, both in males and females. People are living longer, resulting in a rapid growth of the elderly population.

In early 1900, Americans 65 years of age and older comprised only 4% of the total U.S. population. Life expectancies for the average white male and female child in 1900 were 47 and 50 years, respectively. In contrast, the average American white male and female child born today have life expectancies of about 73 and 80 years, respectively (3). In addition, older adults have also increased their longevity. For example, a white female American at age 65 can expect to live, on the average, for another 19 years (3). The result of these demographic changes is an expanding population of elderly persons, not only in the so-called "young-old" age group (65–75 years), but also in the "old-old" age category (75 and older).

Table 1 Infections That Increase in Frequency in Older Adults

Pneumonia
Urinary tract infection
Sepsis
Skin and soft tissue infection
Tuberculosis
Infective endocarditis
Cholecystitis
Diverticulitis
Liver abscess
Herpes zoster

Although the rapid growth of an aging population has resulted in the major causes of death in the United States to shift to such illnesses as arteriosclerotic heart disease, stroke, and cancer, infection nevertheless remains a common and serious cause of death and complications in older adults. Moreover, many common infectious diseases increase significantly in terms of frequency, morbidity, and mortality with advancing age. Thus, it is somewhat ironic that the modern advances of medicine against infections, which served to increase longevity and improve the quality of life of older people, have also facilitated the reemergence of infectious diseases in this population. Infections that increase in frequency with advancing age are shown in Table 1 (4).

B. Predisposition to Infections

What factors ostensibly place the aging person at greater risk for infections? To understand these factors, it is important to be aware of the pathogenesis of infectious diseases. It is beyond the scope of this chapter to describe the details of pathogenetic mechanisms leading to infections. However, simplistically speaking, the risk and severity of infection can be expressed by the following equation (5):

$$\text{Infection (risk or severity)} = \frac{\text{Inoculum} \times \text{Virulence}}{\text{Host Resistance}}$$

That is, the risk or severity of infection is directly proportional or related to the amount of organism exposed (inoculum) and to the invasiveness (virulence) of the organism and inversely related to the integrity of the host's defense mechanism (host resistance).

With aging, physiological changes occur that result in anatomical and physiological decrements. Mechanical barriers such as skin and mucosa—the first line of host resistance to microbes—undergo structural and functional decline with age. Immune dysregulation and immune deficiency are well-described phenomena accompanying aging. Furthermore, age-related chronic diseases may significantly compromise host defenses in older adults. (A detailed discussion on aging and host defenses is found in the following chapter.)

Older persons are hospitalized and institutionalized at higher rates than young adults. They are, thus, at greater risk of exposure to more microorganisms as well as more virulent pathogens. Hospital-acquired and nursing home–acquired infections often occur with such organisms as gram-negative bacilli and methicillin-resistant *Staphylococcus aureus*

Table 2 Relative Death Rates for Infections in Older Versus Young Adults

Infections	Death rate[a]
Pneumonia	3
Kidney infection	5–10
Sepsis	3
Appendicitis	15–20
Cholecystitis	2–8
Tuberculosis	10
Infective endocarditis	2–3
Bacterial meningitis	3

[a]Number of times higher in older versus younger adult.

(MRSA) (6–8). When compared to younger patients, the nosocomial infection rate is approximately threefold higher in elderly patients (9).

II. MORTALITY AND MORBIDITY

A. Increased Mortality with Age

Not only does the frequency of infections rise with age, death rates also increase significantly in older adults with serious infectious diseases (10). Table 2 summarizes the relative death rate of specific infections in older versus younger adults (11–18). Multiple factors contribute to higher mortality in association with aging (19). These factors include:

1. Lack of adequate physiological reserve capacity in various organs and organ systems, which mitigates appropriate responses and recovery from acute stress such as infection
2. Compromised host defense mechanisms, which permit infection to progress locally as well as spread systemically
3. Presence of chronic underlying diseases that invariably accompany aging and themselves will also reduce reserve capacities and host resistance
4. Greater exposure to serious and virulent pathogens through nosocomial exposure, which includes such organisms as gram-negative bacilli and MRSA
5. Delays in diagnosis and treatment because of atypical clinical manifestations of infectious diseases in older adults and reluctance to proceed with invasive diagnostic procedures and potentially toxic therapies
6. Poorer tolerance to invasive diagnostic and therapeutic interventions (e.g., surgery)
7. Delayed and/or poorer responses to antimicrobial therapy with age
8. Higher rate of adverse drug reactions including antibiotics in elderly patients.

B. Increased Morbidity with Age

When compared to younger patients, older adults suffer greater complications when they contract an infectious disease. Those factors that contribute to higher mortality in elderly infected patients also adversely impact on the rate and severity of complications of infections in this population (19).

Several examples of higher morbidity of infections in aging adults can be cited. Pneumonia in older patients is associated with more bacteremia, extrapulmonary sites of infection, delayed resolution, and compromise of pulmonary function (11,20,21). Urinary tract infection is more often complicated by bacteremia and recurrence or persistence with advancing age (22,23). Intraabdominal infections such as appendicitis, cholecystitis, and diverticulitis are more frequently associated with perforation, gangrene, abscess, or sepsis in elderly patients (14). Herpes zoster or shingles not only increases in incidence with age, but the dreaded complication of postherpetic neuralgia occurs primarily in persons 60 years of age and older (24,25). With tuberculosis, disseminated disease appears to occur more often in older adults (16). Dissemination, in turn, results in extrapulmonary forms of tuberculosis (e.g., tuberculous meningitis, skeletal tuberculosis).

III. DIVERSE ETIOLOGY OF INFECTIONS

Although infections in older adults are often caused by pathogens that are commonly isolated in younger patients with the same infection, a significant number of instances occur when the etiology of an infectious disease is quite different or diverse in older persons in comparison to the younger population. These differences must be recognized in infected older patients, especially if they are seriously ill and empiric therapy with antimicrobial agents is contemplated. A few examples of common infectious diseases serve to illustrate these differences.

Community-acquired bacterial pneumonia in the general (younger) population is caused primarily by *Streptococcus pneumoniae*. In contrast, in older patients with bacterial pneumonia, *S. pneumoniae* remains the most common etiology but is less frequently isolated, and such pathogens as *Hemophilus influenzae*, *Staphylococcus aureus*, *Legionella* sp., and enterobacterial gram-negative bacilli are increasingly more common than in younger patients (26–29). Hospital-acquired pneumonia does not appear to be associated with age-related differences in etiology, but good comparison studies are lacking (30). Nursing home–acquired pneumonia is caused predominantly by *S. pneumoniae* and enterobacterial gram-negative bacilli (31). Because young adults comprise only a small percentage of nursing home patients, comparative data on causes of pneumonia are not available.

Urinary tract infection (UTI) in the general population is a disease primarily of sexually active women. In young adults, *Escherichia coli* is overwhelmingly the most common isolate in uncomplicated UTI (32,33). With increasing age, both anatomical and functional abnormalities of the genitourinary tract become more prevalent, and may be one explanation for the high incidence of UTI and bacteriuria in the elderly population. In addition, there is a lesser frequency of isolation of *E. coli* from the urine in noncatheterized older adults, with an increased rate of culturing other gram-negative bacilli as well as *Enterococcus* sp. and coagulase-negative staphylococci (34,35). However, age appears to have no significant impact on the causes of bacteriuria in chronically catheterized patients.

Meningitis is a life-threatening infectious disease with serious complications. Thus, a knowledge of the most frequent meningopathogens is essential for selecting appropriate antimicrobial therapy. In young adults, viruses (e.g., enteroviruses) and such bacteria as *S. pneumoniae* and *Neisseria meningitidis* are the dominant causes of meningitis (37). In adults older than 60 years of age, viral meningitis is relatively uncommon; meningitis is most often caused by *S. pneumoniae*, *Listeria monocytogenes*, and gram-negative bacilli (38,39).

IV. CLINICAL MANIFESTATIONS OF INFECTIONS

Infections, much like other illnesses or diseases in elderly persons, may not manifest clinically with typical or usual symptoms and signs. A review of this topic is discussed in Chapter 3.

V. AGE EFFECTS ON PHARMACOLOGY OF ANTIBIOTICS

Age has an impact on drug pharmacokinetics and pharmacodynamics. Thus, age-related changes in antibiotic pharmacology must be considered when prescribing antimicrobial therapy (see Chap. 4).

VI. APPROACH TO ANTIMICROBIAL THERAPY

Chapter 26 will focus on principles of antimicrobial therapy.

It has already been mentioned that in older adults with infections, mortality and morbidity is greater, clinical manifestations may be atypical, etiology may be diverse, and antibiotic pharmacology may be altered. Given these conditions and circumstances, as well as the need to minimize hospitalization and drug costs, the general approach to antimicrobial therapy in geriatric patients is somewhat different from that of younger patients. There are three important concepts to consider in antimicrobial therapy of elderly patients:

1. Begin empiric antimicrobial therapy sooner because of the higher mortality and morbidity, difficulty in confirming a specific etiological agent, and desire to reduce length of hospitalization.
2. Broad-spectrum antibiotics should be prescribed if there is no specific etiological diagnosis because the pathogens are often diverse and polymicrobial.
3. Aminoglycoside antibiotics should be avoided whenever possible because of their high incidence for untoward renal and otological complications.

Some specific suggestions in the diagnosis and treatment of infectious diseases in older patients are the following:

1. Consider infections in the differential diagnosis of any older patient with a change in functional status or feeling of well-being.
2. Determine the most likely site(s) of infection by history, physical examination, underlying illness, and residential setting (home, hospital, nursing home).
3. Obtain *rapidly* all necessary diagnostic tests, including blood cultures for seriously ill patients.
4. Determine if hospital care is needed or appropriate.
5. If empiric therapy is warranted, beta-lactam antibiotics should be considered in most instances.
6. After culture or other microbiological data become available, appropriate drug changes should be made.
7. Adverse effects should be closely monitored.
8. Oral antibiotics should be prescribed (if the drug is available in oral preparation) as soon as the patient's clinical condition stabilizes.

In summary, infectious diseases are common causes of mortality and morbidity in the geriatric population. The etiology, clinical manifestations, diagnosis, and treatment of infections in older patients present unique challenges and opportunities for practicing clinicians.

REFERENCES

1. Lyons AS, Petrucelli RJ II. Medicine. An illustrated history. New York: Harry N. Abrams Inc. Publishers, 1978.
2. Yoshikawa TT. Geriatric infectious diseases: an emerging problem. J Am Geriatr Soc 1983; 31:34–9.
3. U.S. Senate Special Committee on Aging, American Association of Retired Persons, Federal Council on Aging, U.S. Administration on Aging. Aging america, trends and projections. Washington, DC: DHHS Publication No. (FCOA) 91-28001, 1991.
4. Yoshikawa TT. Important infections in elderly persons. West J Med 1981; 135:441–5.
5. Yoshikawa TT, Norman DC. Predisposing factors to infection. In: Aging and clinical practice: infectious diseases. Diagnosis and treatment. New York: Igaku-Shoin Inc., 1987:8–19.
6. Alvarez S, Shell CG, Woolley TW, Berk SL, Smith JK. Nosocomial infections in long-term facilities. J Gerontol 1988; 1:M9–17.
7. Emore TG, Banerjee SH, Culver DH, Gaynes RP, Horan TC, Edwards JR, Jarvis WR, Tolson JS, Henderson TS, Martone WJ, Hughes JM. Nosocomial infections in elderly patients in the United States, 1986–1990. Am J Med 1991; 91(suppl 3B):289–93.
8. Bradley SF, Terpenning MS, Ramsey MA, Zarins LT, Jorgensen KA, Sottile WS, Schaberg DR, Kauffman CA. Methicillin-resistant *Staphylococcus aureus* colonization and infection in a long-term care facility. Ann Intern Med 1991; 115:417–22.
9. Freeman J, McGowan JE Jr. Risk factors for nosocomial infection. J Infect Dis 1978; 138:811–19.
10. Yoshikawa TT, Norman DC. Aging and infectious diseases. In: Pathy MSJ, ed. Principles and practice of geriatric medicine, 2d ed. Chichester, England: John Wiley & Sons Ltd., 1991:313–18.
11. Marrie TJ, Haldane EV, Faulkner RS, Durant H, Kwan C. Community-acquired pneumonia. Is it different in the elderly? J Am Geriatr Soc 1985; 33:671–80.
12. Kunin CM. Detection, prevention and management of urinary tract infections, 4th ed. Philadelphia: Lea & Febiger, 1987:1–55.
13. Hodgin UG, Sanford JP. Gram-negative rod bacteremia: an analysis of 100 patients. Am J Med 1965; 39:952–60.
14. Norman DC, Yoshikawa TT. Intraabdominal infections: diagnosis and treatment in the elderly. Gerontology 1984; 30:327–38.
15. Fry DE, Cox RA, Harbrecht JB. Gangrene of the gallbladder. South Med J 1981; 74:666–8.
16. Yoshikawa TT. Tuberculosis in aging adults. J Am Geriatr Soc 1992; 40:178–87.
17. Cantrell M, Yoshikawa TT. Aging and infective endocarditis. J Am Geriatr Soc 1983; 31:216–22.
18. Gorse GJ, Thrupp LD, Nudleman KL, Wyle FA, Hawkins B, Cesario TC. Bacterial meningitis in the elderly. Arch Intern Med 1984; 144:1603–7.
19. Yoshikawa TT. Impact of aging on host response to infectious diseases. In: Wood WG, Strong R, eds. Geriatric clinical pharmacology. New York: Raven Press, 1987:107–13.
20. Austrian R, Gold J. Pneumococcal bacteremia with special reference to bacteremic pneumococcal pneumonia. Ann Intern Med 1964; 60:759–76.
21. Chang JI, Mylotte JM. Pneumococcal bacteremia. Update from an adult hospital with a high rate of nosocomial cases. J Am Geriatr Soc 1987; 35:747–54.
22. Gleckman RA, Bradley PJ, Roth RM. Bacteremic urosepsis. A phenomenon unique to elderly women. J Urol 1985; 133:174–5.

23. Gleckman R, Crowley M, Natsios GA. Therapy of recurrent invasive urinary-tract infection. N Engl J Med 1979; 301:878–80.
24. Harnisch JP. Zoster in the elderly: clinical, immunologic and therapeutic considerations. J Am Geriatr Soc 1984; 32:789–93.
25. Schmader KE, Studenski S. Are current therapies useful for the prevention of post-herpetic neuralgia? A critical analysis of the literature. J Gen Intern Med 1989; 4:83–9.
26. Verghese A, Berk SL. Bacterial pneumonia in the elderly. Medicine (Balt.) 1983; 62:271–85.
27. Bentley DW. Bacterial pneumonia in the elderly: clinical features, diagnosis, etiology, and treatment. Gerontology 1984; 30:297–307.
28. Marrie TJ, Durant H, Yates L. Community-acquired pneumonia requiring hospitalization: 5-year prospective study. Rev Infect Dis 1989; 11:586–99.
29. Venkatesan P, Gladman J, MacFarlane JT, Barer D, Berman P, Kinnear W, Finch RG. A hospital study of community acquired pneumonia in the elderly. Thorax 1990; 45:254–8.
30. Bartlett JG, O'Keefe P, Tally FP, Louie TJ, Gorbach SL. Bacteriology of hospital-acquired pneumonia. Arch Intern Med 1986; 146:868–71.
31. Yoshikawa TT. Treatment of nursing home-acquired pneumonia. J Am Geriatr Soc 1991; 39:1040–1
32. Latham RH, Wong ES, Larson A. Laboratory diagnosis of urinary tract infection in ambulatory women. JAMA 1985; 254:3333–6.
33. Stamm WE, Hooton TM, Johnson JR, Johnson C, Stapleton A, Roberts PL, Moseley SL, Fihn SD. Urinary tract infections: from pathogenesis to treatment. J Infect Dis 1989; 159:400–6.
34. Baldassarre JS, Kaye D. Special problems of urinary tract infection in the elderly. Med Clin North Am 1991; 75:375–90.
35. Mims AD, Norman DC, Yamamura RH, Yoshikawa TT. Clinically inapparent (asymptomatic) bacteriuria in ambulatory elderly men: epidemiological, clinical, and microbiological findings. J Am Geriatr Soc 1990; 38:1209–14.
36. Warren JW. The catheter and urinary tract infection. Med Clin North Am 1991; 75:481–93.
37. Broome CV, Schlech WF III. Recent developments in the epidemiology of bacterial meningitis. In: Sande MA, Smith AL, Root RK, eds. Bacterial meningitis. Contemporary issues in infectious diseases, Vol. 3. New York: Churchill Livingstone, 1985:1–10.
38. Karandanis D, Shulman JA. Recent survey of infectious meningitis in adults: review of laboratory findings in bacterial, tuberculous and aseptic meningitis. South Med J 1969; 69:449–57.
39. Choi C. Bacterial meningitis. Clin Geriatr Med 1992; 8:889–902.

2

Age-Related Changes in Host Defenses

Steven C. Castle
University of California, and Veterans Affairs Medical Center—West Los Angeles, Los Angeles, California

I. INTRODUCTION

Dramatic developmental changes occur with the involution of the thymus gland (1–3), which is perhaps the most significant change of any organ postgestation. Thus, it is not surprising that changes in host defenses with aging, and particularly the immune system, are of pivotal importance in understanding the susceptibility of diseases in elderly persons (4). However, the fact that not all older people succumb to an infection or malignancy despite these significant developmental changes in the thymus gland suggests that there are extrathymic sources that begin taking over some of the function of the involuted thymus. Nonetheless, a better understanding of the mechanisms involved in the loss or alteration in immunological response with aging provides some of the most promise in developing strategies to improve health and prevent diseases in older adults.

There is extensive evidence that elderly people, even those with vigorous lifestyles, are at an increased risk for infections, as well as experience more severe complications. While many of the changes in host defenses are thought to be part of "normal aging," the clinical relevance of these changes to the increased risk of infections has remained unclear. At this point in time, it appears that these "normal aging" changes in the immune function predispose and interact with other diseases and external factors, which then results in a shift in the "infection equation" toward a higher incidence and severity of infections (5). Subtle, normal aging changes in the immune system in concert with changes in other factors that might occur in the presence of age-related diseases (e.g., diabetes mellitus, atherosclerosis, or chronic pulmonary disease) or external factors (e.g., invasive procedures or malnutrition) may affect host resistance and hence predispose the older person to an increased risk of infection. Knowledge of age-related changes in host defenses, diseases of aging that adversely affect host resistance, and other factors that compromise the integrity of the immune system may permit clinicians to identify high-risk older patients for infection. Such high-risk patients should be managed more vigorously in preventive interventions (e.g., immunoprophylaxis, chemoprophylaxis, prevention of aspiration), as well as aggressive treatment for their infections.

II. CHANGES IN THE SKIN AND MUCOCUTANEOUS BARRIERS

The skin and mucosal epithelial lining are the first and most important barriers to infection because of their physical obstruction and inherent microbicidal properties. Many of the biological changes of the skin are accelerated and accentuated by photo-aging caused by extensive sunlight exposure (7). Structurally, with aging, the epidermis is thinner, corneocytes are less adherent to each other, and there is a flattening of the epidermal-dermal junction (8). There is a general decline in the cellularity of the epidermis and dermis with a decline in the number of melanocytes and Langerhans cells (local tissue antigen-presenting cells, which are thought to be of monocyte lineage). There are changes in the matrix of the dermis as a result of alteration in the composition of collagen, elastin, and glycosaminoglycans. Subcutaneous tissue is reduced in areas that have the most exposure to the external environment, such as the shins, hands, feet, and the face. The secretory output of most glands, including eccrine, apocrine, and sebaceous glands, is reduced or attenuated with aging. All of these changes result in a decreased rate of growth of the epidermis, hair, and nails; delayed wound healing; reduced dermal clearance of fluids and foreign materials; and compromised vascular responsiveness in older adults. Specific changes in the "skin immune system" are not as well characterized, but they are likely to be significant and contribute to the difficulty in accurately assessing the immunological status of the frail elderly (9). The skin immune system is thought to play a role in the increased incidence of benign or malignant epidermal neoplasm (10). Otherwise, these changes in skin immunity result in an increased susceptibility to blister formation, injury, and a break in the barrier to the dermis and underlying tissue; delayed onset and resolution of blisters and weals; persistent contact dermatitis; and increased risk of wound infections (11). Changes in the skin and the risk of complications, especially skin and soft tissue infections, are much higher in certain disease states and conditions, such as diabetes mellitus, severe peripheral vascular disease, malnutrition, and chronic pulmonary disease, as well as in patients with either reduced sensation in the skin or reduced functional status (12).

III. CHANGES IN PRIMARY IMMUNITY

Primary immunity involves defense mechanisms of tissues or the circulation that are activated without prior exposure to a pathogen. Primary immunity has a cellular (neutrophils, macrophages and monocytes, and natural killer cells) as well as a humoral component (complement cascade) and is extremely important in quickly suppressing the spread of an infection, especially bacterial infections.

A. Phagocytosis (Neutrophils/Macrophages/Monocytes)

Direct engulfing of organisms is frequently the next line of defense after mucocutaneous barriers; phagocytosis can be performed by local tissue macrophages, circulating monocytes, or neutrophils. The efficacy of phagocytosis in defending against invading microbes involves several complex steps, including the number of cells (e.g., neutropenic patients are at great risk for recurrent bacterial infections), the ability of cells to reach the site of infection (adhering to endothelium, moving out of the capillary and moving toward the pathogen by chemotaxis), and the ability to engulf and kill (lysis) the organism (13). With the much higher incidence and mortality of many bacterial infections in elderly persons, such as pneumococcal pneumonia, it would be anticipated that leukocyte function would show deterioration with age. There are a number of studies addressing the integrity of the properties of aging phagocytic cells, but with quite varied results (14,15). Some studies show little impact of age, while others show significant deterioration in leukocyte function. This variability is largely due to differences in populations studied and laboratory methods utilized. Studies on aging mice provide the ability to avoid the confounding influence of chronic diseases and other conditions. Senescent mice (26–28 month C57BL/6) raised in pathogen-free environments showed a greater neutrophil influx to the lungs in response to the deposition of type 3 *Streptococcus pneumoniae* than younger animals (8–10 months), and no difference in survival rates were detected. While there are significant limitations to extrapolating this animal data to human infections, it does not appear that advanced age itself results in an attenuation of the pulmonary inflammatory reaction to infection with type 3 *S. pneumoniae* (16). A study looking at neutrophil function with age in humans also failed to show any difference in in vitro tests (resting adherence to endothelium, random and directed migration, phagocytosis-induced chemiluminescence, and granule secretory behavior) from those of healthy young controls. However, in vivo delivery of neutrophils into skin abrasions was reduced in elderly subjects, and the study also demonstrated a smaller increase in the endothelial adhesion glycoprotein CD11 (17) in the older group. Therefore, it appears that either aging has little clinical impact on neutrophil function, or there are specific functional abnormalities that are difficult to detect, such as the impact of age on neutrophil function in a stressed situation, as in an actual infection. One study that assessed neutrophil function of an ambulatory elderly cohort in a longitudinal manner over 7 years demonstrated a significant deterioration in chemotaxis and elevation of serum lipid peroxidase levels in those who did not survive (18). Macrophage activation is an important step in improving the efficacy of tissue macrophages in engulfing organisms and is especially important in the defense against *Mycobacterium tuberculosis* (19). Macrophage activation has been shown to be facilitated by the cooperation of T lymphocytes via interferon-gamma (20). Other studies on the increased susceptibility of old mice to *M. tuberculosis* suggested that this was due to the inability of aged mice to generate mediator T lymphocytes (T cells), which was based on reciprocal passive cell transfer experiments (21). While phagocytosis and the ability of circulating T cells to secret interferon-gamma generally appear normal with advanced age, perhaps the general age-related decline in T-cell function and, thus, a decrease in T-cell support of local phagocytosis during an infection results in a deterioration of phagocytosis efficiency with age. However, these changes are difficult to measure. Other cytokines may also be involved in modulating primary immunity and may be responsible for some of the changes that have been described. Interleukin-6 has been found to be antagonistic toward tumor necrosis factor alfa (TNF-α)–mediated activation of macrophages (22). Nonetheless, conditions such as diabetes mellitus (decreased neutrophil function) or malnutrition (decreased macrophage function) have shown to have more of an impact on primary immunity than age itself (14).

B. Complement

The limited studies assessing the effects of age on complement activity have not demonstrated a significant decline. However, some investigations have shown an increase in levels of CH50, or total complement activity, as well as an increase in C1q, C4, C3, C5, and C9 (14,17).

C. Natural Killer Cells

Natural killer (NK) cells are immune cells that appear to be primitive cells of either T cell or of monocyte lineage. They are able to provide lysis of foreign organisms or abnormal (infected or malignant) cells without prior exposure. NK cells may represent a phylogenetically old surveillance system and may be of particular importance in the defense against infections such as tuberculosis. NK-cell activity is modulated by many factors, including stress and exercise, and there is considerable variability in the ability to measure NK activity; hence, studies have shown much variability in the impact of age on NK function (23). However, the presence of an acute illness certainly results in a much larger decline in NK activity than does advanced age. This could be particularly relevant to many components of host defense, since NK cells are able to produce large amounts of interferon-gamma and may provide compensation for the decline in T-cell production of interferon-gamma.

IV. CHANGES IN SECONDARY IMMUNITY

Secondary immunity refers to immune function that is activated only after prior exposure to an organism and involves a complex interaction of cells (T cells, bursa-derived lymphocytes or B cells, and antigen-presenting cells—usually monocytes or macrophages) and cytokines (proteins produced by immune cells that act like hormones in regulating the immune response). There is substantial evidence that this component of host defense is the component most affected by aging and age-related diseases (3,23). Studies that use protocols to limit the confounding effects of disease and/or medications have found fewer immunological defects with aging than has been reported in the past (24). However, it must be emphasized that those patients who do show immune dysfunction (e.g., nursing home residents) are of the most clinical relevance because they are the patients who are most at risk of acquiring infections.

A. Cell-Mediated Immunity

Cell-mediated immunity (CMI) is the arm of the immune system that is dependent on T cells and is largely responsible for defense against intracellular pathogens including many viruses (herpes simplex and varicella-zoster viruses), some bacteria (*Legionella* spp. and *Listeria monocytogenes*) and fungi, and mycobacteria (2). Cell-mediated immunity is the component of host defenses that has shown the most consistent changes with aging, in both humans and animals. However, because of the extensive overlap and cross-communication of the various immune cells, deterioration in T-cell function will result in changes in other components of the immune system, especially in the primary antibody response (discussed in more detail later). It should also be emphasized that the spectrum of dysfunction varies from population to population and is more pronounced in the more frail, chronically ill, elderly person. Also, the level of impairment is more varied and less pronounced than the immunodeficiency of the acquired immunodeficiency syndrome (AIDS).

1. Antigen-Presenting Cells

Antigen-presenting cells (APC) include tissue macrophages, circulating monocytes, and occasionally B cells and are extremely important in initiating and amplifying any type of immune response. Therefore, because of the large variability in decline in immune function that is seen with aging, it might be expected that APCs would show definitive changes with aging. Studies have reported some variability of APC activity with advanced age, such as the ability to activate surface antigens (la^+ expression) that are necessary in antigen presentation because these surface markers are recognized by the class II major histocompatibility complex surface marker on T cells, as well as variability in monokine production (2,23). A more pronounced impact of age on APC function is shown following stimulation with phytohemagglutinin (PHA) than with stimulation of APC to the anti-T-cell antibody anti-CD3 (25). A more significant impact of age is also seen when systems are used that require direct T-cell–APC interaction and communication (25–27). Much of the diminished proliferation of peripheral blood mononuclear cells in the aged is abolished by the addition of exogenous interleukin-1 (IL-1) (28) or the addition of exogenous interferon-gamma (IFN-γ) (25). These studies strongly suggest that there is a deterioration of some specific cell–cell interaction. This may be a result of reduced expression and utilization of co-stimulatory pathways that are important in improving the efficiency of T-cell activation by stabilizing intercellular interactions. Adhesion molecules on the APC/T cell, respectively, that have been found to represent the ligand/receptor pair for co-stimulatory pathways include intercellular adhesion molecule-1 (ICAM-1)/leukocyte function–associated antigen-1 (LFA-1), LFA-3/LFA-2, the surface molecules B7/CD28, and vascular cell adhesion molecule-1 (VCAM-1) with the CD49d/CD29 integrin (29,30). Limited data on changes in TNF-$\propto$ suggest this may diminish with aging (31).

2. T-Cell Functional Changes

Despite the previously mentioned involution of the thymus gland with age (T-cell differentiation largely takes place in the thymus gland), elderly people still possess a generative compartment capable of maintaining homeostatic levels of peripheral T cells throughout life (4). Thus, extrathymic T-cell differentiation in older adults is largely taken over by other tissues and may include the bone marrow, liver and lymph nodes (32,44), or even the skin (33). However, there are specific identifiable changes with aging, both clinically and in laboratory indices, in secondary immunity that involve T cells and their ability to respond to stimulation from APCs and cytokines (1–4,23). These changes in T-cell function appear to be of a much larger magnitude than the previously mentioned changes in APCs. The clinical evidence to support these changes in T-cell function in elderly persons includes an increased incidence of infections by intracellular pathogens such as tuberculosis, listeriosis, and herpes zoster. Also, there is a dramatic decline in the delayed-type hypersensitivity (DTH) response, at least in the frail elderly person. Consistent changes in other indices of CMI include a diminished T-cell proliferation in response to certain mitogens. Diminished proliferation is more pronounced in the more chronically ill person, but it is also seen in genetically similar and pathogen-free laboratory animals and, hence, appears to be a consequence of "normal aging," though much heterogeneity has been found. Certain diseases and underlying conditions including depression (34), diabetes mellitus (35), and malnutrition (36) have been found to impair T-cell function in elderly persons. There is also evidence, at least in old (>24-month-old) mice, that there is reduced cytotoxic immune responses of T cells in influenza infection (37,38). Finally, perhaps the most clinically relevant example of a decline in T-cell function is its negative impact on primary antibody response to vaccination, particularly the more T-cell–dependent antibody responses to more complex antigens, such as influenza and hepatitis B (37). Specific potential mechanisms for these functional changes in T cells will be discussed.

3. Changes in T-Cell Phenotype

It has long been hypothesized that decreased T-cell function with aging is a result of less differentiated T cells as an outcome of thymic involution. Much progress has been made in recent years in the immunohistochemical determination of T-cell phenotype because of advances in monoclonal antibody technology. Despite these advances, the ability to detect "dysfunctional" cells based on a specific phenotype has not been successful, probably due to the large variation and confounding variables seen in the elderly population. Some studies have reported a decline in the CD8+ (suppressor/cytolytic) T-cell subset, with a resultant increase in the CD4 (helper)/CD8 T-cell ratio (37–37b). However, other studies, particularly those that carefully exclude patients with chronic disease, have failed to show these changes (38–42). One study, which analyzed results based on various clinical parameters, suggested that patients on multivitamins and mineral supplementation and those who smoked had a higher percentage of CD4+ T cells, while those receiving topical corticosteroids had a decreased percentage of CD8+ T cells (40). Other studies have investigated other phenotypic T-cell markers, including those for so-called "memory" or "educated" T cells. Memory T cells are thought to have a more robust and quicker proliferation response to specific antigens to which these memory T cells have been previously exposed and tend to produce higher levels of IL-2 in comparison with IL-4. (Changes in cytokine production with aging are discussed in more detail in the next section.) These memory T cells (with the Pgp-1+, CDw29+, CD45RO+, and CD45RBlo phenotype) are thought to have been previously activated by exposure to antigen and are thought to represent a higher percentage of T cells in the elderly population, humans as well as mice (41,43). However, despite the apparent accumulation of these cells with advanced age, these cells appear relatively refractory to stimuli in comparison to memory T cells from younger individuals (41). This suggests specific age and age-related disease changes in T-cell activation, especially in memory T cells.

4. Changes in Cytokines

As previously mentioned, there is some evidence suggesting that impaired cell-cell communication is a large contributor to the age-related immune dysfunction. Because of the important regulatory role cytokines play in eliciting an appropriately targeted immunological response, it seems likely that cytokines will be pivotal in understanding as well as developing treatment for age-related immune dysfunction. Since T cells are the immune cells most impacted by aging, T-cell cytokines are expected to be similarly affected. The cytokine that has been studied the most extensively in advanced age is IL-2. It appears that regardless of individuals or populations of young vs. old studied, a decline in the amount of IL-2 produced and a decline in the ability to express the high-affinity (Tac) IL-2 receptor (4,41,42,44–47,50) are found. However, using techniques such as in situ hybridization for IL-2 messenger RNA (50a) and autoradiographic techniques using [125 I]IL-2, the defect of IL-2 associated with aging is more likely to be due to a decline in the proportion of normally responding T cells and not a universal defect in all T cells, or even in the entire population of a specific subset of T cells (44,48). Reduced IL-2 receptor expression has been found to be more pronounced in CD8+ subsets (48,49) and proliferative capacity is most reduced in CD4+ subsets (51). Studies on populations have also shown that many of the functional defects in T cells (ability to proliferate, second messenger signaling, and cytotoxicity) are reversed with exogenous IL-2 added to in vitro systems (52). The clinical importance of these changes in IL-2 production was demonstrated in a study on elderly veterans who had a decline in IL-2 production in response to influenza vaccine (53). Although other cytokines have been less well studied in aging populations, the differential effects of certain cytokines (IL-1, IL-4, and IL-6) on the proliferative response of human CD4+ subsets have been shown (54). Therefore, other cytokines are likely to be involved in the dysfunctional activation of T-cell subsets in immunological responses in elderly persons. While the distinction between helper T-cell subsets is not as clear in humans as it is in mice, there is evidence that changes in the ability to regulate the relative activity of T helper-1 (TH-1), which favor IL-2 and IFNγ production and CMI, and the activity of T helper-2 (TH-2), which favor IL-4, IL-5, and IL-10 production and B-cell activity, are correlated with specific disease states (55–57). Therefore, either the overexpression (IL-6,IL-7?, IL-10) or underexpression (TNF, IL-1, IL-3, IL-12) of specific "regulatory" cytokines in specific tissues may be responsible for a shift toward a TH-2/IL-4–mediated response instead of a TH-1/IL-2–mediated response in older individuals (58).

5. *Changes in T-Cell Activation*

Most studies continue to support the model that the immune system in elderly persons is a mosaic of normal functioning cells (in comparison with cells from young adults) with some percentage of dysfunctional cells instead of the model in which all cells show a lesser, but uniform abnormality (44). As age increases, and more dramatically as disease or frailty increases, the percentage of dysfunctional cells increases in this mosaic model (44). In other words, with aging and age-related diseases, some T cells remain as functionally competent as T cells from young adults, while an increasing percentage of T cells appear refractory to a given stimuli and show specific abnormalities in T-cell activation. Evidence exists that defects in T-cell activation are more profound than changes in cytokine and cytokine receptor levels. That is, when the antigen/T-cell receptor binding is bypassed (using a phorbol ester and a calcium ionophore), T cells from healthy elderly persons can produce equivalent amounts of IL-2 and IL-2 receptors (as in young controls) but still demonstrate impaired proliferation (59).

There appears to be a very specific impairment with advanced age in the ability of T cells to enter the cell cycle. In mice, it has been shown that while 49% of T cells from young mice enter the cell cycle upon stimulation with concanavalin A, 69% of the T cells from old mice were unable to leave the G0-G1 phase and fail to enter into the cell cycle (60). There is evidence that a subset of T cells from aged animals have a reduced rise in intracellular calcium concentration upon stimulation with anti-CD3 (the monoclonal antibody to the T-cell receptor) or with phytohemagglutinin (PHA) (61). These changes in calcium flux appear to be restored with the addition of calcium ionophores and suggest there are some defects in calcium homeostasis, which appeared separate from the inositol phosphate role in determining intracellular calcium mobilization or channel activity since normal levels of inositol phosphates were detected (51,61,62). This reduced intracellular calcium flux has been reported in both CD4+ and CD8+ subsets, though it is also partly due to a reduced number of responding cells (63,64). The defect could also be in other steps involved in increasing cytosolic calcium, such as phospholipase C–induced hydrolysis of phosphoinositol 4,5-biphosphate (PIP2) (59).

With aging it appears that an increasing proportion of the T-cell population shows a general slowing and resistance to moving the cellular machinery to get the cell to enter cell cycle. Some defects in cytosolic second messenger activity have been well described.

Now, nuclear activity responsible for the gene activation from these second messenger steps are being evaluated, and are reviewed more extensively elsewhere (41,42). Studies on DNA methylation, one of the mechanisms involved in the regulation of developmentally relevant genes, have raised the possibility that age-related decreases in T-cell DNA methylation could be contributing to some of these changes in T-cell function (65). An example of this may be a study that showed reduced transcription of the proto-oncogene c-*myc* in the T cells from older individuals (66), which is critical for entry of cells from G0 to G1 phase of the cell cycle. Other evidence of alteration of gene activation of T cells involves studies on the age-related diminished cytotoxic lymphocyte (CTL) activity. Studies suggest that the reduced CTL activity in senescent mice is due to a decline of the expression of the perforin and two serine esterase genes, which appear important in CTL function (67,68).

In summary, whether changes in T-cell function are because of shifts in T-cell subsets (including T-helper "memory" subsets), changes from extrathymic T-cell differentiation, developmental changes of gene regulation of T-cell entry into the cell cycle, or reduced CTL activity, what is apparent is that there is an increasing percentage of "dysfunctional" T cells with advanced age, and especially with increasing frailty and accumulation of chronic diseases. The most dramatic functional impact of these changes described to date includes a decline in both IL-2 production and the ability to respond to IL-2 and a shift toward additional support of B-cell activities (perhaps an increase in IL-3 and IL-4). Clearly, with advanced age and increasing frailty, there is a definite decrease in cell-mediated immune responses along with a less effective primary antibody response and an enhanced autoantibody production. Whether this dysfunctional response is a primary T-cell abnormality or a failed compensation to maintain normal humoral immunity is an intriguing question that is not yet answered.

B. Humoral Immunity

Humoral immunity involves the activation of B cells to produce antibodies, which defend against primarily extracellular pathogens, including most bacterial infections. Age-related changes cause some spectrum of impaired regulation, including both a decreased ability to make specific antibody responses to immunization (and to infections) and an increased expression of autoantibodies. Whether this dysregulation is a consequence of primary B-cell or T-cell changes with aging continues to be debated (1,2,4,41,42). While there are clearly age-related changes in T-cell interaction with B cells, changes in the differential regulation of B-cell autoantibody precursors may also contribute to the rise in autoimmune phenomena and the decline in primary antibody response (41). The increased prevalence in auto-antiidiotypic antibodies in older subjects may result in inhibition of primary antibody formation because the auto-antiidiotypic antibodies bind to surface immunoglobulins on B cells and render them less responsive. However, aging has not been shown to have an effect on the total number of B cells or the total concentration of immunoglobulins, though there tends to be a gradual increase in some classes of immunoglobulins (IgA and IgG) with aging. The most important effect of age on humoral immunity is a general decrease in antibody response to specific antigens (2). Antibody responses can be classified as T-cell–independent (e.g., pneumococcal vaccine) and T-cell–dependent (e.g., influenza and tetanus toxoid vaccines). T-cell–independent response generally involves antibody response to smaller, more simple antigens and does not require as much support from T cells to drive antibody production as is required for more complex antigens. T-cell–independent antibody response tends to be less affected by age, except in the more frail nursing home population. Other confounding conditions such as malnutrition will further depress humoral response and should be corrected, if possible, prior to attempts at immunization procedures.

V. DETECTION OF AGE-RELATED IMMUNE DYSFUNCTION

It can be stated that the usual means to detect the presence of immune dysfunction may be unreliable or are untested in the elderly population, especially the frail nursing home population where the risk of infection is so high. There is substantial clinical and laboratory evidence that suggests DTH testing, the most accepted index of integrity of cell-mediated immunity (CMI), is unreliable in elderly populations (9,69). As stated earlier, this may be due to aging or disease-related changes in both the skin and the skin immune system. Regardless, this results in some difficulty in identifying precisely individuals at risk for infection, applying targeting criteria for measures of immunomodulation, or even accurately identifying specific pathogenetic mechanisms because of the "impure" nature of the study population.

VI. POTENTIAL IMMUNOMODULATION OF AGE-RELATED IMMUNE DYSFUNCTION

A. Hormones/Organ Grafts/Cytokines

Since the most impressive hallmark of immunosenescence is the dramatic decline in thymic hormone levels, it would be reasonable to assume that much of the age-related immune dysfunction could be reversed by thymic hormone replacement. In fact, the subcutaneous implanting of GH3 pituitary adenoma cells reversed thymic atrophy as well as the decline in the mitogenic response of T cells (70). Thymic implants, but only if done with bone marrow implants from 2-month-old mice into old (17 months) mice, normalized many immunological parameters. However, the effect only lasts about one third of the animal's lifespan, but could be boosted by repeated implantation (71). Other studies have shown both potentiation and suppression of immune reactivity to antigenic stimulation, depending on dose and type of thymic hormone (i.e., thymopentin, thymosin-α1, thymulin, THF-γ2) (41,72,73). Another study demonstrated a slight, but not significant, boost in antibody response to influenza vaccination by pretreating with thymosin-α1 (74). The reason thymic hormone replacement has not become widespread practice may be because of the difficulties in showing efficacy; this may be related to subtherapeutic doses, side effects, or an inability to appropriately target patients. With respect to targeting, it may be difficult to show a benefit when thymic hormones are given to a population as a whole because presumably some will not need them, some will be unable to respond to the hormones, and only a fraction will be able to benefit from them. An improved ability to identify patients who would or would not benefit may improve the efficacy of replacement therapy.

Other hormone replacement therapy may also have a role in boosting waning host defenses. Growth hormone therapy has been shown to reverse thymic involution and improve T-cell function in vitro and in vivo, and one study also observed an improvement in in vitro neutrophil activity (75). Cytokine therapy is likely to be developed in the future, because IL-2 has improved T-cell function in vitro in many studies, and IL-3 has been shown to reverse many immune parameters in old murine T cells (76). The use of

IL-2 liposome adjuvants has enhanced vaccine-induced protection of old mice against challenge with a lethal inoculum of influenza A virus (77).

Other methods that have shown or may show a boosting of the immune response involve the timing as well as co-administration of vaccines in an effort to strengthen the immunogenicity of the vaccines and perhaps increase T-helper cell support of the antibody response (78).

B. Pharmacological and Dietary Intervention

Clearly, the correction of specific nutritional deficiencies, especially protein-energy malnutrition and zinc deficiency, may improve immune function and should be considered in any patient who presents with recurrent infections. Also, these patients should be evaluated for any potential drug-induced nutrient depletion, such as caused by cholestyramine, anticonvulsants, thiazide diuretics, alcohol (40,79,80), and possibly benzodiazepines, which have been shown to impact on immune function (81). Taurine, a sulfur-containing amino acid, improved the proliferative response of T cells from old mice, accompanied by a normalization of the cytosolic calcium flux on stimulation (82). Fluorinated 4-quinolones have been shown to increase and prolong IL-2 production of stimulated T cells from healthy young donors (83).

Dietary restriction of rodents has been consistently shown to delay both thymic involution and development of reduced T-cell function (41). While dietary restriction of laboratory animals may actually represent a reversal of the effects of overeating, it nonetheless is a very real, reproducible finding that provides an opportunity to study this phenomenon. The effect of dietary restriction is thought to involve boosting antioxidants, and some people have shown improved T-cell function in vitro and in vivo with antioxidants, such as vitamin C, cysteine, and 2-mercaptoethanol (84). Likewise, the addition of reduced glutathione in vitro totally reversed the defective proliferative response of splenocytes from aged mice (85). This supports the hypothesis that the glutathione peroxidase–dependent detoxification system is defective in T cells from older people or animals.

VII. CONCLUSION

The elderly population is at risk for an increased incidence and severity of many infections. Changes in host defenses with age are only part of the reason for this. The absolute contribution of age-related immune dysfunction to the pathogenesis of these infections is difficult to determine because of the large number of confounding variables associated with aging, and because of different parameters used to assess immune function. Clear impairment of immune function, especially in T-cell function and T-cell–associated antibody production, has been repeatedly demonstrated in healthy elderly subjects as well as laboratory animals. However, these changes are thought primarily to put aged individuals at increased susceptibility to subsequent insults and exposure to environmental factors. Nonetheless, changes in cell-mediated immunity are thought to be a consequence of thymic involution and reduced levels of thymic hormones. This apparently results in a functional impairment of a fraction of T cells, primarily manifested by a delay and inability of cells to enter into the cell cycle as well as delays in other effector cell functions. Humoral immunity is also impaired, both because of these changes in T cells and possibly due to the antiidiotypic response to B cells themselves from immune dysregulation. Ultimately, the accurate identification and subsequent treatment of those frail elderly persons who have significant age- and disease-related immune dysfunction may help reduce the incidence and severity of infections.

REFERENCES

1. Antonaci S, Jirilio E, Bonomo L. Immunoregulation in aging. Diagnost Clin Immunol 1987; 5:55–61.
2. Saltzman RL, Peterson PK. Immunodeficiency of the elderly. Rev Infect Dis 1987; 9:1127–39.
3. Makinodan T, Hahn TJ, McDougall, et al. Cellular immunosenescence: an overview. Exp Gerontol 1991; 26:281–8.
4. Segre D, Miller RA, Abraham GN, et al. Aging and the immune system. J Gerontol 1989; 44:B164–8.
5. Gardener ID. The effect of aging on susceptibility to infections. Rev Infect Dis 1980; 2:801–10.
6. Yoshikawa TT, Norman DC. Predisposing factors to infections. In: Yoshikawa TT, Norman DC, eds. Aging and clinical practice: infectious diseases, diagnosis and treatment. New York: Igaku-Shoin, 1987:8–19.
7. Kligman AM, Balin AK. Aging of human skin. In: Balin AK, Kligman AM, eds. Aging and the skin. New York: Raven Press, 1989:1–34.
8. Branchet MC, Boisnic S, Frances C, et al. Skin thickness changes in normal aging skin. Gerontology 1990; 36:28–35.
9. Castle SC, Norman DC, Perls TT, et al. Analysis of cutaneous delayed-type hypersensitivity reaction and T cell proliferative response in elderly nursing home patients: an approach to identifying immunodeficient patients. Gerontology 1990; 36:217–29.
10. Rogers GS, Gilchrest BA. The senile epidermis: environmental influences on skin ageing and cutaneous carcinogenesis. Br J Dermatol 1990; 122(suppl 35):55–60.
11. Fenske NA, Lober CW. Structural and functional changes of normal aging skin. J Am Acad Dermatol 1986; 15:571–85.
12. Yoshikawa TT, Norman DC, Grahn D. Infections in the aging population. J Am Geriatr Soc 1985; 33:496–503.
13. Lehrer RI, Ganz T, Selsted ME, et al. Neutrophils and host defense. Ann Intern Med 1988; 109:127–42.
14. Antonaci S, Jirillo E, Ventura MT. Non-specific immunity in aging. Deficiency of monocyte and polymorphonuclear cell-mediated functions. Mech Ageing Dev 1984; 24:365–375.
15. Phair JP, Kauffman CA, Bjornson A, et al. Host defenses in the aged: evaluation of components of the inflammatory and immune responses. J Infect Dis 1978; 138:67–73.
16. Esposito AL, Poirier WJ, Clark CA. In vitro assessment of chemotaxis by peripheral blood neutrophils from adult and senescent C57BL/6 mice: correlation with in vivo responses to pulmonary infection with Type 3 *Streptococcus pneumoniae*. Gerontology 1990; 36:2–11.
17. MacGregor RR, Shalit M. Neutrophil function in healthy elderly subjects. J Gerontol 1990; 45:M55–60.
18. Niwa Y, Kasama T, Miyachi Y, et al. Neutrophil chemotaxis, phagocytosis and parameters of reactive oxygen species in human aging: cross-sectional and longitudinal studies. Life Sci 1989; 44:1655–64.
19. Edwards D, Kirkpatrick CH. The immunology of mycobacterial diseases. Am Rev Respir Dis 1986; 134:1062–71.
20. Murray HW. Interferon-gamma, the activated macrophage, and host defense against microbial challenge. Ann Intern Med 1988; 108:595–608.
21. Orme IM. Aging and immunity to tuberculosis: increased susceptibility of old mice reflects a decreased capacity to generate mediator T lymphocytes. J Immunol 1987; 138:4414–18.
22. Bermudez LE, Wu M, Petrofsky M, et al. Interleukin-6 antagonizes tumor necrosis factor-mediated mycobacteriostatic and mycobactericidal activities in macrophages. Infect Immun 1992; 60:4245–52.

23. Proust JJ, Bender BS, Nagel JE, et al. Developmental biology and senescence. Natural Immun 1989; 392–439.
24. Ligthart GJ, Corberand JX, Geertzen HGM, et al. Necessity of the assessment of health status in human immunogerontological studies: evaluation of the Senieur protocol. Mech Ageing Dev 1990; 55:89–105.
25. Beckman I, Dimopoulos K, Xaioning X, et al. T cell activation in the elderly: evidence for specific deficiencies in T cell/accessory cell interactions. Mech Ageing Dev 1990; 51:265–76.
26. Inamizu T, Chang MP, Makinodan T. Influence of age on the production and regulation of interleukin-1 in mice. Immunology 1985; 55:447.
27. Bruley-Rosset M, Vergnon I. Interleukin-1 synthesis and activity in aged mice. Mech Ageing Dev 1984; 24:247–64.
28. Seth A, Nagarkatti M, Nagarkatti P, et al. Macrophages but not B cells from aged mice are defective in stimulating autoreactive T cells in vitro. Mech Ageing Dev 1990; 52:107–24.
29. Damle NK, Klussman K, Linsley PS, et al. Differential costimulatory effects of adhesion molecules B7, ICAM-1, LFA-3, and VCAM-1 on resting and antigen-primed $CD4^+$ T lymphocytes. J Immunol 1992; 148:1985–92.
30. Chang MP, Makinodan T, Peterson WJ, et al. Role of T cells and adherent cells in age-related decline in murine interleukin 2 production. J Immunol 1982; 129:2426–30.
31. Bradley SF, Vibhagool A, Kunkel SL. Monokine secretions in aging and protein malnutrition. J Leuk Biol 1989;45:510–14.
32. Sharp A, Kukulansky T, Malkinson Y, et al. The bone marrow as an effector T cell organ in aging. Mech Ageing Dev 1990; 52:219–33.
33. Stingl G, Hauser C, Tschachler E, et al. Immune functions of epidermal cells. In: Norris DA, ed. Immune mechanisms in cutaneous disease. New York: Marcel Dekker, 1989:3–72.
34. Guidi L, Bartolinia C, Frasca D, et al. Impairment of lymphocyte activities in depressed aged subjects. Mech Ageing Dev 1991; 60:13–24.
35. MacCuish AC, Urbaniak SJ, Campbell CJ. Phytohemagglutinin transformation and circulating lymphocyte subpopulations in insulin-dependent diabetic patients. Diabetes 1974; 23:708–12.
36. Nohr CW, Tchervenkov JI, Meakins JL, et al. Malnutrition and humoral immunity: long-term protein deprivation. J Surg Res 1986; 40:432–7.
37. Walker C, Gauchat J-F, De Weck AL, et al. Analysis of leukocyte markers in elderly individuals. Aging Immunol Infect Dis 1990; 2:31–43.
37a. Jensen TL, Hallgren HM, Yasmineh WG, et al. Do immature T cells accumulate in advanced age? Mech Ageing Dev 1986; 33:237–45.
37b. Powers DC. Immunological principles and emerging strategies of vaccination for the elderly. J Am Geriatr Soc 1992; 40:81–94.
38. Gottesman SRS, Edington J. Proliferative and cytotoxic immune functions in aging mice: V. Deficiency in generation of cytotoxic cells with normal lytic function per cell as demonstrated by the single cell conjugation assay. Aging Immunol Infect Dis 1990; 2:19–28.
39. Deviere J, Kennes B, Closset J, et al. Immune senescence: effect of age, sex and health on human blood mononuclear subpopulations. Arch Gerontol Geriatr 1985; 4:285–93.
40. Dworsky R, Paganini-Hill A, Ducey B, et al. Lymphocyte immunophenotyping in an elderly population: age, sex and medication effects—a flow cytometry study. Mech Ageing Dev 1989; 48:255–66.
41. Miller RA. Aging and immune function. Internat Rev Cytol 1991; 124:187–215.
42. Thoman ML, Weigle WO. The cellular and subcellular bases of immunosenescence. Adv Immunol 1989; 46:221–61.
43. Ernst DN, Hobbs MV, Torbett BE, et al. Differences in the expression profiles of CD45RB, Pgp-1, and 3G11 membrane antigens and in the patterns of lymphokine secretion by splenic $CD4^+$ T cells from young and aged mice. J Immunol 1990; 145:1295–302.
44. Miller RA. The cell biology of aging: immunological models. J Gerontol 1989; 44:B4–8.

45. Robb RJ, Greene WC, Rusk CM. Low and high affinity cellular receptors for interleukin 2. Implications for the level of Tac and antigen. J Exp Med 1984; 160:1126–46.
46. Vie H, Miller RA. Decline, with age, in the proportion of mouse T cells that express IL-2 receptors after mitogen stimulation. Mech Ageing Dev 1986; 33:313–22.
47. Thoman ML. Role of interleukin-2 in the age-related impairment of immune function. J Am Geriatr Soc 1985; 33:781–7.
48. Schwab R, Pfeffer L, Szabo. Defective expression of high affinity IL-2 receptors on activated T cells from aged humans. Int Immunol 1990; 2:329–35.
49. Kubo M, Cinader B. Polymorphism of age-related changes in interleukin (IL) production: differential changes of T helper subpopulations synthesizing IL2, IL3, IL4. Eur J Immunol 1990; 20;1289–96.
50. Nagel JE, Chopra RK, Chrest FJ, et al. Decreased proliferation, interleukin 2 synthesis, and interleukin 2 receptor expression are accompanied by decreased mRNA expression in phytohemagglutinin-stimulated cells from elderly donors. J Clin Invest 1988; 81:1096–102.
50a. Fong TC, Makinodan T. In situ hybridization analysis of the age-related decline in IL-2 mRNA expressing murine T cells. Cell Immunol 1989; 118:199–207.
51. Hertogh-Huijbregts A, Vissinga C, Rozing J, et al. Impairment of CD3-dependent and CD3-independent activation pathways in CD4+ and CD8+ T cells from old CBA/RIJ mice. Mech Ageing Dev 1990; 53:141–55.
52. Candore G, Di Lorenzo G, Caruso C, et al. The effect of age on mitogen responsive T cell precursors in human beings is completely restored by interleukin-2. Mech Ageing Dev 1992; 63:297–307.
53. McElhaney JE, Beattie BL, Devine R, et al. Age-related decline in interleukin 2 production in response to influenza vaccine. J Am Geriatr Soc 1990; 38:652–8.
54. Wasik MA, Morimoto C. Differential effects of cytokines on proliferative response of human $CD4^+$ T lymphocyte subsets stimulated via T cell receptor-CD3 complex. J Immunol 1990; 144:3334–40.
55. Yamamura M, Wang XH, Ohmen JD, et al. Cytokine patterns of immunologically mediated tissue damage. J Immunol 1992; 149:1470–5.
56. Yamamura M, Uyemura K, Deams RJ, et al. Defining protective responses to infectious pathogens: cytokine profiles in leprosy lesions. Science 1991; 254:277–81.
57. Mosmann TR, Moore KW. The role of IL-10 in crossregulation of TH1 and TH2 responses. Immunol Today 1991; 12:A49–53.
58. Zhou D, Munster AM, Winchurch RA. Inhibitory effects of interleukin 6 on immunity. Possible implications in burn patients. Arch Surg 1992; 127:65–9.
59. Chopra RK, Holbrook NJ, Powers DC, et al. Interleukin 2, interleukin 2 receptor, and interferon-γ synthesis and MRNA expression in phorbol myristate acetate and calcium ionophore A23187-stimulated T cells from elderly humans. Clin Immunol Immunopathol 1989; 53:297–308.
60. Miller RA. Immunodeficiency of aging: restorative effects of phorbol esters combined with calcium ionophore. J Immunol 1986; 137:805–8.
61. Whisler RL, Newhouse YG, Donnerberg RL, et al. Characterization of intracellular ionized calcium responsiveness and inositol phosphate production among resting and stimulated peripheral blood T cells from elderly humans. Aging Immunol Infect Dis 1991; 3:27.
62. Franklin RA, Arkins S, Kelley KW. The proliferative response of rat T cells to calcium ionophores increases with age. Cell Immunol 1990; 130:416–28.
63. Philosophe B, Miller RA. Calcium signals in murine T lymphocytes: preservation of responses to PHA and to an anti-Ly-6 antibody. Aging Immunol Infect Dis 1990; 2:11–18.
64. Grossman A, Ledbetter JA, Rabinovitch PS. Aging-related deficiency in intracellular calcium response to anti-CD3 or Concanavalin A in murine T-cell subsets. J Gerontol 1990; 45:B81–6.
65. Golbus J, Palella T, Richardson B. Quantitative changes in T cell DNA methylation occurring during differentiation and ageing. Eur J Immunol 1990; 20:1869–72.

66. Gamble DA, Schwab R, Weksler ME, et al. Decreased steady state c-myc mRNA in activated T cell cultures from old humans is caused by a smaller proportion of T cells that transcribe the c-myc gene. J Immunol 1990; 144:3569–73.
67. Bloom ET, Umehara H, Bleackley RC, et al. Age-related decrement in cytotoxic T lymphocyte (CTL) activity is associated with decreased levels of mRNA encoded by two CTL-associated serine esterase genes and the perforin gene in mice. Eur J Immunol 1990; 20:2309–16.
68. Bloom ET. Functional importance of $CD4^+$ and $CD8^+$ cells in cytotoxic lymphocyte activity and associated gene expression. Impact on the age-related decline in lytic activity. Eur J Immunol 1991; 27:1013–17.
69. Stead W, To T. The significance of the tuberculin skin test in the elderly. Ann Intern Med 1987; 107:837–42.
70. Kelly KW, Brief S, Westly HJ, et al. GH_3 pituitary adenoma cells can reverse thymic aging in rats. Proc Natl Acad Sci (USA) 1986; 83:5663–7.
71. Hirokawa K, Sato K, Makinodan T. Restoration of impaired immune functions in aging animals. V. Long-term immunopotentiating effects of combined young bone marrow and newborn thymus grafts. Clin Immunol Immunopathol 1982; 22:297–304.
72. Duchateau J, Servais G, Vreyens R, et al. Modulation of immune response in aged humans through different administration modes of thymopentin. Surv Immunol Res 1985; 4(suppl 1):94–101.
73. Goso C, Frasca D, Doria G. Effect of synthetic humoral factor (THF-γ2) on T cell activities in immunodeficient ageing mice. Clin Exp Immunol 1992; 87:346–51.
74. Gravenstein S, Duthie EH, Miller BA, et al. Augmentation of influenza antibody response in elderly men by thymosin alpha one. A double-blind placebo-controlled clinical study. J Am Geriatr Soc 1989; 37:1–8.
75. Wiedermann CJ, Neidermühlbichler, Beimpold H, et al. In vitro activation of neutrophils of the aged by recombinant human growth hormone. J Infect Dis 1991; 164:1017–20.
76. Chien YK, Liu YH, Massey DG. Interleukin-3 and anti-aging medication: a review. Hawaii Med J 1990; 49:160–1.
77. Mbawaike I, Wyde P, Anderson P. Enhancement of the protective efficacy of inactivated influenza A virus vaccine in aged mice by IL-2 liposomes. Vaccine 1990; 8:377–82.
78. Bender BS, Tallman E, Johnson MP, et al. Enhancement of anti-influenza cytotoxic T-lymphocyte activity in senescent mice by vaccination early in life. Mech Ageing Dev 1990; 55:1–7.
79. Fillit H. Practical evaluation of secondary immune deficiencies in the elderly. Geriatrics 1991; 46:70–3.
80. Chang MP, Norman DC. Mechanism of ethanol-mediated immunosuppression in mice: ethanol suppresses T-cell proliferation without affecting IL2 production and IL2 receptor expression. Int J Immunopharmac 1992; 14:707–19.
81. Chang MP, Castle SC, Norman DC. Mechanism of immunosuppressive effect of alprazolam: alprazolam suppresses T-cell proliferation by selectively inhibiting the production of IL2 but not acquisition of IL2 receptor. Int J Immunopharmac 1992: 14:227–37.
82. Nishio SI, Negoro S, Hosokawa T, et al. The effect of taurine on age-related immune decline in mice: the effect of taurine on T cell and B cell proliferative response under costimulation with ionomycin and phorbol myristate acetate. Mech Ageing Dev. 1990; 52:125–39.
83. Riesbeck K, Andersson J, Gullberg M, et al. Fluorinated 4-quinolones induce hyperproduction of interleukin 2. Proc Natl Acad Sci USA 1989; 86:2809–13.
84. Heidrick ML, Albright JW, Makinodan T. Restoration of impaired immune functions of aging animals. IV. Action of 2-mercaptoethanol in enhancing age-reduced immune responsiveness. Mech Ageing Dev 1980; 13:107–17.
85. Franklin RA, Yong ML, Arkins S, et al. Glutathione augments in vitro proliferative responses of lymphocytes to Concanavalin A to a greater degree in old than in young rats. J Nutr 1990; 120:1710–17.

3

Clinical Approach to Diagnosis of Infections in Older Patients

Dean C. Norman
University of California, and Veterans Affairs Medical Center—West Los Angeles, Los Angeles, California

I. INTRODUCTION

Clinicians can impact positively on the high morbidity and mortality observed for infections in elderly patients by the following methods:

1. *Identify and reduce risk factors.* For example, clinicians can discourage the use of indwelling bladder catheters unless strict criteria such as inoperable urinary obstruction are met.
2. *Appropriately use antibiotic prophylaxis and maintain vaccination programs.*
3. *Identify infections as early as possible and initiate proper supportive measures and antimicrobial therapy.*

The time between the onset of symptoms and the institution of appropriate therapy is the "diagnostic delay." This chapter will focus on the recognition of potential atypical presentation of infection and the appropriate diagnostic testing necessary to improve the accuracy of diagnosis, both of which impact on the diagnostic delay for infections in older patients. In order to understand the approach to the geriatric patient with infection, it is necessary to briefly review the clinical presentation of infection in this population.

II. CLINICAL MANIFESTATIONS OF INFECTIONS IN ELDERLY PERSONS

A. Atypical Presentation

Infections in elderly persons may present atypically with minimal or subtle findings, often without signs pointing to a specifically involved organ system. For example, an elderly patient with pneumonia may initially complain only of the new onset of falling. In fact,

Table 1 Atypical Presentations of Infection in Elderly Patients

Symptoms
Worsening cognition
Lethargy or agitation
Loss of appetite
Falls
Incontinence
Focal neurological finding
Signs
Blunted temperature
Tachypnea
Abnormal mental status

any unexplained change in functional status should lead the clinician to consider the possibility of infection (see Table 1).

Atypical presentations of infectious diseases are particularly common in those who are very old and/or debilitated. Thus, it is not surprising that nursing home residents present special difficulties in diagnosing infection in a timely manner because most of these residents are frail, over 80 years old, and are likely to suffer from multiple debilitating illnesses as well as cognitive impairments. Resource limitations, ethical considerations, and other factors further hinder the assessment of infection in the long-term care setting (1).

In some cases there may be a disparity between the severity of an acute illness and the clinical presentation of the disease. For example, elderly patients with acute cholecystitis may not exhibit focal peritoneal signs on examination (2), and yet, despite relatively "benign" presentations, the patients' risks of gangrene or perforation of the gallbladder are high, particularly in the extreme of old age (3).

Nonspecific, blunted, or even absent classical signs and symptoms of infection in old age may result from different causes. The most important of these are underreporting of illness, differing etiology, coexisting diseases, and altered response to illness.

B. Underreporting of Illnesses

Underreporting of illnesses is a common problem in geriatric patients and can be expected to be an especially important problem in those with cognitive impairment affecting communication. For certain infections, even in otherwise healthy, independent-living aging adults, underreporting of illnesses results in serious morbidity. This is exemplified by appendicitis. Although only 5% of cases of appendicitis occur in old age, most of the mortality for this disease occurs in elderly persons and is due to the high perforation rates seen in the old compared to the young. The disparity in perforation rates results largely from failure of the older patients to seek timely medical consultation. Failure to consider that abdominal pain may be due to appendicitis and fear of economic loss from hospitalization may contribute to the reluctance by older persons to seek medical evaluation. Finally, other factors play a role as well. Anatomical changes of the appendix with age that leads to vascular compromise, atypical clinical presentations, and over-reliance on laboratory tests may also increase the diagnostic delay for appendicitis (4).

C. Diverse Causes of Infection

Differing etiologies of infections in elderly patients can contribute to the severity of infections observed in this age group. A greater variety of pathogens are encountered in the infections that are seen commonly in older adults compared to the young. Mixed infections involving aerobic or facultative anaerobic gram-negative bacilli and obligate or strict anaerobic bacteria are common in old age (5). These changes in microbial pathogens not only influence the clinical presentation and prognosis of infection, but they have important implications for choice of empiric antimicrobial regimens (see Chap. 26).

D. Coexisting Diseases

Coexisting diseases are common in geriatric patients and may mask infections. For example, the diagnosis of septic arthritis in the elderly patient with chronic gouty arthritis may be overlooked because acute joint symptoms are mistakenly attributed to an exacerbation of gout (6,7). Similarly, the diagnosis of infection in a prosthetic joint may be overlooked because infection may resemble the more common problem of loosening of the prosthesis (8,9).

E. Altered Responses

Altered responses to infections are in part due to the above factors as well as decremental biological changes with age. For example, age-related changes in chest wall expansion and lung tissue elasticity contribute to diminished cough reflex in elderly persons (10). Also, changes in cytokine production and other factors may result in a blunted peripheral blood leukocytosis response to infection.

F. Blunted Fever Responses

Fever, the cardinal sign of infection, may be blunted or absent in up to one third of infected elderly patients (11). This observation is supported by numerous reported studies that show diminished fever responses in the old compared to the young with such infections as bacteremia (12,13), pneumonia (14), tuberculosis (15), and infective endocarditis (16). The blunted fever response may be due in part to factors such as altered production of and response to pyrogens with age and debility such as interleukin 1, interleukin 6, and tumor necrosis factor (11,17,18) or changes in thermogenesis-producing brown fat with age (19,20). Not only does a blunted fever response to infection make the diagnosis of infection difficult, a lack of fever portends a poor prognosis in patients with bacteremias and fungemias (13,21). Moreover, fever is probably an important host defense mechanism (11,22). Recently, it has been reported that residents in long-term care facilities may elevate their temperatures in response to an infection, but their absolute temperatures may not reach 101°F because of lower baseline temperatures (23,24). Thus, in nursing home patients, in the setting of changes in functional status, an increase from baseline temperature of ≥1.4°F or an absolute oral temperature of 100°F is highly suggestive of the presence of a serious infection.

Fever is often indicative of a benign "viral syndrome" or mild bacterial upper respiratory tract infection in children and young adults. However, fever in elderly persons has major clinical implications in that it is usually indicative of a serious infection. This is especially true for persons aged 80 years and older (the "old-old") (25–27). Thus, whenever elderly persons present with fevers (an oral temperature greater than or equal to 100°F) a careful search for infection should be undertaken.

Finally, the syndrome of fever of unknown origin (FUO) does occur in older adults. In the one major series reported in the literature, FUO in elderly patients was usually due to treatable infections such as intraabdominal infection, bacterial endocarditis, and tuberculosis as well as treatable rheumatological diseases such as temporal arteritis (28).

III. HISTORY AND PHYSICAL EXAMINATION OF THE INFECTED ELDERLY PATIENT

Based on the above discussion, the clinician should be aware of the varied clinical presentations of infections in elderly patients.

In all geriatric patients the evaluations should include an assessment of function and mental status. Minimally, functional assessment should focus on activities of daily life (ADL). These are best remembered by the acronym DEATH (dressing, eating, ambulation, toileting, and hygiene). A mini-mental status examination (e.g., Folstein) should also be performed on each patient (29). All historical sources should be utilized (i.e., medical records and interviews with family, friends, and caregivers) in performing functional assessments. This is especially important in order to determine the patient's baseline function. As in younger patients, travel history, tuberculosis exposure history, vaccination history, and risk factors for human immunodeficiency virus (HIV) should be determined in older adults.

IV. LABORATORY EVALUATION OF THE INFECTED ELDERLY PATIENT

The laboratory evaluation of the geriatric patient presents a challenge to clinicians. Before proceeding with any testing, it is important to determine the patient's wishes and expectations. Advanced directives in the form of a living will and durable power of attorney are extremely useful when making decisions about uncomfortable or invasive diagnostic procedure when patients are unable to give informed consent.

Elderly individuals are more likely to develop complications from invasive procedures, such as cardiac arrhythmias due to transtracheal aspirations (30), or morbidity from even some noninvasive procedures (e.g., renal failure from contrast dye). Thus, the potential benefit of any procedure must be carefully weighed against the potential risk. Finally, given limited medical resources, the benefit of a procedure must also be weighed against the potential direct costs of that procedure as well as the indirect costs of complications. An extra day spent in an acute care hospital may cost more than $1000, which, depending on various circumstances, may or may not be reimbursable with the current Diagnosis Related Groups (DRG) system of reimbursement by Medicare.

In some dysfunctional or ill elderly patients, particularly those with cognitive impairments, or those with vague, nonspecific complaints, the cause of incapacity or illness may not be readily apparent. Before beginning an exhaustive diagnostic search for an infection, the clinician should consider that the frequency of certain types or sites of infection varies with the residential status of the patient. Thus, if the initial thorough history and physical examinations do not suggest the source of infection or fever, then further diagnostic tests should focus on the most likely diagnostic possibilities according to residential status. These diagnostic possibilities are depicted in Table 2.

Table 2 Common Types of Infections or Cause of Fever According to Residential Setting

Primary Considerations	Secondary Considerations
Community	
1. Respiratory	4. Infective endocarditis
2. Urinary tract infection	5. Bone and joint
3. Intraabdominal	6. Central nervous system
Nursing Home	
1. Respiratory	4. Tuberculosis
2. Urinary tract infection	5. Intraabdominal
3. Soft tissue	6. Hepatitis
	7. Bone and joint
Acute Care	
1. Pneumonia	4. Pulmonary embolus
2. Urinary tract infection	5. Drug reaction
3. Intravenous catheter site	6. Soft tissue

A. Healthy Community Dwellers

Independent-living, relatively healthy older patients living in a community setting are more likely to have respiratory infections (bacterial pneumonia and bronchitis), genitourinary infections (urinary tract infection and prostatic infection), and intraabdominal infections (diverticulitis, cholecystitis, appendicitis, and abscesses). The initial laboratory evaluation should consist of complete blood count, blood cultures, urinalysis and culture, chest radiograph, and tuberculin skin test. Sputum should be obtained if the patient has a cough or an abnormal chest x-ray, and sputum should be gram-stained, stained for acid-fast bacilli, and processed for bacterial culture. A direct fluorescent antibody examination of sputum for *Legionella* sp. should be done for patients with atypical pneumonia or for those who live in areas in which the prevalence of legionnaires' disease is high. If all of these previously mentioned tests are unrevealing, then a search for an intraabdominal infection should be begun. An ultrasonography of the liver and gallbladder and liver function tests should be the initial tests obtained. If these tests are negative, then a radionuclide scan of the gallbladder and liver or a computed tomographic (CT) scan of the abdomen should be considered. Less common infections such as infective endocarditis (if heart murmurs are heard and/or positive blood cultures are obtained), occult bone or joint infection (if rheumatological complaints or findings are present), and central nervous system infection (if neurological complaints or findings are present) should also be considered. If an infection cannot be found to explain the clinical findings, then a search should be undertaken to look for noninfectious causes such as drug fever, lymphoma, collagen vascular disease, and tumors (e.g, hypernephroma).

B. Nursing Home Residents

Nursing home residents with possible infection should be evaluated for pneumonia, urinary tract infection, and soft tissue infection (especially cellulitis and infected pressure ulcer)

(31). Secondary diagnostic considerations for these patients are shown in Table 2. Certain diagnostic tests may not be readily available in some nursing homes, and it may be necessary to transfer residents to acute care facilities for further evaluation.

C. Hospitalized Patients

Finally, hospitalized elderly patients who are suspected of nosocomial infection in whom the initial examinations are negative should be evaluated for respiratory infections (particularly aspiration pneumonia) and urinary tract infections (especially related to indwelling bladder catheters). Indwelling intravenous catheters are common sources of infection, and therefore, intravenous catheter sites should be carefully inspected, the catheter removed, and the tip of the catheter cultured and gram-stained for bacteria. Other diagnostic possibilities are shown in Table 2. In cases where previous antimicrobial therapy has been given, consideration should be given to the possibility of antibiotic-associated colitis, and stool should be examined for the presence of *Clostridium difficile* toxin.

D. Specimens and Microbiological Tests

Blood cultures are strongly recommended for the evaluation of any elderly patient with a possible infection who is either institutionalized or ill enough to be considered for hospitalization. Standard blood culture methodology consists of obtaining two sets of culture, each from distinct venipuncture sites. In elderly patients with bacterial pneumonia, blood cultures may be positive in 1–20% of cases, while elderly women with pyelonephritis may have positive blood cultures in almost one half of cases (32). One bottle of each set should be capable of sustaining the growth of aerobic and facultative anaerobic bacteria and fungi, and the other bottle in the set should meet the conditions for culturing obligate anaerobic bacteria. In cases of suspected infective endocarditis, three sets of cultures from different venipuncture sites over several hours should be obtained (33).

Urinalysis with examination of urinary sediment is essential in the diagnosis of urinary tract infection in older patients. In elderly men without specific genitourinary complaints, the absence of pyuria virtually excludes the presence of bacteriuria (34).

Other less accessible body fluids such as pleural fluid, joint fluid, ascites, and cerebrospinal fluid (CSF) should be examined if clinically indicated. All body cavity fluids should have complete cell counts, glucose and protein determinations; be stained for bacteria, mycobacteria, and fungi as indicated; and have appropriate (e.g., bacterial, mycobacterial, or fungal) cultures. Both aerobic and anaerobic bacteria cultures as well as a determination of pH should also be performed on all fluids except CSF.

As discussed above, an attempt to examine sputum should be made in all elderly patients with suspected bacterial pneumonia. A gram stain of sputum should be evaluated using the criteria of Murray and Washington (35) to determine the quality of the sample. The presence of more than 25 polymorphonuclear leukocytes and fewer than 10 epithelial cells per low power microscopic field indicates the high probability of a minimally contaminated (by mouth flora) lower respiratory secretion. Such a high-quality sputum sample has the best correlation with the "gold standard" for sputum microbiology, which is culture of a transtracheal aspirate (36).

E. Radiological Tests and Imaging Scans

Plain radiographs are relatively inexpensive, safe, and usually cause little discomfort and are therefore the first choice for radiographical diagnosis. Ultrasonography is probably the best second test to be done if plain films are negative in the search for an occult infection in the abdomen. Two-dimensional ultrasonography is very helpful in imaging cardiac valve vegetations in patients with infective endocarditis (33). CT scans and magnetic resonance imaging (MRI) are certainly useful in the diagnosis of occult infection in the abdomen, particularly if plain films or ultrasonograms suggest a suspicious area in this site (37,38). CT and MRI are very useful in diagnosing central nervous system infection (e.g., brain abscess) and infections of the bone.

Technesium (^{99m}Tc) scanning is frequently used for defining the subphrenic space and for looking for bone infection. ^{99m}Tc-labeled acetanilide iminodiacetic acid (IDA) derivatives are useful for detecting acute cholecystitis. Similarly, gallium (^{67}Ga)- and indium (^{111}In)-tagged leukocytes are at times helpful in locating intraabdominal abscesses and occult bone infection. The use of these scans for the diagnosis of infection in the abdomen has been thoroughly reviewed recently (38).

F. Invasive Tests

Transtracheal aspiration, transbronchial biopsy, pleural biopsy, pulmonary lavage, and open and percutaneous needle biopsy of the lung are some of the invasive tests available for diagnosing the etiology of pulmonary infections. The use of these tests in older patients should be carefully considered, weighing both costs and risks versus potential benefit, remembering that elderly patients are more likely to suffer complications in comparison to younger patients.

Recently, the development of laparoscopy has reduced the risk of direct visualization of an intraabdominal infection. Laparoscopy also allows safer biopsy of the liver, and corrective surgery can be done via the laparoscope. This technique holds a great deal of promise for the diagnosis and treatment of certain intraabdominal infections in elderly patients (39,40).

V. CONCLUSION

Infections in elderly persons present a formidable diagnostic challenge to the clinician. The clinician should be aware of the higher frequency of atypical presentation of infection with old age. Diagnostic testing should be directed toward the common causes of infection in elderly patients. Careful assessment of risk and cost versus benefit should be done before initiating any procedure.

REFERENCES

1. Norman DC, Yoshikawa TT. Clinical features of infection and significance of fever in the nursing home patient. In: Verghese A, Berk SL, eds. Infections in the nursing home. New York: Karger Publishers, Inc., 1990:30–40.
2. Morrow DJ, Thompson J, Wilson SE. Acute cholecystitis in the elderly. A surgical emergency. Arch Surg 1978; 113:1149–52.
3. Fry DE, Cox RA, Harbrecht PJ. Gangrene of the gallbladder: a complication of acute cholecystitis. South Med J 1981; 74:666–8.
4. Norman DC, Yoshikawa TT. Acute appendicitis in the elderly. In: Meakins JL, McClaren J, eds. Surgical care of the elderly. Chicago: Year Book Medical Publications, 1988:386–91.
5. Yoshikawa TT, Norman DC, Grahn D. Infections in the aging population. J Am Geriatr Soc 1985; 33:496–503.
6. Norman DC, Yoshikawa TT. Responding to septic arthritis. Geriatrics 1983; 38:83–91.

7. McGuire NM, Kauffman CA. Septic arthritis in the elderly. J Am Geriatr Soc 1985; 33:170–4.
8. Norman DC. Septic arthritis and osteomyelitis. In: Yoshikawa TT, Norman DC, eds. Aging and clinical practice: infectious diseases. Diagnosis and treatment. New York: Igaku-Shoin, 1987:193–205.
9. Inman RD, Gallegos KV, Brause BD, et al. Clinical and microbial features of prosthetic joint infection. Am J Med 1984; 77:47–53.
10. Pontoppidan H, Beecher MK. Progressive loss of protective reflexes in the airway with the advance of age. JAMA 1960; 174:2209–13.
11. Norman DC, Grahn D, Yoshikawa TT. Fever and aging. J Am Geriatr Soc 1985; 33:859–63.
12. Gleckman R, Hibert D. Afebrile bacteremia: a phenomenon in geriatric patients. JAMA 1981; 248:1478–81.
13. Finklestein MS, Petkun WM, Freedman ML, et al. Pneumococcal bacteremia in adults: age dependent differences in presentation and in outcome. J Am Geriatr Soc 1983; 31:19–27.
14. Marrie TJ, Haldane EV, Faulkner RS, et al. Community-acquired pneumonia requiring hospitalization. Is it different in the elderly? J Am Geriatr Soc 1985; 33:671–80.
15. Alvarez S, Shell C, Berk SL. Pulmonary tuberculosis in elderly men. Am J Med 1987; 82:602–6.
16. Terpenning MS, Bussy BP, Kauffman CA. Infective endocarditis: clinical features in young and elderly patients. Am J Med 1987; 83:626–34.
17. Norman DC, Yamamura R, Yoshikawa TT. Fever response in old and young mice after injection of interleukin 1. J Gerontol 1988; 43:M81–5.
18. Miller D, Castle SC, Yoshikawa TT, et al. Effect of age on fever response to recombinant tumor necrosis factor-alpha in a murine model. J Gerontol 1991; 46:M176–9.
19. Scarpace PJ, Borst SE, Bender BS. The association of *E. coli* peritonitis with an impaired and delayed fever response in senescent rats. J Gerontol 1992; 47:B142–5.
20. Scarpace PJ, Bender BS, Borst SE. *E. coli* peritonitis activates thermogenesis in brown adipose tissue: relationship to fever. Can J Physiol Pharmacol 1991; 69:761–6.
21. Weinstein MP, Murphy JR, Reller RB, et al. The clinical significance of positive blood cultures: a comprehensive analysis of 500 episodes of bacteremia and fungemia II. Clinical observations with special reference to factors influencing prognosis. Rev Infect Dis 1983; 5:54–70.
22. Roberts N. Impact of temperature elevation on immunologic defenses. Rev Infect Dis 1991; 13(3):462–72.
23. Castle SC, Yeh M, Norman DC, et al. Fever response in the elderly. Are the older truly colder? J Am Geriatr Soc 1991; 39:853–7.
24. Castle SC, Yeh M, Toledo S, et al. Lowering the temperature criterion improves detection of infections in nursing home residents. Aging Immunol Infect Dis (in press).
25. Keating MJ III, Klimek JJ, Levine DS, et al. Effect of aging on the clinical significance of fever in ambulatory adult patients. J Am Geriatr Soc 1984; 32:282–7.
26. Mellors JW, Horwitz RI, Harvey MR, et al. A simple index to identify occult bacterial infection in adults with acute unexplained fever. Arch Intern Med 1987; 147:666–71.
27. Wasserman M, Levinstein M, Keller E, et al. Utility of fever, white blood cell, and differential count in predicting bacterial infections in the elderly. J Am Geriatr Soc 1989; 37:534–43.
28. Esposito AL, Gleckman RA. Fever of unknown origin in the elderly. J Am Geriatr Soc 1978; 26:498–505.
29. Folstein MF, Folstein SE, Mchugh PR. "Mini-mental state." A practical method for grading the cognitive state of patients for the clinician. Psychiatr Res 1975; 12:189–98.
30. Unger KM, Moser KM. Fatal complication of transtracheal aspiration. A report of two cases. Arch Intern Med 1973; 132:437–9.
31. Sarubbi FA. Infection control in the nursing-home setting. In: Verghese A, Berk SL, eds. Infections in the nursing home. New York: Karger Publishers, Inc., 1990:55–65.
32. Gleckman RA, Bradley PJ, Roth RM, et al. Bacteremic urosepsis. A phenomenon unique to elderly women. J Urol 1985; 133:174–5.

33. Scheld WM, Sande MA. Endocarditis and intravascular infections. In: GL Mandell, KG Douglas, JE Bennett, eds. Principles and practice of infectious diseases. New York: Churchill Livingstone, 1990:670–5.
34. Norman DC, Yamamura R, Yoshikawa TT. Pyuria: its predictive value of asymptomatic bacteriuria in ambulatory elderly males. J Urol 1986; 135:520–2.
35. Murray PR, Washington JA. Microscopic and bacteriologic analysis of expectorated sputum. Mayo Clin Proc 1975; 50:339–44.
36. Norman DC. Pneumonia. In: Yoshikawa TT, Norman DC, eds. Aging and clinical practice: infectious diseases. Diagnosis and treatment. New York: Igaku-Shoin, 1987:108–26.
37. Norman DC. Intraabdominal infection. In: Yoshikawa TT, Norman DC, eds. Aging and clinical practice: infectious diseases. Diagnosis and treatment. New York: Igaku-Shoin, 1987:151–72.
38. Levison ME, Bush LM. Peritonitis and other intra-abdominal infections. In: GL Mandell, KG Douglas, JE Bennett, eds. Principles and practice of infectious diseases. New York: Churchill Livingstone, 1990:636–69.
39. Dell'Aglio, Parker T., McDonald TJ. Diagnostic experience of laparoscopy in 91 patients at the Guthrie Clinic. Guthrie J 1992; 61(3):111–16.
40. Gadacz TR, Talamini MA, Lillemoe KD, et al. Laparoscopic cholecystectomy. Surg Clin North Am 1990; 70(6):1249–62.

4

Pharmacology of Antimicrobial Agents with Aging

Ingrid Nilsson-Ehle and Bengt Ljungberg
University Hospital, Lund, Sweden

I. INTRODUCTION

When a human being grows old, changes occur in the functions of all body systems as an expression of the natural, physiological aging process. The various organs involved in the disposition of drugs in the body are no exception, and the changes occurring in these systems can have a direct impact on pharmacokinetics. A large proportion of drugs prescribed are consumed by elderly people (1). To calculate optimal dosing regimens for these patients, it is important to consider the influence of normal aging on drug kinetics.

The incidence of infections increases with advancing age, and the use of antibiotics is common in the older age groups (2). The crucial consideration for antibiotic treatment is to give high enough doses for successful infection control, while keeping doses at safe, tolerable levels to avoid concentration-dependent adverse reactions. Frequently, older patients suffer from other diseases that may directly affect organ systems involved in drug disposition. Some of these conditions may be difficult to recognize in elderly persons, but they must be considered when calculating drug dosages. However, many older patients requiring antibiotic treatment for various infections are otherwise healthy and the physiological aging process is the only condition affecting drug disposition. It is still important for the clinician to consider the impact of normal aging on specific drug kinetics to be able to prescribe an optimal dosage.

The processes that determine the disposition of drugs are absorption from the gastrointestinal tract after oral administration or from muscle after intramuscular injection, distribution to various body compartments, and elimination via excretion or metabolic transformation. All these functions may be affected by the physiological changes occurring with increasing age. For some kinetic processes, definite clinical reasons to adjust dosing of antibiotics according to the age of the patient have been documented. For others, experimental evidence of definite impact is lacking and only theoretical speculations can be made. Research concerning the influence of aging on disposition of antimicrobial agents has, since the middle 1970s, been an area of increasing interest to the medical profession, and several studies of specific drugs have been published. However, in many cases it is difficult to directly extract results that show the impact of the aging process in itself, since studies often are done in patients with acute infections and diseases in various body systems that influence drug disposition. This is particularly true for older antibiotics; in recent years it has become more or less mandatory that pharmacokinetic studies in healthy elderly volunteers be included in the documentation of a new antibiotic.

The purpose of this review is to discuss the various processes involved in the disposition of antimicrobial drugs and the evidence available that physiological aging influences these processes.

II. ABSORPTION AND BIOAVAILABILITY

A. Absorption After Oral Administration

Several age-associated changes that have been documented in gastrointestinal functions may have a direct impact on the absorption of drugs. The number of absorbing mucosal cells decreases (3–5), and the blood flow rate in splanchnic vessels is lower in elderly persons (6). Both of these factors may impair the absorption of drugs from the gastrointestinal tract. With aging, the gastric mucosa undergoes atrophic changes, which cause a decrease in the acid-secretory capacity of the stomach (3,7). The resulting rise in pH may affect the solubility and ionization of drugs; that this can be a factor of importance for absorption has been shown in studies of bacampicillin and cefuroxime axetil, in which absorption was impaired at higher pH levels in the stomach (8). The reduced acidity can, furthermore, result in a more rapid emptying of the stomach (9). On the other hand, a general decline in the motility of the gastrointestinal tract has been reported with increasing age (10). It is possible that this lower motility may compensate for the effect of the rise in pH with regard to the rate of gastric emptying. No studies on drug absorption have dealt with this subject. Pathways for active transport of drugs over mucosal membranes may be impaired in aging adults, but since most drugs are absorbed by passive diffusion, this is seldom of any clinical importance.

Very few studies have been performed regarding the influence of aging on intestinal absorption of specific drugs. There is no documented evidence that absorption is impaired (1,11). Theoretically, some drugs may even exhibit a higher bioavailability in older subjects because of impaired first-pass metabolism in the liver (4,12). However, the increased bioavailability after oral administration of ciprofloxacin to elderly volunteers is probably not caused by changes in first-pass elimination but by truly enhanced absorption of the compound (13).

B. Absorption After Intramuscular Administration

Drug absorption from muscular tissue may take place at a lower rate in older persons than in young people. This could be due to decreased muscular blood flow, secondary to a lower level of physical activity. A reduced absorption rate in elderly subjects has been demonstrated for cefuroxime and long-acting penicillin (14,15). However, the absolute bioavailability of cefuroxime was not necessarily decreased (14).

III. DISTRIBUTION

A. General Aspects

The rate and extent of drug distribution to various organs and/or sites of infection are determined not only by the properties of the drug but also by a number of host factors that may be altered in older adults. Advancing age results in histological changes in most tissues, with a decline in cell number, while the remaining cells tend to enlarge causing irregularity of the tissue architecture (16). The mean total body weight is slightly reduced in older persons (17). Changes in body composition are also evident with age, with a reduction in total and intracellular water, a decline in lean body mass, and an increase in absolute and relative fat content (18–21). With no influence of other factors, this age-associated altered body composition would lead to an enlarged volume of distribution of lipophilic drugs but have the opposite effect on the distribution of polar, water-soluble compounds in elderly persons.

Circulatory changes associated with aging may influence drug distribution. Cardiac output decreases by about 1% per year during adult life (6). Alterations in the distribution of the regional blood flow (12) and changes in tissue permeability (22) have also been suggested as being related to aging. Bed rest and reduced physical activity in general is one postulated mechanism for circulatory adjustments and distributional changes in aged subjects. However, the importance of body position for circulation status and drug distribution has still not been clarified (23,24).

Apart from the aging process in itself, many other factors may influence the distribution of drugs. The differences in body composition between men and women may be more pronounced than the age-related changes (1,25). Some phenomena thought to be related to physiological aging may be the result of concurrent disease. For example, after careful exclusion of all subjects with occult or overt heart disease, there seems to be no age-related decline in cardiac output (26). When discussing the distribution of antibiotics, it is especially important to consider the reports from both animal and human studies in which the data indicate that the distribution volume may be altered by acute infectious disease and fever (27–32). This problem of discriminating effects of normal aging from those caused by disease explains some of the confusion in the literature. For instance, the volume of distribution of the same antibiotic is sometimes reported to be increased, unchanged, or reduced in different studies of elderly subjects (30,33,34). Judging from data obtained in healthy volunteers, advancing age imposes no important changes in the distribution volume of water-soluble antibiotics if they are distributed by passive diffusion and the binding to serum proteins and cells is low (29,30,35).

B. Binding to Plasma Proteins and Tissues

The distribution of pharmaceutical compounds is influenced by their binding to biological substances, e.g., serum proteins and red blood cells. There are many reports of a decline of the major carrier protein, albumin, with advancing age (36–38), but it is still unclear whether this is an effect of age as such. Again, immobility has been proposed as the reason for the reduction (39). A definite relationship between age and the concentration of the second important drug binding protein, α_1-acid glycoprotein, has still not been demonstrated, perhaps because of great intrasubject variability in the levels of the protein (40,41). However, some studies show a tendency for higher α_1-acid glycoprotein concentrations in elderly subjects (41). Since albumin tends to be a more efficient carrier of acidic drugs and α_1-acid glycoprotein primarily binds basic drugs, the protein levels alone suggest that the binding of acidic drugs should decrease and of basic drugs should increase in elderly subjects.

Apart from changes in serum protein concentrations, very few causes for altered protein binding have been demonstrable in aging persons. Biological modification of carrier proteins and competition with endogenous substances for binding sites may be mechanisms for the reduced drug binding associated with certain diseases (42–44) but are not applicable to normal aging (36). However, since multiple-drug therapy is common in geriatric patients, the risk for drug interactions at the binding site may be enhanced (45).

A number of factors other than age influence the protein binding of drugs, making it difficult to draw general conclusions from the studies performed so far in elderly subjects (41). Reduced binding with age has been shown for some antibiotics, e.g., cefoxitin (46), ceftriaxone (47), and flucloxacillin (48), while no age-related changes in protein binding could be found in studies of a number of other antimicrobials (33,41). Little is known about the effect of age on binding to cells (17,33), apart from one report on metronidazole showing reduced binding to red blood cells and, thus, a smaller apparent volume of distribution of the drug in older individuals (49). The binding of antibiotics to peripheral tissues is a field open for future study.

IV. ELIMINATION

A. Metabolism

Many pharmaceutical compounds are metabolized, either by metabolic degradation or by synthetic biotransformation, to more water-soluble molecules before excretion of these metabolites from the body. The liver is the dominant organ for the metabolic processes. The weight of the human liver declines with advancing age both in absolute terms and in relation to body weight (3,50). The number of liver cells decreases while the size of the remaining hepatocytes increases (16). The ultrastructure of the hepatocytes is altered with increases in cytoplasm, volume of lysosomes, and surface area of the smooth endoplasmatic reticulum, and a decrease in the number of mitochondria and Golgi apparatus (16).

The hepatic metabolic clearance is determined by the capacity of the transforming enzymes and by the hepatic blood flow. A reduced microsomal enzyme activity of the liver has been demonstrated in old rats (51). In aged humans, antipyrine and other compounds that are cleared by microsomal oxidation have been reported to have a lower elimination rate (50,52–54), although some studies show conflicting data (1,12). Acetylation and other forms of synthetic transformation are considered to be unaffected by old age (55), but a predominance of the slow-acetylator phenotype in elderly subjects was suggested in one report (56). Drugs with a high extraction ratio, i.e., compounds that are rapidly metabolized, depend more on the hepatic blood flow than on the enzymatic capacity for their elimination rate. Since the regional blood flow to the liver is reduced 40–45% between the ages of 25 and 65 (6), it is not surprising that several such drugs have a lower metabolic clearance in older persons (40).

At all ages, there is a large interindividual variation in metabolic drug elimination rate (57,58). Basically, the hepatic enzyme activity is genetically determined (57,58), but it is also affected by liver disease (59) and by several environmental factors, e.g., consumption of coffee (53), tobacco (53,60), alcohol or marijuana (59), and exposure to various chemicals and other drugs (58,59). Differences in hepatic drug metabolism between the sexes may be caused by hormonal influence (61), which is one of several explanations for the age-related decline in microsomal oxidation possibly being more pronounced in men than in women (40).

Much remains to be clarified regarding the influence of age on the metabolic transformation of specific antibiotics (33). The scarce data in the literature support clinical experience that the normal aging process has little impact on the metabolism of most antibiotics and that dose adjustment on that basis alone seldom is necessary (62). However, some of the above-mentioned environmental factors may have a combined effect with age on drug metabolism. For some drugs with mixed elimination mechanisms (i.e., hepatic and renal), maintained or increased nonrenal clearance may compensate for the age-related decline in renal excretion (13,63). The influence of the aging process on enzyme induction is not clearly understood (64).

B. Excretion

Renal excretion of unchanged drug is the most important route of elimination for a number of pharmaceuticals, including most β-lactams and many other antibiotics, such as aminoglycosides. The kidney is also the main excretory organ for the end products of drugs that are metabolized. Renal function may be impaired by diseases such as diabetes mellitus, hypertension, and urinary tract infections, all of which are more common in the geriatric population. Even without obvious disease, a number of morphological and functional alterations occur in the aging kidney: general atrophy (especially of the cortex), reduction in the number of glomeruli, histological abnormalities among the remaining glomeruli, thickening and reduplication of glomerular and tubular basement membranes, fatty degeneration of tubular cells, and development of tubular diverticula (65,66). The proportion of connective tissue increases in the medulla but not in the cortex (65).

Age-related vascular changes include arteriosclerosis of the renal arteries, but the findings in larger vessels are not as clearly related to the morphological and functional changes of the nephron as is the sclerosis of both afferent and efferent arterioli (65). It is unclear whether this arteriolosclerosis is mainly due to disease, e.g., hypertension, or to age alone (66). There is also disagreement on the role of vascular spasm for the decline in renal function; data from one study suggest that resting vasoconstriction in the arteriolar system is increased in elderly subjects (67), while later findings indicate that the vascular changes are structural rather than caused by spasm (68).

Table 1 summarizes the most important functional changes attributed to the aging of the kidneys. Data from a number of cross-sectional studies indicate that the glomerular filtration rate (GFR) decreases with advancing age. One longitudinal study supports these findings in an aging population as a whole, but in one third of the individuals studied for several years, no significant change in renal function was observed (79). Even though a continuous, linear function has been used to describe the relationship between age and GFR from early adulthood (75,80), accumulating evidence suggests that the decline in GFR is rather small at first, to be followed by a more rapid reduction after the age of 50 (69,70,72,74).

During the later decades of life, the decline in renal plasma flow (RPF) is probably slightly more pronounced than the reduction in GFR, resulting in a slow increase in filtration fraction (69,74). It has been suggested that the nephron loses its function as a unit during aging, a hypothesis that is supported by findings of a gradual loss of tubular excretory and reabsorptive capacity paralleling the age-related decline in GFR (70,77). However, there is far less knowledge about the impact of the physiological aging process on tubular than on glomerular function.

Table 1 Functional Changes of the Aging Kidney

Change	Ref.
Reduced glomerular filtration rate	69–74
Decreased renal plasma flow	69,70,74,75
Preferential perfusion to the juxtamedullar region	68
Increased filtration fraction	69,70,74
Altered tubular function	
Decreased maximum secretory transport capacity	70,75
Impaired acid secretion	76
Impaired glucose reabsorption	77
Impaired urine-concentrating ability	78

In view of the described age-related changes in renal function, the many reports on decreased renal clearances of various antibiotics in elderly patients are not surprising. Unfortunately, several of the studies have documented not the kinetic consequences of aging as such, but rather the consequences of various disease states. Subjects with concurrent diseases including renal impairment beyond that caused by physiological aging have often been included in the investigations (33). Nevertheless, data from studies in carefully selected healthy volunteers definitely demonstrate a true relation between advanced age and reduced renal excretion of antibiotics (30,33,35).

The kidneys are not the only excretory organs for antibiotics. Biliary secretion to the intestine is of major importance for some compounds. Animal studies have demonstrated an age-related decline in the efficiency of the hepatobiliary excretory capacity (61), but it is unclear whether these findings are relevant for humans. There are limited data on biliary excretion of antibiotics in healthy volunteers or patients without hepatobiliary disorders because of the difficulty in obtaining samples of bile. Indirect evidence from studies of antibiotics with significant biliary elimination suggests that this pathway is less affected than renal excretion by advancing age (33,62). Some antibiotics may be eliminated via other mechanisms, e.g., direct excretion of quinolones through the enteric mucosa (81), but there is no knowledge of the relation between these mechanisms and age.

V. ADVERSE REACTIONS (see also Chap. 6)

The risk for development of adverse reactions to medical treatment is a clinical problem of some magnitude. Many studies have shown that the frequency of side effects to drugs is higher in patients above 60 years of age (82–84). There is, however, evidence that this higher incidence may not be attributable to the aging process in itself (85); many confounding factors are involved such as concurrent diseases and polypharmacy with risk for interactions with other drugs.

Antibiotics are generally safe to use in the general as well as in a geriatric population. There are, however, some instances where adverse reactions to antimicrobial drugs have been more frequent in older patients, although it is not certain that the higher incidence is a consequence of aging itself.

Reactions in the skin and the lungs due to nitrofurantoin are more common in aging adults as clearly shown in an analysis of 921 reported cases of adverse reactions to this drug (86). It is notable that doses given to older patients were the same as those used in young subjects, and since nitrofurantoin is excreted via the kidneys, the older patients were probably overdosed with regard to their renal function.

Adverse reactions in the central nervous system in patients treated with quinolones (87) are more common in older subjects (88). Confusion and hallucinations seem to be related to relative overdoses of the drugs and to be reversible when therapy is stopped or dosage is reduced.

An increased frequency of *Clostridium difficile*–induced diarrhea has been reported in elderly patients (89,90). This is not necessarily a phenomenon directly related to age; it may be a result of the increased use of antibiotics in the older age groups compared to younger individuals. Alternatively, age-related changes in the colonic microflora have been suggested (91), which may predispose for gastrointestinal disturbances during antibiotic treatment.

There is no evidence that the risk for damage to the kidneys by antibiotics is greater in elderly subjects than in younger age groups. However, great care must be exercised when treatment is initiated with potentially nephrotoxic drugs, since dosing regimens based on pharmacokinetic data from young individuals can result in too large or too frequent doses in elderly patients. This is especially true for antibiotics that are excreted via the kidneys; the physiological decline in renal function with increasing age leads to slower elimination rate, higher area under the curve (AUC), and increased risk for nephrotoxicity. Studies on the nephrotoxicity of certain cephalosporins (92) and aminoglycosides (93,94) support this view. It is true that most often the renal impairment is reversible, but, as exemplified by the ototoxicity of the aminoglycosides and vancomycin, the accumulated levels of a drug in the circulation and in peripheral tissues may induce secondary toxic effects on other organ systems.

VI. INTERACTIONS WITH OTHER DRUGS

With increasing age, medication for a variety of acute or chronic diseases becomes more common. As a consequence, when prescribing antibiotic treatment, especially to an elderly person, it is important to consider what other drugs the patient may be taking. Pharmacokinetic or pharmacodynamic interactions can necessitate dosage adjustments and monitoring of serum levels of different drugs. Drugs that utilize common hepatic metabolic pathways are most likely to interact. There are, however, other examples such as increased risk for nephrotoxicity with specific drug combinations and reduced oral absorption of some antibiotics when combined with certain antacids.

Table 2 shows some clinically important interactions between antibiotics and other commonly used drugs. There are a number of other instances where antibiotics interact pharmacologically, and it must be strongly recommended that the prescription of antibiotics always be done with careful consideration of possible interaction with other medication.

VII. IMPLICATIONS IN CLINICAL PRACTICE

Dose recommendations for many antibiotics in geriatric patients still rely on general experience from related compounds and/or extrapolation of pharmacokinetic information from patients with, for example, mild renal impairment, rather than on actual results from

Table 2 Clinically Important Interactions Between Antibiotics and Other Drugs

Drug	Interaction	Ref.
Antacids containing	Tetracycline absorption is impaired	95
Al, Ca, Mg, and sucralfate	Quinolone absorption is impaired	96
Phenytoin	Doxycycline half-life is reduced	97
	Chloramphenicol inhibits phenytoin metabolism	95
	Trimethoprim inhibits phenytoin metabolism	98
	Rifampicin induces phenytoin metabolism	99
Carbamazepine	Doxycycline half-life is reduced	97
	Erythromycin inhibits carbamazepine clearance	100
Ethacrynic acid	Potentiates ototoxicity of aminoglycosides	95
Furosemide	Potentiates ototoxicity of aminoglycosides	95
Warfarin	Erythromycin reduces warfarin metabolism	100
	Cotrimoxazole reduces warfarin metabolism	101
	Metronidazole reduces warfarin metabolism	102
	Rifampicin increases warfarin metabolism	103
Dicoumarol	Chloramphenicol reduces dicoumarol metabolism	95
	Rifampicin induces dicoumarol metabolism	99
Tolbutamide	Chloramphenicol reduces tolbutamide metabolism	104
	Sulphonamides reduce tolbutamide clearance	105
	Rifampicin induces tolbutamide metabolism	106
Cyclosporin	Erythromycin reduces cyclosporin metabolism	107
	Rifampicin induces cyclosporin metabolism	99
	Gentamicin increases nephrotoxic potential of cyclosporin	108
	Trimethoprim increases nephrotoxic potential of cyclosporin	109
Theophylline	Erythromycin reduces theophylline metabolism	100
	Ciprofloxacin (and other hepatically metabolized quinolones) reduces theophylline clearance	96
Corticosteroids	Rifampicin increases microsomal oxidation of hydrocortisone, methylprednisolone, and prednisolone	99
	Erythromycin reduces methylprednisolone elimination	110

research on elderly subjects (33,62). In order to issue firm guidelines for age-related dosing of individual antibiotics, one would need to study not only the kinetics of the drugs, but also the pharmacodynamics and the clinical efficacy of new dosages in elderly patients. With the present knowledge some general rules can be given but must be used with caution, since even in healthy elderly subjects, interindividual variation of drug disposition is great.

For drugs that have been thoroughly investigated in the elderly population, age-related kinetic changes are usually closely related to alterations in renal elimination, while variations in absorption, distribution, and nonrenal elimination are less conspicuous (33,81). There are important exceptions, however, such as the increased oral bioavailability of ciprofloxacin in older adults (13), which should alert clinicians to the possibility of unexpected age-related pharmacokinetic phenomena occurring with new drugs.

For antibiotics with mainly renal elimination, e.g., many β-lactams, it is reasonable to reduce the daily dose by approximately 50% in patients with healthy kidneys who are older than 70 years. This can be done either by reducing the individual dose or by increasing the dose interval. Many β-lactams are known to be nontoxic, but the toxicity is poorly studied at the serum levels that are reached in elderly patients receiving doses appropriate for younger subjects. Unnecessarily high doses may, theoretically, also increase the ecological consequences of antibiotic use and are certainly uneconomical.

Several drugs with narrow therapeutic ranges, e.g., aminoglycosides and vancomycin, are excreted by the kidneys. Doses should be reduced in elderly patients, but because of inter-subject variation in kinetics and the risk for toxic adverse reactions, serum levels must be monitored regularly to assure efficacy and safety (see Chap. 5).

Since age-related changes in nonrenal elimination routes seem to be of minor or less predictable importance for the gross elimination of antibiotics, compounds that are to a large extent metabolized or excreted by organs other than the kidneys can probably be given at unchanged doses to most elderly patients. However, the influence of age on the kinetics of these drugs is still poorly investigated.

In summary, we would like to stress the necessity to individualize dosage regimens in the elderly patient. Apart from the kinetic changes related to physiological aging, subclinical disorders as well as overt disease affecting the eliminating organs are overrepresented at advanced age. Since the serum creatinine concentration is a poor determinant of renal function in older adults, substantial renal impairment with profound influence on drug elimination may go unrecognized. Approximate creatinine clearance estimation by one of the existing formulas or nomograms based on age, sex, weight, and serum creatinine level (111,112) is a simple and strongly advocated method to overcome this problem.

REFERENCES

1. Greenblatt DJ, Sellers EM, Shader RI. Drug disposition in old age. N Engl J Med 1982; 306:1081–8.
2. Norrby R. Antibiotics in the elderly. In: Butler RN, Bearn AG, eds. The aging process: therapeutic implications. New York: Raven Press, 1984:229–49.
3. Geokas MC, Haverback BJ. The aging gastrointestinal tract. Am J Surg 1969; 117:881–92.
4. Höffler D. Veränderung der Pharmakokinetik im Alter und ihre praktischen Konsequenzen. Z Gerontol 1981; 14:382–7.
5. Warren PM, Pepperman MA, Montgomery RD. Age changes in small-intestinal mucosa. (Letter) Lancet 1978; 2:849–50.
6. Bender AD. The effect of increasing age on the distribution of peripheral blood flow in man. J Am Geriatr Soc 1965; 13:192–8.
7. Kekki M, Samloff IM, Ihamäki T, Varis K, Siurala M. Age- and sex-related behaviour of gastric acid secretion at the population level. Scand J Gastroenterol 1982; 17:737–43.
8. Sommers DK, van Wyk M, Moncrieff J, Schoeman HS. Influence of food and reduced gastric acidity on the bioavailability of bacampicillin and cefuroxime axetil. Br J Clin Pharmacol 1984; 18:535–9.
9. Richey DP, Bender AD. Pharmacokinetic consequences of aging. Annu Rev Pharmacol Toxicol 1977; 17:49–65.
10. Evans MA, Triggs EJ, Cheung M, Broe GA, Creasey H. Gastric emptying rate in the elderly: implications for drug therapy. J Am Geriatr Soc 1981; 29:201–5.
11. Anonymous. Pharmacokinetics in the elderly. Lancet 1983; 1:568–9.
12. Ho PC, Triggs EJ. Drug therapy in the elderly. Aust NZ J Med 1984; 14:179–90.
13. Ljungberg B, Nilsson-Ehle I. Pharmacokinetics of ciprofloxacin in the elderly: increased oral bioavailability and reduced renal clearance. Eur J Clin Microbiol Infect Dis 1989; 8:515–20.

14. Douglas JG, Bax RP, Munro JF. The pharmacokinetics of cefuroxime in the elderly. J Antimicrob Chemother 1980; 6:543–9.
15. Collart P, Poitevin M, Milovanovic A, Herlin A, Durel J. Kinetic study of serum penicillin concentrations after single doses of benzathine and benethamine penicillins in young and old people. Br J Vener Dis 1980; 56:355–62.
16. Ritschel WA. Gerontokinetics. Caldwell, NJ: The Telford Press, 1988.
17. Vestal RE. Drug use in the elderly: a review of problems and special considerations. Drugs 1978; 16:358–82.
18. Bruce Å, Andersson M, Arvidsson B, Isaksson B. Body composition. Prediction of normal body potassium, body water and body fat in adults on the basis of body height, body weight and age. Scand J Clin Lab Invest 1980; 40:461–73.
19. Forbes GB, Reina JC. Adult lean body mass declines with age: some longitudinal observations. Metabolism 1970; 19:653–63.
20. Novak LP. Aging, total body potassium, fat-free mass, and cell mass in males and females between ages 18 and 85 years. J Gerontol 1972; 27:438–43.
21. Shock NW, Watkin DM, Yiengst MJ, Norris AH, Gaffney GW, Gregerman RI, Falzone JA. Age differences in the water content of the body as related to basal oxygen consumption in males. J Gerontol 1963; 18:1–8.
22. Crooks J, O'Malley K, Stevenson IH. Pharmacokinetics in the elderly. Clin Pharmacokinet 1976; 1:280–96.
23. Kates RE, Harapat SR, Keefe DLD, Goldwater D, Harrison DC. Influence of prolonged recumbency on drug disposition. Clin Pharmacol Ther 1980; 28:624–8.
24. Levy G. Effect of bed rest on distribution and elimination of drugs. (Letter) J Pharm Sci 1967; 56:928–9.
25. Wilson K. Sex-related differences in drug disposition in man. Clin Pharmacokinet 1984; 9:189–202.
26. Rodeheffer RJ, Gerstenblith G, Becker LC, Fleg JL, Weisfeldt ML, Lakatta EG. Exercise cardiac output is maintained with advancing age in healthy human subjects: cardiac dilatation and increased stroke volume compensate for a diminished heart rate. Circulation 1984; 69:203–13.
27. Ganzinger U, Haslberger A. Pharmacokinetics of cephalosporins in normal and septicemic rabbits. Antimicrob Agents Chemother 1985; 28:473–7.
28. Ganzinger U, Haslberger A, Sciel H, Omilian-Rosso R, Schütze E. Influence of endotoxin on the distribution of cephalosporins in rabbits. J Antimicrob Chemother 1986; 17:785–93.
29. Ljungberg B, Nilsson-Ehle I. Influence of age on the pharmacokinetics of ceftazidime in acutely ill, adult patients. Eur J Clin Pharmacol 1988; 34:173–8.
30. Ljungberg B, Nilsson-Ehle I. Advancing age and acute infection influence the kinetics of ceftazidime. Scand J Infect Dis 1989; 21:327–32.
31. Pennington JE, Dale DC, Reynolds HY, MacLowry JD. Gentamicin sulfate pharmacokinetics: lower levels of gentamicin in blood during fever. J Infect Dis 1975; 132:270–5.
32. Perfect JR, Durack DT. Pharmacokinetics of cefoperazone, moxalactam, cefotaxime, trimethoprim and sulphamethoxazole in experimental meningitis. J Antimicrob Chemother 1981; 8:49–58.
33. Ljungberg B, Nilsson-Ehle I. Pharmacokinetics of antimicrobial agents in the elderly. Rev Infect Dis 1987; 9:250–64.
34. Ljungberg B, Nilsson-Ehle I. Comparative pharmacokinetics of ceftazidime in young, healthy and elderly, acutely ill males. Eur J Clin Pharmacol 1988; 34:179–86.
35. Ljungberg B, Nilsson-Ehle I. Pharmacokinetics of meropenem and its metabolite in young and elderly healthy men. Antimicrob Agents Chemother 1992; 36:1437–40.
36. Bender AD, Post A, Meier JP, Higson JE, Reichard G Jr. Plasma protein binding of drugs as a function of age in adult human subjects. J Pharm Sci 1975; 64:1711–3.

37. Cammarata RJ, Rodnan GP, Fennell RH. Serum anti-gammaglobulin and antinuclear factors in the aged. JAMA 1967; 199:455–8.
38. Dybkær R, Lautitzen M, Krakauer R. Relative reference values for clinical chemical and haematological quantities in "healthy" elderly people. Acta Med Scand 1981; 209:1–9.
39. Woodford-Williams E, Alvarez AS, Webster D, Landless B, Dixon MP. Serum protein patterns in normal and pathological ageing. Gerontologia 1964/65; 10:86–99.
40. Greenblatt DJ, Abernethy DR, Shader RI. Pharmacokinetic aspects of drug therapy in the elderly. Ther Drug Monit 1986; 8:249–55.
41. Wallace SM, Verbeeck RK. Plasma protein binding of drugs in the elderly. Clin Pharmacokinet 1987; 12:41–72.
42. Anton AH, Corey WT. Interindividual differences in the protein binding of sulfonamides: the effect of disease and drugs. Acta Pharmacol Toxicol 1971; 29(Suppl 3):134–51.
43. Lichtenwalner DM, Suh B, Lorber B, Rudnick MR, Craig WA. Correction of drug binding defects in uremia in vitro by anion exchange resin treatment. Biochem Pharmacol 1982; 31:3483–7.
44. Reitberg DP, Cumbo TJ, Smith IL, Schentag JJ. Effect of protein binding on cefmenoxime steady-state kinetics in critical patients. Clin Pharmacol Ther 1984; 35:64–73.
45. Wallace S, Whiting B, Runcie J. Factors affecting drug binding in plasma of elderly patients. Br J Clin Pharmacol 1976; 3:327–30.
46. Garcia MJ, Garcia A, Nieto MJ, Dominguez-Gil A, Alonso G, Mellado L. Disposition of cefoxitin in the elderly. Int J Clin Pharmacol Ther Toxicol 1980; 18:503–9.
47. Luderer JR, Patel IH, Durkin J, Schneck DW. Age and ceftriaxone kinetics. Clin Pharmacol Ther 1984; 35:19–25.
48. Anderson P, Bluhm G, Ehrnebo M, Herngren L, Jacobson B. Pharmacokinetics and distribution of flucloxacillin in pacemaker patients. Eur J Clin Pharmacol 1984/85; 27:713–9.
49. Ludwig E, Csiba A, Magyar T, Szöcs G, Graber H. Age-associated pharmacokinetic changes of metronidazole. Int J Clin Pharmacol Ther Toxicol 1983; 21:87–91.
50. Bach B, Mølholm Hansen J, Kampmann JP, Rasmussen SN, Skovsted L. Disposition of antipyrine and phenytoin correlated with age and liver volume in man. Clin Pharmacokinet 1981; 6:389–96.
51. Kato R, Vassanelli P, Frontino G, Chiesara E. Variation in the activity of liver microsomal drug-metabolizing enzymes in rats in relation to the age. Biochem Pharmacol 1964; 13:1037–51.
52. O'Malley K, Crooks J, Duke E, Stevenson IH. Effect of age and sex on human drug metabolism. Br Med J 1971; 3:607–9.
53. Vestal RE, Norris AH, Tobin JD, Cohen BH, Shock NW, Andres R. Antipyrine metabolism in man: influence of age, alcohol, caffeine, and smoking. Clin Pharmacol Ther 1975; 18:425–32.
54. Wilkinson GR, Shand DG. A physiological approach to hepatic drug clearance. Clin Pharmacol Ther 1975; 18:377–90.
55. Evans DAP, Manley KA, McKusick VA. Genetic control of isoniazid metabolism in man. Br Med J 1960; 2:485–91.
56. Gachályi B, Vas A, Hajós P, Káldor A. Acetylator phenotypes: effect of age. Eur J Clin Pharmacol 1984; 26:43–5.
57. Evans DAP. Inter-individual differences in metabolism of drugs: the role of genetic factors. Acta Pharmacol Toxicol 1971; 29(Suppl 3):156–63.
58. Sjöqvist F, Alván G. Aging and drug disposition—metabolism. J Chronic Dis 1983; 36:31–7.
59. Jusko WJ, Gardner MJ, Mangione A, Schentag JJ, Koup JR, Vance JW. Factors affecting theophylline clearances: age, tobacco, marijuana, cirrhosis, congestive heart failure, obesity, oral contraceptives, benzodiazepines, barbiturates, and ethanol. J Pharm Sci 1979; 68:1358–66.
60. Hart P, Farrell GC, Cooksley WGE, Powell LW. Enhanced drug metabolism in cigarette smokers. Br Med J 1976; 2:147–9.
61. Schmucker DL. Aging and drug disposition: an update. Pharmacol Rev 1985; 37:133–48.

62. Ljungberg B. Use of antibiotics in the elderly: pharmacokinetics of the most commonly used agents. Geriat Med Today 1988; 7:55–65.
63. Norrby SR, Ljungberg B. Pharmacokinetics of fluorinated 4-quinolones in the aged. Rev Infect Dis 1989; 11(suppl 5):1102–6.
64. Twum-Barima Y, Finnigan T, Habash AI, Cape RTD, Caruthers SG. Impaired enzyme induction by rifampicin in the elderly. (Letter) Br J Clin Pharmacol 1984; 17:595–7.
65. Lindeman RD, Goldman R. Anatomic and physiologic age changes in the kidney. Exp Gerontol 1986; 21:379–406.
66. McLachlan MSF. The ageing kidney. Lancet 1978; 2:143–6.
67. McDonald RF, Solomon DH, Shock NW. Aging as a factor in the renal hemodynamic changes induced by a standardized pyrogen. J Clin Invest 1951; 5:457–62.
68. Hollenberg NK, Adams DF, Solomon HS, Rashid A, Abrams HL, Merrill JP. Senescence and the renal vasculature in normal man. Circulation Res 1974; 34:309–16.
69. Bäck SE, Ljungberg B, Nilsson-Ehle I, Borgå O, Nilsson-Ehle P. Age dependence of renal function: Clearance of iohexol and p-amino hippurate in healthy males. Scand J Clin Lab Invest 1989; 49:641–6.
70. Davies DF, Shock NW. Age changes in glomerular filtration rate, effective renal plasma flow, and tubular excretory capacity in adult males. J Clin Invest 1950; 29:496–507.
71. Gault MH, Cockcroft DW. Creatinine clearance and age. (Letter) Lancet 1975; 2:612–13.
72. Granerus G, Aurell M. Reference values for 51Cr-EDTA clearance as a measure of glomerular filtration rate. Scand J Clin Lab Invest 1981; 41:611–16.
73. Rowe JW, Andres R, Tobin JD, Norris AH, Shock NW. The effect of age on creatinine clearance in men: a cross-sectional and longitudinal study. J Gerontol 1976; 31:155–63.
74. Wesson LG, Jr. Renal hemodynamics in physiological states. In: Physiology of the human kidney, New York: Grune & Stratton, 1969:96–108.
75. Watkin DM, Shock NW. Agewise standard value for C_{In}, C_{PAH}, and Tm_{PAH} in adult males. J Clin Invest 1955; 34:969.
76. Adler S, Lindeman RD, Yiengst MJ, Beard E, Shock NW. Effect of acute acid loading on urinary acid excretion by the aging human kidney. J Lab Clin Med 1968; 72:278–89.
77. Miller JH, McDonald RK, Shock NW. Age changes in the maximal rate of renal tubular reabsorption of glucose. J Gerontol 1976; 31:155–63.
78. Rowe JW, Shock NW, DeFronzo RA. The influence of age on the renal response to water deprivation in man. Nephron 1976; 17:270–8.
79. Lindeman RD, Tobin J, Shock NW. Longitudinal studies on the rate of decline in renal function with age. J Am Geriatr Soc 1985; 33:278–85.
80. Rowe JW, Andres R, Tobin JD, Norris AH, Shock NW. Age-adjusted standards for creatinine clearance. Ann Intern Med 1976; 84:567–9.
81. Nilsson-Ehle I, Ljungberg B. Quinolone disposition in the elderly: practical implications. Drugs Aging 1991; 1:279–88.
82. Fletcher RH, Fletcher SW. Iatrogenic illness and the elderly. In: Petersen MD, White DL, eds. Health care of the elderly: an information sourcebook. Newbury Park, CA: Sage Publications, 1989:451–74.
83. Hurwitz, N. Predisposing factors in adverse reactions to drugs. Br Med J 1969; 1:536–9.
84. Caranasos GJ, Stewart RB, Cluff LE. Drug-induced illness leading to hospitalization. JAMA 1974; 228:713–17.
85. Gurwitz JH, Avorn J. The ambiguous relation between aging and adverse drug reactions. Ann Intern Med 1991; 114:956–66.
86. Holmberg L, Boman G, Böttiger LE, Eriksson B, Spross R, Wessling A. Adverse reactions to nitrofurantoin: analysis of 921 reports. Am J Med 1980; 69:733–8.
87. Monk JP, Campoli-Richards DM. Ofloxacin: a review of its antibacterial activity, pharmacokinetic properties and therapeutic use. Drugs 1987; 33:346–91.

88. National Board of Health and Welfare. Biverkningar av Lexinor—en treårs-uppföljning (in Swedish). Information från Socialstyrelsens läkemedelsavdelning 1989; 14:118–21.
89. Möllby, R, Nord C-E, Aronsson B. Diagnosis of Clostridium difficile-associated enterocolitis in Sweden. Laboratory and epidemiological aspects. Scand J Infect Dis, 1980;(suppl 20):30–6.
90. Mulligan ME, Epidemiology of Clostridium difficile-induced intestinal disease. Rev Infect Dis 1984; 6(suppl 1):222–8.
91. Ljungberg B, Nilsson-Ehle I, Edlund C, Nord CE. Influence of ciprofloxacin on the colonic microflora in young and elderly volunteers: no impact of the altered drug absorption. Scand J Infect Dis 1990; 22:205–8.
92. Foord RD. Cephaloridine, cephalothin and the kidney. J Antimicrob Chemother 1975; 1(suppl):119–33.
93. Moore RD, Smith CR, Lipsky JJ, Mellits ED, Lietman PS. Risk factors for nephrotoxicity in patients treated with aminoglycosides. Ann Intern Med 1984; 100:352–7.
94. Trollfors B, Alestig K, Krantz I, Norrby R. Quantitative nephrotoxicity of gentamicin in nontoxic doses. J Infect Dis 1980; 141:306–9.
95. Bint AJ, Reeves DS. Interactions between antibiotics and other drugs. In Schönfeld H, ed. Antibiotics and chemotherapy. Vol. 25, Pharmacokinetics. Basel: S. Karger, 1978:289–320.
96. Davey PG. Overview of drug interactions with the quinolones. J Antimicrob Chemother 1988; 22(suppl C):97–107.
97. Penttilä O, Neuvonen PJ, Aho K, Lehtovaara R. Interaction between doxycycline and some antiepileptic drugs. Br Med J 1974; 2:470–2.
98. Hansen JM, Kampmann JP, Siersbæk-Nielsen K, Lumholtz IB, Arrie M, Abildgaard U, Skovsted L. The effect of different sulphonamides on phenytoin metabolism in man. Acta Med Scand 1979; 624(suppl):106–10.
99. Dollery C, ed. Therapeutic drugs. Edinburgh: Churchill Livingstone, 1991.
100. Ludden TM. Pharmacokinetic interactions of the macrolide antibiotics. Clin Pharmacokinet 1985; 10:63–79.
101. O'Reilly RA, Motley CH. Racemic warfarin and trimethoprim-sulphamethoxazole interaction in humans. Ann Intern Med 1979; 91:34–6.
102. O'Reilly RA. The stereoselective interaction of warfarin and metronidazole in man. N Engl J Med 1976; 295:354–7.
103. O'Reilly RA. Interaction of rifampicin and long-term anticoagulant therapy. Clin Res 1974; 22:115A.
104. Christensen LK, Skovstedt L. Inhibition of drug metabolism by chloramphenicol. Lancet 1969; 2:1397–9.
105. Christensen LK, Hansen JM, Kristensen M. Sulphaphenazole-induced hypoglycaemic attacks in tolbutamide-treated diabetics. Lancet 1963; 2:1298–1301.
106. Syvälahti EKG, Pihlajamäki KK, Iisalo EJ. Rifampicin and drug metabolism. Lancet 1974; 2:232–3.
107. Larrey D, Funck-Brentano C, Breil P, Vitaux J, Theodore C. Effects of erythromycin on hepatic drug metabolizing enzymes in humans. Biochem Pharmacol 1983; 32:1058–63.
108. Hows JM, Chipping PM, Fairhead S, Baughan A, Gordon-Smith EC. Nephrotoxicity in bone marrow transplant recipients treated with cyclosporin A. Br J Haematol 1983; 54:69–74.
109. Nyberg G, Gäbel H, Althoff P, Björk S, Herlitz H, Brynger H. Adverse effect of trimethoprim on kidney function in renal transplant patients. Lancet 1984; 1:394–5.
110. Laforce CF, Szeffler SJ, Miller MF, Elbing W, Brenner M. Inhibition of methylprednisolone elimination in the presence of erythromycin therapy. J Allergy Clin Immunol 1983; 72:34–9.
111. Cockcroft DW, Gault MH. Prediction of creatinine clearance from serum creatinine. Nephron 1976; 16:31–41.
112. Siersbæk-Nielsen K, Mølholm Hansen J, Kampmann J, Kristensen M. Rapid evaluation of creatinine clearance. (Letter) Lancet 1971; 1:1133–4.

5

Assay Methods for Antimicrobial Therapy

Roger E. Bawdon
The University of Texas Southwestern Medical Center, Dallas, Texas

I. INTRODUCTION

With elderly persons (65 years of age and older) accounting for 25% of health care expenditures and consuming 25% of the prescription drugs dispensed, it is an important consideration that a major portion of this population also requires the use of a large percentage of antimicrobial agents (1,2). Because the elderly person is frequently taking multiple drugs for a variety of illnesses, and because of the physiological changes associated with aging, it is not unusual for at least 10% of older patients to have an adverse drug reaction during their first hospital admission (3). The use of antimicrobials during the hospital stay obviously contributes to these statistics. These antibiotic-related adverse reactions occur for the reasons listed in Table 1.

There are several reasons for the higher incidence of adverse reactions in elderly patients, including decreased renal function, differences in drug absorption caused by changes in gastrointestinal pH, decreased absorption surface, decreases in physical activity, and drug interactions. In addition, the decrease in serum albumin and an increase in body fat associated with aging contribute to elevated serum concentrations of some antimicrobials. Of these pharmacokinetic changes, probably the most important is renal impairment, leading to higher drug levels over longer periods of time (4) (see also Chap. 4). Thus, the clinical laboratory must have the capability to quantitate many of the antimicrobial agents used for the treatment of infections in these patients.

Because of the narrow therapeutic index of some antibiotics and the physiological variability of the elderly patient, there have been rapid advancements in the development of assays for most antibiotics used in geriatric medicine today. The assays that are available range from simple microbiological assays to complex assays using high-pressure liquid chromatography (HPLC) and electrochemical detectors or assays using radiochemicals and immunological complexes. The simplest and most economical method used for quantifying

Table 1 Age-Associated Pharmacokinetic Changes Contributing to Adverse Reactions Related to Antimicrobial Chemotherapy

Antibiotic	Age-associated pharmacokinetic changes
Aminoglycosides	Increased half-life
Tetracyclines	Increased half-life, absorption unchanged with achlorhydria
Penicillins	Increased half-life
Cephalosporins	Increased half-life
Isoniazid	Increased half-life, proportion of rapid acetylators unchanged
5-Flucytosine	Increased half-life

antimicrobial agents is the microbiological assay, which may be used for essentially all antimicrobial agents. This biological method was developed about 30 years ago and is still very useful (5). It can be very accurate when used by experienced laboratory personnel. Although the microbiological method has been replaced by high technology in most instances, the assay remains probably the best assay for macrolide antibiotics.

II. MICROBIOLOGICAL ASSAY

The microbiological assay is based on the simple diffusion of antibiotics through an agar base that has been inoculated with a susceptible strain of bacteria and the inhibition of this microbial growth by antimicrobial diffusion. The size of the zone of inhibition is correlated with known concentrations of a drug in standard samples. Zone sizes are plotted against drug concentrations on semi-log paper. Concentrations of drugs in patient samples are determined by matching the zone size on the graph and ascertaining the corresponding drug concentration. There are three different methods by which the assay may be set up. The first consists of cutting six or eight round holes (about 5 mm in diameter) in the agar of a Petri dish that has been seeded with bacteria and applying both standards and test solutions into these holes. In the second method, stainless steel wells are placed firmly on the agar seeded with the test organism lawn, and the standards and test samples are added to the wells. The last and probably the most common method is the placement of 0.50-cm filter paper discs on the agar inoculated lawn and placing up to 0.015 ml of either standards or patient's samples on the filter paper discs. All methods require incubation for a minimum of 4 h. In general, additional incubation does not alter the results of early measurement of zones of inhibition (6).

A number of variables determine the sensitivity and accuracy of the microbiological methods. In experienced hands the relative standard deviation and percent recovery may be less than 5%. If subtle changes are allowed to occur, errors of up to 30–40% are not uncommon, making the test essentially useless and potentially harmful to the patient (7). One variable that may cause a significant error is the uneven surface in which the agar is allowed to harden. Diffusion of antibiotics in medium with an uneven surface will occur at different rates, which will cause extreme variability in the different zone sizes. Heavily seeded agar may also give erroneous results because the zones of inhibition may be too small, not allowing accurate measurement of the zones. Such inaccuracies translate

Table 2 A Typical Isocratic HPLC System Used for Antibiotic Assays in a Clinical Laboratory

Solvent reservoir → Pump(s) → Sample Processor → Column → Detector → Recorder

into potentially large errors in the quantitation of drugs in either tissue or body fluids. Poor techniques in pipetting may account for significant errors, either in the preparation of the standards or in the addition of the samples to the filter paper discs. Other factors that may contribute to errors include incorrect pH, uremic sera in which the blood urea nitrogen (BUN) is >50 mg/100 ml, combination therapy in which the laboratory is not made aware of the additional antibiotics, and excessive time in the application of the samples to the plate, which allows the antibiotics to diffuse at different times, causing variability in zone sizes.

III. HPLC ASSAYS

The modern HPLC system is an expensive, sophisticated composite of instruments costing approximately $50,000. However, many antibiotic assays may be completed accurately and rapidly on systems costing much less. The basic system consists of a solvent reservoir, pump, injector, column, detector, and recorder. More complex systems may include several pumps, an automated sample processor, a variable wavelength detector, and a microprocessor or integrator system. Table 2 shows one of the systems used for routine drug assays in a clinical laboratory.

An overview of the basic system includes the solvent reservoir or mobile phase, which generally consists of a pH stable buffer, water, and an organic portion consisting of acetonitrile or alcohol in varying percentages. The mobile phase is drawn into the high-pressure pump, which applies up to 3000 psi to the mobile phase to force it and the components of the sample to be separated through the column. Following the pump is the injector, which may either be a hand-operated manual injector or an automated sample processor that may inject up to 100 samples without requiring attention. The simple injector allows the sample to be placed in a sample loop, which permits the injection of a measured sample that is isolated for the pressurized system without the loss of sample or the injection of air into the column or detector.

The column consists of a support matrix of silica that is bound to various octadecylsilane (ODS) groups. The different ODS groups vary in the amount of end capping, chain length, and branching, all of which may contribute to the separation of various compounds. This material is generally packed in a stainless steel column, which has a length of up to 25 cm with an inside diameter of 3–5 mm. The particle size of the packing is generally in the range of 3–5 μm. A wide variety of columns is available for separating different compounds. Probably one of the most important chemical characteristics of a compound is its polarity. Usually reverse-phase chromatography is used for antibiotic assays in which the column support is essentially nonpolar. Compound separation or retention is a function of polar interactions between the stationary phase and the mobile phase. In this situation, reverse-phase chromatography is related to one of the main compounds of the mobile phase, i.e., water, which is the most polar compound. (Water has a polarity index of 9, whereas hexane has a polarity index of 0.) Acetonitrile and methanol are frequently added

Table 3 Physical Chemical Characteristics of Compounds That Result in Separation of Various Antibiotics

Van der Waals forces cause distortion in the electrostatic configuration
Dipole interaction causes an electrostatic attraction
Hydrogen bonding bonds proton donors and proton acceptors
Dielectric interactions result from a solute and a solvent of high dielectric constant

Source: Ref 8.

Table 4 Simple Parameters That Affect Chromatographic Retention Time

Organic modifiers
Temperature
pH
Buffer
Salt concentration
Chain length

Source: Ref. 9.

to water to alter the polarity. Factors contributing to compound separation are depicted in Table 3. Other simple factors that influence the HPLC separation and can be readily altered to change the retention time of an antibiotic are shown in Table 4.

A number of detectors are available, ranging from simple spectrophotometers to sophisticated electrochemical detectors. Table 5 lists the various detectors that are commercially available. The most common detector used in the detection of β-lactam antibiotics is the ultraviolet (UV-Vis) detector because it is simple, inexpensive, stable, and sensitive. In addition, beta-lactam antibiotics have an intrinsic chromophore, which permits the use of UV-Vis detection. Many other antimicrobials have this characteristic, although variable wavelength detection may be required because of different absorption by different chromo-

Table 5 Commercially Available HPLC Detectors

UV-Vis (fixed wavelength)
UV-Vis (variable wavelength)
Electrochemical
Fluorescence
Radioactivity
Refractive index

phores. Concentration of antibiotics may be determined by the relationship established by the Beer-Lambert equation (10):

$$\log(I_0/I) = E \times L \times C$$

where I = transmitted light; I_0 = incident light; E = molar extinction coefficient; L = optical path length; and C = molar concentration.

Detectors vary from fixed-wavelength detectors (FWD) to variable-wavelength detectors (VWD), which have a single light source, and polar filters to accommodate alternate wavelengths. One of the most common light sources is a mercury lamp, which accommodates filters from 254 to 580 nm. More complex systems use a tungsten lamp and a monochromator to select the desired wavelength.

In addition, a photodiode array may be used to select a wavelength, thus allowing continuous monitoring of peaks as they flow through the detector. These VWD detect a wavelength from 190 to 700 nm, thus making the UV-Vis detector very useful in the clinical laboratory.

Fluorescence detectors are used when no chromophore is present. Some antimicrobial compounds such as the quinolones have a natural fluorescence, whereas other compounds such as the aminoglycosides must be derivatized with a derivatizing agent such as orthophthaldehyde before they may be detected. Derivatizing may be done either pre- or postcolumn. However, different mobile phases must be used for each method.

Fluorescence detectors consist of several components: a xenon light source, a series of filters, a photodiode, and a photomultiplier tube. The light source or excitation light is filtered, and the intensity of this light source is used as a reference. This source is again filtered through a series of mirrors while passing through the flow cell in which changes in the mobile phase related to the sample are measured on a photodiode. The emitted energy from the sample passes into the flow cell, through an interference filter, and then into a photomultiplier. The energy of the emitted light can be filtered at a specific wavelength by the introduction of emission filters. As the sample passes through the flow cell, differences in the emitted light are measured on the photomultiplier and diode, and data are calculated electronically to determine the amount of fluorescence in the sample. These data are then transmitted to the recorder for data analysis.

Refractive index detectors measure the difference in the amount of transmitted light as the mobile phase and sample pass through the surface of a glass prism. Two parallel beams of tungsten light are focused through a prism. As the transmitted light is scattered, it is collected by a photo cell so that as the compound to be measured passes through the sample cell, it is refracted and detected by the photo cell. The differences in refractive index are related to sample concentration, and these differences are transmitted electronically to a recorder.

Electrochemical detectors are used primarily for the assay of macrolide antibiotics, such as erythromycin. These detectors may be used for the assay of other antimicrobials, but because of the complexity of these detectors, other methods are used rather than this system. Two different electrochemical detectors are commonly used: the coulometric and the amperometric systems. The theory for these systems is a complex measurement of electron transfer and the oxidation or reduction of the compound to be measured as it passes through a high constant electrical potential. The current resulting from these electrochemical changes is proportional to the amount of the compound present. This difference in signal is recorded on a strip chart recorder or integrator.

Table 6 Classes of Antimicrobials Used by the Geriatric Population and the Most Common Method of Determination

Antibiotic	Method	Detector
Aminoglycosides	FPIA, EMIT	
Amphotericin B	HPLC	UV-Vis
Cephalosporins	HPLC	UV-Vis
Chloramphenicol	HPLC	UV-Vis
Clindamycin	HPLC	UV-Vis
Fluconazole	HPLC	UV-Vis
5-Flucytosine	HPLC	UV-Vis
Ketoconazole	HPLC	UV-Vis
Macrolides	MICRO	
Penicillins	HPLC	UV-Vis
Quinilones	HPLC	FLURO
Tetracyclines	MICRO	
Vancomycin	HPLC EMIT	

FPIA = fluorescences polarization immunoassay; HPLC = high pressure liquid chromatography; MICRO = microbiological assay; UV-Vis = ultraviolet visible light spectrum; FLURO = fluorescence; EMIT = enzyme multiplied immunoassay technique.

Radioactivity detectors are generally not used for the detection of antibiotics in a clinical situation; however, continuous flow radioactivity detectors have been developed for HPLC use but are not applicable in this situation. Antibiotics such as aminoglycosides and vancomycin may be assayed by HPLC, but these assays have been replaced by fluorescence polarization immunoassay (FPIA) and by enzyme multiplied immunoassay techniques (EMIT) (5).

IV. OTHER ASSAYS

The FPIA method involves the polarization of light at an excitation wavelength and a different emission wavelength. The polarization of tracer amounts of fluorescein is attached to the antibiotic, resulting in an increase in emission wavelength excitation time because of the antibody–antibiotic fluorescent complex. When the complex is diluted with patient serum-containing antibiotic (aminoglycoside or vancomycin), there is a corresponding reduction in fluorescence. This reduction in fluorescence relates to the concentration of gentamicin, tobramycin, amikacin, or vancomycin. FPIA used for the estimation of vancomycin is probably not accurate in some situations. The FPIA system overestimates the vancomycin levels in patients with renal failure by as much as 64%—a serious error in these very ill patients (11). The overestimation is related to the accumulation of vancomycin metabolites in the serum of these patients. Therefore, the FPIA method for the estimation of vancomycin should not be used for the assay of this drug in patients with renal disease (11).

The EMIT assay is also available for vancomycin and the aminoglycoside antibiotics (12). The procedure involves the coupling of glucose 6-phosphate dehydrogenase (G6PD)

to the antibiotic and the antibody to the drug. Coenzyme nicotinamide adenine dinucleotide (NAD) from a bacterial source is also involved in the assay. A portion of G6PD is bound to the antibody, while some remains free. The free portion is responsible for the conversion of NAD to NADH, which is spectrophotometrically active. The absorbance measurement from the standard curve is used to determine the concentration of the drug in the patient's serum. G6PD from humans does not cross-react with the bacterial source. The EMIT system provides rapid analysis; however, samples that are lipemic, hemolyzed, or icteric may interfere with the assay.

Table 6 lists antibiotics frequently prescribed in geriatric patients and their most common method of measurement (13–22).

REFERENCES

1. Schmucker DL. Aging and drug disposition: an update. Pharmacol Rev 1985; 37:133–48.
2. Kovar M. Health of the elderly and use of health service. Public Health Rep 1977; 92:9–19.
3. Christopher B, Vallanger R, Shepart A. A survey of hospitals prescribing for the elderly. In: Erato J, Stevenson I, eds. Drugs and the elderly. Baltimore: University Park Press, 1979:321–8.
4. Vestal RE. Drug use in the elderly: a review of problems and special considerations. Drugs 1978; 16:358–82.
5. Edberg SC. The measurement of antibiotics in human body fluids: techniques and significance. In: Lorian V, ed. Antibiotics in laboratory medicine. Baltimore: Williams and Wilkins; 1985:381–476.
6. Sabath LD. The assay of microbiological compound. Human Pathol 1976; 1:287–95.
7. College of American Pathologists. Infectious Disease 1986 Survey. Set 1D-A, p. 6.
8. Fallon A, Booth RFG, Bell LD. Laboratory techniques in biochemistry and molecular biology. In: Burdon RH, Van Knippenberg PH, eds. New York: Elsevier, 1987:73–90.
9. Fallon A, Booth RFG, Bell LD. Laboratory techniques in biochemistry and molecular biology. In: Burdon RH, Van Knippenberg PH, eds. New York: Elsevier, 1987:8–9.
10. Atkins PW, ed. Physical chemistry. San Francisco: W.H. Freeman and Co, 1987:585–90.
11. Morse GD, Narin DK, Bertins JS, Walshe JJ. Overestimation of vancomycin concentrations utilizing fluorescence polarization immunoassay in patients on peritoneal dialysis. Ther Drug Monit 1987; 9:212–15.
12. Yeo KT, Traverse W, Horowitz GL. Clinical performance of the EMIT vancomycin assay. Clin Chem 1989; 35:1504–7.
13. Reeves DS, Ullmann U, eds. High performance liquid chromatography in medical microbiology. New York: Guston Fischer Verlag, 1986.
14. Rudick JT, Bawdon RE. Determination of penicillinase resistant penicillins in serum using high pressure liquid chromatography. J Liquid Chromatogr 1981; 4:1525–45.
15. Rho JP, Jones A, Woo M, Caslle S, Smith K, Bawdon RE, Norman DC. Single dose pharmacokinetics of intravenous ampicillin plus sulbactam in healthy elderly and young adult subjects. J Antimicrob Chemother 1989; 24:573–80.
16. Bawdon RE, Hemsell DL, Hemsell PG. Serum and pelvic tissue concentrations of ceftriaxone and cefazolin at hysterectomy. J Liquid Chromatogr 1984; 7:2011–20.
17. Bawdon RE, Hemsell DL, Guss SP. Comparison of cefoperazone and cefoxitin concentrations in serum and pelvic tissue of abdominal hysterectomy patients. Antimicrob Agents Chemother 1982; 22:999–1003.
18. Bawdon RE, Leveno KL, Cunningham FG, Nobles B, Nelson S. Intrapartum pharmacokinetics of ticarcillin and clavulanic acid in serum as determined by high pressure liquid chromatography. Adv Ther 1984; 1:419–25.
19. Lu YS, Welch WD, Bawdon RE. The pharmacokinetics of procaine penicillin in rabbits infected with *Pasteurella multocida*. J Vet Microbiol 1987; 37:65–8.

20. Nilsson-Ehle I, Yoshikawa TT, Edwards JE, Schotz MC, Guze LB. Quantitation of amphotericin B with use of high pressure liquid chromatography. J Infect Dis 1977; 135:414–22.
21. Swezey SF, Giacomini KM, Borg AA, Brass C, Stevens D, Blaschke TF. Measurement of ketoconazole a new antifungal agent by high-performance liquid chromatography. J Chromatogr 1982; 227:510–15.
22. Lecaillon JB, Febvre N, Metayer JP, Souppart C. Quantitative assay of rifampicin and three of its metabolites in human plasma, urine and saliva by high-performance liquid chromatography. J Chromatogr 1978; 145:319–24.

6

Drug Prescribing, Compliance, and Adverse Reactions

Jay P. Rho
University of Southern California School of Medicine and Shriners Hospital, Los Angeles, California

Mary Y. Ma
Veterans Affairs Medical Center—West Los Angeles, Los Angeles, California

I. INTRODUCTION

Since the introduction of tetracycline and chloramphenicol in the late 1940s, the clinical use of antimicrobial agents has played a major part in reducing overall morbidity and mortality in patients with infection. Advances in the development of antimicrobial agents now allow physicians the opportunity to select from a vast array of more potent and less toxic agents. Despite these pharmacological advances, the appropriate clinical application of antimicrobial agents is much more complex today, and not without inherent risks. The emergence of resistant organisms, observance of untoward toxic effects, and higher medical costs have all been associated with the indiscriminate or misuse of antimicrobial agents (1–3). It is now widely accepted that even the therapeutic use of medications can result in iatrogenic illness or adverse drug reactions, often leading to serious sequelae. Promoting the safe and efficacious use of antimicrobial agents in elderly patients may be even more complicated, in that special attention to the physiological and behavioral changes associated with this age group must be considered in order to prevent unexpected responses. Physiological changes in gastrointestinal, cardiac, and renal function occur as a function of aging and may affect the way certain antimicrobial agents are absorbed, distributed, and excreted (4–6). Pharmacodynamic changes in older adults can alter sensitivities to medications and can dramatically change an expected blood level-dose response curve (7–10).

Because elderly people as a group suffer from a greater number of disease states, they use a disproportionate amount of medication relative to their population size. Although elderly persons comprise approximately an eighth of the U.S. population, they consume almost a third of all medications, placing them at greater risk of drug-related problems (11). The incidence of adverse drug reactions has been noted to increase in relationship to the number of medications taken. Williamson reported that the incidence of adverse drug reactions can increase from 10% in patients receiving one drug to 27% in patients taking six (12). Compliance with medication regimens has been shown to decrease as the complexity of medication regimens increase.

As growth projections indicate, the elderly population will double within the next 50 years, and there is a growing concern about the impending economic consequences. The nation, already reeling from the skyrocketing costs of health care, may not be able to absorb the anticipated economic burden without major changes in medical practice. Rational and judicious use of health care resources must be a first step, but greater emphasis on the prevention of illness will need to be at the heart of our health care solution. The avoidance of adverse drug reactions and improvement in compliance will help to prevent unnecessary hospitalizations. Clearly more research on the influence of age on drug behavior will be needed to help guide drug prescribing. The Food and Drug Administration (FDA), recognizing this need, has recently revised its guidelines on new drug applications by advocating the inclusion of elderly subjects in clinical studies that are intended to measure the effectiveness, adverse effects, dose response, and blood level response to new drugs, particularly if the drug is likely to have significant use in geriatric patients (13). Such measures may help health care practitioners prepare for the increasing needs of an aging nation.

II. ADVERSE DRUG REACTIONS (see also Chap. 4)

An adverse drug reaction can be defined as an unintended, untoward, harmful, or noxious response to a drug occurring at dosage levels used in humans for disease prevention, diagnosis, or therapy. While this definition is considered by many physicians to be ambiguous, it generally serves as an umbrella definition for other terms such as hypersensitivity or allergic reaction, side effect, overdose, or intolerance. It has been well documented that elderly persons experience more adverse drug reactions than their younger counterparts (14–17). One study found that nearly half of all adverse drug reactions reported to the FDA from 1984 to 1989 with age information occurred in patients over the age of 50, and 17.0% of reports were in patients age 70 years or older (14). In a review of spontaneous adverse drug reports filed with FDA's Division of Epidemiology and Surveillance in 1986, investigators compared reporting rates adjusted for population size (15). FDA received 16 reports for every 100,000 U.S. residents aged 65 years or older as compared with 7 per 100,000 U.S. residents under 65 years. The number of drug reactions classified as serious also increased with advancing age. Fifty-three percent of adverse drug reaction reports for patients 85 years or older had a serious outcome, compared with 28% for patients 45–64. Death was noted in 19% of those aged 85 years and older, compared with 6% for the 45- to 64-year age group. The investigators adjusted reporting rates by drug use and found that the percentages were significantly higher in those people 65 years and older versus those 45–64 years for cardiac drugs (12.8 vs. 8.2%), vasodilating agents (6.3 vs. 2.7%), diuretics (5.1 vs. 3.8%), and cephalosporins (4.1 vs. 2.5%) (15). The true incidence of adverse drug reactions in older adults may be even higher than reported, as many signs of adverse reactions such as confusion, weakness, loss of appetite, constipation, diarrhea, tremor, or depression are mistakenly attributed to old age and go unreported.

While many adverse drug reactions are mild in nature and generally self-limiting, many can result in serious illness. It has been estimated that between 3 and 25% of hospital admissions are directly associated with a drug-related problem (16–21). The wide disparity in admission rates between studies may be explained by the differences in study definitions and criteria utilized by investigators. Ives found that 15.4% of admissions to a family medicine inpatient service were identified as drug related. In 9.9% of the above admissions, a drug-related problem was identified as the primary cause of hospitalization. The two most common types of drug-related admissions were adverse drug reactions (37.8%) and drug abuse (31.1%). Adverse drug reactions were most commonly implicated in patients more than 70 years old (16). In a study of iatrogenic admissions to the medical service of a public teaching hospital, 35 of the 45 (78%) noted iatrogenic admissions were considered drug related (19). Among the drug-related causes, 19 (54%) were side effects, 8 (23%) were related to therapeutic overdosage, 7 (20%) were immunological, and 1 was drug-disease interaction. Antibiotics were implicated in two of the reports: one cephalexin-induced pseudomembranous colitis, and one isoniazid- and rifampin-induced hepatitis (19). The role of medication noncompliance and adverse drug reactions in hospitalizations of elderly patients was studied by interviewing 315 consecutively elderly patients admitted to an acute care hospital (20). Eighty-nine of the elderly admissions (28.2%) were drug related, 36 due to noncompliance (11.4%) and 53 due to adverse drug reactions (16.8%). In another study the rate of occurrence of drug-induced illness as a cause of admission to the general medicine service of a community hospital was evaluated. Twenty-three of 244 patients (9.4%) were admitted with drug-induced illness. Patients with drug-induced illness were taking 5.7 medications as compared to 3.2 medications per patient admitted for other reasons (21).

While adverse drug reactions are reported to occur more frequently in aging adults, age in itself may not necessarily be an important risk factor (22–24). Other risk factors such as multiple medication use, types of medications prescribed, multiple disorders, severity of diseases, lengthy hospital stays, and decreased compliance are more likely to account for the increased number of reactions reported in the elderly population. A large multicenter study found that using four or more drugs, staying in a hospital more than 14 days, having more than four active medical problems, staying in a medical ward instead of a geriatric ward, and consuming alcohol to be positively correlated with the occurrence of adverse drug reactions (22). Age, gender, and cigarette smoking, however, were not found to be significant predictors of adverse drug reactions (22).

Numerous studies have linked the incidence of adverse drug reactions with the number of drugs taken. Because the incidence of reactions increases exponentially rather than linearly with the number of drugs given, the effects of multiple drug use may be more than simply additive. This effect may be due in part to the exponential increase in potential drug interaction combinations as additional drugs are added to a regimen. Other studies have shown that the type and dose of drug taken plays a more important role than the actual number of medications. Antimicrobial drugs were reported to be responsible for 22% of adverse drug reactions in one study (25). Drugs with low therapeutic-to-toxicity ratios are more likely to cause reactions. Digoxin, a drug with a low toxicity threshold, has been implicated in over 20% of all adverse drug reactions occurring in hospital inpatients (26). Other commonly implicated drugs include corticosteroids, nonsteroidal anti-inflammatory drugs, anticoagulants, antihypertensives, and psychoactive agents (27).

Certain physiological conditions are known to alter the pharmacokinetics of drugs and can therefore potentiate the occurrence of adverse drug reactions. The clearest association between increased adverse effects and a physiological condition is seen in patients with impaired renal function. One study found that the incidence of adverse effects rose from 9% in patients with a blood urea nitrogen (BUN) less than 20 mg/dl to 24% in patients with an elevated BUN (28). Further damage to kidney function can occur if appropriate adjustments in dosages are not made for nephrotoxic drugs. Nephrotoxicity caused by aminoglycosides and vancomycin has been shown to occur more frequently in elderly patients (29). Hepatic injury such as drug-induced hepatitis appears to be more common in older patients for some hepatotoxic agents such as isoniazid. A decline in cardiac reserve may make elderly persons more susceptible to the effects of tachycardia, sodium overload, and cardiotoxic drugs. Ototoxicity caused by aminoglycosides is also thought to be more common in geriatric patients, although preexisting hearing loss makes actual determination difficult.

While it may be true that adverse drug reactions can occur in patients of any age, the elderly population appears to be particularly susceptible. Although avoidance of adverse drug reactions altogether may not be completely possible, the following steps may help minimize these potential occurrences:

1. Take a careful medication history—this may prevent repetition of a previous untoward experience.
2. Prescribe the minimum number of drugs necessary.
3. Start at conservative dosage levels and titrate gradually to achieve optimal therapeutic benefit.
4. Monitor patients carefully for symptoms or signs of adverse drug reactions, bearing in mind its similarity to disease progression in elderly patients.
5. Monitor appropriate laboratory tests for therapeutic levels.
6. Discontinue any drugs as soon as they are no longer necessary.

III. COMPLIANCE

Noncompliance is generally defined as the extent to which a patient's behavior does not adhere to a medication regimen. Examples of noncompliance may include failure to obtain a prescription, improper administration of a medication, premature discontinuation of a medication, or taking an inappropriate medication. The degree to which noncompliance occurs has been reported to be as low as 25% (30) to as high as 82% (31). As is the case with studies determining adverse drug-reaction rates, determining the incidence of medication noncompliance depends largely on the definitions, criteria, assessment tools, and study populations utilized. Although it may be unrealistic to expect 100% compliance with all instructions, deviation from the medication regimen can have severe consequences, including a worsening of a patient's medical condition. It has been estimated that 125,000 or more deaths and $15 billion lost to the nation's economy each year are attributed directly to illnesses caused by people failing to comply with their prescribed medication regimens (32).

Elderly patients are often perceived as being more noncompliant with medication regimens than are younger patients. However, in a comprehensive review of compliance studies it was found that there was no direct correlation between age and compliance (33). Rather, other age-related factors may contribute to their higher rate of noncompliance such as increased medication use and the complexity of their medication regimen (34,35). Geriatric patients may also have more difficulty complying with their medication regimen because they may have chronic illness (36,37), isolated living situations (38–40), decreased mobility, and limited incomes (41). Memory loss or forgetfulness often associated with aging, however, has not been found to play as large a role in compliance, as is often perceived (42).

Compliance may not necessarily be an all-or-nothing behavior. Some patients do not initially comply, some partially comply, some completely comply, and, finally, some hypercomply. Patients may be compliant with portions of their medication regimen, but noncompliant or hypercompliant with other parts. It has been noted that patients often comply for the few days immediately before and after scheduled visits to a doctor. Of growing concern is the finding by investigators that elderly patients may often be intentionally noncompliant (43–46). A survey by the American Association of Retired Persons reported that 20% of older patients fail to have their prescriptions initially filled and 40% stop taking their medication before they should (45). A recent study showed poor compliance with medication orders among elderly patients after hospital discharge (23). Of the 44 patients surveyed, 64% used at least one medication that was not ordered by the physician at discharge, and 73% failed to use at least one medication according to the way it was ordered. In another investigation, it was found that 70% of noncompliant behavior in a group of elderly patients was deliberate (46). The study also discovered a vast majority of noncompliance to take the form of underuse of a medication. In more than half the cases the reason given for intentional noncompliance was the patient's perception that the drug was not needed in the dosage prescribed (46). Another reason often cited for intentional noncompliance was the attempt to avoid unpleasant side effects. These reasons differ from those of patients who are unintentionally noncompliant, where generally forgetfulness is the primary cause.

Compliance with prescribed treatment is essential for the successful eradication of infection. Unfortunately, compliance with even short-term antibiotic regimens is reported to be poor. Approximately one third of antibiotic prescriptions are often discontinued prematurely soon after patients begin feeling better (46). In one study, investigators examined the contribution of doctor, patient, and consultation interaction patterns to compliance in a general practice (47). Discriminating variables relating to patients included health state, employment state, knowledge of tablet, perception of anxiety level, difficulty in complying, and the patient's observed anger, distance, and assertiveness in the consultation. Discriminating variables relating to doctors included provisions of advice on duration of treatment, complexity of dosage schedule, age of doctor, and number of years in practice. The authors found that multiple factors were relevant to noncompliance (47). In terms of patient variables, significant differences between compliers and noncompliers were determined for employment state and knowledge of the medication name. Consistent with other studies, an association was shown between the complexity of the regimen and compliance (47).

The importance of drug information counseling and its impact on compliance cannot be overstated. In the mid-1980s a FDA-sponsored poll found that about one third of patients do not receive counseling at either the physician's office or the pharmacy unless they asked for this service (48). Directions for use were provided to only 58% of patients at the doctor's office and 23% at the pharmacy. Warnings regarding potential risks were provided to only 30% at a doctor's office (48). The FDA commissioner has urged health care practitioners to communicate better with patients about their medications and has set improvement in the flow of information to consumers as one of the administration's top three priorities, along with enforcing existing food and drug laws and speeding up review of new products (49). Certainly there are many barriers to providing effective communication. Many prescribers believe they do an adequate job of communicating with their patients, only to find out that the patients recall very little. It has been reported that patients arrive at pharmacies knowing only 23% of the information they should about the proper use of their medications.

Recognition of a noncompliant patient is important for targeting counseling. Traits of noncompliant individuals include:

Illness fails to respond to therapy.
Patient is socially isolated.
Patient is forgetful or confused.
Patient has sensory deficits.
Drug therapy is complex.
Patient fails to keep appointments.
Drug therapy is expensive.
Patient fails to obtain timely prescription refills.

Three common methods of measuring medication compliance are serum or urine measurements for drugs or drug products, pill counts, and patient interviews. One study showed that the patient interview may be the most useful method of measuring medication compliance in a clinical setting among chronically ill patients prescribed digoxin (50). Patients admitting noncompliance are more likely to be helped by measures to increase compliance than those who do not.

The following steps may help practitioners maximize compliance:

1. Make medication compliance a priority in patient discussions by specifically and routinely inquiring about it.
2. Monitor the need for medication refills as a crude measure of consumption.
3. Follow up aggressively all patients who drop out of care.
4. Adjust attitude about compliance by never assuming it is satisfactory, by accepting some responsibility for noncompliance, and by refining compliance inquiries to an open, nonjudgmental format.
5. Facilitate compliance by adjusting the regimen to the patient's usual routine, explaining the regimen carefully with written reinforcement, and using available aids such as calendar packaging, when available.

IV. PRESCRIBING ANTIMICROBIALS

Antimicrobials are among the most frequently prescribed drugs in the United States today, second only as a class to cardiovascular drugs. The efficacy of these agents in the treatment of various infectious diseases is indisputable. However, there is a growing concern regarding the manner in which antimicrobial agents are prescribed within hospitals and long-term care facilities today. A review of prescribing practices for systemic antibiotics in the nursing home setting has revealed that antibiotics are frequently prescribed without clear or objective evidence for underlying infection (51). A physician's examination and other features commonly performed in the evaluation of specific infectious diseases were often missing. One fifth of the antibiotics prescribed are for infections not usually thought to require antibiotic therapy, such as viral upper respiratory tract infections and asymptomatic bacteriuria (51,52).

The general problem of antimicrobial misuse has long been recognized. It has been observed that many physicians do not seem to recognize the hazards of the indiscriminate use of antimicrobial drugs and often prescribe them prophylactically for security in treatment (3). Ninety-five percent of physicians surveyed in one study showed that physicians will issue one or more prescriptions to a patient whom they diagnose as having the "common cold." Almost 60% of these prescriptions are for antibiotics, mostly tetracyclines and penicillins (53). Studies evaluating antimicrobial usage in hospitals have shown that more than half of the drugs are used for unjustifiable reasons or that the wrong drug, dose, or duration of therapy is selected. Virtually all the studies identify the same reasons for overuse of antimicrobial agents in the hospitals. They include inappropriate use of agents for prophylaxis of surgical infections and high cost of parenteral agents, particularly the cephalosporins and aminoglycosides. The most representative study of the use of antimicrobial drugs in general hospitals in the United States was conducted by Shapiro et al. (54), who studied 20 short-stay general hospitals, finding that about 30% of the patients received an antimicrobial drug during their hospitalization and about 30% received the drugs for prophylaxis in operations or invasive nonsurgical procedures. Despite indications that prophylaxis may be effective only when given concurrently with and for 24–48 h after an operation, it was usually continued throughout the entire hospitalization (54).

Unnecessary use of antimicrobial drugs is both expensive and potentially dangerous, especially in older patients, who are at greater risk for adverse reactions (see earlier discussion). The rising costs of medical care are aggravated by overuse of these expensive agents, and such costs can only be justified by real need. With the advent of diagnosis-related groups (DRGs) as the basis for reimbursement, hospitals currently face a challenge from both the public and the federal government on the issue of controlling the quality of medical care practiced in hospitals without concurrently increasing costs (55).

Over and above monetary costs, the misuse of antimicrobial agents may alter the older patient's indigenous flora and favor either the emergence of resistant strains or the acquisition of new strains with multiple antimicrobial resistance, which puts patients at greater risk of developing infections that are less amenable to therapy. Antimicrobial agents also may cause such adverse reactions as anaphylaxis with penicillin, aplastic anemia with chloramphenicol, severe diarrhea from lincomycin and clindamycin, and nephrotoxicity combined with ototoxicity from aminoglycosides—deaths attributable to all of these agents have been reported in the literature. Approximately 5% of hospitalized patients who are given antimicrobials will experience some adverse reaction to the particular drug, which approximates the rate of acquisition of nosocomial infection (56). The physician who prescribes an antimicrobial agent in the treatment of a patient in whom no bacterial infection exists must be aware of such risks.

In the current modern antibiotic era, the selection of antimicrobial drugs in clinical practice has become increasingly complex because more patients (especially older adults) are predisposed to infection, a greater diversity of organisms with varying antimicrobial resistance patterns have emerged, and new antimicrobial drugs with unique pharmacological and microbiological properties are available to treat these pathogens.

Attempts to control the inappropriate use of antimicrobial agents have been difficult, according to a recent study, because of the vast array of antimicrobial drugs introduced as well as "the common feeling by many physicians that they should be able to use any antibiotic whenever and however they wish" (57). Misuse of antimicrobial drugs may occur in a number of ways, including selecting an inappropriate drug; incorrect route, dose, or dosing interval; and inappropriate duration of treatment. The results have been the unnecessary or incorrect use of broad-spectrum and expensive antimicrobial drugs with potential adverse effects in numerous patients.

To optimize the use of antimicrobial drugs, several factors are relevant when therapy is considered: (1) site of infection; (2) severity of infection; (3) previous data on clinical efficacy of the drug; (4) culture and sensitivity results or the known antimicrobial susceptibility pattern for suspected organism(s); (5) blood and tissue levels achieved; (6) potential adverse effects of antimicrobial drug selected; (7) patient factors (e.g., age and renal function); and (8) cost of therapy (58).

A. Site of Infection

The site of the infectious process determines the choice of the antimicrobial agent and its dose as well as the route by which it should be administered. For antimicrobial therapy to be effective, an adequate concentration of the drug must be delivered to the site of infection. For example, in the treatment of meningitis, one should select antimicrobial drugs that can rapidly cross the blood-brain barrier and achieve effective cerebrospinal fluid concentrations when given parenterally. If the drug does not cross the blood-brain barrier and alternative agents are not available, it must be given via the intrathecal or intraventricular route.

B. Severity of Infection

The severity of the infection determines the choice of the antimicrobial drug(s) as well as the dose and the route of administration. Oral antimicrobial agents can be prescribed for the management of upper respiratory and urinary tract infections for a relatively short duration. In contrast, pneumonias and nosocomial gram-negative bacillary infections will warrant the use of parenteral broad-spectrum antimicrobial drugs such as third-generation cephalosporins, extended-spectrum penicillins, and aminoglycosides for an extended period of time.

C. Previous Data on Clinical Efficacy

Efficacy should be the first characteristic considered in choosing an antimicrobial agent. If a drug is ineffective, the patient will be needlessly subjected to the risk of toxicity and unwarranted expense. The goal is to prevent infection or to treat an established infection by reducing or eliminating pathogenic organisms. To achieve this goal, the agent must reach the site of infection and be active at that site. Published double-blind controlled comparative studies with good sample sizes that assess the clinical efficacy of the drug should be critically analyzed to determine the role of this particular antimicrobial drug in the treatment of the suspected infection.

D. Culture and Sensitivity Results

Initiation of therapy for a suspected infection cannot always be postponed until results of microbiological studies are available (see Chap. 26). A decision about the likely source or site of infection can usually be made, after which appropriate culture(s) or other diagnostic tests must be performed. The physician should have knowledge of the organisms likely to cause infections in the involved site and the usual antibiotic susceptibility patterns seen in the specific hospital. After empiric therapy is initiated, microbiological data should be carefully reviewed. A positive culture from a usually sterile source is strong evidence that the microorganisms are pathogenic in that setting. The drug susceptibility pattern should serve as a guide to continue or alter the empiric regimen.

E. Blood and Tissue Levels

No antimicrobial agent will be effective if it is not delivered to the site of infection in adequate amounts. In most cases, this means that the local concentration of the antimicrobial agent should be at least equal to or greater than the minimal inhibitory concentration (MIC) of the infecting organism. To determine the doses of antimicrobial agents, combinations of standardized doses and calculations that involve weight or body surface area have been used. In general, those agents with a wide therapeutic index, such as penicillins and cephalosporins, are given as standardized doses. The dose of aminoglycosides, with a narrow margin between therapeutic and toxic levels, is calculated on the basis of ideal or lean body weight. Serum concentrations of antimicrobial agents are relatively easy to determine and therefore are often used as a guide in the therapy. However, except in cases of bacteremia, antimicrobial efficacy is more likely determined by the tissue and body fluid concentrations than by blood levels.

F. Potential Adverse Effects

Toxicity is an unwanted characteristic in any antimicrobial agent used. These drugs affect the patient, the microbial ecology of the hospital and community, and the indigenous microbial flora. Indiscriminate use of antimicrobial agents reduces their subsequent effectiveness by favoring emergence of resistant microorganisms. Individual toxicity may be idiosyncratic, such as allergy, or cumulative to one or more organs as seen with aminoglycosides or amphotericin B. Thus, prescribing the least amount of drug that is effective is the most desirable end point.

G. Patient Factors

Patient age is a major factor to consider in the choice of antimicrobial agents. Gastric acidity declines with age. Penicillin G can be given in lieu of the more expensive acid-resistant penicillin V in elderly patients with achlorhydria. Renal function also varies with age. It is important to recognize that creatinine clearance may be significantly reduced in elderly patients even though they have normal blood urea nitrogen or serum creatinine concentrations. Thus, one must carefully assess the patient's renal and hepatic function since these organs serve as the major routes of excretion and/or inactivation of antimicrobials. Renal excretion is the most important route of elimination for most antimicrobial agents.

H. Cost of Therapy

Cost also must be considered. An inexpensive drug that is ineffective or toxic is no bargain. Considering the price of a single dose of a drug may not be the best way to analyze cost. If a drug must be administered intravenously in frequent doses and numerous tests must be performed to monitor toxicity including serum drug levels, the costs of administration and monitoring must be added to the drug's acquisition price. In contrast, a drug that enables a patient to leave the hospital early, is administered orally, or needs minimal monitoring may be less expensive overall even though the cost of a single dose is more. This is the concept of cost-effective therapy.

In 1990 nonfederal hospitals spent over $2 billion on antimicrobials accounting for 27% of total drug expenditures (59) and is expected to increase at an annual rate of 10–15%. The antimicrobial market is unmistakably the most competitive within the pharmaceutical industry. From 1981 through 1991, 31 antimicrobials received approval for marketing by FDA, 15 of which are cephalosporins. Not surprisingly, cephalosporins were the most frequently prescribed class of antimicrobials during the past decade. Cost-effective therapy will require proper antimicrobial prescribing using an agent that has high efficacy, little adverse impact on the normal human bacterial flora, an acceptable level of adverse effects, and low cost. The quest in the 1990s is for cost effectiveness to control costs.

Under cost containment, alternative drugs are compared based on price and the least costly one is chosen. The goal is to minimize the dollars spent on drugs. In contrast, under cost effectiveness, the least expensive drug is not necessarily the most cost effective. A drug with a greater expense may be preferable if it also offers greater benefit. The goal is to minimize the overall health care dollars spent to achieve the outcome (60).

Many hospitals are still concentrating on cost containment, which limits the money spent on drugs and focuses on drug price, pharmacy budget, and drug therapy in isolation. On the other hand, cost effectiveness limits the money spent by the entire hospital to achieve a therapeutic outcome. It focuses on utilization of all health care resources, the hospital budget, and drug therapy as an integral component of health care. Cost effectiveness focuses on achieving the best value for the money spent by all functions within the hospital system as a direct result of using a particular drug therapy, while cost containment focuses on minimizing the amount spent on drugs (61).

Cost effectiveness is then an economic technique used to compare the negative consequences and positive outcomes that result from a drug therapy. The cost effectiveness of a drug therapy is then a measure of its impact on the cost of providing health care relative to its contribution to improving patient health. The components of cost include direct costs of the antimicrobial regimen such as acquisition cost, storage costs, and administration costs, while indirect costs include emergence of resistance and adverse drug reactions. Typically, a drug therapy involves costs and benefits that extend beyond pharmacy. Once drug therapy is initiated, it often requires monitoring and clinical testing to avoid adverse reactions. On the other hand, when the drug yields the intended benefits, it may help reduce the length of stay in the hospital, because illness may be managed on an outpatient basis.

To provide the best possible medical care in keeping with hospital fiscal constraints, the following strategies to achieve cost-effective antimicrobial therapy are proposed (2,57,62).

1. Antimicrobial Formulary

A formulary is a list of drugs, chosen by a committee of physicians, pharmacists, dentists, and nurses, based on their effectiveness, safety, and cost. A viable formulary should continually be revised to add important new drugs when they become available and delete older products no longer considered useful. Each hospital should have a drug formulary to promote safe and cost-effective drug therapy. A well-structured formulary of antimicrobial agents should be assembled to meet the therapeutic needs of the medical staff. A formulary decreases confusion among physicians as to which agent among a group of equally effective agents should be selected, promotes educational programs, and decreases pharmacy expense. The formulary should contain a basic minimum of antimicrobial agents. For example, it is recommended that there be one antistaphylococcal penicillin (nafcillin or oxacillin), one antipseudomonal penicillin (piperacillin), one first-generation cephalosporin (cefazolin), one cephalosporin for anaerobic infections (cefoxitin or cefotetan), one extended-spectrum third-generation cephalosporin (ceftizoxime or cefotaxime), and one antipseudomonal cephalosporin (ceftazidime). The selection of aminoglycoside antibiotics depends on the overall patterns of resistance in the medical center. In general, gentamicin can be used as the first-line agent in areas where gentamicin resistance is low and amikacin can be reserved for the management of gentamicin- and tobramycin-resistant gram-negative bacteria.

The formulary should be updated periodically so that the best antimicrobial agents can be represented. It should also list additional antimicrobial agents whose use is restricted because of special indications, toxicity, or significant cost. These drugs may be released for use when preapproved protocols are followed (e.g., treatment of febrile neutropenic patient, diabetic foot, or suspected *Pneumocystis carinii* pneumonia) or after consultation with an infectious disease consultant.

Physicians should be encouraged to prescribe formulary antimicrobial drugs because they are usually the best and most cost-effective available. If a particular drug is not on the formulary, this means generally that equally effective, less costly alternatives are available. A nonformulary drug theoretically has no clinical advantage over a formulary drug that provides the same therapeutic value.

The most formidable challenge facing pharmacy and therapeutics committees in the 1990s is to ensure the rational, reasonable, and fiscally sound use of drugs. This has also been the oldest challenge.

2. *Antibiotic Order Forms*

Controversy exists over the value of the antibiotic order form as a method of cost containment and quality assurance. Simplified forms that are easy to complete may result in retrieval of insufficient clinical information to assess the appropriateness of antimicrobial usage. The more elaborate antibiotic order form is rarely completed by the physicians because it is too time consuming. In one hospital pharmacy in Rhode Island, the information from the antimicrobial order sheets were used to generate a variety of computerized reports that monitor trends in the use of antimicrobial agents and identify potential areas of misuse. This was a clinical intervention strategy that resulted in a $700,000 reduction in antimicrobial expenditures over a 2-year period (62).

3. *Automatic Stop Orders*

Antimicrobial agents are often needed for a limited period of time. The implementation of automatic stop orders may help to curtail needless use of antimicrobial agents. Orders for antimicrobials used for treatment of documented infection can have a 7-day stop order. The drug will automatically be discontinued unless the physician renews the order. For surgical prophylaxis, the automatic stop date may be 24–48 h depending on the consensus of the surgery department. There is no evidence that continuation of the antimicrobial agent beyond the completion of the operation achieves any better protection against infection than does one dose given at the proper time before the operation. In fact, not only does the continuation of prophylactic antimicrobials beyond 2 days add unnecessary costs, it may be harmful by selecting resistant organisms and increasing the chances for an adverse drug reaction. Considerable cost savings can be realized by restricting the use of prophylactic antimicrobial drugs to no more than 2 days postoperatively, since inappropriate usage is so frequent.

4. *Limited Susceptibility Reporting*

The microbiology laboratory should use generic class antibiotic disks in their sensitivity tests. The results of in vitro susceptibility tests should be limited to antimicrobial agents that are currently on the hospital formulary. Susceptibility to nonformulary antimicrobial drugs should only be reported under special circumstances when multiple resistance is noted. The goal of the microbiology laboratory is to provide reports that are clinically meaningful as well as encourage therapy with the least expensive and least toxic agent.

5. *Concurrent Monitoring*

The Joint Commission on Accreditation of Health Organizations (JCAHO) requires that medical staff develop criteria based on ongoing, planned, and systematic process for monitoring and evaluating the prophylactic, therapeutic, and empiric use of drugs effectively. The clinical pharmacist in conjunction with the infectious disease specialist can set up a program of concurrent antimicrobial surveillance. The program has the potential to (1) improve the quality of medical care for patients through promotion of better usage of antimicrobial agents; (2) ensure the safe and rational use of antimicrobial agents by improving prescribing practices through an educational approach; (3) prevent or delay the emergence of resistant organisms in the medical center; and (4) reduce the cost for treatment and hospitalization due to misuse of antimicrobial agents.

In the course of evaluating the patient's antimicrobial therapy, the clinical pharmacist can identify problem areas in antimicrobial prescribing that may be corrected by performing a drug usage evaluation (audit), educational program, or modification of the hospital formulary. During the 1990s, health care professionals will need to be creative in their approach to deliver the best possible medical care while limited by fiscal constraints.

REFERENCES

1. Caldwell JR, Leighton EC. Adverse reactions to antimicrobial agents. JAMA 1974; 230:77–80.
2. Kunin, CM. Problems in antibiotic usage. In: Mandell GL, Douglas RG Jr, Bennett JE, eds. Principles and practice of infectious diseases. New York: Churchill Livingstone, 1990:427–34.
3. Simmons HE, Stolley PD. This is medical progress? trends and consequences of antibiotic use in the United States. JAMA 1974; 227:1023–8.
4. Lamy PP, ed. Prescribing for the elderly. MA: PSG Publishing Company, Inc., 1990.
5. Simonson W, ed. Medications in the elderly. Rockville, MD: Aspen Systems Corporation. 1984.
6. Sumner ED, ed. Handbook of geriatric drug therapy for health care professionals. Philadelphia: Lea and Febiger, 1983.
7. Vestal RE, Wood AJJ, Shand DG. Reduced beta-adrenoceptor sensitivity in the elderly. Clin Pharmacol Ther 1979; 26:181–6.
8. O'Malley K, Stevenson IH, Ward CA, et al. Determinants of anticoagulant control in patients receiving warfarin. Br J Clin Pharmacol 1977; 4:309–14.
9. Shepherd AMM, Hewick DS, Moreland TA, et al. Age as a determinant of sensitivity to warfarin. Br J Clin Pharmacol 1977; 4:315–20.
10. Cook PJ, Flanagan R, James IM. Diazepam tolerance: effect of age, regular sedation and alcohol. Br Med J 1984; 289:351–3.
11. Health Care Financing Administration Office of National Cost Estimates. National health expenditures, 1988. Health Care Financing Rev 1990; 11:1–41.
12. Williamson J, Chopin JM. Adverse reactions to prescribed drugs in the elderly: a multicenter investigation. Age Ageing 1980; 9:73–80.
13. Center for Drug Evaluation and Research Food and Drug Administration Department of Health and Human Services. Guideline for the study of drugs likely to be used in the elderly. J Geriatr Drug Ther 1990; 5:5–17.
14. Faich GA. National adverse drug reaction reporting. Arch Intern Med 1991; 151:1645–7.
15. Tanner LA, Baum C, Prela CM, et al. Spontaneous adverse reaction reporting in the elderly for 1986. J Geriatr Drug Ther 1989; 3:31–54.
16. Ives TJ, Bentz EJ, Gwyther RE. Drug-related admissions to a family medicine inpatient service. Arch Intern Med 1987; 147:1117–20.
17. Fincham JE. Adverse drug reaction occurrence in elderly patients. J Geriatr Drug Ther 1991; 5:3–50.

18. Grymonpre RE, Mitenko PA, Sitar DS, et al. Drug-associated hospital admissions in older medical patients. J Am Geriatr Soc 1988; 36:1092–8.
19. Lakshmanan MC, Hershey CO, Breslau D. Hospital admissions caused by iatrogenic disease. Arch Intern Med 1986; 146:1931–4.
20. Col N, Fanale JE, Kronholm P. The role of medication noncompliance and adverse drug reactions in hospitalizations of the elderly. Arch Intern Med 1990; 150:841–5.
21. Colt HG, Shapiro AP. Drug-induced illness as a cause for admission to a community hospital. J Am Geriatr Soc 1989; 37:323–26.
22. Carbonin P, Pahor M, Bernabei R, et al. Is age an independent risk factor of adverse drug reactions in hospitalized medical patients. J Am Geriatr Soc 1991; 39:1093–9.
23. Beers MH, Sliwkowski J, Brooks J. Compliance with medication orders among the elderly after hospital discharge. Hosp Formul 1992; 27:720–4.
24. Bryant SG, Fisher S, Prinsley DM, et al. Effects of age on reporting of adverse clinical events: results from two postmarketing surveillance methods. Pharmacotherapy 1991; 11:249–55.
25. Mulroy R. Iatrogenic disease in general practice: its incidence and effects. Br Med J 1973; 2:407–10.
26. Melmon KL. Preventable drug reactions—causes and cures. N Engl J Med 1971; 284:1361–8.
27. Korrapati MR, Loi C, Vestal R. Adverse drug reactions in the elderly. Drug Ther 1992; 22:21–30.
28. Smith JW, Seidl LG, Cluff LE. Studies on the epidemiology of adverse drug reactions. Ann Intern Med 1966; 65:629–40.
29. Yoshikawa TT. Antimicrobial therapy for the elderly patient. J Am Geriatr Soc 1990; 38:1353–72.
30. Stewart RB, Cluff LE. A review of medication errors and compliance in ambulant patients. Clin Pharm Ther 1972; 13:463–8.
31. Evans L, Spelman M. The problem of noncompliance with drug therapy. Drugs 1983; 25:63–76.
32. Clepper I. Noncompliance the invisible epidemic. Drug Topics 1992; 136:44–65.
33. Haynes RB. A critical review of the determinants of patient compliance with therapeutic regimens. In: Sackett DL, Haynes RB, eds. Compliance with therapeutic regimens. Baltimore: Johns Hopkins University Press, 1976:26–39.
34. Kendrick R, Bayne JR. Compliance with prescribed medication by elderly patients. Can Med Assoc J 1982; 127:961–2.
35. Smith SE, Stead KC. Noncompliance or misprescribing. Lancet 1974; 1:937.
36. Butler RN, Lewis MI, eds. Aging and mental health. St Louis: CV Mosby Co., 1977.
37. Fries JF, Crapo LM, eds. Vitality and aging. San Francisco: WH Freeman and Company, 1981.
38. Haynes RB, Sackett DL, Taylor DW. How to detect and manage low patient compliance in chronic illness. Geriatrics 1980; 355:91–7.
39. Porter AMW. Drug defaulting in a general practice. Br Med J 1969; 1:218–22.
40. Schwartz D, Wang M, Zeitz L. Medication errors made by elderly, chronically ill patients. Am J Public Health 1962; 52:2018–29.
41. Brand RN, Smith RT, Brand P. Effect of economic barriers to medical care on patient's noncompliance. Public Health Rep 1977; 92:72–8.
42. Norell SE. Memory and medication compliance. J Clin Hosp Pharm 1985; 10:107–9.
43. Fincham JE, Wertheimer AI. Initial drug noncompliance in the elderly. J Geriatr Drug Ther 1986; 1:19–29.
44. Fincham JE, Wertheimer AI. Elderly patient initial noncompliance: the drugs and the reasons. J Geriatr Drug Ther 1988; 2:53–62.
45. American Association of Retired Persons. A Survey of Consumer Use, Attitudes and Behavior. Washington, D.C.: AARP 1984:3–5.
46. Cooper, JK, Love, DW, Raffoul, PR. Intentional prescription nonadherence (noncompliance) by the elderly. J Am Geriatr Soc 1982; 30:329–33.

47. Cockburn J, Gibberd RW, Reid AL, et al. Determinants of non-compliance with short term antibiotic regimens. Br Med J 1987; 295:814–8.
48. Morris LA, Grossman R, Barkdoll GL, et al. A national survey of prescription drug information provided to patients. Rockville, MD: Food and Drug Administration, 1986.
49. Kessler DA. Communicating with patients about their medications. N Engl J Med 1991; 325:1650–2.
50. Fletcher SW, Pappius EM, Harper SJ. Measurement of medication compliance in a clinical setting comparison of three methods in patients prescribed digoxin. Arch Intern Med 1979; 139:635–8.
51. Warren JW, Palumbo FB, Fitterman L, et al. Incidence and characteristics of antibiotic use in aged nursing home patients. J Am Geriatr Soc 1991; 39:963–72.
52. Katz PR, Beam TR, Brand F, et al. Antibiotic use in the nursing home. Arch Intern Med 1990; 150:1465–8.
53. Stolley PD, Becker MH, McEvilla JD, et al. Drug prescribing and use in an American community. Ann Intern Med 1972; 76:537–40.
54. Shapiro M, Townsend TR, Rosner B, et al. Use of antimicrobial drugs in general hospitals. N Engl J Med 1979; 301:351–5.
55. Ma MY. Meeting the challenge of rising antibiotic costs. VA Practitioner 1984; 1:63–5.
56. Caldwell JR, Leighton EC. Adverse reactions to antimicrobial agents. JAMA 1974; 230:77–80.
57. Qunitiliani R, Nightingale CH, Crowe HM, et al. Strategic antibiotic decision-making at the formulary level. Rev Infect Dis 1991; 13(suppl 9):770–7.
58. Wilkowske CJ. General principles of antimicrobial therapy. Mayo Clin Proc 1991; 66:931–41.
59. Miwa LJ, Kennedy DL, Freiman JP. US hospital anti-infective use from 1985 to 1990. P&T 1992; 17:983–93.
60. Dao TD. Cost-effectiveness of drug therapy: the basic ingredients. Hospital Therapy 1990; 15:39–45.
61. Jolicoeur LM, Jones-Grizzle AJ, Boyer JG. Guidelines for performing a pharmacoeconomic analysis. Am J Hosp Pharm 1992; 49:1741–7.
62. Hess DA, Mahoney CD, Johnson PN, et al. Integration of clinical and administrative strategies to reduce expeditures for antimicrobial agents. Am J Hosp Pharm 1990; 47:585–91.

7

Penicillins

Ronald A. Sherman and Maury Ellis Mulligan
Veterans Affairs Medical Center, Long Beach, and University of California—Irvine, Orange, California

Penicillin was first isolated from *Penicillium notatum* in 1929 (1) but was not available for clinical use until the end of World War II (2,3). Commercial production of penicillin increased when *Penicillium chrysogenum* was found to produce larger quantities of the drug. When grown in different media, *Penicillium* produced different forms of the antibacterial agent, eventually designated as penicillin F, G, K, N, and X. The early preparations were actually mixtures of several penicillin compounds along with a number of impurities introduced during the fermentative process. Many patients who developed allergic reactions to penicillins during the 1940s and 1950s may actually have reacted to these impurities rather than to the penicillin itself. Thus, a history of penicillin allergy in an elderly individual should be scrutinized carefully. Penicillin G (benzylpenicillin) is the most potent of these early penicillins and is now the form produced; impurities are no longer present. The penicillins continue to demonstrate significant utility for the treatment of infections in elderly patients, due to their high toxic:therapeutic ratios, the wide choice of administration modalities, and the practical range of antibacterial spectra (both narrow- and relatively broad-spectrum penicillins are currently available). The vast varieties of penicillins are summarized by biochemical characteristics (by class) in Table 1.

I. CHEMISTRY

The fundamental penicillin structure is a four-membered β-lactam ring fused to a five-membered thiazolidine ring (Fig. 1), with an acyl side chain. The major determinant of the penicillin's antibacterial spectrum is the side chain. The β-lactam ring is required for antibacterial activity, and disruption of this ring by β-lactamases inactivates the compound.

Synthesis of the penicillin nucleus has been achieved, but it is not commercially practical; fermentation remains the method of production for penicillin G. Penicillins generally exist as salts, in combination with sodium or potassium. These two salts are

Table 1 Penicillins by Class

Antibiotic Class	Generic name	Proprietary name
Natural penicillins	Penicillin G	Pentids, Pfizerpen, Crysticillin, Duracillin, Wycillin, Bicillin L-1 A
	Penicillin V	Betapen VK, Ledercillin VK, Penpar VK, Pen Vee K, Robicillin VK, Uticillin VK
	Phenethicillin	Darcil, Maxipen, Syncillin
Penicillinase-resistant penicillins	Methicillin	Celbenin, Dimocillin, Metin, Staphcillin
	Nafcillin	Nafcil, Unipen
Isoxazolyl penicillins	Oxacillin	Bactocill, Prostaphlin, Resistopen
	Cloxacillin	Tegopen, Austra-Staph, Orbenin
	Dicloxacillin	Dycill, Dynapen, Pathocil, Veracillin
	Flucloxacillin	Floxapen, Ladropen, Stafoxil, Staphcil
Aminopenicillins	Ampicillin	Ampen, Amcill, Omnipen, PenA, Penbritin, Pensyn, Polycillin, Principen, Probampacin, Supen, Totacillin, Vidapen
	Amoxicillin	Amoxil, Larotid, Polymox, Moxacin, Robamox, Trimox
	Epicillin	
	Cyclacillin	Calthor, Cyclopen
	Hetacillin	Versapen, Versapen K, Phenazacillin
	Pivampicillin	Pondocillin
	Talampicillin	Talpen
	Bacampicillin	Spectrobid
	Metampicillin	
Carboxypenicillins	Carbenicillin	Geopen, Pyopen, Carbapen
	Indanylcarbenicillin	Geocillin
	Ticarcillin	Ticar
Acylamino penicillins	Apalcillin	
Ureidopenicillins	Piperacillin	Pipracil, Pipril
	Mezlocillin	Mezlin, Baypen
	Azlocillin	Azlin
	Furazlocillin	
Amidino penicillins	Amdinocillin (Mecillinam)	Selexidin
	Pivamdinocillin (Pivmecillinam)	Selexid

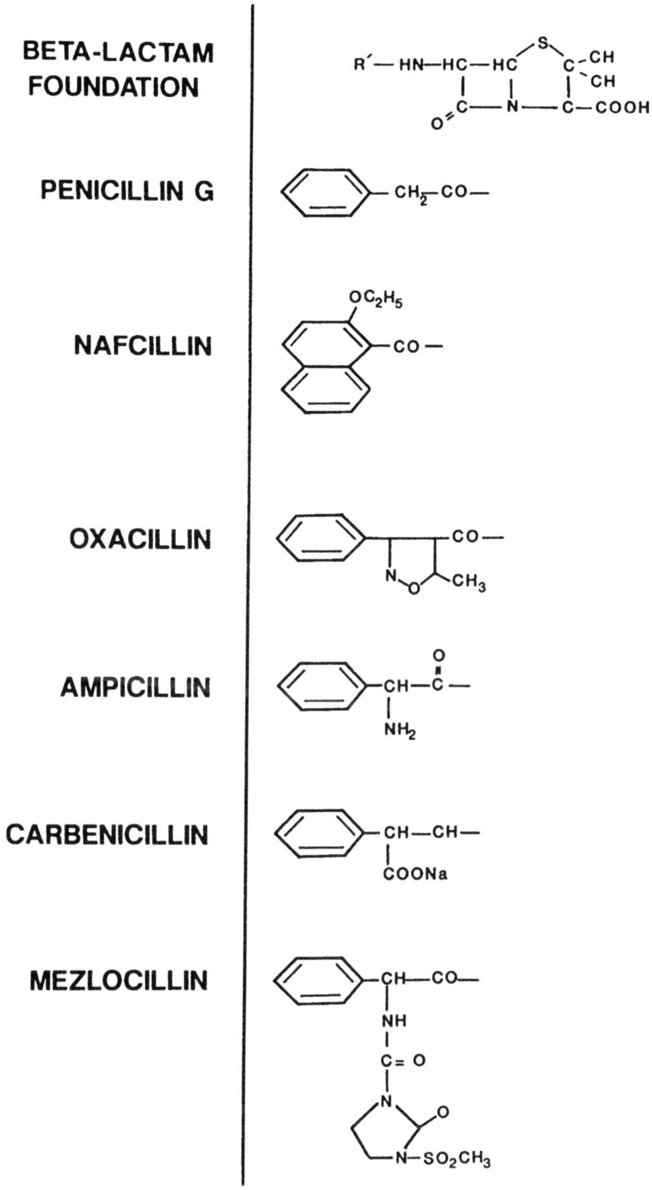

Figure 1 Chemical structure of the penicillin nucleus and representative side chains.

sometimes referred to as "crystalline" penicillin; however, the other penicillin G preparations in use today are also crystalline, unlike the earlier impure compounds. Procaine penicillin G (procaine benzylpenicillin) and benzathine penicillin G (di-benzylethylene-diamine penicillin) are suspensions with low solubility, formulated for slow release after intramuscular injection.

Efforts to develop penicillins with activity against gram-negative organisms or with resistance to β-lactamases led to the development of methicillin in 1960, ampicillin in 1961, and carbenicillin in 1967. These drugs remain major landmarks in penicillin development and are the foundations upon which most current penicillins are built.

Successful antibacterial activity of the penicillins is dependent upon adequate penetration of the cell wall, resistance to enzymatic destruction (usually in the form of β-lactamases), and satisfactory binding to the penicillin binding proteins (PBPs). Chemical alterations of the penicillin molecule are aimed at improving one or more of these attributes. Sometimes one factor may be improved at the expense of another, resulting in several changes in the antibiotic spectrum of the new drugs.

Semisynthetic penicillinase-resistant penicillins, for example, have an acyl side chain that inhibits the ability of penicillinase to open the β-lactam ring. These drugs include methicillin, nafcillin, and oxacillin as well as orally active cloxacillin and dicloxacillin. This alteration allows activity against β-lactamase–positive staphylococci (although not against so-called methicillin-resistant strains). The alteration, however, is associated with decreased activity against certain other organisms (4). Thus, these drugs should not be used against enterococci or for therapy of most anaerobic bacterial infections.

The substitution of a carboxy group for the amino group on the acyl side chain of ampicillin produces carbenicillin and ticarcillin, which, because of increased penetration of these drugs through the bacterial cell wall, have increased activity against gram-negative bacilli including *Pseudomonas aeruginosa* (5). However, this alteration decreases binding to the PBPs of *Enterococcus faecalis*. Substitution of ureido groups for the carboxy group increases bacterial cell wall penetration as well as affinity for PBPs; these ureidopenicillins—azlocillin, mezlocillin, and piperacillin—therefore have increased activity against gram-negative bacilli and anaerobes while remaining relatively active against enterococci (6).

II. MECHANISMS OF ACTIONS

Although studies of the interactions between penicillins and bacteria have taught us much about bacterial growth and biochemistry, detailed knowledge regarding the mechanisms by which penicillins affect bacteria is still incomplete. In order to understand the basic principles of penicillin activity upon bacterial cell wall synthesis, it is necessary first to review the composition of the bacterial envelope.

The bacterial cell (cytoplasm) is surrounded by a multilayered envelope, comprised of the cellular or cytoplasmic membrane, the cell wall, and an outer protein or carbohydrate coat (Fig. 2). The cell wall of gram-positive organisms consists largely of a network of cross-linked polysaccharide strands (the peptidoglycan, murein, or mucopeptide layer), forming one baglike macromolecule ("sacculus") surrounding the cell (7). This peptidoglycan cell wall may be 15–80 nm thick (8). The cell wall of gram-negative organisms, by contrast, is composed of a very thin peptidoglycan layer (2 nm thick), covered by an outer membrane of phospholipids, lipopolysaccharides, and matrix proteins. Because the cell wall is rigid, the bacteria cannot grow or divide unless the peptidoglycan layer is lysed and more peptidoglycan polymers are inserted into the wall. This cleaving process is performed by periplasmic-residing "autolysins."

The peptidoglycan consists predominantly of two amino sugars—glucosamine and muramic acid—arranged alternatingly (β-1, 4-linked) as *N*-acetyl-D-glucosamine and *N*-acetylmuramic acid. Synthesis of the peptidoglycan involves the production of the nucleotide precursors, translocation across the cytoplasmic membrane, and then transglycosylation into the peptidoglycan polymer. A transpeptidase is responsible for assembly of the

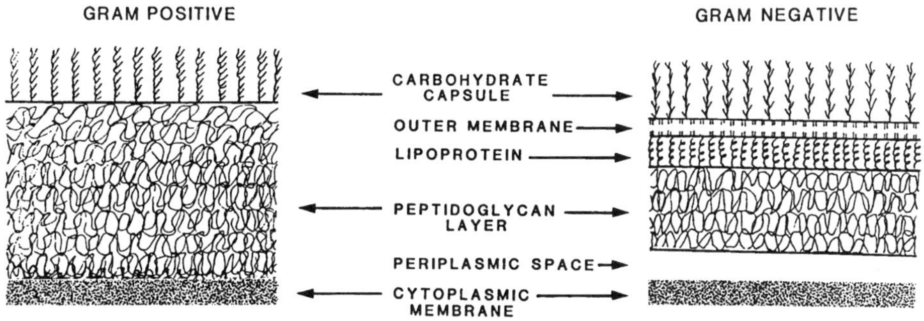

Figure 2 Cellular envelope surrounding gram-positive and gram-negative bacteria.

new polymer into the previously established peptidoglycan saccule (transpeptidation). This is the step previously thought to be the major site of penicillin action. It is now known that penicillin's mechanism of action is much more complex. Not only does penicillin appear to affect earlier steps in cell wall synthesis, but it also binds with the PBPs in the cell membrane, inhibits RNA synthesis, and interacts with products of the bacteria and the host (9–11).

The PBPs are enzymes located on the bacterial cell membrane. They include transpeptidases, carboxypeptidases, and endopeptidases and are essential for maintaining the bacterial cell wall integrity. The specific effects of the different β-lactam antimicrobial agents depend upon the specific PBPs for which they have affinity. Inactivation of some PBPs is lethal for the bacteria, whereas other PBPs are not crucial for cell viability.

Ideally, once the cell wall is weakened, the organisms will rupture under mechanical pressure. However, the bacteria may simply alter their shape without rupturing or may cease growing only while the antibiotic is present. The lethal effect of penicillins may be due, in part, to the release of autolysins that are no longer inhibited after binding of the β-lactam agent to the PBPs. Indeed, some organisms that lack autolysins can be inhibited but not lysed by penicillins; they are said to be "tolerant." Penicillin G, combined with heterologous autolysins in the growth medium, is capable of killing penicillin G–tolerant strains of *Streptococcus sanguis*, indicating that host products may also contribute to the action of penicillin therapy in vivo (12).

Penicillins may act synergistically with other classes of agents. For example, the ability to alter bacterial wall permeability (even without causing cell death) can allow other antibiotics such as aminoglycosides to enter the cell. This type of synergistic interaction can be used effectively against tolerant organisms that would not be killed by either drug alone. The mode of action of most penicillins appears to be similar to that of penicillin G, with the exception of amdinocillin (which has a few differences in its action, including a very delayed killing of certain organisms). The broader antibacterial spectrum of some of the penicillins is due in large part to their increased ability to penetrate the outer membrane of various gram-negative bacteria.

Bacterial resistance to the penicillins may occur if there is an alteration in the binding properties of the PBPs or a decrease in the penetrability of the cellular envelope (13). Both of these mechanisms are uncommon. Bacteria that have demonstrated resistance to β-lactam agents because of altered PBPs include *Escherichia coli*, *Enterococcus faecium*,

Haemophilus influenzae, *Streptococcus pneumoniae*, and methicillin-resistant *Staphylococcus aureus* (14). Decreased permeability of the bacterial cell wall is the most important mechanism of resistance for gram-negative organisms (11). These bacteria have a complex outer cell wall with channels called porins through which antibacterial agents can pass. The third and most common mechanism of bacterial resistance to penicillins is the production of a β-lactamase, which inactivates the penicillin by hydrolyzing the β-lactam ring of the antibiotic.

The β-lactamases produced by gram-positive organisms are usually plasmid-mediated and inducible (15). Furthermore, the enzyme may be released into the environment, thereby inactivating the penicillin before it ever reaches this or neighboring bacteria. In gram-negative bacteria, the β-lactamases may be chromosomal or plasmid-mediated (16). They generally exist in the periplasmic space and may be inducible or constitutive. The ability of certain genera such as the *Enterobacter* spp. to produce specific classes of β-lactamases has contributed to their importance as nosocomial pathogens that can be selected by the widespread use of antimicrobial agents (17).

III. ANTIMICROBIAL SPECTRUM

Of course, the selection of an agent with appropriate antimicrobial activity does not assure a therapeutic cure. An intact immune system is also required to eradicate many organisms; and waning of immunity is an expected accompaniment of old age. Recent investigations into the antibacterial effects of human serum have indicated that serum from elderly subjects, like that from patients with diabetes and cancer, showed less antibacterial activity than did the serum from younger controls (18). Therefore, one should never assume that the initiation of an appropriate antibiotic obviates the need for close observation and continued support.

Penicillins have a wide spectrum of activity depending on the specific class of the drug. All penicillins have some similar antimicrobial activity, but still retain unique antimicrobial characteristics. Table 2 summarizes the antibacterial spectrum of the major penicillins that are used clinically.

A. Natural Penicillins

1. Gram-Positive Cocci

Although penicillin G was initially very active against *S. aureus*, resistance developed quickly. Any isolate of *S. aureus* should now be assumed to be resistant to this agent—especially if it is from an institutionalized patient—unless susceptibility testing demonstrates otherwise. Coagulase-negative staphylococci, too, are now generally resistant to penicillin. The so-called "methicillin-resistant" staphylococci should be considered to be resistant to all penicillins. These multiresistant staphylococci are increasingly important pathogens, especially in institutional settings (18).

Most streptococci have remained exquisitely susceptible to penicillin G, although foci of resistance are now reported in certain parts of the world. *Streptococcus pyogenes* (group A β-hemolytic *Streptococcus*) appears to be demonstrating an increased virulence during the final decade of this century; yet it remains susceptible to penicillin G. The group B (*Streptococcus agalactiae*), C, D, F, and G streptococci, too, have remained susceptible to penicillin G. However, some of these organisms are penicillin tolerant (20–22) and are killed more effectively by the synergistic action of penicillin plus an aminoglycoside (23–25). *S. agalactiae* tends to be more susceptible to penicillin G than to the other

Table 2 In Vitro Activity of Penicillins Against Selected Organisms[a]

	Penicillin G	Oxacillin	Ampicillin	Carbenicillin, ticarcillin	Azlocillin, mezlocillin, piperacillin
Streptococcus pneumoniae	+[b]	+[b]	+[b]	+[b]	+[b]
Staphylococcus aureus (not methicillin-resistant)	0[c]	+	0	0	0
Coagulase-negative staphylococci	0	+/−	0	0	0
Enterococcus spp.	+[b]	0	+[b]	+/−	+[b]
Listeria monocytogenes	+	0	+	+	+
Enterobacteriaceae	0	0	+/−	+[b]	+[b]
Pseudomonas aeruginosa	0	0	0	+/−	+[b]
Bacteroides fragilis group	0	0	0	+/−	+/−
Fusobacterium spp.	+[b]	0	+[b]	+[b]	+[b]
Anaerobic cocci and gram-positive bacilli	+	+/−	+	+	+
Other *Bacteroides/ Prevotella*	+/−	0	+/−	+/−	+/−

+ = active; − = variable activity; 0 = inactive.
[a]Organisms and drugs selected to be representative; exceptions can occur. In vitro activity does not necessarily equate with clinical efficacy or appropriateness.
[b]Occasional or rare resistance.
[c]Can be useful if organisms are susceptible, but most are resistant.

penicillins. Relatively resistant and highly resistant strains of *Streptococcus pneumoniae* now exist. Inhibition of relatively resistant isolates requires 5–100 times the concentration of penicillin needed to inhibit susceptible strains. Highly resistant strains, resistant to all β-lactam agents, account for 50% of all pneumococci isolated in Johannesburg (11). Fortunately, spread to other parts of the world has not been a significant problem. A few such strains have been isolated in the United States (26) and the United Kingdom (27), often from asymptomatic carriers, from international travelers, from institutionalized individuals, or from patients treated with frequent and long courses of antibiotics. The elderly population has not yet been a notable target of this strain of *S. pneumoniae*, but older adults may fall into several potential risk groups. The viridans streptococci are usually susceptible to penicillin G (28), although tolerant (29) and resistant strains (30) have been encountered occasionally. Enterococci (*Enterococcus faecalis*, *Enterococcus faecium*) are usually penicillin tolerant (31) and sometimes resistant to the drug. The degree of synergy achieved with the addition of an aminoglycoside is variable (11), but combination therapy is almost always recommended for serious infections. High-level resistance to penicillins is an increasingly common and serious problem, especially in large tertiary care hospitals. Infections due to strains of enterococci resistant to one or more classes of drugs can be very difficult to manage.

Several species of *Peptostreptococcus* (anaerobic gram-positive cocci) are important pathogens in many infections due to "oral flora." Penicillin remains the drug of choice for these organisms (32).

2. *Gram-Negative Cocci*

Within the past 20 years, penicillin-resistant *Neisseria gonorrhoeae* has become a significant problem throughout the world (33–37), with the result that penicillin is no longer appropriate empiric therapy for gonorrhea. Gonococci may have a variety of mechanisms for penicillin resistance; penicillin-resistant strains are often resistant to multiple other classes of agents as well (38). *Neisseria meningitidis* is nearly always susceptible to penicillin G (39), although it is theoretically possible for this organism to acquire plasmids from *N. gonorrhoeae* that confer penicillin resistance (40).

Many strains of *Moraxella* (*Branhamella*) *catarrhalis* now produce a β-lactamase (41,42). *Kingella*, a recently recognized cause of infective endocarditis, is usually susceptible to penicillin. The anaerobic gram-negative cocci (i.e., *Veillonella*) are predictably susceptible to penicillin (32).

3. *Gram-Negative Bacilli*

Although penicillin is never considered for therapy of infections due to the common gram-negative bacilli such as the Enterobacteriaceae or *P. aeruginosa*, many gram-negative bacillary pathogens are penicillin susceptible. Some of these organisms cause infective endocarditis; these include the genera *Haemophilus* (species other than *H. influenzae*), *Actinobacillus*, *Cardiobacterium*, and *Eikenella*. *Eikenella* (part of the human oral flora) is often associated with human bite wound infections. *Pasteurella multocida* and *Capnocytophaga canimorsus* (normal feline and canine flora, respectively) often infect cat and dog bite wounds.

The anaerobic gram-negative bacilli include a diverse group of organisms. Some, such as the *Bacteroides fragilis* group and *Bacteroides gracilis*, must be assumed to be penicillin resistant. Other *Bacteroides* species, as well as some that have been recently renamed *Porphyromonas* and *Prevotella*, are variably susceptible to penicillin. In contrast, penicillin remains a drug of choice for therapy of most infections caused by *Fusobacterium* other than *F. varium* (32).

4. *Gram-Positive Bacilli*

Listeria monocytogenes, an important pathogen in elderly patients, is predictably susceptible to penicillin G (43–45). Laboratory sensitivity testing occasionally and inaccurately reports *Listeria* as being penicillin resistant (46). Ampicillin is the drug of choice for treating infections caused by this organism; aminoglycosides act synergistically with penicillin or ampicillin (43).

The activity of penicillins against anaerobic gram-positive bacilli is very important. *Clostridium tetani*, *C. perfringens*, *C. septicum*, and the other clostridia are nearly always susceptible to penicillin (32,47,48), although penicillin-tolerant and penicillin-resistant strains have been identified (49). Fecal isolates of *C. difficile* are also often reported as susceptible to penicillin; however, penicillins are never appropriate therapy for infections due to this pathogen.

Penicillin is a first-line drug for therapy of actinomycosis. Although *Actinomyces* are frequently grouped with the anaerobic gram-positive bacilli, they are often microaerophilic and, as such, resistant to other drugs commonly used to treat anaerobic infections. Penicillin also has excellent activity against other non–spore-forming anaerobic gram-positive bacilli (32).

Some species of corynebacteria, as well as *Bacillus* species, are almost always sensitive to penicillin G (50,51). These genera include some very important but presently uncommon pathogens such as *Corynebacterium diphtheriae* and *Bacillus anthracis*.

5. *Other Microorganisms*

The family Spirochaetaceae consists of several pathogenic species, including *Treponema pallidum* (the etiologic agent of syphilis), other treponemes, *Leptospira* spp., *Borrelia burgdorferi* (the causative agent of Lyme disease), and the causative agents of rat-bite fever—*Spirillum minus* and *Streptobacillus moniliformis*. All are highly susceptible to penicillin.

Phenoxypenicillins include penicillin V (phenoxymethyl penicillin) and phenethicillin (phenoxyethyl penicillin), which have a spectrum of activity very similar to that of penicillin G. However, they are less active against most of the streptococci (including *S. pneumoniae*), enterococci, the penicillin-susceptible staphylococci, as well as *Neisseria* spp.

B. Penicillinase-Resistant Penicillins

The major improvement in activity of the penicillinase-resistant penicillins (i.e., methicillin and nafcillin) over penicillin is their stability in the presence of the β-lactamases produced by staphylococci (52). Thus, they are effective in treating infections due to penicillinase-producing staphylococci, but not methicillin-resistant *Staphylococci*. Methicillin-resistant staphylococci are resistant to all known penicillins as a consequence of the organisms' altered PBPs. Methicillin-tolerant organisms are inhibited by low levels of methicillin, but are killed only by very high levels, due to the absence of autolysins, which are necessary for the penicillins to exert their cidal effect. The clinical significance of this variant is questionable; these strains may respond no differently from methicillin-susceptible strains (53), or they may be more effectively killed with the addition of an aminoglycoside (54,55).

The structural modification of methicillin which protects the β-lactam ring from attack by penicillinases also obstructs the molecule's ability to penetrate the cellular envelope of enterococci and certain gram-negative cocci. In fact, methicillin is "20 to 50 times less active than penicillin G against bacteria sensitive to both drugs" (11).

The antimicrobial activity of nafcillin against staphylococci is similar to that of methicillin; enterococci are also resistant to nafcillin (56). Nafcillin is more effective than methicillin or the isoxazolyl penicillins against *S. pneumoniae* and the β-hemolytic streptococci, but still not as effective as penicillin G.

The isoxazolyl penicillins (oxacillin, cloxacillin, dicloxacillin, and flucloxacillin) are very similar to methicillin and nafcillin in their antimicrobial activity (57). They are effective in treating penicillin-resistant, methicillin-susceptible staphylococci; they are effective against most streptococci, but only at much higher concentrations than penicillin G itself. The enterococci are resistant to this group of agents.

C. Aminopenicillins

Ampicillin and the other aminopenicillins are effective against all bacteria for which penicillin G is also effective. Some strains of pneumococci and enterococci may be slightly more susceptible to ampicillin than to penicillin (11). Like penicillin, ampicillin is destroyed by β-lactamase–producing bacteria.

The aminopenicillins are effective against some gram-negative bacilli, including some strains of *E. coli* and *Proteus mirabilis* (58–60). Ampicillin-resistant strains of these organisms, still more common in hospitals than in the community, are encountered with increasing frequency in both settings. *Salmonella* spp. and *H. influenzae* are no longer reliably susceptible to ampicillin, either. Penicillin-susceptible *N. meningitidis* and *N. gonorrhoeae* are also susceptible to ampicillin. Isolates of *M. catarrhalis* are often resistant because of β-lactamase production. The gram-negative and gram-positive anaerobes susceptible to penicillin G are also susceptible to ampicillin (32).

D. Carboxypenicillins

The advantage of carboxypenicillins is their activity against *P. aeruginosa*. *P. aeruginosa* produces a chromosomally mediated β-lactamase, which is responsible for inactivating most penicillins and cephalosporins (16); carbenicillin and ticarcillin are not disrupted by this enzyme. Some strains, however, carry a plasmid-coded β-lactamase, which can destroy the carboxypenicillins. Other strains are intrinsically resistant to the carboxypenicillins as a result of altered PBPs. Ticarcillin demonstrates greater activity against *P. aeruginosa* than does carbenicillin (61), but organisms resistant to one are resistant to the other (62). Activity of the carboxypenicillins against gram-positive cocci and gram-negative bacilli is similar to that of ampicillin (5). Carbenicillin and ticarcillin are active against streptococci but not against penicillin-resistant staphylococci. They are not as effective against enterococci as penicillin G or ampicillin.

E. Acylamino Penicillins

The acylamino penicillins are also effective against many strains of *Pseudomonas aeruginosa*. In fact, they are often more effective, and are destroyed by fewer strains, than the carboxypenicillins (6). Mezlocillin, piperacillin, azlocillin, ureidopenicillins, and the other members of this group are also more effective against *Klebsiella pneumoniae* and other Enterobacteriaceae, as well as *H. influenzae*. These drugs approach ampicillin in efficacy against the gram-positive cocci, including enterococci.

F. Amidino Penicillins

The amidino penicillins (amdinocillin and pivamdinocillin) are markedly different from the other penicillins in that they are more active against gram-negative bacilli than against gram-positive organisms (63–66). Amdinocillin (also called mecillinam) is much less active against staphylococci and streptococci than is ampicillin, although the relatively high concentrations reached in the urine may be effective in eradicating gram-positive urinary tract organisms (67). Amdinocillin and pivamdinocillin are very active against most Enterobacteriaceae, but they are somewhat less active against *Morganella* spp. and *Providencia* spp. *P. aeruginosa* and *Acinetobacter* spp. are resistant to the amidino penicillins, as are *Serratia marcescens* and *H. influenzae*. The gram-negative and gram-positive anaerobic bacteria are resistant to amdinocillin and pivamdinocillin.

IV. CLINICAL PHARMACOLOGY

As a group, the penicillins differ from each other in their bioavailability, but they are relatively similar in their distribution and elimination.

A. Oral Absorption

Orally absorbed penicillins are especially valuable antimicrobial agents for many elderly patients who are not appropriate candidates for parenteral drugs. Penicillin G, methicillin, and the antipseudomonal penicillins are not stable in acid environments, and are therefore not useful as oral preparations. Penicillin V is stable, however, and is well absorbed, especially as the potassium salt. Compared to young adults, higher serum concentrations at 30 and 90 min and 3 and 6 h were noted in one study of hospitalized elderly patients after administration of oral penicillin (68), although another smaller study did not detect such differences for ambulatory older patients (69). Any difference may be more a function of renal clearance rather than directly the result of age. Ampicillin is only 30–60% absorbed. Absorption of the drug does not appear to be decreased in elderly persons, although its clearance has been reported to be less than in the young (70). Structural modification to form amoxicillin or the preampicillins (bacampicillin and pivampicillin) increases absorption significantly (60,71). Because amoxicillin can be given three times a day, this may make it especially useful for some elderly patients. The oral esters of carbenicillin, such as indanyl carbenicillin, also have increased absorption so that they can be used as oral agents for urinary tract infections (the achievable serum levels are not high enough to treat systemic infections). The penicillinase-resistant isoxazolyl penicillins, cloxacillin, and dicloxacillin are the most commonly used oral antistaphylococcal penicillins. Renal excretion of these drugs is important, but hepatic metabolism also occurs, especially in the setting of renal impairment (57), making these suitable drugs for use in elderly persons.

Those penicillins that are not destroyed in the stomach are absorbed in the duodenum (72). Peak serum levels are usually reached within 1–2 h after ingestion on an empty stomach; ingestion with food results in peak serum levels that are lower and delayed (2–3 h). Peak serum levels of isoxazolyl penicillins persist for 2–3 h (57).

B. Intramuscular Injection

Some penicillins are, of course, routinely given intramuscularly (IM) regardless of the patient's age. Occasionally lack of other suitable access may make IM therapy with other penicillins of special value for the elderly patient. Relative lack of muscle mass is, however, also a concern. Following IM injection of 1 million units (MU) penicillin G, peak serum levels reach a maximum of 12 μg/ml within 30 min, and then fall rapidly over the next 4–6 h (11); higher serum concentrations may occur in elderly as compared to younger patients given the same doses (68). Intramuscular procaine penicillin G reaches its peak serum level in about 2 h and rapidly falls to undetectable levels within 24 h. Benzathine penicillin G, given IM, maintains low drug levels for 1–3 weeks (following 2.4 MU IM, levels of 0.2 μg/ml at 48 h, 0.05 μg/ml at 1 week, and 0.02 μg/ml at 2 weeks were detected) (11). Benzathine penicillin administered to elderly patients produced serum levels twice as high, which persisted twice as long, as those measured in younger adults (73). Procaine and benzathine penicillin preparations should never be administered intravenously (IV).

Intramuscular injections of the antipseudomonal penicillins result in peak levels 30–60 min following injection. Peak levels of the isoxazolyl penicillins are twice as high following IM injection as those achieved with the same dose given orally (57).

Procaine or lidocaine may be combined with intramuscularly administered antipseudomonal penicillins, but this does not result in prolonged drug levels (15). Diabetic patients appear to absorb intramuscularly administered penicillin more slowly than nondiabetic patients (74).

C. Intravenous Administration

Intravenously administered penicillin G can produce high serum concentrations rapidly, making it a mainstay of therapy for many serious infections. A dose of 2 MU IV every 2 h yields a constant serum level of 20 μg/ml (75). Penicillin is unstable in solution at room temperature, so it not only loses activity but may also lead to penicillin sensitization due to the potent antigenic degradation products (76). Therefore, intravenous penicillin should be freshly prepared and administered intermittently rather than as a constant infusion (77).

There are relatively few studies of the more broad-spectrum penicillins in elderly patients. In elderly patients with varying degrees of renal dysfunction, the half-life of mezlocillin was minimally affected except with severe renal impairment (78). Both mezlocillin and azlocillin pharmacokinetics were studied in elderly patients with biliary disease; serum half-life was related to renal function but age as an independent factor was unrelated to drug half-life, renal clearance, or biliary concentrations (79). Healthy ambulatory elderly subjects given mezlocillin had decreased renal clearance but increased nonrenal clearance with resultant serum half-lives similar to younger persons (80).

The carboxypenicillins reach a constant state by the end of a 30-min infusion, which lasts about 7 h (81). Serum levels of the ureidopenicillins are not as high and do not last as long.

D. Other Routes

Other routes of penicillin administration include intraperitoneal, intrathecal, and ophthalmic. These are not known to be influenced by age.

E. Distribution

Distribution of the penicillins is relatively extensive. The penicillins penetrate most tissues sufficiently to treat susceptible organisms. Entry into abscesses, the middle ear, and pleural, peritoneal, and synovial fluid are adequate in the presence of inflammation (5,82–84,). Although levels in the brain, cerebrospinal fluid (CSF), eye, and prostate are negligible in the absence of inflammation (85), inflammation alters drug clearance and makes penicillins very useful for infections at some of these sites. There is no intracellular activity.

Urinary drug levels are very high, even in the presence of significant renal insufficiency, although with creatine clearance less than 10 ml/min, concentrations are comparable to blood levels (86). Even those penicillins with minimal biliary elimination can be found in the bile at levels in excess of 10 times the serum levels; however, levels are markedly reduced in the presence of common duct obstruction (79).

Protein binding (primarily to albumin) varies from 15% for aminopenicillins to 97% for dicloxacillin. It is the free drug that is felt to be the active molecule, the protein-bound fraction having no antibacterial effect (87,88). The clinical significance of this observation is open to question, however, since the binding is readily reversible. Drugs that compete with penicillins for albumin-binding sites will raise the free (active) serum level of the antibiotic. This is one of the mechanisms by which probenecid raises the serum level of penicillin. Very high levels of the penicillins may surpass the binding capability of albumin, leading to larger proportions of unbound drug. Additionally, renal failure decreases the binding of a drug to albumin, probably as a result of the accumulation of other metabolites that compete for binding sites, and possibly as a result of structural changes of the albumin itself (89).

F. Excretion

Urinary excretion via renal tubular cells is the major route of elimination for all penicillins. Rapid renal excretion gives the penicillins a relatively short half-life: 30–60 min. Hepatic metabolism and elimination is minimal except for nafcillin, oxacillin, and the ureidopenicillins (90). Therefore, doses of most penicillins require adjustment in patients with significant renal impairment. It appears that the major factor influencing dosing of penicillins in elderly patients is their relative renal insufficiency rather than any other attribute directly related to age. Decreased renal function is especially important for carbenicillin, ticarcillin, and temocillin. Except with severe impairment, doses of the ureidopenicillins require minimal adjustment; doses of nafcillin and the isoxazolyl penicillins require no adjustment. Probenecid prolongs the serum half-life (91) and raises the serum levels of all the penicillins by blocking renal excretion and competing for binding sites on albumin.

All but the penicillinase-resistant penicillins are substantially removed by hemodialysis (92); removal by peritoneal dialysis is more variable.

G. Pharmacokinetics in Elderly Patients

In most elderly patients, penicillin may be used in standard doses unless there is relatively severe renal dysfunction. However, there are certain special considerations. Elderly patients frequently have multiple medical illnesses, requiring multiple medications. Additionally, alterations in renal and hepatic function, integrity of the gastrointestinal tract, gastric acidity and blood flow, and circulatory competence often accompany advanced age (93–96). These factors may impact on penicillin pharmacokinetics and thus influence the choice of drug or the dose or route to be used. Most often these are theoretical considerations with unknown clinical consequence. For example, the semisynthetic penicillins such as carbenicillin can inactivate aminoglycosides (see Chap. 13). This effect is increased with increased dose and exposure time (97,98); this might therefore be more likely in the elderly patient with renal impairment.

The likelihood that older patients may be receiving more drugs may also be a concern. As stated earlier, drugs that compete with the penicillins for albumin-binding sites may cause elevated levels of free (active) antimicrobial agent. Heparin raises the level of circulating free fatty acids, which reduces protein binding of some penicillins (i.e., dicloxacillin) while increasing the binding of others (i.e., penicillin G) (99). The fraction of unbound antibiotic may be unusually high if hypo-albuminemia results from malnutrition, nephrotic syndrome, hepatic insufficiency, or other causes. This, too, is a theoretical concern.

The short half-life of the penicillins necessitates frequent administration. When administered by nursing personnel or in a supervised setting, this may not be a problem. However, self-administration of antibiotics every 4–6 h by older patients who are already taking multiple other medications, or who are developing memory difficulties, may result in profound administration errors.

The number of studies evaluating penicillins in elderly persons is unfortunately small, despite the long history of these commonly prescribed drugs. The future will see more pharmacological investigations, with consequent improved understanding of their action and utility in older individuals.

V. CLINICAL INDICATIONS

When penicillin was first introduced, a wide range of organisms, including many gram-negative bacilli, were susceptible in vitro and responded to clinical therapy. Over the past several decades, resistance has appeared in many bacteria. Some organisms, such as *S. pneumoniae*, have remained susceptible except in very limited circumstances; others, such as *S. aureus*, rapidly displayed widespread resistance. To minimize further development of resistance, if the causative pathogen is known, it is important to use an agent with the most narrow spectrum of activity whenever possible. Narrow-spectrum therapy is especially beneficial for older individuals who have frequent or recurrent infections.

Antimicrobial agents can be administered for empiric therapy, for definitive therapy, or for prophylaxis. For an established infection, after a specific organism and its antimicrobial susceptibility pattern have been determined, selecting appropriate therapy can be a relatively simple matter. However, it is often necessary to begin antimicrobial therapy before the infecting organism and its susceptibilities are known. Prompt initiation of therapy is essential in elderly patients (100) because the initial manifestations of infection are often less dramatic; consequently the infection may be more advanced by the time it is recognized (101). In addition, the infectious process may spread more rapidly in the relatively immunocompromised aged individual (102). Another concern is that appropriate clinical specimens are sometimes difficult to obtain. The elderly patient is thus more likely to be maintained on the initial empiric regimen because there are no culture results to allow therapy to be adjusted. If the laboratory is able to identify and characterize the specific infecting organisms, then the therapeutic regimen should be appropriately altered as much as possible. When an infecting organism is susceptible to several antibiotics, the choice should almost always be made for the antibiotic with the least toxicity and most narrow or directed spectrum of activity (103). This is often a penicillin. Continued use of antibiotics with coverage broader than necessary simply leads to the emergence of resistant organisms, which themselves may eventually cause infection.

In addition to their low toxicity, their bactericidal activity, and their availability in a wide selection of broad and narrow formulations, the penicillins are easy to administer via a wide variety of routes and are of relatively low cost. Indeed, in the nursing home, they are one of the most commonly prescribed groups of antibiotics (104).

A. Natural Penicillins

Penicillin is the drug of choice for most streptococcal infections, regardless of site. Despite the availability of pneumococcal vaccine, *S. pneumoniae* remains a common cause of pneumonia and meningitis in the elderly population and is still associated with high mortality in this group. The development of relatively resistant strains of pneumococcus is of great concern; because the concentration of penicillin in the cerebral spinal fluid is only a fraction of that achieved in serum, penicillin is not the drug of choice when relative (or full) resistance is suspected. Nevertheless, if bacterial resistance is not a concern, penicillin is still a valuable drug as it penetrates the blood-brain barrier (in the presence of inflammation) better than most of the alternative drugs.

Penicillin has long been one of the drugs used for meningitis because many pathogens have been susceptible. Nearly all strains of *N. meningitidis* remain susceptible, but β-lactamase production has made penicillin unreliable for therapy of *H. influenzae* infections. *Listeria monocytogenes* is not susceptible to the newer cephalosporins frequently used for therapy of meningitis. *L. monocytogenes* remains susceptible to penicillin and ampicillin, the latter being the drug of choice. Penicillin is also a first-line drug for treating a variety of other streptococcal infections including those due to *S. pyogenes*, *S. agalactiae*, viridans streptococci, and the enterococci. Serious or life-threatening enterococcal infections, however, should never be treated with a single agent if an aminoglycoside can be added to achieve a synergistic effect. Because the various streptococci are relatively common etiological agents of infective endocarditis, penicillin is often part of the therapeutic regimen. In many cases combination therapy that includes an aminoglycoside is used. Penicillin (or ampicillin) plus gentamicin remains the standard therapy for most cases of enterococcal endocarditis. Infective endocarditis caused by susceptible strains of staphylococci and streptococci should be treated with penicillin plus an aminoglycoside in certain circumstances (105). Although shorter-term therapy is sometimes used for younger patients with infective endocarditis due to penicillin-susceptible strains of streptococci, it is probably not wise to attempt short-term therapy for most older patients.

Penicillin has traditionally been used for therapy of infections derived from the endogenous oral flora (so-called "above-the-diaphragm" anaerobic infections). Although the organisms that make up the normal oral flora are usually thought of as anaerobic, many of the streptococci and some of the other genera are not obligate anaerobes. Penicillin has remained a common therapy for aspiration pneumonia that occurs outside the institutional setting. It may be inadequate therapy for the seriously ill patient (106) because some oral anaerobes produce β-lactamases. It is also insufficient as a single-agent therapy unless the presence of aerobic or facultative gram-negative bacilli, as well as staphylococci, have been excluded. Penicillin can be used alone or in combination with other drugs for periodontal infections and other infections derived from the oral flora, such as deep neck space infections and brain abscesses. For serious infections, it is almost always used in combination with other agents because of the possibility of β-lactamase–producing organisms. Penicillin continues to be an excellent drug when other specific "anaerobic" pathogens such as clostridia and *Actinomyces* spp. are detected.

Penicillin remains the drug of choice for the treatment of treponemal infections, although it should no longer be used to treat gonococcal infections or other sexually transmitted diseases.

Penicillins are often used for prophylaxis. Oral or intramuscular penicillin has been effective in preventing recurrences of rheumatic fever and in controlling outbreaks of infections due to *S. pyogenes*. Alone or in combination, penicillin is also useful for the prevention of infective endocarditis in specific circumstances.

B. Penicillinase-Resistant Penicillins

1. Methicillin, Nafcillin

The penicillinase-resistant penicillins are active against many β-lactamase producing gram-positive cocci, as well as some of the same organisms as the natural penicillins. The alterations that make these agents penicillinase resistant, however, are associated with decreased activity against many other organisms including the streptococci (especially enterococci) and anaerobes. Thus, these drugs are neither substitutes for nor broader spectrum than penicillin itself. The appropriate clinical use of methicillin or nafcillin is limited to suspected or proven infections caused by penicillinase-producing *S. aureus* that are not intrinsically resistant to β-lactam agents. Actually, methicillin is rarely used—especially in elderly patients—due to the frequency of the side effect of interstitial nephritis, although some clinicians feel that the lower level of protein binding could make the drug more effective in treating infections of the central nervous system. Oral nafcillin is not recommended due to the unreliable nature of its absorption from the alimentary tract; intramuscular injection of nafcillin leads to low blood levels. Administered intravenously, nafcillin is the standard agent for therapy of infections due to susceptible β-lactamase–producing staphylococci. Nafcillin should not be used for empiric therapy of hospital-acquired infections due to coagulase-negative staphylococci, since more than 50% of strains may be resistant. When initial empiric therapy consists of another agent such as vancomycin (because of the concern for resistance) the regimen should be changed if cultured specimens demonstrate the presence of staphylococci that are susceptible to the penicillinase-resistant penicillins. Organisms sensitive to penicillin should be treated with that drug, as it is generally more effective.

2. *Isoxazolyl Penicillins*

The isoxazolyl penicillins include oxacillin and two drugs used only for oral administration—cloxacillin and dicloxacillin. One other drug, flucloxacillin, is not currently available in the United States. All of these drugs are considered to have the same spectrum of activity as nafcillin and can be used when oral therapy is adequate.

C. Aminopenicillins

These penicillins all have a similar spectrum of activity. They can be substituted for penicillin G in most cases (unlike the penicillinase-resistant penicillins), but they are not themselves resistant to β-lactamases. Because of their increased activity against gram-negative bacteria, they also are effective in settings in which penicillin G would not be used; these include infections of the gastrointestinal and urinary tracts.

Ampicillin, given intravenously or orally, is useful for treating a variety of infections. Ampicillin is more active than penicillin G against enterococci and is also effective, especially in high concentrations, against many strains of *E. coli* and *Proteus* species. It is therefore an excellent antibiotic for uncomplicated urinary tract infections due to susceptible organisms. Even when the in vitro susceptibility tests indicate resistance, ampicillin may be effective at the high levels attained in the urine (11). Ampicillin is safe, even in the presence of renal insufficiency. Because of its relatively narrow spectrum of activity and low toxicity, it is often a good therapeutic choice for infections in older patients. Ampicillin is appropriate for the treatment of all infections [including life-threatening ones) caused by *L. monocytogenes* as well as susceptible strains of enterococci (in combination with an aminoglycoside such as gentamicin for serious infections (107)], *E. coli* and *Proteus mirabilis*. Severe infections caused by pneumococcus are better treated with penicillin because it is more active against the organism and also is a more narrow-spectrum drug. Enteric infections due to susceptible strains of *Salmonella* spp. and *Shigella* spp. can be treated with ampicillin, but resistance due to β-lactamase production is now common among many of these pathogens. Ampicillin may be effective in treating biliary tract infections caused by susceptible organisms (108); however, susceptibility testing should be completed before using ampicillin as a single agent. Ampicillin is used less often than in the past for therapy of respiratory infections because of the increased frequency of resistance. *H. influenzae*, even the nontypable strains that are more common in older individuals, may produce β-lactamase. Other pulmonary pathogens such as *M. catarrhalis* are usually resistant. Ampicillin should no longer be used for the treatment of sexually transmitted diseases. Syphilis is best treated with penicillin; *N. gonorrhoeae* strains are frequently resistant to both penicillin and ampicillin.

The clinical indications for amoxicillin are similar to those for ampicillin. However, because it is administered only three times per day, improved compliance may offer an advantage for this drug; also important are the higher blood levels achieved after oral administration. Amoxicillin appears to be better absorbed into the pulmonary tissue (109,110), making it a better antimicrobial for treating respiratory infections. It should not be used for therapy of shigellosis. The other aminopenicillins have demonstrated no superiority to ampicillin or amoxicillin, except perhaps in having a slightly different constellation of adverse reactions.

D. Carboxypenicillins

The major advantage of the carboxypenicillins (carbenicillin, ticarcillin) is their activity against *P. aeruginosa* and certain other gram-negative bacilli. For life-threatening *P. aeruginosa* infections, carboxypenicillins should be combined with other antipseudomonal agents. Even after susceptibility has been demonstrated, use of two antipseudomonal agents is often appropriate for certain serious infections (72). Carboxypenicillins may be used for treating specific *P. aeruginosa* respiratory infections, such as those in chronic bronchitic patients previously treated with multiple other agents. These agents may also be used for the treatment of pseudomonal urinary tract infections. However, as *P. aeruginosa* in the urine may indicate an anatomical abnormality, eradication with these agents alone is not always achieved. Although there is activity against most organisms susceptible to ampicillin, the carboxypenicillins are less effective against *E. faecalis*, some of the other streptococci, and *L. monocytogenes*. These agents should rarely be used to treat infections due to organisms, including gram-negative bacilli, for which more narrow-spectrum antimicrobials exist. Widespread use may lead to drug resistance, often making other antipseudomonal agents ineffective as well. Carbenicillin and ticarcillin are usually administered intravenously. Indanyl carbenicillin, an oral agent, is recommended for treating chronic bacterial prostatitis. It is sometimes used to treat *P. aeruginosa* urinary tract infection. However, because urine levels are lower when renal function is decreased, this agent may be ineffective for this latter indication.

E. Acylamino Penicillins

The acylamino penicillins have more in vitro antipseudomonal activity than do the carboxypenicillins on a gram per gram basis; however, this may not be clinically relevant (111–115). In fact, their use as single agents for febrile neutropenic patients, or for therapy of *P. aeruginosa* infections, often results in the development of resistance (6,116,117). When combined with aminoglycosides for these purposes, they have proven to be quite effective (118).

Because the acylamino penicillins maintain much more of their antistreptococcal activity than the carboxypenicillins, they are much more valuable for treating mixed gram-positive and gram-negative infections, such as intraabdominal and hepatobiliary infections. Complicated polymicrobial urinary tract infections and respiratory infections have also responded well to this group of agents. However, for most single pathogen infections, they are no more effective than the older, less expensive, and more narrow-spectrum penicillins. Not unexpectedly, when infections with susceptible organisms have not been eradicated by these drugs, the causes have generally been inadequate drainage of abscesses, obstructions of the urinary tract, or other mechanical impediments (6,119).

F. Amidino Penicillins

Amdinocillin and pivamdinocillin have been used successfully in treating uncomplicated urinary tract infections caused by susceptible gram-negative bacilli with efficacy equaling that of ampicillin or trimethoprim sulfamethoxazole (120–123). The effectiveness in treating some gram-positive urinary tract infections (especially those due to enterococci or *Staphylococcus saprophyticus*) is questionable (67,124,125). Because of their different sites of action, the amidino penicillins have been used in combination with other β-lactams for their synergistic effect. The combination of amoxicillin and pivamdinocillin for the treatment of exacerbations of chronic bronchitis was reported to be beneficial compared to amoxicillin alone, in terms of faster response and fewer relapses (126). Benefit from these types of combination regimens, however, has not been universally demonstrated.

VI. ADMINISTRATION OF DRUG

The wide choice of administration modalities makes penicillins a useful group of antimicrobial agents for treating infections in elderly patients. Because of rapid urinary excretion, most penicillins require only minor adjustments when administered to patients with creatinine clearances as low as 10 ml/min.

Table 3 lists dosages that are recommended for the penicillins. Table 4 provides recommended dosages for patients with moderate to severe renal failure.

Penicillin itself is relatively unstable, but its salts (usually sodium or potassium) are available in oral solid and liquid formulations and in parenteral preparations. Intravenous penicillin should be administered as an intermittent infusion over 30 minutes, soon after preparation. When allowed to flow as a continuous infusion, the penicillin is unstable at room temperature and may be inactivated by constituents of other IV solutions (76). The degradation products of penicillin are not only less potent, but also more allergenic.

Orally active penicillins that are available include the sodium or potassium salts of phenoxymethylpenicillin (penicillin V), phenethicillin, nafcillin (oral absorption is erratic, however, and use of this agent is therefore not recommended), the isoxazolyl penicillins, ampicillin and the other aminopenicillins, indanylcarbenicillin, and pivamdinocillin. Many of these, and all of the remaining penicillins, are available as parenteral preparations for IV or IM administration.

Concurrent administration of probenecid will prolong the half-life and raise the serum levels of all of the penicillins (91). Procaine penicillin G, given as an IM injection, produces sustained drug levels for several days. Procaine or lidocaine can be added to the antipseudomonal penicillins for IM administration, but will not prolong the half-lives of these drugs. Benzathine penicillin G, administered by the IM route, achieves a significantly lower serum level of active drug, but maintains that level for 1–3 weeks. Procaine and benzathine preparations of penicillin should never be administered intravenously.

VII. DRUG MONITORING AND ADVERSE EFFECTS

Penicillins have been associated with a wide array of adverse reactions. Nevertheless, their toxic:therapeutic ratio, or margin of safety, is quite high, especially compared with many other antimicrobials. Elderly individuals, compared to younger patients, tend to be more susceptible to the adverse effects of penicillins, as they are to the effects of many other drugs. Contributing factors include renal insufficiency (with subsequently elevated drug levels), polypharmacy (leading to increased opportunities for drug–drug interactions), and multiple medical problems (making, for example, the sodium load of the carboxypenicillins more of a problem for a patient with congestive heart failure). In addition to polypharmacy, preexisting dementia has a major impact on the capacity for self-administra-

Table 3 Recommended Dosages of Penicillins and Available Preparations

Antibiotic	Route of administration	Average daily dose	Frequency	Available preparations
Amoxicillin	PO	0.75–1.5 g	q 8 h	Cap: 125, 250, 500 mg, Tab: 3 g Susp: 125 or 250 mg/5 ml
	IM,IV	1.5–4 g	q 6–8 h	Vial: 0.25, 0.5, 1.0 g
Ampicillin	PO	2–4 g	q 6 h	Cap: 250, 500 mg, Tab: 125 mg Syrup: 125 or 250 mg/5 ml
	IM,IV	2–12 g	q 6 h	Vial: 0.25, 0.5, 1 g
Bacampicillin	PO	0.8–1.6 g	q 12 h	Tab: 400 mg Susp: 125 mg
Carbenicillin	IM,IV	30–40 g	q 4–6 h	Vials: 1.5 g
Cloxacillin	PO	2–4 g	q 6 h	Cap: 250, 500 mg, Syrup: 125 mg/ml
	IM,IV	1–3 g	q 6 h	Vial: 0.25, 0.5 g
Cyclacillin	PO	1–2 g	q 6 h	Tab: 250, 500 mg Susp: 125–250 mg/5 ml
Dicloxacillin	PO	1–2 g	q 6 h	Cap: 125, 250, 500 mg Syrup: 62.5 mg/5 ml
Flucloxacillin	PO	1–2 g	q 6 h	Cap: 250, 500 mg Syrup: 125 or 250 mg/5 ml
	IM,IV	1–4 g	q 6 h	Vial: 0, 25, 0.5, 1.0 g
Hetacillin	PO	0.9–1.8 g	q 6 h	Cap: 250 mg Susp: 125–250 mg/5 ml
Indanycarben-icillin	PO	4–8 tabs	q 4–6 h	Tab: 382 mg
Methicillin	IM,IV	4–12 g	q 4–6 h	Vial: 1 g
Nafcillin	PO[a]	2–4 g	q 6 h	Cap: 250 mg, Tab: 500 mg Susp: 250 mg/5 ml
	IV	2–9 g	q 6 h	Vial: 0.5, 1.0, 2.0 g
Oxacillin	PO	2–4 g	q 6 h	Cap: 250, 500 mg Syrup: 250 mg/5 ml
	IV	2–12 g	q 6 h	Vial: 0.25, 0.5, 1.0, 2.0, 4.0 g
Penicillin G	PO	1.2 g	q 6 h	Tab: 125, 250, 500 mg
	IM,IV	1.2–24 MU	q 2–12 h	Vials: 0.5, 1.0, 2.0, 5.0, 10.0 MU (0.3, 0.6, 1.2, 3.0, 6.0 g)
Penicillin G, Benzathene	IM	2.4 MU		Syringe, disposable: 0.3, 0.6, 1.2 MU
Penicillin G, Procaine	IM	0.3–4.8 MU	q 24 h	Syringe, disposable: 0.6, 1.2, 2.4 MU
Penicillin V	PO	1–2 g	q 6 h	Cap, Tab: 125, 250, 500 mg Susp: 125–250 mg/5 ml

Table 3 Continued

Antibiotic	Route of administration	Average daily dose	Frequency	Available preparations
Phenethicillin	PO	1–2 g	q 6 h	Cap, Tab: 125, 250, 500 mg Susp: 125–250 mg/5 ml
Pivampicillin	PO	1 g	q 8–12 h	Tab: 500 mg Susp: 162 mg/5 ml Sachets: 162 mg/sachet
Talampicillin	PO	0.75–1.5 g	q 8 h	Tab: 250 mg Syrup: 125 mg/5 ml
Ticarcillin	IM,IV	200–300 mg/kg	q 4–6 h	Vial: 1.5 g

tion of all antimicrobial agents. For patients administering their own medications, the penicillins still offer a relatively wide margin of safety.

A. Hypersensitivity Reactions

Hypersensitivity reactions usually result from prior exposure to the drug. Allergic reactions were more common when early penicillin preparations were used, because they contained

Table 4 Recommended Dosages of Penicillins in Patients with Renal Failure

Antibiotic	Dose	Frequency		Dose following hemodialysis (supplemental to anuric dose)
		CrCl=10–50	CrCl<10 (anuric)	
Amdinocillin (Mecillinam)	10 mg/kg	q 6 h	q 8 h	
Amoxicillin	250–500 mg	q 12 h	q 12–24 h	250 mg
Ampicillin	1–2 g	q 8 h	q 12 h	0.5 g
Azlocillin	2–4 g	q 8 h	q 12 h	3 g
Bacampicillin	400–800 mg	q 12 h	q 24 h	
Carbenicillin	2–3 g	q 6 h	q 8–12 h	2 g
Cloxacillin	0.5–1.0 g	q 6 h	q 6 h	
Cyclacillin	250–500 mg	q 12–24 h	q 24 h	
Dicloxacillin	250–500 mg	q 6 h	q 6 h	
Methicillin	1–2 g	q 8 h	q 12 h	2 g
Mezlocillin	1.5–4 g	q 6–8 h	q 8–12 h	2–3 g
Nafcillin	0.5–1.0 g	q 6 h	q 6 h	
Oxacillin	0.5–1.0 g	q 6 h	q 6 h	
Penicillin G	0.5–2.5 MU	q 6 h	q 6 h	0.5 MU
Penicillin V	250–500 mg	q 6 h	q 6 h	250 mg
Piperacillin	3–4 g	q 6–12 h	q 12 h	2 g q 8 h + 1 g after HD[a]
Ticarcillin	2–3 g	q 6–8 h	2 g q 12 h	3 g

[a]HD = hemodialysis.

many impurities (127,128). Therefore, many patients who developed their "allergies" during the 1940s and 1950s may not actually be hypersensitive to the penicillin used in formulations today. Occasionally a hypersensitivity reaction develops without a known exposure to the drug. It has been shown, at least for some of the cases, that blood transfusions from patients who were taking penicillin, or bovine milk from animals receiving penicillin, may be the initial source of drug exposure (129).

Penicillin degradation products—which rapidly develop as penicillin remains in solution at room temperature—are more antigenic than the penicillin molecule itself. Penicilloyl, formed upon breaking the β-lactam ring, acts as a hapten by attaching to protein via the amino group. This conjugate of penicilloyl with body proteins is called the major determinant of penicillin allergy, since it is quantitatively the major antigenic metabolite. Minor determinants include penicilloic acid and penilloic acid.

Anaphylactic shock is rare, reported to occur in no more than 0.01–0.10% of all recipients (127,130,131); but it is associated with a 10% mortality (132,133). Mediated by IgE antibodies, anaphylaxis is most often associated with parenteral penicillin G, but it has also occurred after oral administration and following the use of other penicillin analogs. Serum sickness, a late onset hypersensitivity reaction, has been reported in 2% of penicillin G recipients (132). Onset of symptoms, probably due to IgG antibodies, generally occurs 3–10 days following administration and may consist of fever, malaise, arthralgias, urticaria, and angioedema. Exfoliative dermatitis and Stevens-Johnson syndrome are rare but severe allergic reactions. Contact dermatitis from topical penicillin and local swelling at the site of injections have also been reported. The most common allergic reaction is rash, which is probably IgM-mediated. It may disappear with continued treatment but has the potential to progress to the more severe dermatological reactions.

Patients with a history of "penicillin allergy" must be considered allergic to all penicillins. Some authorities advise against using cephalosporins as well in patients with a history of anaphylaxis or severe immediate penicillin hypersensitivity (134), although cross-reactivity is not complete (135,136). However, it must also be remembered that not all penicillin-related drug reactions are truly allergic (137–139). Even true hypersensitivity reactions may represent allergies to contaminants rather than to the penicillin itself. This is particularly true for patients whose reactions occurred over 30 years ago.

B. Other Immune-Mediated Reactions

The Jarisch-Herxheimer reaction has been correlated with release of endotoxin or other pyrogens when microorganisms are killed. Seen as early as 1–2 h following penicillin administration and lasting 8–24 h, this reaction consists of fever, chills, malaise, sore throat, myalgias, headache, and tachycardia. It is primarily associated with penicillin treatment of syphilis (140), but may occur in patients with leptospirosis, yaws, rat-bite fever, anthrax, and, rarely, meningococcal meningitis (11,141).

1. Renal

Interstitial nephritis can occur with use of any of the penicillins but is particularly associated with methicillin (142–148). Typically, fever, rash, albuminuria, uremia, and eosinophilia are seen 1 week into the course of therapy. Prompt discontinuation of the drug generally leads to resolution of the nonoliguric renal failure, but this process can progress to anuria. Although this reaction will not necessarily recur with the administration of a different penicillin, it is nevertheless prudent to at least temporarily avoid all penicillins and cephalosporins immediately following a case of penicillin-induced nephritis, as it occasionally recurs with the administration of a second β-lactam (149).

2. *Neurological*

Despite the relatively high margin of safety, very high doses of penicillin can lead to drowsiness, myoclonus, seizures, or coma (150). These effects are associated with CSF levels greater than 5 μg/ml (11), which may result from total daily doses in excess of 100,000,000 units IV, smaller doses in the presence of renal failure, meningitis (which increases the permeability of the blood brain barrier), or intrathecal doses above 20,000 units per day (151). Mental status changes may be more common in individuals with preexisting mental disorders (152), but their frequency in individuals with dementia is not known.

3. *Hematological*

Hemolytic anemia, although uncommon, may occur as a result of the penicillin metabolites acting as haptens as they coat red blood cells. This phenomenon is dose related, usually occurring only with doses of more than 10,000,000 units per day. It is reversible but can recur due to cross-reactivity with the semisynthetic penicillins and cephalosporins (153,154). The direct Coombs' test is positive.

Neutropenia (155,156) and agranulocytosis (157) have also been described. Pancytopenia may result when the normal release of mature cells from the bone marrow is blocked (158).

Coagulopathy may occur as a result of platelet dysfunction (159,160), disturbed conversion of fibrinogen to fibrin (161), increased antithrombin III activity (162), or specific clotting factor inhibitors (163). Vitamin K, administered intramuscularly, has successfully prevented carbenicillin-associated bleeding in a series of elderly patients (164).

C. Rashes and Other Soft Tissue Reactions

Ampicillin is commonly associated with rashes, often of the maculopapular type rather than true urticaria. Rashes appear to be associated with ampicillin more than any other penicillin, having an incidence of 7.7% vs. 2.7%, respectively (165). Such rashes may be particularly more common in patients with certain leukemias and lymphomas (166). Many of these rashes are probably toxic rather than allergic, since (1) they have been observed to be dose-related (167), (2) ampicillin-specific antibodies are not always present (168), (3) patients whose rash occurred during infection with mononucleosis did not have a recurrence after the resolution of their viral illness (169), and (4) patients with a history of ampicillin-associated rash have subsequently received other penicillins without developing a rash or any other hypersensitivity (170). Therefore, ampicillin-associated rashes may not always be a contraindication to receiving other penicillins (11).

Subcutaneous extravasation of nafcillin has been demonstrated to cause significant tissue necrosis (171).

D. Gastrointestinal Effects

Nausea, vomiting, and diarrhea are seen most frequently with oral ampicillin therapy and least commonly with the more readily absorbable oral preparations, such as amoxicillin (172,173), epicillin (174), and cyclacillin (175). Pivampicillin is associated with minimal diarrhea, but relatively frequent nausea and vomiting (176). All penicillins have been associated with the development of pseudomembranous colitis (177,178). The most appropriate treatment for antimicrobial agent-associated colitis is complete discontinuation of the agents, whenever possible. If infection persists, or if continued antimicrobial therapy for an underlying infection is required, then specific therapy effective against *C. difficile* may be necessary.

E. Other Adverse Reactions

Drug fevers without any other symptoms have been described. These may recur when other penicillins are substituted (149).

Reactions to procaine have been observed and are believed to result from intravascular entry of the procaine. These include anxiety, mental lability, fever, vomiting, hallucinations, convulsions, tachycardia, hypertension, hypotension, and cardiac arrest (179).

Cation intoxication may be an important issue in patients with congestive heart failure, renal insufficiency, or electrolyte disturbance. Each gram of carbenicillin is administered with 4.7 meq of Na^+. Being a weak acid, carbenicillin can also cause a mild acidosis, as well as hypokalemia. Sodium load is also great for ticarcillin.

REFERENCES

1. Fleming A. On the antibacterial action of culture of a penicillin, with special reference to their use in the isolation of B. influenzae. Br J Exp Pathol 1929; 10:226–36.
2. Chain E, Florey HW, Gardner AD, et al. Penicillin as a chemotherapeutic agent. Lancet 1940; 2:226–8.
3. Abraham EP. Flemings' discovery. Rev Infect Dis 1980; 2:140–1.
4. Barber M, Waterworth PM. Penicillinase-resistant penicillins and cephalosporins. Br Med J 1964; 2:344–9.
5. Neu HC. Carbenicillin and ticarcillin. Med Clin North Am 1982; 66:61–77.
6. Drusano GL, Schimpff SC, Hewitt WL. The acylampicillins: mezlocillin, piperacillin, and azlocillin. Rev Infect Dis 1984; 6:13–32.
7. Tomasz A. Surface components of *Streptococcus pneumoniae*. Rev Infect Dis 1981; 3:190–211.
8. Joklik WK, Willett HP, Amos DB. Zinsser microbiology, 17th ed. New York: Appleton-Century-Crofts, 1980.
9. Mychajlonka M, McDowell TD, Shockman GD. Inhibition of peptidoglycan ribonucleic acid and protein synthesis in tolerant strains of *Streptococcus mutans*. Antimicrob Agents Chemother 1980; 17:572–82.
10. Mychajlonka M. Effects of low penicillin concentrations on cell morphology and on peptidoglycan and protein synthesis in a tolerant streptococcus strain. Antimicrob Agents Chemother 1981; 19:972–9.
11. Kucers A, Bennett N McK. The use of antibiotics, 4th ed. Philadelphia: J. B. Lippincott Co., 1987.
12. Horne D, Tomasz A. Lethal effect of a heterologous murein hydrolase on penicillin-treated *Streptococcus sanguis*. Antimicrob Agents Chemother 1980; 17:235–46.
13. Dever LA, Dermody TS. Mechanisms of bacterial resistance to antibiotics. Arch Intern Med 1991; 151:886–95.
14. Donowitz GR, Mandell GL. Beta-lactam antibiotics (part 1). N Engl J Med 1988; 318:419–26.
15. Neu HC. Penicillins. In: Mandell GL, Douglas RG, Bennett JE, eds. Principles and practice of infectious diseases, 3rd ed. New York: Churchill Livingstone, 1990:230–46.
16. Sanders CC, Sanders WE Jr. Type I β-lactamases of gram-negative bacteria: interactions with β-lactam antibiotics. J Infect Dis 1986; 5:792–800.
17. Chow JW, Fine MJ, Shlaes DM, et al. *Enterobacter* bacteremia: clinical features and emergence of antibiotic resistance during therapy. Ann Intern Med 1991; 115:585–90.

18. Yotsuji A, Takahata M, Yasuda T, et al. Studies on the sub-MIC of beta-lactam antibiotics—bactericidal activity in compromised host's serum. Kansenshogaku Zasshi 1990; 64:1499–1506.
19. Brumfitt W, Hamilton-Miller J. Methicillin-resistant *Staphylococcus aureus*. N Engl J Med 1989; 320:1188–96.
20. Kim KS, Anthony BF. Penicillin tolerance in group B streptococci isolated from infected neonates. J Infect Dis 1981; 144:411–19.
21. Portnoy D, Prentis J, Richards GK. Penicillin tolerance of human isolates of group C streptococci. Antimicrob Agents Chemother 1981; 20:235–8.
22. Moellering RC Jr, Watson BK, Kunz LJ. Endocarditis due to group D streptococci. Am J Med 1974; 57:239–50.
23. Baker CN, Thornsberry C, Facklam RR. Synergism, killing kinetics and antimicrobial susceptibility of Group A and B streptococci. Antimicrob Agents Chemother 1981; 19:716–25.
24. Lam K, Bayer AS. *In vitro* bactericidal synergy of gentamicin combined with penicillin G, vancomycin, or cefotaxime against group G streptococci. Antimicrob Agents Chemother 1984; 26:260–2.
25. Swingle HM, Bucciarelli RL, Ayoub EM. Synergy between penicillins and low concentrations of gentamicin in the killing of group B streptococci. J Infect Dis 1985; 152:515–20.
26. Centers for Disease Control. Isolation of multiple antibiotic-resistant pneumococci—New York. MMWR 1985; 34:545–6.
27. George RH, Mulligan EAR, Roycroft CA, et al. Multiresistant pneumococci. Lancet 1981; 2:751–2.
28. Bourgault AM, Wilson WR, Washington JA II. Antimicrobial susceptibilities of species of viridans streptococci. J Infect Dis 1979; 140:316–21.
29. Holloway Y, Dankert J, Hess J. Penicillin tolerance and bacterial endocarditis. Lancet 1980; 1:589.
30. Phillips I, Warren C, Harrison JM, et al. Antibiotic susceptibilities of streptococci from the mouth and blood of patients treated with penicillin or lincomycin and clindamycin. J Med Microbiol 1976; 9:393–404.
31. Moellering RC Jr, Korzeniowski OM, Sande MA, et al. Species-specific resistance to antimicrobial synergism in *Streptococcus faecium* and *Streptococcus faecalis*. J Infect Dis 1979; 140:203–8.
32. Sutter VL, Finegold SM. Susceptibility of anaerobic bacteria to 23 antimicrobial agents. Antimicrob Agents Chemother. 1976; 10:736–52.
33. Finger A, Handke G. Antibiotic sensitivity of gonococci in South Australia (1974–1975). Med J Aust 1977; 1:133–6.
34. Seth AD, Kolator B, Wilkinson AE. Sensitivity of *Neisseria gonorrhoeae* to antibiotics in London (1976–1978). Br J Vener Dis 1979; 55:325–8.
35. Jaffe HW, Biddle JW, Johnson SR, et al. Infections due to penicillinase-producing *Neisseria gonorrhoeae* in the United States (1976–1980). J Infect Dis 1981; 144:191–7.
36. Yoshida SI, Vrabe S, Mizuguchi Y. Antibiotic sensitivity patterns of penicillinase-positive and penicillinase-negative strains of *Neisseria gonorrhoeae* isolated in Fukuoka, Japan. Br J Vener Dis 1982; 58:305–7.
37. Liebowitz LD, Ballard RC, Koornohf HJ. In vitro susceptibility and cross-resistance of South African isolates of *Neisseria gonorrhoeae* to 14 antimicrobial agents. Antimicrob Agents Chemother 1982; 22:598–602.
38. Powell JT, Bond JH. Multiple antibiotic resistance in clinical strains of *Neisseria gonorrhoeae* isolated in South Carolina. Antimicrob Agents Chemother 1976; 10:639–45.
39. Peltola H. Meningococcal disease: still with us. Rev Infect Dis 1983; 5:71–91.
40. Dillon JR, Pauze M, Yeung KH. Spread of penicillinase-producing and transfer plasmids from the gonococcus to *Neisseria meningitidis*. Lancet 1983; 1:779–81.

41. Doern GU, Tubert TA. In vitro activities of 39 antimicrobial agents of *Branhamella catarrhalis* and comparison of results with different quantitative susceptibility test methods. Antimicrob Agents Chemother 1988; 32:259–61.
42. Sarubbi FA, Verghese A, Caggiano C, et al. *In vitro* activity of cefpodoxime proxetil (U76,252; CS-807) against clinical isolates of *Branhamella catarrhalis*. Antimicrob Agents Chemother 1989; 33:113–114.
43. Wiggins GL, Albritton WL, Freeley JC. Antibiotic susceptibility of clinical isolates of *Listeria monocytogenes*. Antimicrob Agents Chemother 1978; 13:854–60.
44. Prichard MG, Miles HM, Pavillard ER. Listeria meningitis—in vitro sensitivities to co-trimoxazole, penicillins and gentamicin. Aus NZ J Med. 1983; 13:76–7.
45. Auwera P Van Der, Grenier P, Glupczynski Y, et al. In vitro activity of lomefloxacin in comparison with pefloxacin and ofloxacin. J Antimicrob Chemother 1989; 23:209–19.
46. Winslow DL, Damme J, Dieckman E. Delayed bactericidal activity of β-lactam antibiotics against *Listeria monocytogenes*: antagonism of chloramphenicol and rifampin. Antimicrob Agents Chemother 1983; 23:555–8.
47. Gabay EL, Rolfe RD, Finegold SM. Susceptibility of *Clostridium septicum* to 23 antimicrobial agents. Antimicrob Agents Chemother 1981; 20:852–3.
48. Swenson JM, Thornsberry C, McCrosckey LM, et al. Susceptibility of *Clostridium botulinum* to thirteen antimicrobial agents. Antimicrob Agents Chemother 1980; 18:13–19.
49. Silpa DE, Bulloch GF, Silverman ME, et al. *Clostridium perfringens* empyema unresponsive to penicillin. JAMA 1982; 247:2568.
50. Weber DJ, Sabiteer SM, Rutala WA, et al. In vitro susceptibility of *Bacillus* spp. to selected antimicrobial agents. Antimicrob Agents Chemother 1988; 32:642–5.
51. Smith RP, Baltch AL, Hammer MC, et al. In vitro activities of PD 117,596 and reference antibiotics against 448 clinical bacterial strain. Antimicrob Agents Chemother 1988; 32:1450–5.
52. Rolinson GN, Stevens S, Batchelor FR, et al. Bacteriological studies on a new penicillin—BRL 1241. Lancet 1960; 2:564–7.
53. Drake TA, Sande MA. Studies of the chemotherapy of endocarditis: Correlation of in vitro, animal model and clinical studies. Rev Infect Dis 1983; 5(suppl):345–55.
54. Mayhall CG, Medoff G, Marr JJ. Variation in the susceptibility of strains of *Staphylococcus aureus* to oxacillin, cephalothin and gentamicin. Antimicrob Agents Chemother 1976; 10:707–12.
55. Svenungsson B, Kalin M, Lindgren LG. Therapeutic failure in pneumonia caused by a tolerant strain of *Staphylococcus aureus*. Scand J Infect Dis 1982; 14:309–11.
56. Molavi A, LeFrock JL. Antistaphylococcal penicillins. In: Ristuccia AM, Cunha BA, eds. Antimicrobial therapy. New York: Raven Press, 1984:183–92.
57. Marcy SM, Klein JO. The isoxazolyl penicillins: oxacillin, cloxacillin, and dicloxacillin. Med Clin North Am 1970; 54:1127–43.
58. Neu HC. Antimicrobial activity and human pharmacology of amoxicillin. J Infect Dis 1974; 129(suppl):123–31.
59. Rolinson GN. Laboratory evaluation of amoxicillin. Rev Infect Dis 1974; 129(suppl):139–45.
60. Neu HC. Amoxicillin. Ann Intern Med 1979; 90:356–60.
61. Prior RB, Fass RJ. Comparison of ticarcillin and carbenicillin activity against random and select populations of *Pseudomonas aeruginosa*. Antimicrob Agents Chemother 1978; 13:184–7.
62. Kalkani E, Marketos N. Comparative in vitro evaluation of the effects of ticarcillin and carbenicillin upon *Pseudomonas aeruginosa*. Antimicrob Agents Chemother 1976; 9:89–90.
63. Greenwood D, Brook HL, Gargan R, et al. Activity of FL 1060, a new β-lactam antibiotic, against urinary tract pathogens. J Clin Path 1974; 27:192–7.
64. Reeves DS, Wise R, Bywater MJ. A laboratory evaluation of a novel β-lactam antibiotic mecillinam. J Antimicrob Chemother 1975; 1:337–44.

65. Tybring L. Mecillinam (FL 1060), A 6-β-amidinopenicillanic acid derivative; in vitro evaluation. Antimicrob Agents Chemother 1975; 8:266–70.
66. Steinkraus GE, McCarthy LR. In vitro activity of mecillinam against anaerobic bacteria. Antimicrob Agents Chemother 1980; 17:954–6.
67. Anderson JD, Adams MA, Wilson LC, et al. Studies on the effect of mecillinam upon micrococcaceae and faecal streptococci under conditions simulating urinary tract infections. J Antimicrob Chemother 1976; 2:351.
68. Leikola E, Vartia KO. On penicillin levels in young and geriatric subjects. J Gerontol 1956; 11:48–52.
69. Dube AH. A comparison of serum concentrations produced by phenethicillin, penicillin V, and penicillin G after oral and intramuscular administration in geriatric patients. Antibiot Chemother 1961; 11:625–9.
70. Triggs EJ, Johnson JM, Learoyd B. Absorption and disposition of ampicillin in the elderly. Eur J Clin Pharmacol 1980; 18:195–8.
71. Neu HC. The pharmacokinetics of bacampillin. Rev Infect Dis 1981; 3:110–16.
72. Wright AJ, Wilkowske CJ. The penicillins. Mayo Clin Pro 1991; 66:1047–63.
73. Collart P, Poitevin M, Milovanovic A, et al. Kinetic study of serum penicillin concentrations after single doses of benzathine and benethamine penicillins in young and old people. Br J Vener Dis 1980; 56:355–62.
74. Weinstein L, Dalton AC. Host determinants of response to antimicrobial agents. N Engl J Med 1968; 279–524.
75. Bryan CS, Stone WJ. Comparably massive penicillin G therapy in renal failure. Ann Intern Med 1975; 82:189–95.
76. Neftel KA, Walti M, Spengler H, et al. Effect of storage of penicillin-G solutions on sensitization to penicillin-G intravenous administration. Lancet 1982; 1:986–8.
77. Plaut ME, O'Connell CJ, Pabico RC, et al. Penicillin handling in normal and azotemic patients. J Lab Clin Med 1969; 74:12–18.
78. Frimodt-Moller N, Maigaard S, Toothaker RD, et al. Mezlocillin pharmacokinetics after single intravenous doses to patients with varying degrees of renal function. Antimicrob Agents Chemother 1980; 17:599–607.
79. Gundert-Remy U, Weber E. Elimination of azlocillin in patients with biliary T-tube drainage. Eur J Clin Pharmacol 1982; 435–9.
80. Meyers BR, Sabbaj J, Weinstein L. Bacteriological, pharmacological, and clinical studies of carbenicillin. Arch Intern Med 1970; 125:282–6.
81. Meyers BR, Hirschman SZ, Strougo L, et al. Comparative study of piperacillin, ticarcillin, and carbenicillin pharmacokinetics. Antimicrob Agents Chemother 1980; 17:608–611.
82. Parker RH, Schmid FR. Antibacterial activity of synovial fluid during therapy of septic arthritis. Arthritis Rheum 1971; 14:96–104.
83. Barza M, Weinstein L. Penetration of antibiotics into fibrin loci in vivo. I. Comparison of penetration of ampicillin into fibrin clots, abscesses and interstitial fluid. J Infect Dis 1974; 129:59–65.
84. Taryle DA, Good JT Jr, Morgan EJ III, et al. Antibiotic concentrations in human parapneumonic effusions. J Antimicrob Chemother 1981; 7:171–7.
85. Strausbaugh LJ, Murray TW, Sande MA. Comparative penetration of six antibiotics into the cerebrospinal fluid of rabbits with experimental staphylococcal meningitis. J Antimicrob Chemother 1980; 6:363–71.
86. Whelton A, Carter GG, Bryant HH, et al. Carbenicillin concentrations in normal and diseased kidneys. A therapeutic consideration. Ann Intern Med 1973; 78:659–62.
87. Rolinson GN, Sutherland R. The binding of antibiotics to serum proteins. Br J Pharmacol 1965; 25:638–50.
88. Merrikin DJ, Briant J, Rolinson GN. Effect of protein binding on antibiotic activity in vivo. J Antimicrob Chemother 1983; 11:233–8.

89. Lindup WE, Orme MCLE. Clinical pharmacology: plasma protein binding of drugs. Br Med J. 1981; 282:212–14.
90. Acocella G, Mattiussi R, Nichols FB, et al. Biliary excretion of antibiotics in man. Gut 1968; 9:536–45
91. Gibaldi M, Schwartz MA. Apparent effect of probenecid on the distribution of penicillins in man. Clin Pharmacol Ther 1968; 9:345–9.
92. Appel GB, Neu HC. Infections and antibiotic usage in patients with renal diseases. In: Martinez-Maldonado, ed. Handbook of renal therapeutics. New York: Plenum, 1983:227–62.
93. Yoshikawa TT. Physiology of aging: impact on pharmacology. Semin Anesth 1986; 5:8–13.
94. Ljungberg B, Nilsson-Ehle I. Pharmacokinetics of antimicrobial agents in the elderly. Rev Infect Dis 1987; 9:250–64.
95. Yoshikawa TT. Antimicrobial therapy for the elderly patient. J Am Geriatr Soc 1990; 38:1353–72.
96. Feely J, Coakley D. Altered pharmacodynamics in the elderly. Clin Geriatr Med 1990; 6:269–83.
97. Pickering LK, Rutherford I. Effect of concentration and time upon inactivation of tobramycin, gentamicin, netilmicin and amikacin by azlocillin, carbenicillin, mecillinam, mezlocillin and piperacillin. J Pharmacol Exp Ther 1981; 217:345–9.
98. Ervin FR, Bullock WE Jr, Nuttall CE. Inactivation of gentamicin by penicillins in patients with renal failure. Antimicrob Agents Chemother 1976; 9:1004–11.
99. Suh B, Craig WA, England AC, et al. Effect of free fatty acids on protein binding of antimicrobial agents. J Infect Dis 1981; 143:609–16.
100. Norman DC. Pneumonia in the elderly: Empiric antimicrobial therapy. Geriatrics 1991; 46:26–32.
101. Owens RE, Allen DM. Infections in the elderly. Singapore Med J 1991; 32:179–82.
102. Cummings DM, Uttech KM. Antibiotics for common infections in the elderly. Primary Care 1990; 17:883–903.
103. Yoshikawa TT, Norman DC, Grahn D. Infections in the aging population. J Am Geriatr Soc 1985; 496–503.
104. Warren JW, Palumbo FB, Fitterman L, et al. Incidence and characteristics of antibiotic use in aged nursing home patients. J Am Geriatr Soc 1991; 39:963–72.
105. Friedlander AH, Yoshikawa TT. Pathogenesis, management, and prevention of infective endocarditis in the elderly dental patient. Oral Surg Oral Med Oral Pathol 1990; 69:177–81.
106. Finegold SM. Therapy for infections due to anaerobic bacteria: an overview. J Infect Dis 1977; 135(suppl):25–9.
107. Mandell GL, Kaye D, Levison ME, et al. Enterococcal endocarditis. Arch Intern Med 1970; 125:258–64.
108. Kune GA, Burdon JGW. Are antibiotics necessary in acute cholecystitis? Med J Aust 1975; 2:627–30.
109. May JR, Ingold A. Amoxicillin in the treatment of chronic non-tuberculous bronchial infections. Br J Dis Chest 1972; 66:185–91.
110. May JR, Ingold A. Amoxicillin in the treatment of infections of the lower respiratory tract. J Infect Dis 1974; 129(suppl):189–93.
111. Bodey GP, Bolivar R, Fainstein V, et al. Infections caused by *Pseudomonas aeruginosa*. Rev Infect Dis 1983; 5:279–313.
112. Ellis CJ, Geddes AM, Davey PG, et al. Mezlocillin and azlocillin; an evaluation of two new β-lactam antibiotics. J Antimicrob Chemother 1979; 5:517–25.
113. Ellis CJ, Walter PH. *Pseudomonas* meningitis treated with azlocillin. Br Med J 1979; 2:767.
114. Eykyn SJ. Azlocillin in the treatment of serious infection with *Pseudomonas aeruginosa*. J Antimicrob Chemother 1982; 9:395–403.

115. Norden CW, Shaffer M. *In vitro* synergism between mezlocillin and isoxazolyl penicillins against β-lactamase-producing gram-negative organisms. J Antimicrob Chemother 1983; 11:377–80.
116. Wade JC, Schimpff SC, Newman KA, et al. Potential of mezlocillin as empiric single-agent therapy in febrile granulocytopenic cancer patients. Antimicrob Agents Chemother 1980; 18:299–306.
117. Gribble MJ, Chow AW, Naiman SC, et al. Prospective randomized trial of piperacillin monotherapy versus carboxypenicillin-aminoglycoside combination regimens in the empirical treatment of serious bacterial infections. Antimicrob Agents Chemother 1983; 24:388–93.
118. Hughes WT, Armstrong D, Bodey GP, et al. Guidelines for the use of antimicrobial agents in neutropenic patients with unexplained fever. J Infect Dis 1990; 161: 381–96.
119. Baldassarre JS, Kaye D. Special problems of urinary tract infections in the elderly. Med Clin North Am 1991; 75:375–90.
120. Bentzen AJ, Vejlsgaard R, Jacobsen J, et al. Clinical evaluation of a novel β-lactam antibiotic: pivmecillinam (FL 1039). Infection 1975; 3:154–60.
121. Verrier Jones ER, Asscher AW. Treatment of recurrent bacteriuria with pivmecillinam (FL 1039) (1975). J Antimicrob Chemother 1975; 1:193–6.
122. Damsgaard T, Jacobsen J, Korner B, et al. Pivmecillinam and trimethoprim/sulfamethoxazole in the treatment of bacteriuria. J Antimicrob Chemother 1979; 5:267–74.
123. Cox CE. Parenteral amdinocillin for treatment of complicated urinary tract infections. Am J Med 1983; (Amdinocillin symposium):82–4.
124. Guttmann D. A comparison of pivmecillinam and cotrimoxazole in the treatment of simple cystitis in general practice. J Antimicrob Chemother 1977; 3(suppl B):137–40.
125. Granlund M, Landgren E, Henning C. Pivmecillinam in the treatment of *Staphylococcus saprophyticus* urinary tract infections. Scand J Infect Dis 1983; 15:65–9.
126. Pines A, Nandi AR, Raafat H, et al. Pivmecillinam and amoxicillin as combined treatment in purulent exacerbations of chronic bronchitis. J Antimicrob Chemother 1977; 3(suppl B):141–8.
127. Idsoe O, Guthe T, Willcox RR, et al. Nature and extent of penicillin side-reactions, with particular reference to fatalities from anaphylactic shock. Bull WHO 1968; 38:159–88.
128. Idsoe O, Guthe T, Willcox RR. Penicillin in the treatment of syphilis. The experience of three decades. Bull WHO 1972; 47(suppl):1–68.
129. Michel J, Sharon R. Non-haemolytic adverse reactions after transfusion of a blood unit containing penicillin. Br Med J 1980; 280:152–3.
130. Porter J, Jick H. Drug-induced anaphylaxis, convulsions, deafness and extrapyramidal symptoms. Lancet 1977; 1:587–8.
131. Rudolph AH, Price EV. Penicillin reactions among patients in venereal disease clinics: A national survey. JAMA 1973; 223:499–501.
132. Polk IJ. Penicillin allergy skin tests. JAMA 1982; 247:1745.
133. Erffmeyer JE. Penicillin allergy. Clin Rev Allergy 1986; 4:171–88.
134. Petz LD. Immunologic cross-reactivity between penicillins and cephalosporins: a review. J Infect Dis 1978; 137(suppl):74–9.
135. Blanca M. Fernandez J, Miranda A, et al. Cross-reactivity between penicillins and cephalosporins: clinical and immunologic studies. J Allergy Clin Immunol 1989; 83:381–5.
136. Blanca M, Vega JM, Garcia J, et al. Allergy to penicillin with good tolerance to other penicillins; study of the incidence in subjects allergic to β-lactams. Clin Exp Allergy 1990; 20:475–81.
137. Surtees SJ, Stockton MG, Gietzen TW. Allergy to penicillin: fable or fact? Br Med J 1991; 302:1051–2.
138. Lin RY. A perspective on penicillin allergy. Arch Intern Med 1992; 152:930–7.
139. Sogn DD, Evans III R, Shephard GM, et al. Results of the National Institute of Allergy and Infectious Diseases collaborative clinical trial to test the predictive value of skin testing with

major and minor penicillin derivatives in hospitalized adults. Arch Intern Med 1992; 152:1025–32.
140. Gelfand JA, Elin RJ, Berry FW Jr, et al. Endotoxemia associated with the Jarisch-Herxheimer reaction. N Engl J Med 1976; 295:211–13.
141. Friedland JS, Warrell DA. The Jarisch-Herxheimer reaction in leptospirosis: possible pathogenesis and review. Rev Infect Dis 1991; 13:207–10.
142. Baldwin DS, Levine BB, McCluskey RT, et al. Renal failure and interstitial nephritis due to penicillin and methicillin. N Engl J Med 1968; 279:1245–52.
143. Parry MF, Ball WD, Conte JE, et al. Nafcillin nephritis. JAMA 1973; 225:178.
144. Woodroffe, AJ, Thomson NM, Meadows R, et al. Nephropathy associated with methicillin administration. Aust NZ J Med 1974; 4:256–61.
145. Ditlove J, Weidmann P, Bernstein M, et al. Methicillin nephritis. Ann Intern Med 1977; 80:483–91.
146. Galpin JE, Shinaberger JH, Stanley TM, et al. Acute interstitial nephritis due to methicillin. Am J Med 1978; 65:756–65.
147. Barriere SL, Conte Jr JE. Absence of nafcillin-associated nephritis. A prospective analysis of 210 patients. West J Med 1980; 133:472–7.
148. Castot A, Carlier P, Bidault I. The kidney and synthetic penicillins, apropos of 62 cases. Cooperative evaluation of French Drug surveillance centers. Therapie 1988; 43:399–403.
149. Yow MD, Taber LH, Barrett FF, et al. A ten-year assessment of methicillin-associated side-effects. Pediatrics 1976; 58:329–34.
150. Bloomer HA, Barton LJ, Maddock Jr RK. Penicillin-induced encephalopathy in uremic patients. JAMA 1967; 200:131–3.
151. Barrons RW, Murray KM, Richey RM. Populations at risk for penicillin-induced seizures. Ann Pharmacother 1992; 26:26–9.
152. Menke HE, Pepplinkhuizen L. Acute non-allergic reaction to acqueous procaine penicillin. Lancet 1974; 2:723–4.
153. White JM, Brown DL, Hepner GW, et al. Penicillin-induced haemolytic anaemia. Br Med J. 1968; 3:26–9.
154. Kerr RO, Cardamone J, Dalmasso AP, et al. Two mechanisms of erythrocyte destruction in penicillin-induced hemolytic anemia. N Engl J Med 1972; 287:1322–5.
155. Corbett GM, Perry DJ, Shaw TRD. Penicillin-induced leukopenia. N Engl J Med 1982; 307:1642–3.
156. Lang R, Lishner M, Ravid M. Adverse reactions to prolonged treatment with high doses of carbenicillin and ureidopenicillins. Rev Infect Dis 1991; 13:68–72.
157. Markowitz SM, Rothkopf M, Holden FD, et al. Nafcillin-induced agranulocytosis. JAMA 1975; 232:1150–2.
158. Joorabachi B, Kohout E. Apparent penicillin-induced arrest of mature bone marrow elements. Br Med J 1973; 2:26–7.
159. Brown CH III, Natelson EA, Bradshaw MW, et al. Study of the effects of ticarcillin on blood coagulation and platelet function. Antimicrob Agents Chemother 1975; 7:652–7.
160. Fass RJ, Copelan EA, Brandt JT, et al. Platelet-mediated bleeding caused by broad-spectrum penicillins. J Infect Dis 1987; 155:1242–8.
161. Shevchuk YM, Conly JM. Antibiotic-associated hypoprothrombinemia: a review of prospective studies, 1966–1988. Rev Infect Dis 1990; 12:1109–25.
162. Andrassy K, Scherz M, Ritz E, et al. Penicillin-induced coagulation disorder. Lancet 1976; 2:1039–41.
163. Orris DJ, Lewis JH, Spero JA, et al. Blocking coagulation inhibitors in children taking penicillin. J Pediatr 1980; 97:426–9.
164. McCue, JD, Brown RB. Preventing antibiotic-associated bleeding in elderly patients. Adv Ther 1988; 5:283–9.

165. Shapiro S, Slone D, Siskind V, et al. Drug rash with ampicillin and other penicillins. Lancet 1969; 2:969–72.
166. Potter, JPL. Skin reactions to ampicillin. Br Med J 1972; 1:749.
167. Sleet RA, Sangster G, Murdoch JMcC. Comparison of ampicillin and chloramphenicol in treatment of paratyphoid fever. Br Med J 1964; 1:148–50.
168. Kluge RM, Waldman RH, Delafuente JC, et al. Ampicillin-specific antibody and delayed hypersensitivity skin tests to ampicillin in patients with acute infectious mononucleosis. J Infect Dis 1982; 145:397.
169. Nazareth I, Mortimer P, McKendrick GDW. Ampicillin sensitivity in infectious mononucleosis—temporary or permanent? Scand J Infect Dis 1972; 4:229–30.
170. Report of a collaborative study group. Prospective study of ampicillin rash. Br Med J 1973; 1:7–9.
171. Tilden SJ, Craft JC, Cano R, et al. Cutaneous necrosis associated with intravenous nafcillin therapy. Am J Dis Child 1980; 134:1046–8.
172. Wise PJ, Neu HC. Experience with amoxicillin: An overall summary of clinical trials in the United States. J Infect Dis 1974; 129 (suppl):266–71.
173. Knudsen ET. Amoxil and talpen. Br Med J 1977; 1:442–3.
174. Limson BM, Siasoco RF, Dial FP. The effect of combined sodium epicillin injection and orally administered epicillin in the treatment of acute infective illness. Med J Aust 1972; 2:1348–51.
175. Gold JA, Hegarty CP, Deitch MW, et al. Double-blind clinical trails of oral cyclacillin and ampicillin. Antimicrob Agent Chemother 1979; 15:55–8.
176. Neringer R, Stromberg A. A comparison of the side-effects of amoxicillin and pivampicillin. Scand J Infect Dis 1980; 12:133–5.
177. Bartlett JG. Antimicrobial agents implicated in *Clostridium difficile* toxin associated diarrhea or colitis. Johns Hopkins Med J 1981; 149:6–9.
178. Thomas DR, Bennett RG, Laughon BE, et al. Postantibiotic colonization with *Clostridium difficile* in nursing home patients. J Am Geriatr Soc 1990; 38:415–20.
179. Silber TJ, D'Anglo L. Psychosis and seizures following the injection of penicillin G procaine. Am J Dis Child 1985; 139:335–7.

8

Cephalosporins

Jack D. McCue
Baystate Medical Center, Springfield, and Tufts University School of Medicine, Boston, Massachusetts

Edward G. Tessier
Baystate Medical Center, Springfield, and Massachusetts College of Pharmacy and Allied Health Sciences, Boston, Massachusetts

I. INTRODUCTION

The cephalosporins are the most numerous (25 compounds are currently approved for use in the U.S.) and commonly used class of parenteral and oral antimicrobials. They are easy to dose in elderly patients because of their wide margin of safety, and idiosyncratic toxicity is uncommon and reversible. Because the cephalosporin C molecule has been so amenable to chemical manipulation, they are available in remarkably diverse formulations that are active against most important bacterial pathogens.

The major use of the parenteral forms of cephalosporins in geriatric patients is in empiric therapy of undefined but presumed bacterial infection. The safety of cephalosporins and their simplicity of dosing for empiric regimens, however, have often overshadowed their utility as definitive therapy that can avoid more expensive, toxic combination antibiotic regimens. The oral formulations of cephalosporins, by comparison to parenteral forms, yield relatively low serum concentrations and have a relatively limited spectrum of activity. They are useful predominantly in pediatric infections and are not as useful for treating infections in elderly patients as other oral antimicrobials such as trimethoprim-sulfamethoxazole or the fluoroquinolones.

II. CHEMISTRY

The cephalosporins are semisynthetic antibiotics derived from the natural product of the fungus *Cephalosporium acremonium*, cephalosporin C. They share the basic cephalosporin structure (1), which has a β-lactam six-member dihydrothiazine ring, similar to the five-member thiazolidine ring of the penicillin class of antibiotics. Chemical alterations at R1 or position 7 of the β-lactam ring are associated with alterations in antimicrobial activity, and structures added at position 3 (R2) modify pharmacokinetic properties (1). Strictly

Table 1 Parenteral and Oral Cephalosporins

Generic name	U.S. proprietary names
PARENTERAL FORMS	
FIRST GENERATION	
Cefazolin	Ancef, Kefzol
Cephapirin	Cephadyl
Cephradine	Velocef
Cephalothin	Keflin
SECOND GENERATION	
Cefamandole	Mandol
Cefmetazole	Zefazone
Cefonicid	Monocid
Ceforanide	Precef
Cefotetan	Cefotan
Cefoxitin	Mefoxin
Cefuroxime	Kefurox, Zinacef
THIRD GENERATION	
Cefoperazone	Cefobid
Cefotaxime	Claforan
Ceftazidime	Fortaz, Tazicef, Tazidime
Ceftizoxime	Cefizox
Ceftriaxone	Rocephin
Moxalactam	Moxam
ORAL FORMS	
FIRST GENERATION	
Cefadroxil	Duricef, Ultracef
Cephalexin	Keflex
Cephapirin	Cefadyl
Cephradine	Anspor, Velocef
SECOND GENERATION	
Cefprozil	Cefzil
Cefuroxime axetil	Ceftin
Loracarbef (carbacephem)	Lorabid
Cefaclor	Ceclor®
THIRD GENERATION	
Cefixime	Suprax
Cefpodoxime	Vantin

speaking, cefoxitin, cefmetazole, and cefotetan are cephamycins, created from a parent compound derived from a *Streptomyces* species; moxalactam is totally a synthetic oxa-β-lactam and is not, therefore, a cephalosporin. The similarity of the cephamycins and moxalactam to cephalosporins, however, has led clinicians to consider them as a single group.

Table 1 lists the parenteral and oral cephalosporins currently available in the United States and Canada by generation. First-generation cephalosporins are active against methicillin-sensitive staphylococci and streptococci, but are susceptible to hydrolysis by many β-lactamases produced by gram-negative bacteria and therefore have relatively limited activity against gram-negative bacilli. Second-generation cephalosporins are more resistant to β-lactamases and have broader activity that includes Enterobacteriaceae and respiratory gram-negative bacilli, *Neisseria* spp., and variable anaerobic activity, including activity of some drugs against *Bacteroides fragilis*. The third-generation cephalosporins have variable activity against staphylococci and anaerobic bacteria, but because they are resistant to β-lactamase hydrolysis, have considerably enhanced activity against streptococci and gram-negative bacilli, including in some cases activity against antibiotic-resistant organisms such as *Pseudomonas aeruginosa* (2).

III. MECHANISM OF ACTION

Cephalosporins bind to and inactivate specific bacterial targets called penicillin-binding proteins (PBPs), which are enzymes located on the inner aspect of the bacterial cell membrane. The various cephalosporins bind to or inactivate different PBPs and have dissimilar affinities for the PBPs that they do bind, thus accounting for their different in vitro activity against various bacterial species. Some PBPs are essential to survival of the bacterium, so that inactivation will lead to cell lysis; other PBPs are not essential, and binding leads to nonlethal changes, inhibition of growth, or distorted shapes (3). Nonlethal changes may also affect bacterial virulence, may lead to a phenomenon called "tolerance" in which bacteria (inhibited but not killed by antibiotic) survive in altered forms that may or may not be virulent, or may be indirectly beneficial by enhancing phagocytosis.

Because cephalosporins vary greatly in how they manifest bactericidal and bacteriostatic activity by binding different PBPs, arguments for the use of combination β-lactam antibiotics for synergistic effect have been advanced in some circumstances (4).

Cephalosporin resistance may occur by three mechanisms (5). Gram-negative bacteria have an outer cell wall that includes a lipopolysaccharide and lipoprotein membrane exterior to the peptidoglycan layer that resists penetration of antibiotic, which is true for *P. aeruginosa* or *Enterobacter cloacae*. Cephalosporins must penetrate the membrane through channels called porins, and success of penetration depends on their relative size, charge, and hydrophilic properties (6). Second, PBPs may become altered after exposure of a bacterial species to an antibiotic, leading to lowering of binding affinity, which occurs with methicillin-resistant *S. aureus* (MRSA) (7). Third, the bacterium may produce enzymes called β-lactamases that bind to or destroy the cephalosporin molecule by hydrolyzing the β-lactam ring, which may be true of organisms such as *Serratia marcescens* or *Citrobacter* spp. (3). There are many β-lactamases—some are located on chromosomes, some on plasmids, and some are inducible; β-lactamases produced by gram-positive bacteria are excreted extracellularly, but gram-negative bacteria retain their β-lactamases in the periplasmic space between the cytoplasmic and outer membranes, a strategic location to cleave the β-lactam ring before the cephalosporin can reach the PBPs (8).

Despite concern that the widespread use of broad-spectrum cephalosporins would lead to increased resistance of common pathogens, development of resistance to second- or third-generation cephalosporins has been largely confined to special environments such as intensive care or burn units or "problem" organisms such as *P. aeruginosa* or *Enterobacter cloacae*. Strains of *Enterobacter* and *Klebsiella* spp. with plasmid-mediated β-lactamase production that hydrolyze third-generation cephalosporins have raised concern, however, that greater resistance of Enterobacteriaceae to cephalosporins will emerge in the future (9).

Table 2 Bacteria Against Which Cephalosporins Have Little or No Reliable Activity

Methicillin-resistant *Staphylococcus aureus*
Methicillin-resistant *Staphylococcus epidermidis*
Enterococcus faecalis
Penicillin-resistant Streptococcus pneumoniae
Corynebacterium jekeium
Listeria monocytogenes
Legionella pneumophila and *L. micdadei*
Clostridium difficile
Xanthomonas maltophila
Pseudomonas putida and *P. cepacia*
Acinetobacter calcoaceticus
Campylobacter jejuni

IV. ANTIMICROBIAL SPECTRUM

While the various cephalosporins have activity against most of the bacterial pathogens encountered in clinical infectious diseases including geriatric practice, there are some bacteria against which these drugs, as a class, do not have reliable activity (Table 2). In addition, they are not reliably active against intracellular pathogens such as chlamydia, mycoplasma, or ureaplasma—organisms not commonly isolated from infected elderly patients. Although some cephalosporins have some antimycobacterial activity, they are inactive against *Mycobacterium tuberculosis*. They are not active against fungi or viruses.

Table 3 Typical In Vitro Antibacterial Activity of Selected Parenteral Cephalosporins

Bacteria	Cefazolin	Cefoxitin	Cefuroxime	Cefoperazone	Ceftriaxone	Ceftazidime
S. aureus	0.5	3.1	1.4	4	4	16
S. epidermidis	0.5	12.5	1.0	8	16	32
S. pneumoniae	0.12	0.5	0.12	0.25	0.03	0.25
E. coli	5	8	4	2	0.1	0.5
K. pneumoniae	6	5	4	4	0.1	0.5
E. cloacae	>100	>100	>100	8	16	16
S. marcescens	>100	>100	>100	16	4	1
P. aeruginosa	>100	>100	>100	32	>32	32
Indole + *Proteus*	>100	>100	>100	4	0.12	0.12
Proteus mirabilis	4	5	3	0.5	0.01	0.06
H. influenzae	10	6	2	0.06	0.1	0.1
B. fragilis	>100	16	>100	>64	>64	>64

MIC 90 in μg/ml.
Source: Adapted from Refs. 2, 86.

Table 4 Typical In Vitro Antibacterial Activity of Selected Oral Cephalosporins

Bacteria	Cephalexin	Cefaclor	Cefprozil	Cefuroxime	Cefpodoxime	Cefixime
S. aureus	2	2	1	1	4	16
S. pneumoniae	4	4	0.25	0.25	0.06	0.25
E. coli	16	8	8	4	1	0.12
K. pneumoniae	16	8	4	4	0.25	0.12
Proteus mirabilis	16	2	1	0.5	0.12	0.06
H. influenzae	8	4	4	0.25	0.12	0.06
M. catarrhalis	4	2	4	0.25	0.12	0.25

MIC 90 in μg/ml.
Source: Adapted from Refs. 86–90.

Tables 3 and 4 summarize the antimicrobial activity of selected parenteral and oral cephalosporins against common pathogens found in infections of older patients (5,9,10).

A. Gram-Positive Bacteria

First- and some second-generation cephalosporins—cefuroxime and cefamandole—have good to excellent activity against methicillin-sensitive *S. aureus* and *S. epidermidis*. Other second-generation cephalosporins have less activity, with cefotetan having the least. The third-generation cephalosporins vary widely: cefotaxime has the greatest in vitro activity, ceftriaxone and cefoperazone are intermediate, and ceftazidime has the least antistaphylococcal activity. All the cephalosporins are active against streptococcal species (excluding enterococci, now renamed *Enterococcus* spp.), with the third-generation compounds having the greatest activity. Steptococcal species, *Enterococcus* spp., and staphylococci are important pathogens in the geriatric population.

B. Gram-Negative Bacteria

Most community-acquired strains of *E. coli*, *P. mirabilis*, *Klebsiella* spp., and *Citrobacter diversus* that infect older patients are sensitive to first-generation cephalosporins. Because of the potential for β-lactamase production, they are not reliably active against *Haemophilus*, *Neisseria*, or *Moraxella* organisms; second- and third-generation cephalosporins are, however, active against these clinically important bacteria. Second-generation cephalosporins, in addition to greater activity against community-acquired strains of *E. coli*, *P. mirabilis*, *Klebsiella* spp., and *Citrobacter diversus*, have variable activity against nursing home– and hospital-acquired strains, as well as variable activity against *P. vulgaris*, *Morganella* spp., *S. marcescens*, *E. aerogenes*, and *Providencia* spp. Cefotetan has the greatest in vitro gram-negative activity among the second-generation cephalosporins.

Except for unusual hospital-acquired strains and some strains of *E. cloacae* and *C. freundii*, Enterobacteriaceae are usually sensitive to third-generation cephalosporins; resistance of nursing home–acquired Enterobacteriaceae to these drugs would be very unusual. Only cefoperazone and ceftazidime are active in vitro against *P. aeruginosa*; however, most clinicians prefer ceftazidime for treatment of *P. aeruginosa* tissue infections in both young and older patients, often in combination with another antipseudomonal drug.

Table 5 Pharmacokinetics of Oral Cephalosporins

Agent	Beta elimination $t_{\frac{1}{2}}$ (h) Norm	ESRD	>60 y	Plasma protein bound (%)	Excretion (%)	Typical adult dose range
FIRST GENERATION						
Cephalexin	0.5–1	20–40	[c]	15	R (90–96)	250–500 mg q 6 h
Cephradine	0.7–2.0	6–15	1.7	10	R (100)	250–500 mg q 8 h
Cefedroxil	1.1–2.1	20–25	4.3–10.5[d]	20	R (70–90)	500 mg–1 g q 12 h
SECOND GENERATION						
Cefuroxime axetil	1.0–2.0	17	[c]	33	R (90–100) (Cefuroxime)	250–500 mg q 12 h
Cefaclor	0.5–1	3	[c]	25	R (70–90%)	250–500 mg q 8 h
THIRD GENERATION						
Cefixime	2.4–4.0	12	3.9–4.2	35–70	R(40) H(50–60)	400 mg q 24 h
Cefpodoxime	2.5–2.7	7.7	3.1–3.7	20	R(80)	200 mg q 12 h

[a]Dose adjustment (method); D = dose (% normal dose), I = interval (h).
[b]Assumes typical 50-kg 80-year-old female with CrCl = 50 ml/min.
[c]No published studies.
[d]Includes patients with CrCl < 10 ml/min.
Norm = normal renal function; ESRD = end stage renal disease; UTI = urinary tract infection; R = renal; H = hepatobiliary.
Source: Adapted from Refs. 24, 91, 92.

C. Anaerobes

A variety of anaerobic bacteria cause in elderly patients such serious infections as aspiration pneumonia, intraabdominal sepsis (e.g., diverticulitis), skin and soft tissue infections (e.g., infected pressure ulcers), and brain abscess. Activity against anaerobic bacteria does not follow the generation classification. All cephalosporins except ceftazidime are active against the usual anaerobic pathogens (*Peptococcus* spp., *Peptostreptococcus* spp., *Fusobacterium* spp., nonfragilis *Bacteroides* spp., and nondifficile *Clostridium* spp.). Activity against *B. fragilis* is variable, with the cephamycins—cefoxitin, cefotetan, and cefmetazole—having the greatest activity.

V. CLINICAL PHARMACOLOGY

A. Pharmacokinetics

1. Absorption

The orally administered cephalosporins (cephalexin, cephradine, cefadroxil, cefuroxime axetil, cefaclor, and cefixime) are relatively well absorbed (11). Utility of the orally administered agents, however, is still limited by gastrointestinal intolerance of higher

Dose adjust for renal dysfunction[a]	creatinine clearance (CrCl) (ml/min)			Typical frail elderly[b]		Addt'l
Method	>50	10–50	<10	doses	Comment	ref.
I	6	6–8	12–24[a]	Same	Usual dose to treat UTI, give before meals	
I	6	6–8	12	Same		12
D	100	50	25			
I	12	12–24	24–48	Same	Give with meals	14
I	12	12	(?24)	Same	↓Absorption with reduced gastric acidity ↑Absorption after meals	17
I	8	8–12	12–24	Same	Give before meals	
D	100	50–100	33–50			
I	24	24	48	Same	Not affected by food	13, 93
I	12	12–24	24	Same	↑Absorption with meals	15, 16, 94

doses, resulting in relatively lower serum levels compared to parenterally administered cephalosporins.

The rate and extent of absorption of oral cephalosporins in elderly persons has not been well studied, but there appears to be little difference in oral absorption: the bioavailability and time to peak serum levels of oral cephradine is virtually identical in young and older patients (12). Peak cefixime levels are similar in young and elderly patients, with older patients achieving peak levels slightly later than younger counterparts (13). Peak cefadroxil and cefpodoxime levels appear higher and later in older patients compared to younger patients (14–16); this may be caused by impaired renal function in older patients, resulting in reduced elimination during the absorption phase. While cefuroxime axetil absorption is impaired with reduced gastric acidity (17), the clinical significance of this finding in older patients, who may have achlorhydria, is not clear.

Intramuscular (IM) administration is often the only parenteral route of administration readily accessible for many older patients. The rate of IM absorption is slower and the peak concentration is lower for older patients compared to younger patients for a number of drugs (18,19) including cefoxitin (20) and cefuroxime (21). This delay in absorption may be related to reduced regional blood flow due to reduced physical activity in elderly persons (18,19).

Intraperitoneal absorption of cephalosporins is efficient; this mode of administration may be useful in older patients undergoing peritoneal dialysis (22).

2. *Distribution*

Antimicrobial agents with minimal protein binding usually have greater tissue penetration than highly protein-bound agents (23). With few exceptions, cephalosporins are not significantly protein bound and are distributed well in many tissues, penetrating into pleural

Table 6 Pharmacokinetics of First-Generation Parenteral Cephalosporins

Agent	Beta elimination $t_{\frac{1}{2}}$ (h) Norm	ESRD	>60 y	Plasma protein bound (%)	Excretion (%)	Typical adult dose range
Cefazolin	1.2–2.2	40–70	3.5–4.8	80	R(90–96)	500 mg–1 g q 8 h IM, IV
Cephapirin	0.4–0.8	2.4–2.7	c	45–60	R(50)	500 mg–2 g q 4–6 h IM, IV
Cephradine	0.7–2.0	6–15	1.7	10	R(100)	500 mg–2 g q 6 h IM, IV
Cephalothin	0.5–1	3–18	c	65	R(60–90) H(10–40)	500 mg–2 g q 4–6 h IM, IV

[a]Dose adjustment (method): D = dose (% normal dose), I = interval (h).
[b]Assumes typical 50-kg 80-year-old female with CrCl = 50 ml/min.
[c]No published studies.
Norm = normal renal function; ESRD = end stage renal disease; UTI = urinary tract infection; R = renal; H = hepatobiliary
Source: Adapted from Refs. 24, 91, 92.

fluid, ascites, synovial fluid, aqueous humor, and bone (24–29). Adequate distribution into bile and cerebrospinal fluid (CSF) is limited for most cephalosporins: cefoperazone, ceftriaxone, and cefixime achieve high concentrations in the bile (30,31); with inflamed meninges, parenteral administration of third-generation agents (except cefoperazone) may give adequate CSF concentrations for the treatment of some types of meningitis (2,3).

Albumin and other plasma protein levels are often reduced in older patients (32) giving the potential for decreased protein binding or increased "free" or unbound drug. Antibiotics with a low degree of protein binding are excreted more quickly, because a greater amount of unbound drug is available not only for distribution to tissue sites, but for renal or hepatic elimination as well. Increased excretion, however, is usually counterbalanced by reduced renal drug elimination in most older patients (33–35). As noted in Tables 5–8, most drugs with minimal protein binding have increased clearance, as demonstrated by fairly short β-elimination half-lives, but their half-lives are generally increased in older patients and in patients with end-stage renal disease. The net result for older patients is often a positive one, i.e., prolonged, elevated unbound drug levels are available for improved tissue penetration (18). It is unlikely that elevated free levels predispose to greater risk of adverse effects.

The more highly protein bound cephalosporins (those with greater than 85% protein binding) include cefonicid, cefotetan, cefoperazone, and ceftriaxone. The protein binding of ceftriaxone is concentration-dependent, in which higher concentrations yield an increase in the percentage of unbound drug. Even for the highly protein-bound ceftriaxone, however, older patients have an increase in relative unbound drug compared to their younger counterparts (36).

Dose adjust for renal dysfunction[a]						
	CrCl(ml/min):					
Method	>50	10–50	<10	Typical frail elderly doses[b]	Comment	Addt'l ref.
I	8	12	24–48[a]	1 g q 8–12 h	Ineffective for UTI if CrCl <10 ml/min May falsely raise creatinine by interference with assay	95
I	6	6–8	12	1 g q 6–8 h		
I	6	6–8	12	1 g q 6–8 h		12
D	100	50	25			
I	6	6–8	12	1 g q 6 h	Seizure risk with high doses. May falsely raise creatinine by interference with assay. ↑Local irritation or thrombophlebitis after injection.	

3. *Elimination*

Most cephalosporins are eliminated renally by glomerular filtration and/or tubular secretion. Elimination half-lives vary, but generally are prolonged in older patients due to reduction in renal clearance (37). Many studies of the pharmacokinetics of cephalosporins in older patients have been conducted exclusively in patients under the age of 80 (13,15,38,39) or have not stratified the elderly populations by age (15,20,40–42), and have often revealed only modest reductions in cephalosporin clearance. Studies examining pharmacokinetic parameters in patients over 80 years of age often reveal a more significant deterioration in clearance of drug (36,43–45). Whether deterioration in renal function in frail elderly persons can fully explain this phenomenon or whether other factors are involved, however, is not clear. For most cephalosporins, a reduction in dosage or increase in interval between doses is generally recommended for very old patients (over 80 years) and in patients with reduced renal function.

B. Pharmacodynamics

Unlike some antimicrobials such as the fluoroquinolones, the rate and extent of bactericidal activity of the cephalosporins is not concentration-dependent, i.e., bactericidal activity does not increase in rapidity or extent with increasing concentrations of antibiotic, an observation that has clinical relevance to dosing recommendations. There is a postantibiotic inhibitory effect on gram-positive cocci for about 2 h (in which the effect of the cephalosporin on bacteria persists after the antibiotic has been removed), but little or no such effect is seen with gram-negative bacilli (46).

C. Drug-Drug Interactions

Cephalosporins have remarkably few significant drug interactions. This is particularly relevant because elderly patients are frequently taking several medications. A disulfiramlike reaction consisting of weakness, headache, nausea, vomiting, and flushing has

Table 7 Pharmacokinetics of Second-Generation Parenteral Cephalosporins

	Beta elimination $t_{\frac{1}{2}}$ (h)			Plasma protein bound	Excretion	Typical adult dose
Agent	Norm	ESRD	>60 y	(%)	(%)	range
Cefamandole	0.5–2.1	11	[c]	75	R(100)	500 mg–1 g q 4–6 h IM, IV
Cefmetazole	0.8–1.5	24	1.5	65	R(80)	1 g q 6–8 h IV
Cefonicid	3.5–5.8	17–56	9.6	96 (concentration dependent)	R(90–99) t	1 g q 24 h IM, IV
Ceforanide	2.2–3.3	25	[c]	80	R(85–90) t/g	500 mg–1 g q 12 h IM, IV
Cefotetan	2.8–4.6	13–25	[c]	85	R(75) g/t H(20)	1–2 g q 12 h IM, IV
Cefoxitin	0.6–1.1	13–23	1.3	41–75	R(77–90) g/t	1–2 g q 6–8 h IM, IV
Cefuroxime	1.0–2.0	17	2.0–2.7	33	R(90–100) g/t	750 mg–1.5 g q 8 h IM, IV

[a]Dose adjustment (method): D = dose (% normal dose), I = interval (h)
[b]Assumes typical 50-kg 80-year-old female with CrCl = 50 ml/min.
[c]No published studies.
Norm = normal renal function; ESRD = end stage renal disease; R = renal (%); t = tubular secretion; g = glomerular filtration; H = hepatobiliary.
Source: Adapted from Refs. 24, 91, 92.

been noted when agents with the *N*-methylthiotetrazole (NMTT) side chain (moxalactam, cefoperazone, cefotetan, and cefamandole) are administered to patients with recent alcohol ingestion, or when alcohol is ingested up to 24 h after a dose of antibiotic. Concurrent use of anticoagulants in older patients receiving these same agents may significantly increase the risk for bleeding diathesis (see Sec. VIII). Concurrent use of cephalothin and aminoglycosides reportedly resulted in additive nephrotoxicity (47). Use of furosemide with cephaloridine (no longer available in the United States) has been associated with nephrotoxicity (47), but increased risk of furosemide use and other cephalosporins has not been demonstrated. Probenecid increases serum levels of most cephalosporins eliminated by tubular secretion (Tables 7 and 8). Finally, agents increasing gastric pH (H_2 antagonists, omeprazole, antacids) may result in reduced absorption of orally administered cefuroxime axetil (17).

D. Drug-Laboratory Interactions

High concentrations of some cephalosporins (including cefoxitin, cephalothin, cefamandole, cefazolin) may variably but falsely elevate serum or urine creatinine levels when specific analytic methods utilizing the Jaffé reaction or alkaline picrate are employed (48,49). Because serum creatinine in elderly persons does not always accurately reflect renal function, caution should be exercised when interpreting the serum creatinine results

Dose adjust for renal dysfunction[a]						
	CrCl (ml/min)					
Method	>50	10–50	<10	Typical frail elderly doses[b]	Comment	Addt'l ref.
I	6	6–8	12	1 g q 6–8 h	May falsely elevate creatinine by interference with assay	
I	6–8	12	24	1 g q 8–12 h		39,85,96
I	24	24–72	72–120	500 mg–1 g q 24 h		97
D	50	10–50	5–20			
I	12	24–48	48–72	1 g q 12–24 h		
I	12	12–24	48	1 g q 12 h	Active metabolite in ESRD	98
D	100	50	25			
I	8	8–12	24–48	1 g q 8–12 h	Active metabolite in ESRD May falsely elevate creatinine by interference with assay.	20
I	8	8–12	24	750 mg q 8 h		21,40

in such patients who are receiving these cephalosporins. Cefotaxime has increased serum glucose, albumin, electrolyte (calcium, magnesium, phosphate, potassium, sodium), creatine kinase, iron, and iron saturation results in laboratories utilizing the Parallel method (48). Cephalexin has resulted in false-positive urine glucose testing utilizing the Benedict's, Fehling's, and Clinitest® methods (48). Cephalothin and cephaloridine increase urine 17-ketogenic steroid levels (48).

VI. CLINICAL INDICATIONS

The third-generation and to a lesser degree the second-generation cephalosporins are useful empiric agents in the types of common infections that afflict debilitated elderly patients, e.g., lower respiratory, complicated urinary tract, and skin/soft tissue infections (37,50–56).

A. Parenteral First-Generation Cephalosporins

The spectrum of activity of the first-generation cephalosporins limits their usefulness in the treatment of infections in elderly patients. Cefazolin is an appropriate alternative to penicillin or penicillinase-resistant penicillins, such as nafcillin for the treatment of older patients with gram-positive coccal infections, and may offer advantages over penicillins because of less frequent dosing and lower toxicity. Although cefazolin is active against the majority of Enterobacteriaceae that cause urinary tract infections (UTIs), it should not be used empirically as a single agent for serious UTIs, whether community-acquired or institutionally acquired, because at least 30% of *E. coli* and other urinary pathogens are resistant to first-generation cephalosporins in most settings. Similarly, because it is not

Table 8 Pharmacokinetics of Third-Generation Parenteral Cephalosporins

Agent	Beta elimination $t_{\frac{1}{2}}$ (h)					Plasma protein bound (%)	Excretion
	Norm	ESRD	>60 y[a]	60–80 y	>80 y		
Cefoperazone	1.3–2.6	2.1–2.9	2.1	2.1–10.3	[d]	90	H(75–80) R(20) g/t
Cefotaxime	0.8–1.7	2.6–15	1.2–2.9	1.2–2.0	2.3–2.6	37	R(50–60) t/?g H(40)
desacetyl-cefotaxime	1.4–1.9	8.2–57					
Ceftazidime	1.2–2	13–25	2.9–3.1	2.6–3.7	3.5–3.9	17	R(60–90) g
Ceftriaxone	5.4–10.9	12–24	[d]	Age 60–70: 7.4 Age 70–80: 11.2	14.2	85–95 (concentration dependent)	R(30–65) g H(30–65)
Ceftizoxime	1.3–1.9	[d]	2.2	3.5	[d]	30	R(60–92) g/t
Moxalactam	2.0–3.5	18–23	[d]	[d]	[d]	35–50	R(61–97) g

[a]Data not stratified beyond age > 60–65.
[b]Dose adjustment (method): D = dose (% normal dose), I = interval (h).
[c]Assumes typical 50-kg 80-year-old female with CrCl = 50 ml/min.
[d]No published studies.
Norm = normal renal function; ESRD = end stage renal disease; R = renal (%); g = glomerular filtration; t = tubular secretion; H = hepatobiliary.
Source: Adapted from Refs. 24, 91, 92.

reliably active against *H. influenzae* and *M. catarrhalis*, two major respiratory pathogens in elderly patients, it should not be used for empiric therapy for presumed bacterial bronchitis or pneumonia. Cefazolin remains the preferred antibiotic for surgical prophylaxis, to reduce the frequency of postoperative infection; other cephalosporins may have similar efficacy but usually at a greater cost.

In summary, the major uses of cefazolin for geriatric patients are for defined bacterial infections in which the pathogen is known with reasonable certainty to be sensitive to first-generation cephalosporins and for surgical prophylaxis (57). Its role as an empiric agent is limited to use as an alternative to penicillin, ampicillin, or nafcillin. Other first-generation cephalosporins have shorter half-lives than cefazolin and offer no compensating advantages.

B. Oral First-Generation Cephalosporins

There are no clinically important differences among these drugs. They are more limited in usefulness in elderly patients than parenteral first-generation cephalosporins because

Typical adult dose range	Dose adjust for renal dysfunction[b] Method	CrCl (ml/min): >50	10–50	<10	Typical frail elderly doses[c]	Comment	Additional ref.
1–2 g q 12 h IM, IV	I	12	12	12	1 g q 12 h	Bleeding due to hypo-prothrombinernia. Good penetration into bile. In hepato-billary disease, renal excretion up to 90%.	30, 37, 99, 100–102
1–2 g q 6–8 h IV	I	6–8	8–12	24	1–2 g q 12 h		37, 41,43, 103, 104
						Active metabolite. Accumulates in ESRD, patients > 80.	
1–2 g q 8–12 h IM, IV	I	8–12	24	48	1–2 g q 12 h		37, 38, 42, 44, 67, 105, 106
1–2 g q 24 h IM, IV	I	24	24	24	500 mg–1 g q 24 h	Good penetration into bile. Add 1% lidocaine for IM injection.	30, 36, 37, 45, 107, 108
1–2 g q 8–12 h IM, IV	I	8–12	12	24–48	1 g q 8–12 h		37, 102
500 mg–2 g q 8 –12 h IM, IV	I	8	12–24	12–48	1 g q 12 h	Significant risk of bleeding due to hypoprothrombinemia.	

of their relative lack of activity against gram-negative bacilli and low serum concentrations after oral administration of tolerable doses. Their major indications in older patients are for the treatment of upper respiratory or skin/soft tissue infections in which penicillin, amoxicillin, or dicloxacillin cannot be used. They should not be used for empiric therapy of serious infections, especially in elderly patients in whom infections tend to be polymicrobial and involve a broad range of pathogens. Because they are excreted renally, they achieve adequate urinary levels for the treatment of UTIs caused by sensitive bacteria; they give, however, lower cure rates in the treatment of complicated UTI than trimethoprim-sulfamethoxazole or quinolones.

In summary, oral first-generation cephalosporins are relatively expensive, overused antibiotics that have limited utility for geriatric patients. They should be primarily viewed as alternatives to penicillin, amoxicillin, or dicloxacillin for penicillin-allergic patients, or second-line agents in the treatment of UTI.

C. Parenteral Second-Generation Cephalosporins

Because of their broader spectrum of activity, cefuroxime or cefoxitin are useful as empiric therapy for community-acquired or nursing home–acquired infections—in which the antibiotic-resistant bacteria that cause hospital-acquired infections are unlikely to be present—such as UTI, lower respiratory infections, and skin/soft tissue infections. Cefuroxime has activity against gram-positive cocci that approaches that of the first-generation agents.

Cefoxitin and cefotetan are, in addition, active against *B. fragilis* and are therefore useful in the treatment of abdominal infections; they have less activity against gram-positive cocci, however, and cefotetan has marginal antistaphylococcal activity, similar to ceftazidime. Cefotetan has a longer half-life and somewhat better activity against gram-negative bacilli than cefoxitin and may offer cost and administration advantages that offset its in vitro differences in activity against staphylococci.

In summary, second-generation cephalosporins are reasonable choices for empiric treatment of common community-acquired or nursing home–acquired infections of the elderly patients, and cefoxitin or cefotetan have a special role in the treatment of mixed anaerobic-aerobic infections such as abdominal or complicated skin/soft tissue infections. Their indications overlap considerably those of the third-generation cephalosporins, and they offer no consistent cost advantages.

D. Oral Second-Generation Cephalosporins

The relatively poor absorption (30–50%) of the axetil of cefuroxime, which is metabolized to cefuroxime after absorption, results in relatively low serum concentrations and tissue concentrations. It cannot, therefore, be viewed as equivalent to the parenteral form and should not be used as empiric therapy for most serious infections in elderly patients. Because cefuroxime is concentrated in the urine, it is a reasonable second-line agent for the treatment of UTI. It is an option for the treatment of mild to moderate respiratory or skin/soft tissue infections in which nosocomial pathogens or *B. fragilis* is not a likely pathogen.

In summary, cefuroxime axetil is not a first-line choice for moderate to severe infections, but may have limited usefulness in penicillin-allergic older patients in the treatment of some respiratory, urinary tract, or skin/soft tissue infections. When they can be used, amoxicillin-clavulanate, quinolones, or trimethoprim-sulfamethoxazole are preferable options. Cefaclor, loracarbef, and cefprozil offer no advantages over cefuroxime. Loracarbef, a carbacephem, has in vitro antibacterial activity similar to that of cefaclor or cefprozil and an elimination half-life of about 1.2 h in young adults, slightly longer than that of cefaclor.

E. Parenteral Third-Generation Cephalosporins

Although third-generation cephalosporins are less active against staphylococci than first- or second-generation cephalosporins, with the exception of ceftazidime they provide adequate empiric coverage against *S. aureus* in suspected sepsis (9). Third-generation cephalosporins are highly active against respiratory pathogens such as ampicillin-resistant *H. influenzae* or *M. catarrhalis*. They are highly active against all community-acquired Enterobacteriaceae, including nursing home strains; hospital-acquired strains of Enterobacteriaceae, however, may be resistant. Unlike other cephalosporins, cefoperazone and ceftazidime have in vitro activity against *P. aeruginosa*; however, serious pseudomonas tissue infections are usually treated in combination with an aminoglycoside or aztreonam.

In addition to the advantage of breadth of spectrum, the third-generation cephalosporins have some clinical uses conferred by their greater in vitro activity against gram-negative organisms. For example, central nervous system infections, ophthalmic infections, and cardiac infections caused by susceptible gram-negative bacteria, which might otherwise require multiple-drug therapy or the use of more toxic antibiotics, may be successfully treated with a third-generation cephalosporin. Ceftriaxone is the drug of choice for treatment of the central nervous system complications of Lyme disease (58).

Cefotaxime and ceftizoxime have similar antimicrobial activity to ceftriaxone, but shorter half-lives, necessitating more frequent dosing. Moxalactam is rarely used because of its toxicity.

A major unresolved, and perhaps unresolvable, issue that arises in discussions of third-generation cephalosporins is whether physicians should use narrower-spectrum cephalosporins, e.g., a second-generation drug such as cefuroxime rather than a third-generation cephalosporin such as ceftriaxone, for empiric therapy of community- or nursing home–acquired infections. This approach sacrifices probably unnecessary breadth of coverage in the hope that the pressure for emergence of resistant organisms within the nursing home or hospital will be less. It is certain that no simple answer to this question is possible, however, and physicians should also consider cost, frequency of dosing, and the possibility that elderly patients are more often infected with multiple pathogens or antibiotic-resistant bacteria when choosing a cephalosporin for empiric or definitive therapy.

F. Oral Third-Generation Cephalosporins

In vitro activity of cefixime against Enterobacteriaceae is similar to parenteral third-generation cephalosporins and exceeds that of other oral cephalosporins. There is no activity against *P. aeruginosa*, *Enterobacter* spp., or *Acinetobacter calcoaceticus*, however. Atypically for oral cephalosporins, cefixime has no activity against staphylococci. It may be useful as a broad-spectrum alternative to quinolones or amoxicillin-clavulanate for empiric oral therapy for UTI or respiratory infection in elderly patients.

Being intermediate between antibacterial activity typical for second- and third-generation cephalosporins, cefpodoxime is less active than cefixime against gram-negative bacilli, but it is more active against gram-positive cocci. Its half-life is shorter than cefixime.

G. Specific Clinical Indications

The waggish comment that cephalosporins are alternative drugs for most infections but are the drugs of first choice for none ignores their utility in the types of circumstances encountered specifically and commonly in the debilitated elderly patient—atypical clinical presentations, poor or no culture data, ill-defined clinical syndromes, susceptibility to nephrotoxicity or neurotoxicity from drugs such as vancomycin or the aminoglycosides, and polymicrobial infection and colonization. Table 9 illustrates the wide range of infections in geriatric patients in which cephalosporins may be *reasonably* used as empiric or definitive therapy; therapy must, of course, be individualized, and there are many alternatives to cephalosporin therapy that are less expensive and equally safe.

1. UTI

Oral cephalosporins—except for cefixime, cefpodoxime, and cefuroxime axetil—are not ideal UTI drugs even for community-acquired urinary infections. In general, trimethoprim-sulfamethoxazole and the systemic quinolones offer comparable empiric coverage for complicated infections and probably superior cure rates. Similarly, parenteral second- or third-generation cephalosporins are reasonable choices for seriously ill elderly patients with UTI, although parenteral therapy is uncommonly needed once the septic phase of UTI is stabilized, since most oral antibiotics that might be considered for therapy are highly concentrated in urine.

2. Respiratory Infections

Second- or third-generation cephalosporins are the cornerstone of empiric therapy of the elderly patient with bacterial bronchitis or pneumonia. The majority of these patients do

Table 9 Infections in Elderly Patients in Which Cephalosporins May Be Indicated

Infections	Community-acquired	Nursing home–acquired	Hospital-acquired
Febrile urinary tract infection	Oral second/third	Oral third	Cefoperazone/ Ceftazidime[a]
Febrile lower respiratory infection	Oral third or parenteral second/third	Parenteral second/third	Cefoperazone/ Ceftazidime[a]
Simple skin/soft tissue infection	Oral/parenteral first	Oral/parenteral first	Oral/parenteral first
Complicated skin/soft tissue infection	Parenteral second	Parenteral second/third	Parenteral second/ third
Presumed diverticulitis or pelvic infection	Cefoxitin/Cefotetan	Cefoxitin/Cefotetan	Cefoxitin/Cefotetan or parenteral third plus Metronidazole/ Clindamycin
Cholangitis/ Cholecystitis	Parenteral second/ third	Parenteral second/third	Cefoperazone/ Ceftazidime[a]
Meningitis	Ceftriaxone plus Ampicillin	Ceftriaxone plus Ampicillin	Ceftriaxone/ Ceftazidime plus Ampicillin
Sepsis of unclear cause	Parenteral second/ third	Parenteral third	Parenteral third
Sinus, middle ear, or periorbital tissue infection	Parenteral or oral second/third	Parenteral or oral second/third	Parenteral third
Bone/Joint infection	Parenteral second	Parenteral second/third	Parenteral third

[a]Or other third-generation cephalosporin in combination with antipseudomonas coverage.

not have a reliably identifiable pathogen, and when a pathogen is cultured most often it is a gram-negative bacillus such as *H. influenzae* or *M. catarrhalis* or a mixed infection. Hospital-acquired infections may be caused by antibiotic-resistant pathogens such as *P. aeruginosa*, especially following exposure to an intensive-care unit environment.

3. Simple Skin/Soft Tissue Infections

Regardless of the site at which these infections are acquired, the most common pathogens are *S. aureus* and streptococci. Oral or parenteral first-generation cephalosporins, oral second-generation cephalosporins such as cefuroxime axetil, or parenteral cefuroxime or cefamandole are appropriate therapy.

4. Complicated Skin/Soft Tissue Infections

Cellulitis-complicating pressure sores, diabetes mellitus, or peripheral vascular disease, or infections at feeding-tube sites, which are common in older patients, may involve a variety of pathogens, including anaerobic bacteria. In addition, reliable culture data are difficult to obtain because these wounds typically become colonized with gram-negative organisms such as *P. aeruginosa*. Whether coverage for *B. fragilis* is helpful or necessary is controversial, and such coverage complicates empiric therapy decisions. It is unlikely, however, that a properly debrided nonnecrotic wound would support active bacteroides infection, or that specific coverage for bacteroides would improve clinical response. It may be relevant that quinolones, which have minimal anaerobic activity and little or no activity against *B. fragilis*, have been successfully employed in diabetic foot infections or infected pressure sores (59–61).

5. Diverticulitis/Pelvic Infections

Conventional wisdom holds that activity against *B. fragilis* is helpful, although it is probable that any second- or third-generation cephalosporin will give comparable results in these ill-defined syndromes. If abscess is suspected, however, antibacteroides coverage (e.g., cefoxitin or cefotetan) is an important component of therapy.

6. Cholangitis/Cholecystitis

Cephalosporins, in particular cefoperazone and ceftriaxone (30), achieve therapeutic levels in the bile. Gallbladder abscess may complicate cholecystitis in geriatric patients when therapy is delayed, and coverage for bacteroides may be important in such circumstances. Hospital-acquired biliary infection is usually postoperative in origin and may be caused by a variety of gram-negative and gram-positive bacteria.

7. Meningitis

Only third-generation cephalosporins achieve adequate concentrations in cerebrospinal fluid for treatment of meningitis. Although pneumococcal meningitis is the most common central nervous system infection in elderly patients, gram-negative meningitis (often as a complication of trauma or surgery) becomes more common. Ceftriaxone (or ceftazidime if *P. aeruginosa* is a possible pathogen) in combination with ampicillin for *L. monocytogenes* is the regimen of choice.

8. Sepsis of Unclear Cause

Febrile elderly patients usually have a bacterial rather than viral source of their fever, and the cause of infection is usually a common one that responds well to cephalosporin therapy. If a cephalosporin is chosen, choice of a drug is determined primarily by the microbial flora to which the patient is exposed: a parenteral second-generation cephalosporin is sufficient for community-acquired infection and perhaps for nursing home–acquired infection. A third-generation cephalosporin is reasonable in all circumstances. Oral cephalosporins should not be used for suspected serious infection of unknown source: oral trimethoprim-sulfamethoxazole or a quinolone may, however, be reasonable empiric therapy in some circumstances.

9. Sinus, Middle Ear, or Periorbital Tissue Infection

The second-generation oral cephalosporins have a long history of pediatric use for these infections. They may similarly be considered for these uncomplicated infections in elderly patients as part of empiric therapy. The lack of staphylococcal activity of cefixime must be considered when it is chosen, especially in nursing home settings where staphylococcal infections may be common.

10. Bone/Joint Infections

Although most bone and joint infections in younger persons involve staphylococci and *N. gonorrhoeae*, the range of pathogens is far greater in the complicated elderly patient. It is appropriate to broaden the range of pathogens to include the gram-negative bacilli, as well as anaerobic pathogens; while disseminated gonococcal infections certainly do occur in the independently living elderly persons, they are uncommon and are likely to respond to a parenteral second- or third-generation cephalosporin.

Table 10 Cephalosporin Empiric Alternatives in the Penicillin-Allergic Patient

Penicillin	Oral alternative	Parenteral alternative
Penicillin G or V	First	First
Aminopenicillin	Second	Second
Aminopenicillin with clavulanate or sulbactam	Third for UTI or bronchitis	Cefoxitin or Cefotetan or Third
Penicillinase-resistant penicillin	First or second	First
Extended-spectrum parenteral penicillin (with or without clavulanate)	—	Ceftazidime plus metronidazole or clindamycin

UTI = urinary tract infection.

11. Other Infections

The elderly patient is more likely to develop complicated infections that require the expertise of an infectious disease consultant. Broad generalizations, such as those in Table 9, do not apply to many of these patients, and specially designed multiple-drug regimens may be needed. For example, Gleckman (62) listed his preferences for initial and alternative empiric antibiotic regimens for 17 community-acquired infections of elderly patients: only 3 of the possible 34 regimens were single-drug cephalosporin regimens!

In many clinical syndromes, the circumstances of the infection are more important than age or age-related issues. For example, the young and elderly patient with cancer and leukopenia, a postoperative infection, infection of a prosthetic heart valve or other foreign body, bacterial diarrhea, or head and neck infections are usually treated similarly because the syndrome itself dictates the therapy. For the elderly person with one of the common infections such as those listed in Table 9, however, therapy may be more influenced by age and age-related conditions, and empiric cephalosporin regimens may be more useful.

12. Penicillin Allergy

An important indication for oral and parenteral cephalosporin use is as an alternative to penicillins in the penicillin-allergic patient (62). Cross-sensitivity occurs in only a few percent, and reactions such as rash or drug fever are usually minor and resolve with drug discontinuation. A history of an immediate hypersensitivity reaction is usually considered a contraindication to use of any β-lactam drug, although monobactams appear to be safe. Table 10 lists possible cephalosporin alternatives for the penicillin-allergic patient.

VII. ADMINISTRATION OF DRUG

Since cephalosporins are associated with minimal dose-related toxicities, recommendations for reduction in dosage are generally limited to patients with significant renal insufficiency (creatinine clearance < 30 ml/min) or in frail elderly patients older than 80 years.

The efficacy of β-lactams and cephalosporins may be related to the amount of time that serum or tissue concentration exceeds the minimal inhibitory concentration (MIC) of a drug against a pathogen (18). An ideal regimen for cephalosporin dosing in elderly patients would maintain antibiotic concentrations above the MIC for as much of the dosage interval as possible since, unlike aminoglycosides, cephalosporins have minimal if any postantibiotic effect (18,63). Because of the minimal toxicity of cephalosporins, negligible age-related differences in absorption, and often reduced drug clearance in elderly persons, increasing dosing intervals may be better than lowering the dose. This approach provides higher peak levels, may reduce development of resistant organisms (64–66), and may increase tissue concentrations. When studied with ceftazidime, this strategy appears efficacious and maintains serum trough concentrations above the MIC for 90% of the pathogens (67). It is also more cost effective in that readily available dosage preparations can be used, and it reduces drug acquisition, preparation, and administration costs (68). In addition, reduced frequency of dosing may allow for continued care in the home with support from home health care agencies. Dosing recommendations for cephalosporins in elderly patients are listed in Tables 5–8. If there is doubt about the proper cephalosporin dose for an acutely ill elderly patient, however, it is always safe to give a 24-h course of younger-adult dose, then reassess the appropriateness of a reduced dose or lengthened dose interval.

VIII. DRUG MONITORING AND ADVERSE EFFECTS

A clear advantage of cephalosporin therapy for older patients is the wide margin of safety in comparison to non–β-lactam antimicrobials. Adverse effects are primarily limited to hypersensitivity reactions, coagulopathies, and gastrointestinal symptoms.

A. Hypersensitivity Reactions

Maculopapular rashes occurring after several days of therapy are the most frequent hypersensitivity reactions reported with cephalosporins. Serious hypersensitivity reactions, including IgE-mediated bronchospasm, urticaria, and anaphylaxis are uncommon. Patients hypersensitive to penicillins develop cross-hypersensitivity at a frequency of less than 5–10% (69–71). The degree of cross-reactivity may be related to the presence or absence of side chains on the cephalosporin molecule (72,73). Cephalosporin use should, however, be avoided in patients with a history of immediate IgE-mediated hypersensitivity reactions to penicillins; when use of cephalosporins is necessary in such patients, desensitization is prudent (74).

B. Bleeding Reactions

Coagulopathies and bleeding have been associated with moxalactam, cefoperazone, cefotetan, and cefamandole, all of which contain an *N*-methylthiotetrazole (NMTT) side chain (75). Moxalactam is implicated most often and is best avoided in older patients. Ceftriaxone contains a methylthiotriazone side chain, which may be related to bleeding diathesis, but clinical significance is not clear. Other third-generation cephalosporins have also been implicated in bleeding disorders (76).

The mechanism of coagulopathies associated with cephalosporins appears to be primarily related to interference with intestinal synthesis of vitamin K_2 or with inhibition of hepatic carboxylation of vitamin K (76). Malnourished patients and patients receiving vitamin K–deficient enteral/parenteral feedings—typical of many older patients—appear to be at increased risk for bleeding disorders (75). Whether clinically significant age-related changes in vitamin K metabolism exist is debatable (77,78). Vitamin K supplementation should be considered in older patients receiving moxalactam, cefoperazone, or other cephalosporins known to affect vitamin K levels significantly. Other mechanisms of cephalosporin-related bleeding diathesis include irreversible inhibition of platelet function, thrombocytopenia, inhibition of fibrin polymerization, potentiation of warfarin effects, and eradication of vitamin K producing flora in the gut (76,79). Third-generation cephalosporins should be used cautiously if at all in older patients receiving concurrent anticoagulant therapy.

C. Hematological Reactions

Direct and/or indirect Coombs' tests are occasionally positive for patients receiving cefamandole, cefoxitin, cephalexin, cephaloridine, cephalothin, and moxalactam (48), but only rarely result in clinically significant hemolytic anemia (70,79). Immune-mediated thrombocytopenia has been rarely reported with cephalosporins (79), including ceftriaxone and cefotaxime (76). Neutropenia has occasionally been reported with cephalosporins (48,79,80), and this risk may be increased with use of high doses or use for extended periods of time (80,81). Most immune-mediated hematological reactions reverse upon discontinuation of the cephalosporin (69,80).

D. Nephrotoxicity

Cephalosporins are rarely associated with clinically significant injury to the kidney. Cephaloridine (not available in the United States) and cephalothin have been infrequently reported to induce nephrotoxicity in high doses or when dosed with aminoglycosides. Modest reductions in renal function have been associated with standard doses of ceftazidime in patients with preexisting renal impairment (47). Proposed mechanisms of nephrotoxicity include high intracellular levels of drug in the renal tubule and concentration-dependent mitochondrial injury (82).

E. Gastrointestinal Effects

Gastrointestinal disturbances include nausea, vomiting, anorexia, and diarrhea. Diarrhea appears to be more frequent with orally administered agents and those with high biliary excretion (cefoperazone, ceftriaxone). All cephalosporins have been implicated as a cause of pseudomembranous colitis due to *Clostridium difficile*, a particularly hazardous complication in frail elderly patients.

F. Hepatic/Biliary Effects

Clinically significant hepatobiliary toxicity is rare with cephalosporin therapy (83). Ceftriaxone has been reported to produce pseudolithiasis in the gallbladder when administered quickly, but primarily in children (76). Elevated liver enzymes and reversible hepatotoxicity have been reported rarely with cefamandole, cefazolin, ceftizoxime, and cephaloridine; elevated liver enzymes in the absence of hepatotoxicity have been noted with cefoperazone, cefoxitin, cephalothin, and moxalactam. (48)

G. Neurological Effects

Seizure activity has very rarely been reported with cephalosporin therapy and is usually limited to patients with underlying severe renal impairment (84). Headaches and paresthesia have been reported (76).

H. Local Effects

The irritant effects of intravenously administered cephalosporins may cause thrombophlebitis, and intramuscular injection may be painful, although not consistently so (69). Cephalothin, cefoperazone, cefotaxime, and moxalactam have been associated with a higher frequency of thrombophlebitis than other injectable cephalosporins (85).

REFERENCES

1. Barza M, Miao VW. Antimicrobial spectrum, pharmacology and therapeutic use of antibiotics. Part 3: Cephalosporins. Am J Hosp Pharm 1977; 34:621–9.
2. Donowitz GR, Mandell GL. β-Lactam antibiotics. N Engl J Med 1988; 318:490–500.
3. Donowitz GR, Mandell GL. Cephalosporins. In: Mandell GR, Douglas RG, Bennett JE, eds. Principles and practice of infectious diseases, 3d ed. New York: Churchill Livingstone, 1989:246–57.
4. Tomasz A. Penicillin-binding proteins in bacteria. Ann Intern Med 1982; 96:502–4.
5. Molavi A. Cephalosporins: rationale for clinical use. AFP 1991; 43:937–48.
6. Livermore DM. Permeation of β-lactam antibiotics into Escherichia coli, Pseudomonas aeruginosa and other gram-negative bacteria. Rev Infect Dis 1988; 10:691–8.
7. Hartman B, Tomasz A. Altered penicillin-binding proteins in methicillin-resistant strains of Staphylococcus aureus. Antimicrob Agents Chemother 1981; 19:726–35.
8. Bauernfeind A. Classification of β-lactamases. Rev Infect Dis 1986; 8(suppl 5):470–80.
9. Neu H. Pathophysiologic basis for the use of third-generation cephalosporins. Am J Med 1990; 88:3s–11s.
10. Thornsberry C. Review of in vitro activity of third-generation cephalosporins and other newer β-lactam antibiotics against clinically important bacteria. Am J Med 1985; 79:14–20.
11. Wise R. The pharmacokinetics of oral cephalosporins—a review. J Antimicrob Chemother 1990; 26(suppl E):13–20.
12. Schwinghammer TL, Norden CW, Gill E. Pharmacokinetics of cephradine administered intravenously and orally to young and elderly subjects. J Clin Pharmacol 1990; 30:893–9.
13. Faulkner RD, Bohaychuk W, Lanc RA, et al. Pharmacokinetics of cefixime in the young and elderly. J Antimicrob Chemother 1988; 21:787–94.
14. Cutler RE, Blair AD, Kelly MR. Cefadroxil kinetics in patients with renal insufficiency. Clin Pharmacol Ther 1979; 25:514–21.
15. Tremblay D, Dupront A, Ho C, Coussediere D, et al. Pharmacokinetics of cefpodoxime in young and elderly volunteers after single doses: J Antimicrob Chemother 1990; 26(suppl E):21–8.
16. Backhouse C, Wade A, Williamson P, Tremblay D, et al. Multiple dose pharmacokinetics of cefpodoxime in young adult and elderly patients. J Antimicrob Chemother 1990; 26(Suppl E):29–34.
17. Sommers DK, van Wyk M, Moncrieff J, et. al. Influence of food and reduced gastric acidity on the bioavailability of bacampicillin and cefuroxime axetil. Br J Clin Pharmacol 1984; 18:535–9.
18. Meyers BR, Wilkinson P. Clinical pharmacokinetics of antibacterial drugs in the elderly—implications for selection of dosage. Clin Pharmacokinet 1989; 17:385–95.
19. Ljungberg B, Nilsson-Ehle I. Pharmacokinetics of antimicrobial agents in the elderly. Rev Infect Dis 1987; 9:250–64.
20. Garcia MJ, Garcia A, Mieto MJ, et al. Disposition of cefoxitin in the elderly. Int J Clin Pharmacol Ther Toxicol 1980; 18:503–9.
21. Douglas JG, Bax RP, Murnro JF. The pharmacokinetics of cefuroxime in the elderly. J Antimicrob Chemother 1980; 6:543–9.
22. Imada A, Itagaki N, Hasegawa H, et al. Comparative study of the pharmacokinetics of various β-lactams after intravenous and intraperitoneal administration in patients undergoing continuous ambulatory peritoneal dialysis. Drugs 1988; 35(suppl 2):82–7.

23. Scheife RT. Protein binding: what does it mean? DICP Ann Pharmacother 1989; 23(suppl):27–31.
24. McEvoy GK, Litvak K, Welsh O, et al., eds. Cephalosporins. American Hospital Formulary Service Drug Information 92. Bethesda, MD: American Society of Hospital Pharmacists, Inc., 1992:90–5.
25. Van Gossum A, Quenon M, Van Gossum M, et al. Penetration of cefoperazone into ascites. Eur J Clin Pharmacol 1989; 37:577–80.
26. Gobeaux D, Ambart L, Couderc JL, et al. Ceftriaxone diffusion from blood to aqueous humour in man. Br J Ophthal 1989; 73:574–5.
27. Sharir M, Triester G, Kneer J, et al. The intravitreal penetration of ceftriaxone in man following systemic administration. Invest Ophthalmol Vis Sci 1989; 30:2179–83.
28. Leigh DA. Determination of serum and bone concentrations of cephradine and cefuroxime by HPLC in patients undergoing hip and knee joint replacement surgery. J Antimicrob Chemother 1989; 23:877–83.
29. Makiyama T, Asai T. Study on transfer of cefotaxime into bone tissue. Drugs 1988; 35(suppl 2):88–92.
30. Berger S, Levy Y, Halevy A, et al. Penetration of cefazolin, ceftriaxone, cefoperazone, and ceftazidime into human gallbladder tissue and bile. World J Surg 1988; 12:641–4.
31. Moorthi K, Fleckenstein G, Nies B. Concentration of cefixime in bile, gallbladder wall and serum after preoperative administration in patients undergoing cholecystectomy. Meth Find Exp Clin Pharmacol 1990; 12:287–90.
32. Cooper JK, Gardner C. Effect of aging on serum albumin. J Am Geriatr Soc 1989; 37:1039–42.
33. Brown WW, Davis BB, Spry LA, et al. Aging and the kidney. Arch Intern Med 1986; 146:1790–6.
34. Lindeman RD, Tobin J, Shock N. Longitudinal studies on the rate of decline in renal function with age. J Am Geriatr Soc 1985; 33:278–85.
35. O'Connell MB, Dwinell AM, Bannick-Mohrland SD. Predictive performance of equations to estimate creatinine clearance in hospitalized elderly patients. Ann Pharmacother 1992; 26:627–35.
36. Luderer JR, Patel IH, Durkin J, et al. Age and ceftriaxone kinetics. Clin Pharmacol Therapeut 1984; 35:19–25.
37. Deeter RG, Weinstein MP, Swanson KA, et al. Crossover assessment of serum bactericidal activity and pharmacokinetics of five broad-spectrum cephalosporins in the elderly. Antimicrob Agents Chemother 1990; 34:1007–13.
38. Ljungberg B, Nilsson-Ehle I. Advanced age and acute infection influence the kinetics of ceftazidime. Scand J Infect Dis 1989; 21:327–32.
39. Borin MT, Peters GR, Smith TC. Pharmacokinetics and dose proportionality of cefmetazole in healthy young and elderly volunteers. Antimicrob Agents Chemother 1990; 34:1944–8.
40. Broekhuysen J, Deger F, Douchamps J, et al. Pharmacokinetic study of cefuroxime in the elderly. Br J Clin Pharmacol 1981; 12:801–5.
41. Sugihara H, Yoneyama K, Sorimachi H, et al. Pharmacokinetics of cefotaxime on elderly patients. Drugs 1988; 35(suppl 2):93–6.
42. Ljungberg B, Nilsson-Ehle I. Comparative pharmacokinetics of ceftazidime in young, healthy and elderly, acutely ill males. Eur J Clin Pharmacol 1988; 34:179–86.
43. Ludwig E, Szekely E, Csiba A, et al. Pharmacokinetics of cefotaxime and desacetylcefotaxime in elderly patients. Drugs 1988; 35(suppl 2):51–6.
44. Ljungberg B, Nilsson-Ehle I. Influence of age on pharmacokinetics of ceftazidime in acutely ill, adult patients. Eur J Clin Pharmacol 1988; 34:173–8.
45. Hayton WL, Stoeckel K. Age-associated changes in ceftriaxone pharmacokinetics. Clin Pharmacokinet 1986; 11:76–86.
46. Levison ME, Bush LM. Pharmacodynamics of antimicrobial agents. Bactericidal and postantibiotic effects. Infect Dis Clin North Am 1989; 3:415–21.

47. Zhanel GG. Cephalosporin-induced nephrotoxicity: does it exist? DICP Ann Pharmacother 1990; 24:262–5.
48. Young DS. Effects of drugs on clinical laboratory tests, 3d ed. Washington, DC: American Association for Clinical Chemistry Press, 1990.
49. Young DS. Effects of drugs on clinical laboratory tests, 1991 supplement to third edition. Washington, DC: American Association for Clinical Chemistry Press, 1991.
50. Scheckler WE, Peterson PJ. Infections and infection control among residents of eight rural Wisconsin nursing homes. Arch Intern Med 1986; 146:1981–4.
51. Setia U, Serventi I, Lorenz P. Bacteremia in a long-term care facility. Spectrum and mortality. Arch Intern Med 1984; 144:1633–5.
52. Rudman D, Hontanosas A, Cohen Z, et al. Clinical correlates of bacteremia in Veterans Administration extended care facility. J Am Geriatr Soc 1988; 6:726–32.
53. Garibaldi RA, Brodine S, Matsumiya S. Infections among patients in nursing homes: Policies, prevalence, and problems. N Engl J Med 1981; 305:731–5.
54. Muder RR, Brennan C, Wagener MM, et al. Bacteremia in a long-term care facility: a five-year prospective study of 163 consecutive episodes. Clin Infect Dis 1992; 14:647–54.
55. Jacobson C, Strausbaugh LJ. Incidence and impact of infection in a nursing home care unit. Am J Infect Control 1990; 18:151–9.
56. Modai J. Empiric therapy of severe infections in adults. Am J Med 1990; 88(suppl 4):12–17.
57. Gorbach SL. The role of cephalosporins in surgical prophylaxis. J Antimicrob Chemother 1989; 23:61–70.
58. Steere AC. Lyme disease. N Engl J Med 1990; 321:586–96.
59. Andriole VT. The quinolones. New York: Academic Press, 1988.
60. Hooper DC, Wolfson JS. Fluoroquinolone antimicrobial agents. N Engl Med 1991; 324:94.
61. Wolfson JS, Hooper DC. Quinolone antimicrobial agents. Washington, DC: American Society for Microbiology, 1989.
62. Gleckman RA. Antibiotic use in the elderly. Infect Dis Clinic North Am 1989; 3:507–15.
63. Shentag JJ, Ballow CH, Paladino JA, et al. Dual individualization with antibiotics: integrated antibiotic management strategies for use in hospitals. In: Evans WE, Schentag JJ, Jusko WJ, eds. Applied pharmacokinetics: principles of therapeutic drug monitoring, 3d ed. Vancouver, WA: Applied Therapeutics, Inc., 1992:17.1–17.20.
64. Pechere JC. Resistance to third generation cephalosporins: the current situation. Infection 1989; 5:333–7.
65. Nightingale CH. Interaction of microbiology and pharmacokinetics in the selection of appropriate antibiotic therapy. DICP Ann Pharmacother 1989; 23:S16–20.
66. Dudley MN. Commentary on dual individualization with antibiotics. In: Evans WE, Schentag JJ, Jusko WJ, ed. Applied pharmacokinetics: principles of therapeutic drug monitoring, 3d ed. Vancouver, WA: Applied Therapeutics, Inc., 1992:18.1–18.13.
67. Sirgo MA, Norris S. Ceftazidime in the elderly: appropriateness of twice-daily dosing. DICP Ann Pharmacother 1991; 25:284–8.
68. McCue JD. Cost conscious use of cephalosporins. New York: Raven Press, 1987.
69. Cephalosporins and related agents. AMA Drug Evaluations. Chicago: American Medical Association, 1990:2.1–2.58.
70. Saxon A. Immediate hypersensitivity reactions to β-lactam antibiotics. Rev Infect Dis. 1983; 5(suppl 2):368–79.
71. Anderson JA. Cross-sensitivity to cephalosporins in patients allergic to penicillin. Pediatr Infect Dis J 1986; 5:557–61.
72. Blanca M, Fernandez J, Miranda A, et al. Cross-reactivity between penicillins and cephalosporins: clinical and immunologic studies. J Allergy Clin Immunol 1989; 83:381–5.
73. Uno K, Yamasaku F. Structural correlations with cross-reactivity of β-lactam antibiotics in delayed type hypersensitivity. Cross-allergenicity in hypersensitivity to cephems with a tetrazolyl group in the C-3 side chain. J Antimicrob Chemother 1989; 24:251–64.

74. Sanford JP. Penicillin desensitization. J Crit Illness 1992; 7:791–5.
75. Shearer MJ, Bechtold H, Andrassy K, et al. Mechanism of cephalosporin-induced hypoprothrombinemia: relation to cephalosporin side chain, vitamin K metabolism, and vitamin K status. J Clin Pharmacol 1988; 28:88–95.
76. Fekety FR. Safety of parenteral third generation cephalosporins. Am J Med 1990; 88(suppl 4A):38–44.
77. Uehara S, Honjo K, Hirayama A, et al. Effects on the urinary level of γ-carboxylglutamic acid caused by the administration of antibiotics with N-methyl thiotetrazole side chains to patients with infectious diseases. Chemotherapy 1989; 35:254–59.
78. Gurwitz JH, Avorn J, Ross-Degnan D, et al. Aging and the anticoagulant response to warfarin therapy. Ann Intern Med 1992; 116:901–4.
79. Bang NU, Krammer RB. Hematologic complications associated with β-lactam antibiotics. Rev Infect Dis 1983; 5:s380–93.
80. Neftel KA, Hauser SP, Muller MR. Inhibition of granulopoiesis in vivo and in vitro by β-lactam antibiotics. J Infect Dis 1985; 152:90–8.
81. Pan CV, Quintela AG, Garcia JR et al. Cephapirin-induced neutropenia. Chemotherapy 1989; 35:449–53.
82. Tune BM, Hsu CY. Mechanisms of β-lactam antibiotic nephrotoxicity. Toxicol Lett 1990; 53:81–6.
83. Neu HC. Third generation cephalosporins: safety profiles after 10 years of clinical use. J Clin Pharmacol 1990; 30:396–403.
84. Uchihara T, Tsukagoshi H. Myoclonic activity associated with cefmetazole, with a review of neurotoxicity of cephalosporins. Clin Neurol Neurosurg 1988; 90:369–71.
85. Sanford JP. Guide to antimicrobial therapy, 1992. Dallas: Antimicrobial Therapy, Inc., 1992.
86. Reese RE, Betts RF, eds. A practical approach to infectious diseases, 3rd ed. Boston: Little, Brown, 1991.
87. Smith GH. Oral cephalosporins in perspective. DICP Ann Pharmacother 1990; 24:45–51.
88. Klein JO. Evaluation of new oral antimicrobial agents and the experience with cefprozil—a broad-spectrum oral cephalosporin. Clin Infect Dis 1992; 14(suppl 2):183–272.
89. Sheppard M, King A, Phillips I. In vitro activity of cefpodoxime, a new oral cephalosporin, compared with that of nine other antimicrobial agents. Eur J Clin Microbiol Infect Dis 1991; 10:573–81.
90. Moore EP, Speller DCE, White LO, et al., eds. Cefpodoxime proxetil: a third-generation oral cephalosporin. J Antimicrob Chemother 1990; 26(suppl E):1–101.
91. Gilbert DN, Bennett WM. Use of antimicrobial agents in renal failure. Infect Dis Clin North Am 1989; 3:517–31.
92. Bennett WM. Guide to drug dosage in renal failure. Clin Pharmacokinet 1988; 326–54.
93. Fillastre JP, Singlas E. Pharmacokinetics of newer drugs in patients with renal impairment (part I). Clin Pharmacokinet 1991; 20:293–310.
94. Borin MT. A review of the pharmacokinetics of cefpodoxime proxetil. Drugs 1991; 42(Suppl 3):13–21.
95. Bergan T, Digranes A, Schreiner A. Absorption, distribution, and elimination of cefazolin in patients with normal renal function. Chemotherapy 1978; 24:277–82.
96. Halstenson CE, Guay DR, Opsahl JA, et al. Disposition of cefmetazole in health volunteers and patients with impaired renal function. Antimicrob Agents Chemother 1990; 34:519–23.
97. Trang JM, Monson TP, Ackerman BH, et al. Effect of age and renal function on cefonicid pharmacokinetics. Antimicrob Agents Chemother 1989; 33:142–6.
98. Ripa S, Mignini F, Prenna M. Pharmacokinetics of cefotetan in elderly subjects after intramuscular administration. Chemiotherapia 1987; 6:59–63.
99. Schwartz JI, Jauregue LE, Bachmann KA, et al. Multiple-dose pharmacokinetics of intravenously administered cefoperazone and sulbactam when given in combination to infected, seriously ill, elderly patients. Antimicrob Agents Chemother 1988; 32:730–5.

100. Meyers BR, Mendelson MN, Deeter RG et al. Pharmacokinetics of cefoperazone in ambulatory elderly volunteers compared with young adults. Antimicrob Agents Chemother 1987; 31:925–9.
101. Matsuzaki Y, Kitahara Y, Hara N et al. Clinical evaluation of cefoperazone in lower respiratory tract infections. Jpn J Antibiot 1986; 39:2780–94.
102. Horiuchi I, Kawamoto T, Tokumo H, et al. Therapeutic effect of ceftizoxime on infections in aged patients. Jpn J Antibiot 1986; 39:1671–80.
103. Jones RN. A review of cephalosporin metabolism: a lesson to be learned for future chemotherapy. Diagn Microbiol Infect Dis 1989; 12:25–31.
104. Jonsson M, Malder M. Pharmacokinetics of intravenous antibiotics in acutely ill elderly patients. Eur J Clin Microbiol 1986; 621–33.
105. Ljungberg B, Nilsson-Ehle I. Pharmacokinetics of ceftazidime in elderly patients and young volunteers. Scand J Infect 1984; 16:325–6.
106. Naber KG, Kees F, Grobecker H. Ceftazidime: pharmacokinetics in young volunteers versus elderly patients and therapeutic efficacy with complicated urinary tract infections. J Antimicrob Chemother 1983; 12A:41–5.
107. Yuk JH, Nightingale CH, Quintaliani R. Clinical pharmacokinetics of ceftriaxone. Clin Pharmacokinet 1989; 17:223–35.
108. Brogden RN, Ward A. Ceftriaxone—a reappraisal of its antibacterial activity and pharmacokinetic properties, and an update on its therapeutic use with particular reference to once-daily administration. Drugs 1988; 35:604–45.

9

Monobactams

John S. Czachor
Wright State University School of Medicine and Miami Valley Hospital, Dayton, Ohio

Richard A. Gleckman
Boston University School of Medicine and Carney Hospital, Boston, Massachusetts

I. INTRODUCTION

*Mono*cyclic *bac*terial-produced β-lac*tam* (monobactam) antibiotics were originally recovered from gram-negative soil bacteria. These initial compounds did not provide impressive antibacterial activity, but they have formed the basic structure from which current monobactams are synthesized. These agents possess improved antibacterial activity over the naturally occurring monobactams, and they also possess enhanced stability from β-lactamase attack (1–3). Aztreonam is the first monobactam antibiotic released for clinical use, though several other related compounds (carumonam, tigemonam) are being evaluated. The addition of aztreonam to the antibiotic armormentarium has allowed physicians the luxury of an alternative to the traditional agents used to treat patients with gram-negative bacillary infections, particularly the penicillin-allergic individual and the elderly patient. This chapter will focus exclusively on aztreonam, since it is the only currently available monobactam.

II. CHEMISTRY

The monobactams have a four-membered ring with a nitrogen at position 1 (Fig. 1). The various substitutions at the R positions impart unto the compound unique biological activities. In general, the side chain substitution at C-4 increases resistance to β-lactamase degradation, while antibacterial activity and potency is governed by biochemical modifications at C-3 (1–5). The structure-activity relationships of aztreonam, accomplished by substitutions at all four R positions, are depicted in Figure 1.

Aztreonam demonstrates a high degree of stability to β-lactamases. It is not inactivated by the most common plasmid-mediated TEM-1, TEM-2, and SHV-1 enzymes, as well as most chromosomally mediated β-lactamases. Aztreonam is not hydrolyzed by gram-

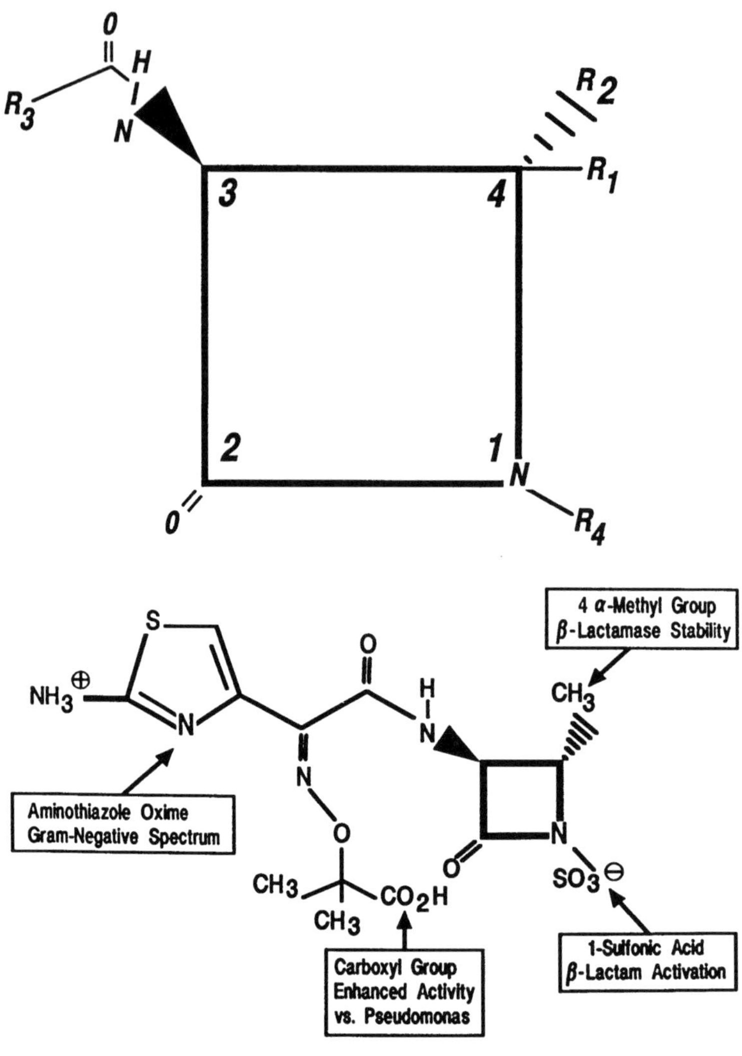

Figure 1 Monobactam structure-activity relationships. (Modified from Ref. 5.)

positive, β-lactamases or most β-lactamases produced by anaerobic bacteria, particularly *Bacteroides* species (1–5). Aztreonam is, however, degraded by several cephalosporin-hydrolyzing plasmid-mediated β-lactamases such as TEM-3, TEM-5, TEM-7, and SHV-2 (5). The appearance of several new broad-spectrum plasmid-mediated cephalosporinases has reduced the ability of aztreonam to resist enzymatic degradation (7,8). These β-lactamases are related to TEM-1, TEM-2, SHV-1, and K-1 varieties, structurally differing by as few as one amino acid, yet producing greater activity against many β-lactam compounds including aztreonam. Another type of β-lactamase related to TEM or SHV remains susceptible to cephamycins and β-lactamase inhibitors, but not to aztreonam or other cephalosporins. *Klebsiella* spp. generally produce these new β-lactamases, although other Enterobacteriaceae have been isolated bearing this plasmid as well. Aztreonam may serve as a weak inducer to some chromosomally mediated β-lactamases (1–6). One such inducible β-lactamase found in many Enterobacteriaceae is regulated by the AMP-C gene along with promoter (AMP-R, AMP-G) regions and a regulator (AMP-D) portion of the chromosome. This enzyme can undergo a single-step mutation, presumably at the AMP-D regulator gene, forming a large amount of constitutively produced β-lactamase, which results in resistance to aztreonam and other β-lactam agents.

III. MECHANISM OF ACTION

As with other β-lactam antibiotics, the monobactams interfere with the biosynthesis of bacterial cell walls. Aztreonam targets penicillin-binding protein 3 (PBP-3) as an attachment site to produce cell lysis or the formation of elongated, filamentous, nonviable bacteria. In addition, the sulfonic acid group at the N-1 position activates the β-lactam ring, which assists in the acetylation and destruction of key enzymes that septate cell walls (see Fig. 1).

The bactericidal concentration of aztreonam approximates its inhibitory concentration. There is no change in the minimal inhibitory concentration (MIC) of aztreonam when the inoculum size (IS) is increased from 10^4 to 10^6 colony-forming units (cfus), although when the IS is extended to 10^7 or 10^8 cfus, a marked increase in aztreonam concentration is required to kill or inhibit bacterial growth (9). The addition of varying amounts of human serum has little, if any, overall effect on the MIC or minimal bactericidal concentration (MBC) for susceptible bacteria (9). There is no postantibiotic effect (PAE) for aztreonam.

IV. ANTIMICROBIAL SPECTRUM

The antimicrobial spectrum of aztreonam is directed exclusively against facultative and aerobic gram-negative organisms, as the compound binds to PBP-3 in Enterobacteriaceae, *Pseudomonas*, and other bacteria. Aztreonam has no significant antibacterial activity against gram-positive or anaerobic organisms because of little or no affinity for PBP-3 in these species. Some nonfermentative aerobic gram-negative bacilli, such as *Acinetobacter* spp., *Enterobacter* spp., *Citrobacter* spp., *Xanthomonas maltophilia*, and the nonaeruginosa *Pseudomonas* spp., demonstrate considerable resistance to aztreonam.

Aztreonam possesses very good inhibitory activity against members of the Enterobacteriaceae class: most are killed by concentrations two to four times the MIC, with the MIC_{90}* value $\leq 1\ \mu g/ml$ (3,5). The side chains added to the core monobactam molecule provide aztreonam with improved inhibitory power against gram-negative bacilli, including antipseudomonal activity (see Fig. 1). Against *P. aeruginosa*, aztreonam has generally been similar in activity to ceftazidime and piperacillin, but consistently less active than impenem/cilastatin (9). Other gram-negative microorganisms that aztreonam effectively inhibits include *Neisseria meningitidis*, *N. gonorrhoeae* (including penicillinase-producing strains), β-lactamase and non–β-lactamase strains of *H. influenzae*, and *Aeromonas* species.

Aztreonam acts synergistically with the aminoglycosides against *P. aeruginosa* and some members of the Enterobacteriaceae class, though synergy with other β-lactam agents has not been demonstrated. Antagonism with some β-lactam compounds has been noted, presumably caused by the β-lactamase production induced by the co-administered antibiotic (10,11).

*Minimum concentration of drug at which 90% of organisms (growth) are inhibited.

V. CLINICAL PHARMACOLOGY

Therapeutic levels of aztreonam are readily achieved with parenteral administration, though oral absorption is almost negligible, with less than 1% of an enteral dose available to the systemic circulation (9,12). The mean plasma concentration following aztreonam administration adheres to linear kinetics. There is little difference in measured peak serum levels after single bolus intravenous administration over 10 min or single prolonged infusion over 30 min (9). Whether intramuscular (IM) or intravenous (IV) routes are used, the serum concentrations of aztreonam approximate each other within 1 h of administration (9,12). Average serum levels following 0.5, 1.0, and 2.0 g IV infusion of aztreonam at 5 min are 58 ± 3 μg/ml, 125 ± 3 μg/ml, and 242 ± 20 μg/ml, respectively (12). After 8 h, the serum concentrations decrease to 1.3 ± 0.1 μg/ml, 2.7 ± 0.1 μg/ml, and 6.0 ± 0.6 μg/ml. Serum half-life ranges from 1.5–2.1 h in normal and infected subjects (13). A metabolite of aztreonam, SQ 26,992, has an elimination half-life of 26 h, 10 times greater than the parent compound (13). Repeated parenteral administrations at 8-h intervals maintain therapeutic levels. There is no evidence for the accumulation of aztreonam after repeated dosings in healthy or infected patients with normal renal function (2,9).

Aztreonam is widely distributed throughout the body, penetrating with therapeutic levels into various tissues and fluids. Concentrations useful in treating infection are achieved in adipose tissue, gallbladder, liver, intestinal tissue, peritoneal fluid, kidney, prostatic tissue, lungs, heart, aqueous humor, and bone (9,12). Studies specifically in elderly patients reveal therapeutic concentrations of aztreonam in bronchial secretions (14–16) and genitourinary tract tissues (17). When meningitis occurs, aztreonam penetrates into the cerebrospinal fluid (CSF) in concentrations well above the MIC/MBC of most gram-negative bacilli (18).

The major route of aztreonam excretion is via the urinary system, by both glomerular filtration and tubular excretion. Though the majority of the drug (60–75%) is excreted unchanged in the urine, a small amount (<10%) is metabolized into an opened-ring form (9,12). Nearly 25% of aztreonam is cleared from the serum by nonrenal mechanisms, with fecal elimination of both unchanged and metabolized compounds occurring in small percentages (9,12,19). Approximately 55–70% of the drug is protein bound (13). The elimination of aztreonam is reduced in patients with alcoholic cirrhosis due to greater protein binding (20).

Subtle physiological changes associated with aging may affect the pharmacokinetic properties of aztreonam (21). Often in elderly persons, a reduced glomerular filtration rate (GFR) is offset by a reduction in lean body mass. The result is often a normal serum creatinine level despite a reduced GFR. By measuring creatinine clearance or estimating renal function using the Cockcroft and Gault equation

$$\text{Creatinine clearance} = \frac{(140 - \text{age}) \times \text{body weight in kg}}{72 \times \text{serum creatinine in mg/dl,}} \quad \text{women multiply by 0.85}$$

basic dosages for drugs such as aztreonam that are excreted renally can then be more accurately determined. Healthy elderly males with normal renal function who receive aztreonam experience no changes in its pharmacokinetic properties despite their age (22). However, aztreonam and its metabolites accumulate in the serum of elderly patients with renal insufficiency (20). Therefore, age, in the absence of renal dysfunction, does not alter the behavior of aztreonam (20,22,23). Aztreonam can be administered safely in elderly patients with decreased renal function, but dosages need to be reduced accordingly,

(20,24). For those patients with renal failure, aztreonam is effectively removed by hemodialysis, and less efficiently by peritoneal dialysis (12,19).

VI. CLINICAL INDICATIONS

Aztreonam is clinically indicated for the treatment of both mild and life-threatening infections caused by susceptible facultative and aerobic gram-negative bacilli, including *P. aeruginosa* (1–3,9,25,26). Infectious diseases in older adults, however, pose difficult and unique challenges for clinicians. Antimicrobial agents may not behave pharmacokinetically or pharmacologically similarly in elderly and nonelderly patients; infections may not manifest in traditional fashion in an aging population; physiological changes of aging may alter the choice of antibiotic therapy in an elderly patient; and concomitant illnesses, as well as coexistent medications, can also influence antibiotic selection in geriatric patients.

A number of studies have established the effectiveness of aztreonam in treating elderly patients with serious infections. Gram-negative bacteremia and gram-negative sepsis have been successfully treated using aztreonam in this population (27–30). Lower respiratory infections, including bronchitis, tracheobronchitis, and pneumonia, have been eradicated using aztreonam by itself or in combination with other antimicrobial agents (14–16,27,29–31). Aztreonam administered as a single agent has been invaluable for the treatment of elderly patients with pyelonephritis, as well as complicated and uncomplicated urinary tract infections (UTIs) (27–30,32,33). When prescribed as a single-dose IM injection prior to Foley catheterization in older patients, aztreonam reduced the number of catheter-associated UTIs (34). Elderly patients with intraabdominal/intrapelvic infections, including abscesses, peritonitis, and biliary tract infections, have responded favorably to aztreonam therapy (27–29).

Other potential therapeutic uses for aztreonam in the geriatric patient include a component of initial empiric combination therapy for the treatment of infection in the febrile neutropenic patient (35) and therapy for gram-negative meningitis (18). Aztreonam is currently being investigated for the treatment of traveler's diarrhea, employing a poorly absorbed oral form of the drug (36).

Aztreonam has also been a useful addition to the antibiotic spectrum for surgical prophylaxis. When combined with clindamycin during high-risk colorectal surgery in elderly patients, aztreonam reduced the incidence of postoperative abdominal wound infections (37). It has also proven to be an effective prophylactic agent when administered prior to transurethral resection of the prostate (38).

VII. ADMINISTRATION OF DRUG

Aztreonam can be administered parenterally to any patient without documented hypersensitivity to this compound. The ability to administer aztreonam intramuscularly provides an alternative to the intravascular route. This becomes particularly important in those older patients lacking intravenous access, such as nursing home residents, who may be infected yet do not require hospitalization. An oral preparation of aztreonam has not yet been released.

Perhaps the elderly penicillin-allergic patient poses the greatest dilemma to the clinician. Often the exact nature of the adverse reaction to penicillin (and related compounds) is unknown or unavailable, resulting in a conundrum of which antibiotic to prescribe. Physicians faced with the possibility of an immediate or accelerated hypersensitivity reaction

Table 1 Aztreonam and the Elderly Paatient

Advantages	Concerns
Can administer to penicillin-allergic patients	Limited spectrum of activity (facultative and aerobic gram-negative baccilli only)
Active against *Pseudomonas aeruginosa*	No oral preparation
Mild adverse reactions	Expense (however, no serum monitoring needed)
No significant drug interactions	Superinfection
No pharmacokinetic effect from aging	
Poor inducer of β-lactamase and resistant bacteria	

are reluctant to infuse a cephalosporin with cross-reactivity rates known to be between 5 and 15%. Aztreonam, though similar in structure to other β-lactam agents, does not demonstrate any cross-reactivity with these compounds and can be safely administered to the penicillin-allergic individual (39–41).

The dosage and route of administration for aztreonam should be determined by the following factors: severity of infection, general condition of the elderly patient, renal function, and in vitro susceptibility of the isolated pathogen(s). General dosage guidelines for aztreonam range from 1.5 to 8 g per day in divided doses. Low doses (0.5–1.0 g IV or IM q 8–12 h) are useful for the treatment of UTIs. Traditional doses (1–2 g IV q 8–12 h) are applicable for severe infections such as pneumonia, intraabdominal infections, bacteremia, sepsis, or skeletal infections not involving *P. aeruginosa*. Higher doses of aztreonam (2 g IV q 6–8 h) are reserved for serious infections caused by *P. aeruginosa* or for patients with gram-negative meningitis (9,18).

For elderly patients with reduced renal function (creatinine clearance > 10 ml/min but ≤ 30 ml/min), the usual dose of aztreonam should be halved following an initial loading dose of 1–2 g (9,28). For those elderly patients undergoing hemodialysis or peritoneal dialysis, the same loading dose of 1–2 g is followed by one half to one quarter of the loading dose every 24 h, administered after dialysis (42). There is no dosage adjustment for age with aztreonam (9,12).

VIII. DRUG MONITORING AND ADVERSE EFFECTS

Aztreonam has been widely prescribed over a number of years for the therapy of facultative and aerobic gram-negative bacillary infections with only minor untoward and toxic effects reported in elderly patients (20,24,27–30,43–45). An additional benefit is that there are no clinically significant drug interactions between aztreonam and other therapeutic agents, including antibiotics (9,46). Aztreonam may also be administered to the elderly penicillin-allergic patient, as no hypersensitivity or cross-reactivity exists between these compounds (39–41).

Aztreonam is often compared to the aminoglycosides since both share a similar spectrum of inhibition primarily directed against facultative and aerobic gram-negative bacilli. Aztreonam is an alternative to the aminoglycosides for therapy of mild to severe infections due to susceptible organisms, but significant differences exist between the untoward effects of these two antibiotic classes. While aztreonam possesses the relatively nontoxic profile of a β-lactam agent, aminoglycosides are ototoxic and nephrotoxic, especially in the elderly patient with preexisting renal dysfunction, hepatic disease, or eighth cranial nerve damage. Serum drug concentration monitoring is recommended for the aminoglycosides because of their narrow therapeutic/toxic ratios, but it is unnecessary when administering aztreonam. Even though acquisition costs for aztreonam are higher, some cost equality is achieved through the added expenses of serial renal function determinations and serum peak/trough levels needed during aminoglycoside infusion. Overall costs of aminoglycoside therapy certainly can exceed those of aztreonam if an adverse reaction, particularly nephrotoxicity, occurs (47).

Adverse effects with aztreonam in the elderly patient population do not occur more frequently than in younger individuals (9,24,27–30,43–46,48–52). Overall, 6.2–7.4% of patients who receive aztreonam encounter untoward effects, though only 2.1–2.4% will necessitate discontinuance of the drug (44,48,49). Local reactions to IM injection are found between 3.1 and 10% of elderly patients (24,28,30), while only 1.3–3.2% suffer ill effects at IV infusion sites (9,29,44,48,49). Skin rash with or without pruritus is uncommon, occurring in only 0.7–1.8% (9,29,30,44,48,49). Diarrhea may be common (0.8–16.3%) with aztreonam administration, but antibiotic-associated pseudomembranous colitis secondary to *Clostridium difficile* is rare (approximately 0.2%) (9,43,44,48,49). Elevations in liver function tests (1.3–14.2%) are mild, usually transient, and resolve after the aztreonam administration is terminated (9,24,28–30).

Coagulation disorders are very uncommon with aztreonam administration; changes in prothrombin time (PT) are found in less than 0.1% (44). Laboratory tests of renal function are abnormal infrequently during aztreonam therapy (1–4%), and in some instances, renal function actually improves in elderly patients receiving a treatment course of aztreonam (20,24,28,30,44,45). Hematological abnormalities include changes in hemoglobin (7%), elevation of eosinophil count (11%), thrombocytosis (9%), thrombocytopenia (0.7–4.7%), and neutropenia (1 patient) (29,30,44,48,49,52). Superinfection has been demonstrated in 2–6% of elderly patients who are prescribed aztreonam, though some studies report rates as high as 38% (28–30,43,44,48,49,51). Enterococci are the most frequently identified superinfecting microorganisms, though other aerobic gram-positive cocci, resistant aerobic gram-negative bacilli, anaerobes, and fungi have also caused superinfection in elderly patients.

REFERENCES

1. Sanders CC, Thomson KS, Sanders Jr. WE. Other β-lactam antibiotics. In: Gorbach SL, Bartlett JG, Blacklow NR, eds. Infectious diseases. Philadelphia: W.B. Saunders, 1992:182–8.
2. Neu HC. Other β-lactam antibiotics. In: Mandell GL, Douglas Jr. RG, Bennett JE, eds. Principles and practice of infectious diseases. New York: Churchill Livingstone, Inc., 1990:257–63.
3. Brewer NS, Hellinger WC. The monobactams. Mayo Clin Proc 1991; 66:1152–7.
4. Sykes RB, Bonner DP. Discovery and development of the monobactams. Rev Infect Dis 1985; 7(suppl 4):579–93.
5. Sykes RB, Bonner DP. Aztreonam: the first monobactam. Am J Med 1985; 78(suppl 2A):2–10.

6. Bush K, Sykes RB. Interaction of new β-lactams with β-lactamases and β-lactamase-producing gram-negative rods. In: Neu HC, ed. New β-lactam antibiotics: a review from chemistry to clinical efficacy of the new cephalosporins. Philadelphia: Francis Clark Wood Institute for the History of Medicine, College of Physicians of Philadelphia, 1982:47–64.
7. Jacoby GA, Archer GL. New mechanisms of bacterial resistance to antimicrobial agents. N Engl J Med 1991; 324:601–12.
8. Sanders CC. β-Lactamases of gram-negative bacteria: new challenges for new drugs. Clin Infect Dis 1992; 14:1089–99.
9. Brogden RN, Heel RC. Aztreonam: a review of its antibacterial activity, pharmacokinetic properties and therapeutic use. Drugs 1986; 31:91–130.
10. Stutman HR, Welch DF, Scribner RK, et al. In vitro antimicrobial activity of aztreonam alone and in combination against bacterial isolates from pediatric patients. Antimicrob Agents Chemother 1984; 25:212–15.
11. Buesing MA, Jorgensen JH. In vitro activity of aztreonam in combination with newer β-lactams and amikacin against multiply resistant gram-negative bacilli. Antimicrob Agents Chemother 1984; 25:283–5.
12. Swabb EA. Review of the clinical pharmacology of the monobactam antibiotic aztreonam. Am J Med 1985; 78(suppl 2A):11–18.
13. Swabb EA, Singhvi SM, Leitz MA, et al. Metabolism and pharmacokinetics of aztreonam in healthy subjects. Antimicrob Agents Chemother 1983; 24:394–400.
14. Boccazzi A, Langer M, Mandelli M, et al. The pharmacokinetics of aztreonam and penetration into the bronchial secretions of critically ill patients. J Antimicrob Chemother 1989; 23:401–7.
15. Miglioli PA, Pivetta P, Fantoni, V, et al. Penetration of aztreonam in pleural exudate following rapid intravenous bolus or constant infusion. Chemotherapy 1990; 90:321–4.
16. Velluti G, Capelli O, Bonucchi ME, et al. Aztreonam activity in pneumology. Part 1: Clinical activity and pulmonary bioavailability of two different administration regimens. J Chemother 1991; 3:30–8.
17. Whitby M, Hempenstall J, Gilpin C, et al. Penetration of monobactam antibiotics (aztreonam, carumonam) into human prostatic tissue. Chemotherapy 1989; 35:7–11.
18. Duma RJ, Berry AJ, Smith SM, et al. Penetration of aztreonam into cerebrospinal fluid of patients with and without inflamed meninges. Antimicrob Agents Chemother 1984; 26:730–3.
19. Mihindu JC, Scheld WM, Bolton ND, et al. Pharmacokinetics of aztreonam in patients with various degrees of renal dysfunction. Antimicrob Agents Chemother 1983; 24:252–61.
20. Sattler FR, Schramm M, Swabb EA. Safety of aztreonam and SQ 26,992 in elderly patients with renal insufficiency. Rev Infect Dis 1985; 7(suppl 4):622–7.
21. Gleckman RA, Czachor JS. Reviewing the safe use of antibiotics in the elderly. Geriatrics 1989; 44:33–9.
22. Creasey WA, Platt TB, Frantz M, et al. Pharmacokinetics of aztreonam in elderly male volunteers. Br J Clin Pharmacol 1985; 19:233–7.
23. Yoshikawa TT. Antimicrobial therapy for the elderly patient. J Am Geriat Soc 1990; 38:1353–72.
24. Sion ML, Pyrpasopoulos M, Nicolaidis P, et al. Efficacy and safety of aztreonam in the treatment of patients with renal failure. Rev Infect Dis 1991; 13(suppl 7):652–4.
25. Neu HC, ed. Aztreonam: a monocyclic β-lactam antibiotic. Am J Med 1985; 78(suppl 2A):1–80.
26. Rubinstein E, Isturiz R, eds. Aztreonam: the expanding clinical profile. Rev Infect Dis 1991; 13(suppl 7):581–654.
27. Knockaert DC, Dejaeger E, Nestor L, et al. Aztreonam-flucloxacillin double beta-lactam treatment as empirical therapy of serious infections in very elderly patients. Age Aging 1991; 20:135–9.
28. Deger F, Douchamps J, Freschi E, et al. Aztreonam in the treatment of serious gram-negative infections in the elderly. Internat J Clin Pharmacol Ther Toxicol 1988; 26:22–6.

29. Clergeot A, Steru D, Rosset MA, et al. Efficacy and safety of low-dose aztreonam in the treatment of moderate to severe infections due to gram-negative bacilli. Rev Infect Dis 1991; 13(suppl 7):648–51.
30. DeMaria Jr. A, Treadwell TL, Saunders CA, et al. Randomized clinical trial of aztreonam and aminoglycoside antibiotics in the treatment of serious infections caused by gram-negative bacilli. Antimicrob Agents Chemother 1989; 33:1137–43.
31. Colardyn F, Gala JL, Verschraegen G, et al. Infections in patients in intensive care units: Can the combination of a monobactam and a penicillin replace the classic combination of a β-lactam agent and an aminoglycoside? Rev Infect Dis 1991; 13(suppl 7):640–4.
32. Jones SR, Kimbrough R. UTIs and two new antibiotics in the elderly. Geriatrics 1988; 43:49–58.
33. Friman G, Cars O, Bäck E, et al. Randomized comparison of aztreonam and cefuroxime in Gram-negative upper urinary tract infections. Infection 1989; 17:284–9.
34. Romanelli G, Giustina A, Cravarezza P, et al. A single dose of aztreonam in the prevention of urinary tract infections in elderly catheterized patients. J Chemother 1990; 2:178–81.
35. Jones PG, Rolston KVI, Fainstein V, et al. Aztreonam therapy in neutropenic patients with cancer. Am J Med 1986; 81:243–8.
36. Dupont HL, Ericsson CD, Mathewson JJ, et al. Oral aztreonam, a poorly absorbed yet effective therapy for bacterial diarrhea in US travelers to Mexico. JAMA 1992; 267:1932–5.
37. Dionigi R, Mozzillo N, Ventriglia L. Comparative multicenter study on efficacy and safety of aztreonam and gentamicin in prophylaxis of high-risk colorectal surgery. J Chemother 1989; 1(suppl 2):22–7.
38. Rosetti SR, Boccafoschi C, Pellegrini A, et al. Aztreonam monotherapy as prophylaxis in transurethral resection of the prostate: a multicenter study. Rev Infect Dis 1991; 12(suppl 7):626–8.
39. Saxon A, Swabb E, Adkinson F. Investigation into the immunologic cross-reactivity of aztreonam with other beta-lactam antibiotics. Am J Med 1985; 78(suppl 2A):19–26.
40. UCLA Conference. Immediate hypersensitivity reactions to beta-lactam antibiotics. Ann Intern Med 1987; 107:204–15.
41. Saxon A, Hassner A, Swabb EA, et al. Lack of cross-reactivity between aztreonam, a monobactam antibiotic, and penicillin in penicillin-allergic subjects. J Infect Dis 1984; 149:16–22.
42. Gerig JS, Bolton ND, Swabb EA, et al. Effect of hemodialysis and peritoneal dialysis on aztreonam pharmacokinetics. Kidney Int 1984; 26:308–18.
43. LeFrock JL, Smith BR, Chandrasekar P, et al. Efficacy and safety of aztreonam in the treatment of serious gram-negative bacterial infections. Arch Intern Med 1987; 147:325–8.
44. Newman TJ, Dreslinski GR, Tadros SS. Safety profile of aztreonam in clinical trials. Rev Infect Dis 1985; 7(suppl 4):648–55.
45. Moore RD, Lerner SA, Levine DP. Nephrotoxicity and ototoxicity of aztreonam versus aminoglycoside therapy in seriously ill non-neutropenic patients. J Infect Dis 1992; 165:683–8.
46. Creasey WA, Adamovies J, Dhruv R, et al. Pharmacokinetic interaction of aztreonam with other antibiotics. J Clin Pharmacol 1984; 24:174–80.
47. Eisenberg JM, Koffer H, Glick HA, et al. What is the cost of nephrotoxicity associated with aminoglycosides? Ann Intern Med 1987; 107:900–9.
48. Henry SA, Bendush CB. Aztreonam: worldwide overview of the treatment of patients with gram-negative infections. Am J Med 1985; 78(suppl 2A):57–64.
49. Bendush CB, Henry SA, Newman TJ, et al. Aztreonam: worldwide clinical experience with the first monobactam. NJ Med 1986; Jan. (special issue):30–6.
50. Sakata H, Kakehashi H, Fujita K, et al. Effects of aztreonam on fecal flora and on vitamin K metabolism. Antimicrob Agents Chemother 1990; 34:1045–7.
51. Chandrasekar P, Smith B, LeFrock JL, et al. Enterococcal superinfection and colonization with aztreonam therapy. Antimicrob Agents Chemother 1984; 26:280–2.
52. Dallal MM, Czachor JS. Aztreonam-induced myelosuppression during treatment of *Pseudomonas aeruginosa* pneumonia. DICP Ann Pharmacother 1991; 25:594–7.

10

Carbapenems

Lynette H. Posorske and Fred M. Gordin
Veterans Affairs Medical Center, Washington, D.C.

I. CHEMISTRY

Carbapenems are a new class of broad-spectrum antibiotic, of which imipenem is the first one available for clinical use (1). The carbapenems are another class of β-lactam antibiotics that differ from the penicillins by the substitution of a carbon atom for a sulfur atom at the 1 position and the addition of a double bond in the five-membered ring (2). Additionally, penicillins and cephalosporins contain an acylamino side chain at the R_1 position, whereas imipenem contains a hydroxyethyl group at this position. The hydroxyethyl group assumes a *trans* position (1).

Imipenem is a synthetic derivative of the naturally occurring compound thienamycin (2). Thienamycin was discovered in the 1970s during a screening process of various microorganisms for their ability to inhibit peptidoglycan synthesis. In this screening, a new species of *Streptomyces*, termed *Streptomyces cattleyea* because of its distinct orchid color, was identified. Culture broths of this organism were active in peptidoglycan synthesis inhibition; the active agent was found to be thienamycin (3).

Thienamycin proved to be chemically unstable, due to a reaction of the side-chain amine with the β-lactam ring of a second molecule, thus forming an inactive dimer. A systematic search for a more stable derivative was therefore undertaken, which resulted in the synthesis of an amidine derivative, *N*-formimidoyl thienamycin, subsequently renamed imipenem. Imipenem exhibited the requisite chemical stability in both solution and solid form and retained the antimicrobial spectrum of the parent compound (3).

Numerous other carbapenems, both synthetic and naturally occurring, have been discovered. Examples of naturally occurring carbapenems are carpetimycins and asparenomycins (3). None of these other carbapenems have been developed for clinical use; hence, imipenem is the only clinically available carbapenem at this time.

In addition to the chemical instability of thienamycin, metabolic instability of imipenem was encountered in clinical trials. Despite the fact that the drug was known to be renally excreted, low and variable urinary recovery was observed (2). An enzyme found in the brush border of the renal proximal tubule, a zinc-containing dipeptidase, termed dehydropeptidase I, was found to be the active agent in imipenem's destruction (3). The enzyme was active against all other carbapenems, which were, in fact, metabolized more extensively than imipenem. This enzyme has no effect on any of the penicillins or cephalosporins (3).

The extensive urinary metabolism of imipenem posed some obvious problems in development of the drug for clinical use. If the drug is extensively inactivated in urine, then its use in infections of the urinary tract would be limited and therapeutic failure might be expected (1). A search was undertaken for a specific inhibitor that could (1) be co-administered with imipenem and (2) selectively inhibit the enzyme that caused the destruction of imipenem while minimizing destruction of physiologic peptides. The most successful compounds were the Z-2-acylamino-propenoate class of compounds; maximal activity was found with the acylamino moiety S(+) dimethylcyclo-propyl-amido moiety combined with the L-cysteine moiety. This compound is cilastatin, which is very specific for dehydropeptidase I and shows less affinity for other zinc metalloenzymes. It has neither inherent antibacterial activity nor activity against bacterial β-lactamases. There is no synergistic or antagonistic interaction with imipenem (3).

Imipenem and cilastatin are administered in equal amounts by weight under the brand name of Primaxin® (2). Unless otherwise stated for the rest of this discussion, imipenem/cilastatin will be simply referred to as imipenem.

II. MECHANISM OF ACTION

Imipenem's mechanism of action is similar to that of other β-lactam antibiotics. All drugs of this class function by binding bacterial transpeptidases, a series of proteins on or near the cell surface of bacteria (2). These peptidases, known as penicillin-binding proteins (PBPs), are involved in the cross-linking and elongation of the bacterial cell wall. Binding of the antibiotic leads to impairment of cell wall construction, inhibition of bacterial cell growth, and, often, lysis and death of the cell (2,4). In gram-positive organisms, the PBPs are located at the cell surface, while in gram-negative organisms, they are found in the periplasmic space (2). (See also Chap. 7.)

Imipenem has the broadest antimicrobial spectrum of all available antibiotics. It owes its broad spectrum of activity to its affinity for PBPs from a wide variety of bacteria. It has been shown to bind PBPs from *Staphylococcus*, *Enterococcus*, and gram-negative organisms. Of the six PBPs of gram-negative bacilli, PBPs 1 to 3 are essential for cell survival. The carbapenems bind preferentially to PBP-2, the protein thought to be most involved in maintaining cell shape. With higher concentrations of drug, PBP-1b, followed by PBP-3, is bound, thus producing cell death by alternative mechanisms (5).

Another reason for imipenem's broad spectrum of activity is the ability of the drug to efficiently reach its site of action. In gram-positive bacteria, antibiotics can relatively easily traverse the loosely connected peptidoglycan outer cell wall. Gram-negative bacteria, however, possess a complex lipopolysaccharide outer membrane. Substances traverse this outer membrane and reach the periplasmic space by means of channels called porins. Some cephalosporins and penicillins, because of bulky acyl side chains, cannot readily enter the periplasmic space, and many are weak anions. Imipenem, in contrast, is a relatively small molecule and exists in a zwitterion state; the compact structure and zwitterion state are thought to permit more rapid passage through porin channels (5,6).

Imipenem is resistant to a large number of β-lactamases from both gram-positive and gram-negative bacteria (1). This resistance extends to both chromosomal and plasmid-mediated β-lactamases (5). As previously discussed, the hydroxyethyl side chain is in a *trans* configuration; this conformation is responsible for imipenem's stability to β-lactamases. Most other β-lactam antibiotics possess the side chain in a *cis* configuration (1). Also, the S-configuration at C-8, as found in the epithienamycins, seems to confer β-lactamase susceptibility. The C-8 of imipenem is in the R configuration (3).

There is evidence that imipenem can function as an inhibitor of β-lactamases, particularly the Richmond-Sykes type found in *Enterobacter*, *Citrobacter freundii*, *Morganella*, and *Providencia*. One report showed that imipenem functioned as a suicide inhibitor; that is, after the enzyme had interacted with imipenem, it no longer was able to hydrolyze other compounds (5).

Thus, imipenem is a β-lactam antibiotic with an unusually broad spectrum of activity, which can be attributed to its ability to bind a wide variety of PBPs, and its favorable stereochemistry, which allows ready penetration to the site of action and resistance to β-lactamase degradation.

III. ANTIMICROBIAL SPECTRUM

Imipenem has the broadest antibacterial spectrum of all the antibiotics currently available for human use. Common and serious bacterial infections in older adults involve gram-positive cocci, facultative and aerobic gram-negative bacilli and anaerobes (see Chap. 26). Thus, imipenem is potentially a useful drug for geriatric patients in select circumstances.

Like all β-lactams, imipenem is bactericidal (1), and for most organisms the minimal inhibitory concentration (MIC) is close to the minimal bactericidal concentration (MBC). In addition, culture medium and pH have little influence on susceptibility patterns (1). In the following discussion, an MIC of ≤4 μg/ml will be considered susceptible, MIC 4–8 μg/ml moderately susceptible, and >8 μg/ml will be considered resistant.

Imipenem has good activity against most gram-positive bacteria, as shown in Table 1. It is very active against methicillin-sensitive *Staphylococcus aureus*; *Streptococcus pyogenes*; β-hemolytic *Streptococcus* groups A, C, and G; viridans group streptococci; *Streptococcus bovis* (1,7), and *Streptococcus agalactiae* (7). It is very active against *Streptococcus pneumoniae*, but penicillin-resistant strains of this organism may be 8- to 16-fold less susceptible than penicillin-sensitive strains (7). Unlike the cephalosporins, imipenem has good activity against *Listeria monocytogenes*; the MBC, however, ranges from 5 to 32 μg/ml (vs. MIC_{90} of 0.13–1). The clinical significance of this is uncertain (7). Some, but not all, strains of *Staphylococcus epidermidis* are sensitive to imipenem with MICs ranging from <0.1 to 4.5 μg/ml. Other strains, usually methicillin-resistant *Staphylococcus epidermidis*, have MICs up to 50 μg/ml. In one report, 8 of 10 studies showed MICs of >8 μg/ml. The mechanism of resistance is probably altered penicillin-binding proteins (7). *Enterococcus faecalis* is usually sensitive to imipenem, which is consistent with its similarity to penicillins, but there are a small number of uniformly resistant strains. A significant increase between MIC_{90} and MBC is also seen (1). Similar phenomena are also seen with use of penicillin and ampicillin for this organism (7).

Imipenem has good activity against most facultative and aerobic gram-negative bacilli (Table 1). It is highly active against *Escherichia coli*, *Citrobacter diversus* and *C. freundii*,

*The lowest drug concentration(s) at which 90% of all strains of organism are inhibited.

Table 1 Antimicrobial Activity of Imipenem

Organism	MIC_{90} (μg/ml)
Staphylococcus aureus (not MRSA)	0.12
Staphylococcus epidermidis	<0.1–4.5
Streptococcus pneumoniae	0.01
Streptococcus pyogenes	0.01–0.1
Viridans streptococci	0.1
Streptococcus bovis	0.1
Enterococcus faecalis	0.8
Streptococcus agalactiae	0.07
Listeria monocytogenes	0.1–1
Escherichia coli	0.5
Citrobacter freundii	0.5
Citrobacter diversus	0.5
Klebsiella pneumoniae	0.5
Klebsiella oxytoca	0.5
Salmonella spp.	0.1–1.0
Shigella spp.	0.5–1
Yersinia enterocolitica	0.1
Enterobacter aerogenes	2
Enterobacter cloacae	4
Serratia marcescens	1–8
Proteus mirabilis	1–4
Proteus vulgaris	1–4
Providencia stuartii	2
Morganella morganii	2
Pseudomonas aeruginosa	2–5
Acinetobacter calcoaceticus	1–4
Aeromonas hydrophila	0.5–1
Haemophilus influenzae	1
Neisseria meningitidis	0.1–0.25
Neisseria gonorrhoeae	0.25
Bacteroides fragilis	0.5–1
Bacteroides melaninogenicus	0.1
Bacteroides disiens	0.03
Bacteroides thetaiotaomicron	1
Bacteroides vulgatus	1
Fusobacterium nucleatum	0.5
Veillonella	1
Peptostreptococcus	0.1
Peptococcus	1
Clostridium perfringens	1–4
Propionibacterium	0.01
Eikenella corrodens	0.25
Campylobacter fetus	0.12
Brucella melitensis	2.0
Nocardia asteroides	3.9
Erysipelothrix	0.015
Pasturella multocida	1.0
Actinomyces species	0.12

Source: Refs. 1,2,13.

Hafnia alvei, *Klebsiella oxytocia* and *K. pneumoniae*, *Salmonella spp.*, *Shigella* spp., *Yersinia enterocolitica*, and *Aeromonas hydrophilia* (1,2,7). *Enterobacter cloacae* and *Enterobacter aerogenes* have MIC_{90} in the 1–4 μg/ml range. An occasional *Enterobacter* isolate has MICs >8 μg/ml (7). For both *Enterobacter* species and *Citrobacter freundii*, imipenem is useful when resistance to aminothiazoyl cephalosporins (i.e., cefotaxime, ceftazidime) is encountered, as imipenem is resistant to the β-lactamases these organisms produce (1). *Serratia* species are also susceptible to imipenem (1,2,7). The least susceptible Enterobacteriaceae are those of the *Proteus-Providencia-Morganella* group, with MIC_{90} of *Proteus mirabilis*, *Proteus vulgaris*, *Proteus* spp., *Providencia stuartii*, *Providencia rettgeri*, and *Providencia* spp., and *Morganella morganii* ranging from 2–5 μg/ml. The etiology of this group's relative resistance is poorly understood (7). Imipenem has good activity against many non-Enterobacteriaceae gram-negative bacilli. MICs of 2–5 μg/ml are reported for *Pseudomonas aeruginosa* (1,2,7). Sensitivity to imipenem does not correlate with sensitivity to other β-lactam antibiotics or aminoglycosides (1). An MBC/MIC of greater than 8 has been shown for many *Pseudomonas* isolates (6). If used as single-agent therapy in the treatment of pseudomonal infections, resistance may develop (1,2). The role of combination therapy will be addressed in the next section. Other pseudomonads (*Pseudomonas fluorescens* and *Pseudomonas stutzeri*) are usually sensitive to imipenem (1,7). *Acinetobacter calcoaceticus*, *A. anitratus*, and *A. Lwoffii* (1,7) are generally sensitive, as are *Achromobacter* isolates (1,7). Imipenem has excellent activity against *Hemophilus influenzae*, *Neisseria meningitidis*, *Neisseria gonorrhoea*, and *Moraxella* species (1,2,7).

A very important aspect of the antimicrobial spectrum of imipenem is its activity against anaerobic bacteria. It is active against nearly all gram-positive and gram-negative anaerobes. Its activity exceeds that of all other β-lactam antibiotics and is considered in the range of metronidazole, clindamycin, and chloramphenicol (1). It is active against most *Bacteroides* species, including *B. fragilis*, *B. bivius*, *B. melaninogenicus*, *B. disiens*, *B. thetaiotaomicron*, *B. vulgatus*, and *B. ovatus* (1,2,7). Rarely, *Bacteroides fragilis* group isolates are resistant to imipenem (8). Activity is also seen against *Fusobacterium* spp., *Veillonella* spp., anaerobic gram-positive cocci, including *Peptostreptococcus* and *Peptococcus*, *Clostridium perfringens*, *Propionibacterium*, *Eikenella corrodens*, and *Campylobacter fetus*, including *C. fetus* subsp. *fetus** (formerly subspecies *intestinalis*) and *C. jejuni* subsp. *jejuni* (1,2,7).

Imipenem has also been shown to have activity against some infrequently isolated species, which may occasionally be seen in elderly persons, including *Bordetella bronchiseptica*, *Brucella melitensis*, *Nocardia asteroides*, *Erysipelothrix rhusiopathiae*; *Pasteurella multocida*, and *Actinomyces* spp. (7).

Relatively few organisms are resistant to imipenem, but this short list (Table 2) includes some important pathogens. Activity against methicillin-resistant *S. aureus* (MRSA) has been variable, with some studies showing good activity against this organism, while other studies show most isolates to be resistant (7). Imipenem cannot be considered reliably active against MRSA (1) and should not be considered as an alternative to vancomycin. *Enterococcus faecium* is always resistant to imipenem, probably on the basis of poor binding to penicillin-binding proteins. *Corynebacterium* JK is also resistant to imipenem (1). Very few gram-negative bacteria are resistant to imipenem. The antibiotic is not active against *Xanthomomas maltophilia*; the mechanism is thought to be a zinc metallo β-lactamase highly active against imipenem (6). *Pseudomonas cepacia* and *Flavobacterium* are also resistant (1,2).

*Based on *Manual of Clinical Microbiology*, 5th ed., 1991.

Table 2 Organisms Resistant to Imipenem

Staphylococcus aureus (methicillin-resistant)
Corynebacterium jeikeium
Xanthomonas maltophilia
Pseudomonas cepacia
Flavobacterium
Enterococcus faecium
Clostridium difficile
Chlamydia spp.
Mycoplasma spp.
Mycobacteria spp.
Legionella spp.

Clostridium difficile is the only anaerobic bacterium with significant resistance to imipenem (1,2,7). Good in vitro activity against *Legionella pneumophila* has been observed, but the drug is probably not a good choice for clinical use, as the organism is intracellular and the drug does not penetrate well (2). Imipenem does not have good activity against *Chlamydia trachomatis* and other *Chlamydia* spp. or *Mycoplasma* spp. (1,2,7). It is not considered adequate therapy for *Mycobacteria* spp. (1,2,7).

IV. CLINICAL PHARMACOLOGY

Neither imipenem nor cilastatin are absorbed after oral administration, so the drug must be given parenterally by either the intravenous or intramuscular route (9). The pharmacological properties of imipenem are somewhat similar to those of third-generation cephalosporins, namely, in its renal clearance and low protein binding (2). In normal adults of average size and normal renal function, a 1000-mg dose administered intravenously over 30 min produces peak levels of 55–65 μg/ml (2). Six hours later, levels are approximately 1 μg/ml (9). Serum levels are linearly related to dosage. In persons with normal renal function, the drug does not accumulate when given at 6-h intervals (2). A 500-mg dose (the usual dose) produces a peak serum level of approximately 35 μg/ml (1). The half-life of imipenem is 1 h (1), and protein binding is approximately 20% (2). Imipenem is widely distributed throughout the body, and following a standard dose of imipenem, levels that are therapeutic have been measured in serum, sputum, lung, skin, muscle, bone, abdominal viscera, peritoneal and pleural fluid, and both aqueous and vitreous humor (2,6). Cerebrospinal fluid levels of imipenem in patients with inflamed meninges have been variable, ranging from 0.5–11 μg/ml (2).

Imipenem is nearly completely eliminated by the kidney (2). In the presence of cilastatin, approximately 70% of the drug is recovered in the urine in 6 h. Most of the remaining drug (20%) is recovered from the urine over the next 120 h as an inactive metabolite (2). Renal handling is through both glomerular filtration and tubular secretion. There is also a nonrenal component that can be unmasked with probenecid, which produces a shift to nonrenal handling of the drug (3). One percent of the drug is excreted in the bile (2). Less than 1% is recovered in the feces, which may account for the minimal effect imipenem has on normal fecal flora. In addition, the intestine has a brush border peptidase that hydrolyzes imipenem, which may function in nonrenal metabolism of the drug (1).

Pharmacokinetic parameters for cilastatin, when given to individuals with normal renal function, are similar to those for imipenem; this includes peak serum levels, volume of distribution, and serum half-life. Cilastatin also undergoes tubular secretion. Approximately 20–30% of administered cilastatin is converted to the *N*-acetyl conjugate, which is twice as active as the parent compound, but whose serum half-life is too short to allow its use in place of cilastatin (9).

Renal clearances of imipenem and cilastatin differ markedly in the presence of renal failure. With a glomerular filtration rate (GFR) of <10 ml/min/1.73 m^2, the serum half-life of imipenem is prolonged from 1 to 3.69 h, but that of cilastatin increases to 17 h. There are no reports of adverse effects from the increase in cilastatin levels. In patients on hemodialysis, the serum half-life of imipenem decreases from 3.69 to 2.45 h and that of cilastatin decreases from 17 to 3.86 h (2).

For glomerular filtration rates of <30 ml/min/1.73 m^2 the dose should be reduced by 50%. If the glomerular filtration rate is <10 ml/min/1.73 m^2, the recommended dosage is 500 mg intravenously every 12 h. If the patient is on hemodialysis, supplemental doses should be administered after each dialysis. No modification of drug dosage is necessary in the presence of hepatic failure (2). Finch et al. (10) have studied the pharmacokinetics of imipenem and cilastatin in six elderly men, ages ranging from 68 to 83, and with creatinine clearances ranging from 31 to 80 ml/min. Half-lives of imipenem and cilastatin were 1.6 ± 0.72 h and 2.1 ± 2.14 h, respectively. Plasma clearances were similar to younger subjects with mild to moderate renal insufficiency. Overall pharmacokinetic parameters correlated with renal function, not age per se (10).

Reported drug interactions with imipenem are limited to interactions with other antibiotics. Synergy with aminoglycosides against *S. aureus*, *Enterococcus*, and *P. aeruginosa* has been reported. Another study has shown synergistic activity of imipenem and amikacin against *P. aeruginosa* in a neutropenic rat model (5,7).

A theoretical consideration is imipenem's role as a potent inducer of chromosomal cephalosporinases. Antagonism of cefoperazone by imipenem has been shown for *S. marcescens* in vitro but not demonstrated in an animal model. The clinical significance of this observation is unknown (5). There are no known interactions with any other class of drugs.

V. CLINICAL INDICATIONS

While ambulatory elderly persons have a lower incidence of acute infections than children or younger adults, they are more at risk for severe complications of infection (11). In addition, once elderly patients enter the hospital they are at a higher risk for nosocomial infection than are younger patients (12). High rates of infection are also reported from other types of institutions, such as skilled nursing facilities and other types of extended care facilities (11). In terms of microbial pathogens, a more diverse variety of pathogens is seen in older patients; aerobic and facultative gram-negative bacilli are seen more often, and there is a higher incidence of mixed infections, that often include anaerobes (13).

Predominant sites of infection in elderly patients vary with the setting. For functional elderly patients in the community, bacterial pneumonias, urinary tact infection and intraabdominal sepsis are seen most commonly. In the chronic care patient, pneumonia, skin and soft tissue infection, and urinary tract infection predominate. The full range of nosocomial infections seen in younger patients—pneumonia, urinary tract infection, wound sepsis, and bacteremia—also occurs in hospitalized elderly patients, but at a higher rate (13).

The diversity of infected sites and microbial pathogens present a wide variety of situations where imipenem could be potentially useful.

A. Respiratory Tract Infection

Pneumonia is a particularly important infection, as it is the leading infectious cause of death in elderly persons (14). Elderly patients presenting with community-acquired pneumonia are most likely to be infected with *Streptococcus pneumoniae*, which accounted for 30–60% of isolates in several reports (12,14). Next in frequency was *H. influenzae*, which represented 2.5–20% of isolates, with increasing incidence in the patient population with chronic lung diseases (14). *S. aureus* was seen in 2–10% of cases in the older patients (14), and gram-negative bacilli show considerable variability in frequency, ranging from 6–37% of isolates (12,14). In patients with nosocomial pneumonias, gram-negative bacilli are the most frequently encountered organisms. Verghese et al. reported a 13% incidence of *Klebsiella pneumoniae* isolates, and a 10–12% incidence of *Pseudomonas aeruginosa* isolates in elderly patients with pneumonia (14). Also important are the other Enterobacteriaceae, *S. aureus*, and *S. pneumoniae*. The true incidence of anaerobic infection is difficult to calculate due to the difficulty of obtaining noncontaminated sputum specimens, but aspiration is felt to play an important role in the more debilitated elderly population (14). Depending on the geographic region, *Legionella pneumophila* takes on varying importance. Its incidence ranges from 0–22% in series of community and nosocomial pneumonia cases (13,14).

The use of imipenem as monotherapy in the treatment of pneumonia has been evaluated in several studies. Salata et al. (15) examined the use of imipenem in 43 patients with pneumonia. Mean patient age was 59.4 years with a range of 28–89. All 14 patients with community-acquired infection obtained either a clinical or microbiological cure. Infectious agents in this series were *H. influenzae*, *S. pneumoniae*, *Enterobacter*, *S. aureus*, and *E. coli*. Of the 29 patients with nosocomial infection, 90% were either clinically or microbiologically cured; 10% failed therapy. All organisms except one *Proteus mirabilis* were initially susceptible to imipenem, but some isolates of *Pseudomonas aeruginosa* developed resistance during therapy (15). In Acar's (16) study of patients with lower respiratory tract infection, 173 of 204 patients were either cured or improved using imipenem. Pathogens in this study were similar to those above: of 31 patients in whom treatment failed, 16 were infected with *P. aeruginosa*. Other treatment failures included pneumonias caused by *H. influenzae*, *Klebsiella pneumoniae*, *S. aureus*, *P. mirabilis*, *Acinetobacter*, and *Enterobacter* (16).

Other investigations utilizing imipenem in open-label trials have included patients with respiratory tract infections (17–21). These studies have shown results comparable to the two studies just discussed with 60–100% of patients either cured or improved. None of the studies have specifically dealt with elderly patients, but the mean ages of the subjects ranged from 54–60 years and the ages of the oldest patient ranged from 70–99 years in these series. Overall, excellent results were obtained with imipenem use in pneumonias caused by the usual community pathogens and the less resistant gram-negative bacilli. *Pseudomonas aeruginosa* isolates were more commonly resistant and accounted for many treatment failures.

With its broad spectrum of antimicrobial activity, imipenem could be a reasonable choice as empiric therapy in the treatment of pneumonia in seriously ill elderly patients, particularly if an anaerobic component or an Entrobacteriaceae species is suspected. This would be most important for the hospitalized patient or person living in a chronic care facility who develops pneumonia. However, most elderly patients with nosocomial or nursing home–acquired pneumonias may be effectively treated with other less potent and less expensive antibiotics (see Chap. 26). Imipenem should be reserved for pneumonias caused by organisms susceptible only to imipenem or for pneumonia in which other drugs have failed (13). If *Pseudomonas aeruginosa* is a prevalent colonizing organism in a hospital and/or the older patient is known to be colonized with this organism, then one of the standard antipseudomonal regimens should be used instead of imipenem. Similarly, the drug is not reliably active against MRSA, and an agent such as vancomycin should be used if this organism is suspected. Imipenem is not active against *Legionella*, so if clinical or epidemiological considerations include this organism in the differential diagnosis, usually erythromycin must be used. This also applies to suspected infections with *Mycoplasma* and *Chlamydia*, including TWAR species.

B. Urinary Tract Infection

While pneumonia is the leading infectious cause of death in elderly people, the most common infectious problem in this population is urinary tract infection (UTI) (22). The urinary tract is the most common site of origin for gram-negative sepsis in geriatric patients (12). The incidence of bacteriuria (bacteriuria may be symptomatic, i.e., UTI, or asymptomatic) rises with age and is seen in at least 10% of men and 20% of women aged 65 and older (12). In nursing homes, the prevalence of UTI and bacteriuria is even higher; frequencies for elderly men are 15%–20% and for elderly women, 25–50% This includes bacteriuria and UTI together (22).

In younger and functionally independent adults, *E. coli* accounts for over 80% of all cases of bacteriuria. However, in the nursing home population, a larger variety of gram-negative bacilli is seen, including *Klebsiella* spp., *Proteus* spp., *Enterobacter* spp., *Citrobacter* spp., *Serratia* spp., and *Pseudomonas* spp. In patients with chronic indwelling urinary catheters, the organisms may be polymicrobial and may include *Enterococcus* (22). *Enterococcus* is particularly a problem in elderly men with chronic indwelling urinary catheters.

Cox and Corrado studied the use of imipenem in 43 patients with complicated urinary tract infection (23). The age of patients ranged from 24–91 years. The most commonly isolated organism in this series was *P. aeruginosa* (25 patients). Other gram-negative bacilli were also seen, and one patient had *Enterococcus*. All patients had good clinical responses and eradication of their organisms (23). In other multicenter studies on imipenem in serious infections, patients with urinary tract infections have been included. Cure rates have been high. In cases where microbiological cure was not achieved, clinical response was usually seen. Organisms associated with relapse were *Serratia marcescens* and *P. aeruginosa* (17–21,24).

In addition to its broad spectrum, imipenem offers the advantage of almost complete urinary excretion, which can allow for low doses in urinary tract infection. Its use can be considered in seriously ill older patients, particularly those with complicated urinary tract infection caused by organisms susceptible only to imipenem.

C. Skin and Soft Tissue Infection

Skin and soft tissue infections, principally infected pressure ulcers, are common in the nursing home population (13). Estimates of pressure sore prevalence range from 3–11% of patients in acute care hospitals to 24–35% of patients in extended care facilities (22).

Culture of these wounds usually shows a variety of skin organisms, such as *S. aureus*, coagulase-negative staphylococci, and diphtheroids. Deeper ulcers are usually colonized by gram-negative bacilli and anaerobic bacteria (22). Although many pressure ulcers do not produce systemic illness or require antibiotics, pressure sores have been shown as a probable cause for 49–76% of bacteremias in two studies (22). Furthermore, pressure ulcer wounds that appear superficial may be covering an active deeper infection and require aggressive therapy.

There are no studies evaluating the role of imipenem strictly in pressure ulcers, but Marier has studied the use of the drug in skin and soft tissue infections, which included carbuncles, abscess, cellulitis, surgical wound infection, and skin ulcers (25). The median age of the patients in the study was 44 years, with a range from 14–89 years. Of 243 patients, 230 had either a clinical cure (56%) or improvement (38%). A variety of gram-positive, gram-negative, and anaerobic etiological agents were isolated. Eight *P. aeruginosa* isolates and one *Enterococcus* isolate acquired resistance to imipenem during treatment. This resistance was associated with clinical failure in two patients. In multicenter studies of imipenem use, comparable results have been seen. Iannini et al. treated 17 patients with skin and soft tissue infection; cure was achieved in 10 of 17 and improvement in 6 other patients. One patient with *Pseudomonas* did not respond (17). Trambore et al. treated nine patients with soft tissue infections. Three of these patients were considered to have failed therapy; of these, two patients had persistent *P. aeruginosa* and another had persistent *Serratia* (18). Nielson et al. studied six patients; cure was achieved in only one, but four were considered clinically improved (20).

The limited use of imipenem in elderly patients with skin and soft tissue structure infection would appear to be as part of empiric therapy in an acutely ill patient in whom drug-resistant bacteria are suspected or in whom other antibiotics have failed. It should probably be used in conjunction with another agent, as some gram-positive organisms may not be sensitive. This is particularly important for methicillin-resistant *S. aureus*, which is usually imipenem-resistant and a major problem in nursing home facilities. Other gram-positive organisms such as *S. epidermidis* and diphtheroid are also resistant to imipenem. Also, it is important to note that antibiotic therapy alone is not likely to be effective in the treatment of an infection that requires surgical debridement, such as a deep pressure ulcer.

D. Intraabdominal Infections

Intraabdominal infections, while not as common as lower respiratory or urinary tract infections in elderly persons, are a particularly important problem because of their associated high mortality rate in this population. This increased mortality is probably due to a variety of factors including atypical and subtle clinical presentations, delay in diagnosis, and, often, a reluctance to perform surgery on elderly individuals who may have multiple underlying medical problems (12,26). Important infections in this group include biliary sepsis, appendicitis, diverticulitis, and intraabdominal abscesses (26).

The incidence of gallstones increases with age (30% of individuals over 70); in addition, the incidence of bacteria in bile increases. Approximately 55% of cultures of bile yield aerobic bacteria only, and 45% of cultures grow both aerobes and anaerobes. Bacteria most commonly encountered are *E. coli*, *K. pneumoniae*, *Enterococcus*, *Enterobacter*, *Bacteroides fragilis*, and *Clostridium* species. Appendicitis in older adults carries an increased incidence of perforation and gangrene. The microbiology is not well studied, but generally in acute uncomplicated appendicitis facultative and aerobic gram-negative bacilli predominate, while in a perforated or gangrenous appendix, increased numbers of anaerobes are isolated. Diverticulitis is a disease of elderly persons, given the increasing incidence of diverticular disease in this age group. Pathogens in this condition are a mixture of aerobic and anaerobic organisms, with anaerobes predominating, reflecting the normal flora of the large bowel. Hepatic abscesses have become primarily a disease of geriatric patients and may be associated with biliary sepsis, diverticulitis, or bowel carcinoma with perforation. Pathogens are therefore associated with these prior conditions and include gram-negative bacilli, anaerobes, and streptococci. Nonhepatic intraabdominal abscesses, however, account for most cases of intraabdominal abscess in elderly patients; pathogens again include gram-negative bacilli, anaerobes, and streptococci (26).

Imipenem has been well studied in intraabdominal sepsis. Kager and Nord evaluated 164 patients with the following types of infection: peritonitis, appendicitis, abscess, and heptobiliary infection (27). An overall clinical cure or improvement was seen in 91% of patients treated with imipenem. Only 3 of 416 bacterial isolates were resistant to imipenem (one *S. epidermidis*, one *Morganella morganii*, one *Fusobacterium*). Three strains of *P. aeruginosa* became resistant during treatment. Comparable results were seen in large studies evaluating imipenem's use in serious infections (17,19–21).

Imipenem has been compared to tobramycin/clindamycin for the treatment of intraabdominal infection. Solomkin (28) compared these two regimens for the treatment of 162 evaluable patients, 43 of whom were $\geq$70 years old. Sites of infection included the biliary tract and large and small bowel. Pathogens were consistent with those previously described. A significant improvement in outcome was seen in the imipenem patients, which was due to fewer failures in patients with gram-negative infection (28). In a similar study, Poenaru et al. found that patients with intraabdominal infections treated with imipenem had fewer febrile episodes and occurrences of breakthrough bacteremia (29). Two cases of *Xanthomonas maltophilia* resistant to imipenem were seen.

These and other studies indicate a potential role for imipenem in the treatment of intraabdominal infection in elderly patients, particularly in patients who acquire their infections in the community. It may be considered as an alternative agent for initial therapy prior to obtaining the results of culture and sensitivity data. Currently, initial empiric therapy is generally with a second- or third-generation cephalosporin, ampicillin-sulbactam, or a combination of clindamycin or metronidazole plus an aminoglycoside or quinolone (see Chap. 26). An important aspect of imipenem is its lack of nephrotoxicity. This is particularly important in the elderly group of patients, who may have other medical conditions that place them at increased risk for aminoglycoside toxicity.

E. Bacteremia

Although bloodstream infections must be considered in the context of the underlying etiology, some special considerations apply to bacteremic infections in the elderly patient. As with other infections, physiological responses may be blunted, making diagnosis more difficult (12). Mortality from bloodstream infection is high; up to 34% mortality from community-acquired infection and 47% from nosocomial bacteremia have been reported (16). McCue, in a study of gram-negative bacteremia in elderly patients, found no overall age-related increase in mortality, but did document increased mortality from bacteremia when underlying disease was present (30). Mortality from bacteremia occurring in elderly patients increases when one or more of the following is present: *S. aureus* bacteremia, bacteremia secondary to pneumonia, age >85, and total peripheral white blood cell count <5000/mm^3 (12).

In one study of 100 community-acquired bloodstream infections in elderly patients, the urinary tract was the most common focus (34%), followed by the biliary tract (20%), lung (13%), and abdomen (8%). In 11% of cases no source was documented. The authors found that only three organisms—*S. aureus*, *E. coli*, and *K. pneumoniae*—accounted for 73% of the total number of bacteremias (31).

Eron (32) has evaluated the use of imipenem in 135 patients with bacteremia and signs of infection. In this study, the ages ranged from 15–91 years, with a mean age of 50. The most common pathogens were *S. aureus*, *Streptococcus* spp., and *E. coli*. Imipenem produced clinical cure or improvement in 90% of patients. Only one patient's isolate broke through therapy—a susceptible *Clostridium septicum*; resistance developed in two *P. aeruginosa* isolates (32).

As with other infections, imipenem can be considered in the initial management of an elderly patient with suspected bacteremia of unknown cause or as therapy in patients with proven bacteremia in which final culture and susceptibility results indicate imipenem as the only effective drug.

F. Meningitis

Imipenem has excellent antimicrobial activity against the most common causes of meningitis: *S. pneumoniae*, *H. influenzae*, and *N. meningitidis*, as well as *Listeria monocytogenes* and most gram-negative bacilli, the latter two organisms assuming greater importance in elderly patients. However, due to the increased incidence of imipenem-related seizures in patients with ongoing central nervous system (CNS) disease, the use of imipenem as antibiotic therapy in meningitis should probably be avoided.

VI. ADMINISTRATION OF DRUG

The usual dose of imipenem/cilastatin is 500 mg every 6–8 h (1). For an elderly patient of small body weight, the total dose should be 25 mg/kg/day, given in four divided doses (2). The dosage range, in normal renal function, depending upon the severity of infection, is 250–1000 mg every 6 h (2).

Imipenem can also be given intramuscularly. This route of delivery could be potentially useful for some elderly patients if early discontinuation of intravenous therapy could lead to earlier discharge to home or an extended care facility. Garau and Calandra studied 20 patients with mild to moderate infections using imipenem 500 mg two to three times a day. All patients responded to and tolerated therapy well (33). Only parenteral dosage is used; the drug is not absorbed from the gastrointestinal tract (9).

VII. DRUG MONITORING AND ADVERSE EFFECTS

The reported adverse effects of imipenem are few and generally minor, with the exception of seizures. Other reported adverse reactions are nausea, vomiting, diarrhea, phlebitis at the infusion site, and allergic reactions (1).

As with all β-lactam antibiotics, hypersensitivity is a consideration. In a study of the first 2516 patients to receive imipenem, no anaphylactic reactions were reported. Rash or drug fever occurred in 2.7% of the 2516 patients. However, patients with a history of severe β-lactam allergy were excluded from the study (2). Although the degree of cross-reactivity between imipenem and the other classes of β-lactam antibiotics has not been determined, this cross-reactivity is felt to be similar to that of penicillins and cephalosporins. Patients having IgE-mediated responses to minor penicillin determinants also have reactivity to the analogous imipenem determinants (34). It is recommended that imipenem not be used in the severely penicillin-allergic patient.

Nausea and vomiting were observed in 4% of patients receiving imipenem. When these reactions occurred, it was most often during infusion of the drug. Nausea may be relieved by slowing down the infusion rate, but can be so severe that the drug must be discontinued (35). Diarrhea was observed in 3% of patients in the initial studies (2), and only 0.16% of the total patient population had documented pseudomembranous colitis (35). The low incidence of diarrhea and *Clostridium difficile* may be due to the low levels of antibiotic that reaches the stool. Approximately 5% of patients experienced phlebitis at the infusion site (35).

The most serious adverse effect associated with imipenem has been seizures. In the original clinical studies, 1.5% of patients treated with imipenem developed seizures (35). In other studies, the incidence has ranged from 1 to 3% (35,36). Although the reported initial incidence of seizures was no worse than the incidence in patients receiving other β-lactam antibiotics (1), imipenem has been considered to be more epileptogenic by some investigators.

Calandra et al. (36) retrospectively analyzed seizures in patients receiving imipenem. Of 1700 patients, seizures occurred in 52 (3%). Nine of these patients also had seizures while on other drugs. Types of seizures included tonic/clonic, focal, and myoclonic. The average time of seizure onset was 7 days after beginning imipenem therapy. Patient characteristics associated with seizure development were decreased creatinine clearance, lower body weight, older age group, and CNS abnormalities. However, when a stepwise regression analysis was performed, age was not a factor. The following factors were significant: prior history of seizures, other CNS lesions, excess imipenem dosage, renal insufficiency, and *Pseudomonas aeruginosa* infection (independent of imipenem dosage). There was no association with age, sex, and concurrent aminophylline or cimetidine administration. No apparent interaction with electrolyte abnormalities, prior burn injury, ethanol consumption, or use of hyperbaric oxygen therapy was seen. The highest incidence of seizures is seen in patients with decreased renal functions. The reasons for this association are incompletely understood, but include a theoretical increase in permeability of the blood-brain barrier and increasing quantitative significance of a cilastatin insensitive nonrenal dipeptidase. The metabolite of this process has been proposed as a causative factor (36).

A number of minor laboratory test abnormalities in association with imipenem use have been seen in initial clinical studies. These include minor liver function test abnormalities, eosinophilia, a positive Coombs' test, elevated prothrombin time, thrombocytopenia, leukopenia, thrombocytosis, and increased blood urea nitrogen. It should be emphasized that all of the abnormalities were mild and were reversible upon discontinuation of the drug. No significant bleeding diatheses were observed (35).

In rabbit studies acute proximal tubular necrosis was seen when doses exceeding 100 mg/kg were used. It is postulated that a toxic metabolite, as yet unidentified, accumulates in the renal tubular epithelium. The histological damage is similar to the damage seen with cephaloridine. The nephrotoxicity of imipenem is, however, completely eliminated with the co-administration of cilastatin. Presumably the mechanism is through preventing metabolism of the drug to its toxic metabolite(s). Thus the combined imipenem/cilastatin preparation in current clinical use does not cause nephrotoxicity (3). As with other β-lactam antibiotics, it is not necessary to monitor drug levels.

REFERENCES

1. Lipman B, Neu HC. Imipenem: A new carbapenem antibiotic. Med Clin North Am 1988; 72:567–79.
2. Hellinger WC, Brewer NS. Imipenem. Mayo Clinic Proc 1991; 66:1074–81.
3. Birnbaum J, Kahan FM, Kropp H, et al. Carbapenems, a new class of β-lactam antibiotics. Discovery and development of imipenem/cilastatin. Am J Med 1985; 78(suppl 6A):3–21.
4. Mandell GL, Sande MA. Penicillins, cephalosporins, and other β-lactam antibiotics. In: Gilman A, Rall T, Nies A, Taylor P, eds. The pharmacological basis of therapeutics. New York: Pergamon Press, 1991:1065–97.
5. Neu HC. Carbapenems. Special properties contributing to their activity. Am J Med 1985; 78(suppl 6A):33–40.
6. Rice LB, Eliopoulos GM. Imipenem and aztreonam: current role in antimicrobial therapy. In: Remington J, Swartz M, eds. Current clinical topics in infectious diseases. Cambridge, MA: Blackwell Scientific, 1989:109–20.
7. Jones RN. Review of the in vitro spectrum of activity of imipenem. Am J Med 1985; 78(suppl 6A):22–32.
8. Hureburt S, Cuchural GJ, Tally FP. Imipenem resistance in *Bacteriodes distasonis* mediated by a novel β-lactamase. Antimicrob Agents Chemother 1990; 34:117–20.
9. Drusano GL, Standiford HC. Pharmacokinetic profile of imipenem/cilastatin in normal volunteers. Am J Med 1985; 78(suppl 6A):47–53.
10. Finch RG, Craddock C, Kelly J, et al. Pharmacokinetic studies of imipenem/cilastatin in elderly patients. J Antimicrob Chemother 1986; 18(suppl E):103–7.
11. Garibaldi RA, Nurse BA. Infections in the elderly. Am J Med 1986; 81(suppl 1A):53–8.
12. Bryan CS. Serious infection in the elderly. Update an septicemia, pneumonia, meningitis, endocarditis, GI infections, UTI, and FUO. Consultant 1989; 29:41–53.
13. Yoshikawa TT. Antimicrobial therapy for the elderly patient. J Am Geriatr Soc 1990; 38:1353–72.
14. Verghese A, Berk SL. Bacterial pneumonia in the elderly. Medicine (Balt.) 1983; 62:271–85.
15. Salata RA, Gebhart RL, Palmer DL, et al. Pneumonia treated with imipenem/cilastatin. Am J Med 1985; 78(suppl 6A):104–9.
16. Acar JF. Therapy for lower respiratory tract infections with imipenem/cilastatin: a review of worldwide experience. Rev Infect Dis 1985; 7(suppl 3):513–17.
17. Iannini PB, Kunkel MJ, Hilton E, et al. Imipenem/cilastatin: general experience in a community hospital. Am J Med 1985; 78(suppl 6A):122–6.
18. Trambore D, Pontzer R, Levison ME, et al. Multicenter study of the clinical efficacy of imipenem/cilastatin for treatment of serious infections. Rev Infect Dis 1985; 7(suppl 3):S476–81.
19. Brooks RG, McCabe RE, Vosti KL, et al. Open trial of imipenem/cilastatin therapy for serious bacterial infections. Rev Infect Dis 1985; 7(suppl 3):496–505.
20. Nielson DM, Katz JR, AhLoy RD, et al. Imipenem/cilastatin therapy for serious bacterial infections. Rev Infect Dis 1985; 7(suppl 3):S506–12.
21. Shah PR. Clinical experience with imipenem/cilastatin: analysis of a multicenter study. Rev Infect Dis 1985; 7(suppl 3):471–5.
22. Norman DC, Castle SC, Cantrell M. Infections in the nursing home. J Am Geriatr Soc 1987; 35:796–805.
23. Cox CE, Corrado ML. Safety and efficacy of imipenem/cilastatin in treatment of complicated urinary tract infections. Am J Med 1985; 78(suppl 6A):92–4.
24. Chiodini PL, Geddes AM, Smith EG, et al. Imipenem/cilastatin in the treatment of serious bacterial infections. Rev Infect Dis 1985; 7(suppl 3):490–5.

25. Marier RL. Role of imipenem/cilastatin in the treatment of soft tissue infections. Am J Med 1985; 78(suppl 6A):140–4.
26. Norman DC, Yoshikawa TT. Intraabdominal infections in the elderly. J Am Geriatr Soc 1983; 37:677–84.
27. Kager L, Nord CE. Imipenem/cilastatin in the treatment of intraabdominal infections: a review of worldwide experience. Rev Infect Dis 1983; 7(suppl 3):518–21.
28. Solomkin JS. Results of a multicenter trial comparing imipenem/cilastatin to tobramycin/clindamycin for intraabdominal infection. Ann Surg 1990; 212:581–91.
29. Poenaru D, DeSantis M, Christou NV. Imipenem versus tobramycin—antianaerobe antibiotic therapy in intra-abdominal infections. Can J Surg 1990; 33:415–22.
30. McCue JD. Gram-negative bacillary bacteremia in the elderly: incidence, ecology, etiology, and mortality. J Am Geriatr Soc 1987; 35:213–18.
31. Esposito AL, Gleckman RA, Cram S, et al. Community-acquired bacteremia in the elderly: analysis of one hundred consecutive episodes. J Am Geriatr Soc 1980; 28:315–19.
32. Eron LJ. Imipenem/cilastatin therapy of bacteremia. Am J Med 1985; 78(suppl 6A):95–9.
33. Garau J, Calandra GB. Intramuscular imipenem/cilastatin in multiple-dose treatment regimens: review of the worldwide clinical experience. Chemotherapy 1991; 37(suppl 2):44–52.
34. Sadon A, Gilden BN, Bohr AS, et al. Immediate hypersensitivity reactions to β-lactam antibiotics. Ann Intern Med 1987; 127:204–15.
35. Calandra GB, Brown KR, Grad LC, et al. Review of adverse experiences and tolerability in the first 2,516 patients treated with imipenem/cilastatin. Am J Med 1985; 78(suppl 6A):73–8.
36. Calandra G, Lydick E, Carrigan J, et al. Factors predisposing to seizures in seriously ill infected patients receiving antibiotics: experience with imipenem/cilastatin. Am J Med 1988; 84:911–18.

11

Beta-Lactamase Inhibitors

Jay P. Rho
University of Southern California School of Medicine and Shriners Hospital, Los Angeles, California

Fawn C. S. Takemoto and Ariane An
Veterans Affairs Medical Center—West Los Angeles, Los Angeles, California

Dean C. Norman
University of California and Veterans Affairs Medical Center—West Los Angeles, Los Angeles, California

I. INTRODUCTION

Almost immediately after the introduction of penicillin in the early 1940s, bacterial strains of *Bacillus coli* (now referred to as *Escherichia coli*) with the ability to produce enzymes capable of inactivating the penicillin molecule were discovered. Identified as penicillinase, the enzyme catalyzed the hydrolysis of the β-lactam nucleus of penicillin, which resulted in the antibiotic's inactivation (1). Penicillinase was also identified by Kirby in 1944 as the principal reason for penicillin resistance in an extract of *Staphylococcus* (2). Since these early discoveries of "penicillin-inactivating enzymes," bacteria capable of producing these β-lactamases have become more widespread. In response to this epidemiological problem, numerous attempts to counteract the actions of β-lactamases have been investigated. Generally, two approaches have been taken to protect β-lactam antibiotics against the actions of β-lactamases: (1) β-lactam antibiotics are chemically modified to improve stability against β-lactamase hydrolysis, which has resulted in the development of the semisynthetic penicillins (e.g., oxacillin, nafcillin) and, more recently, monobactams (e.g., aztreonam) and carbapenems (e.g., imipenem), or (2) protective, nonantimicrobial drugs (e.g., clavulanic acid, sulbactam, and tazobactam) capable of inhibiting β-lactamase activity are coadministered with a β-lactam antibiotic.

The focus of this chapter will be on the latter approach—the coadministration of β-lactamase inhibitors. In discussing the merits of various inhibitors, both commercially available and in development, one must consider the characteristics or properties that an ideal β-lactamase inhibitor should exhibit: (1) activity against a wide range of β-lactamase enzymes, (2) activity at physiologically attainable tissue and fluid concentrations, (3) pharmacology similar to that of the partner antimicrobial, (4) minimal intrinsic toxicity, and (5) reasonable cost (3).

While β-lactam antimicrobials may be inactivated by enzymes other than β-lactamases, such as acylases and esterases, bacterial production of β-lactamases remains the single most important mechanism of resistance (4). Specifically, β-lactamases inactivate β-lactam antibiotics by hydrolyzing the cyclic amide bond in the β-lactam ring to form acidic derivatives that have no antibacterial properties (5). All gram-negative and certain gram-positive organisms are capable of producing β-lactamase. Beta-lactamases produced by gram-negative organisms are usually concentrated in the periplasmic space and not excreted. Beta-lactamases produced by gram-positive bacteria may be excreted extracellularly (6–8).

Genetic information for encoding β-lactamase production may reside on the bacterial chromosome or on plasmids. Beta-lactamases may be also be subclassified as inducible or constitutively produced. Inducible β-lactamases are produced after exposure to a β-lactam, whereas constitutive β-lactamases are not affected by β-lactam exposure. Gram-negative bacteria can produce both chromosomally mediated and plasmid-mediated β-lactamases. Gram-positive bacteria usually produce plasmid-mediated β-lactamases (5,7,9).

A variety of microbial β-lactamases exist and different classification schemes have been reviewed (10,11). One of the earliest attempts to classify β-lactamases was by Sawai et al. in 1968, who listed three types of β-lactamases: penicillinases (enzymes that prefer to hydrolyze penicillins), inducible cephalosporinases (enzymes that prefer to hydrolyze cephalosporins), and broad-spectrum β-lactamases (enzymes that hydrolyze both selected penicillins and cephalosporins) (12). In 1973, Richmond and Sykes outlined a scheme designating five classes of β-lactamases from gram-negative bacteria (I–V) based on substrate profiles, isoelectric points, inhibition data, and genetic origin (13). Neu describes a sixth class of β-lactamase isolated from *Bacteroides* which hydrolyze cephalosporins better than penicillins (14). While the Richmond classification scheme has gained widespread acceptance, one major limitation has been the exclusion of β-lactamases produced from gram-positive bacteria. Ambler proposed, in 1980, a new classification scheme consisting of two classes of β-lactamases, A and B, based on amino acid sequences and molecular structure (15). A third class of β-lactamases, C, was subsequently added to the Ambler scheme by Jaurin and Grundström in 1981 (16).

II. CHEMISTRY

Produced by the fermentation of *Streptomyces clavuligerus*, clavulanic acid is a naturally occurring bicyclic β-lactam structurally similar to the penicillin nucleus. Chemically, clavulanic acid is 3-(2-hydroxyethylidene)-7-oxo-4-oxa-1-azabicyclo [3.2.0] heptane-2-carboxylic acid and has a molecular weight of 199.16. Clavulanic acid differs from penicillin in that it does not have an acylamino side chain, substitutes an oxygen atom in place of the sulfur, and has a hydroxyethylidene substituent in the oxazolidine ring (17). While clavulanic acid is a potentially useful agent in combination with a variety of penicillins and cephalosporins, it is currently marketed in combination with amoxicillin (Augmentin®) for oral administration and ticarcillin disodium (Timentin®) for parenteral administration.

Sulbactam is a semisynthetic β-lactamase inhibitor chemically described as (2S-cis)-3,3-dimethyl-7-oxo-4-thia-1-azabicyclo[3.2.0]heptane-2-carboxylic acid 4,4-dioxide and has a molecular weight of 233.24. Sulbactam, a penicillanic acid sulfone, is a simple derivative of the basic penicillin nucleus. Commercially, sulbactam is available in combination with ampicillin sodium (Unasyn®) for parenteral administration. Investigationally, sulbactam has been combined with cefoperazone as a parenteral agent.

Tazobactam is a triazolymethyl penicillanic acid sulfone. The chemical name for tazobactam is [2s-(2α,3β,5α)]-3-methyl-7-oxo-3-(1H-1,2,3-triazol-1-ylmethyl)-4-thia-1-azabicyclo-[3.2.0]-heptane-2-carboxylic acid 4,4-dioxide and has a molecular weight of 300.30. Tazobactam was developed by Taiho Pharmaceutical Company, Ltd., Tokyo, Japan, and is often designated as YTR830 in clinical trials. Investigationally, tazobactam has been paired primarily with piperacillin as a parenteral agent.

III. MECHANISMS OF ACTION

The interaction between a β-lactamase inhibitor and β-lactamase enzyme may be described as reversible competitive, irreversible competitive, or noncompetitive. Noncompetitive inhibitors bind the β-lactamase enzyme at a site away from the catalytic site and cause the enzyme to lose its function by changing its conformation. In contrast to the noncompetitive inhibitors, competitive inhibitors compete with the substrate (β-lactams susceptible to β-lactamase) for the active site of the β-lactamase. With reversible competitive inhibitors, no permanent chemical interaction takes place, so its removal from the active site of the β-lactamase enzyme results in a freed β-lactamase that can again act upon the substrate. Irreversible competitive inhibitors inactivate β-lactamases through covalent chemical interactions that eventually result in the destruction of both enzymatic activity and the inhibitor itself. The β-lactamase is not regenerated upon removal of the inhibitor (3,11).

Clavulanic acid, sulbactam, and tazobactam share similar inhibitory profiles and are examples of irreversible competitive inhibitors (14). Clavulanic acid penetrates through the bacterial cell wall and is able to enter the periplasmic space of gram-negative bacteria where it interacts with the β-lactamases. Clavulanic acid has been shown to bind to both intracellular and extracellular β-lactamases. In contrast, sulbactam, a penicillanic acid sulfone, is limited by a decreased ability to enter the bacterial cell wall. Clavulanic acid, sulbactam, and tazobactam generally have poor intrinsic antimicrobial activity at physiologically achievable concentrations, and therefore their usefulness is dependent entirely on their ability to inhibit β-lactamases.

In vitro studies indicate that clavulanic acid generally inhibits β-lactamases that are produced by *Staphylococcus*, *Bacteroides fragilis*, and *Moraxella catarrhalis*, as well as Richmond-Sykes types II, III, IV, and V β-lactamases. Clavulanic acid generally does not inhibit inducible, chromosomally mediated cephalosporinases classified as Richmond-Sykes type I. Clavulanic acid's specific mechanism of inactivation can vary among the different systems. When clavulanic acid (I) reacts with a β-lactamase to form an acyl enzyme (E-I), there are several potential fates for this entity, including (1) an enzyme-substrate complex with eventual destruction of clavulanate to a hydrolysis product (P) and release of free enzyme (E), (2) transiently inhibited forms (E-T), or (3) an irreversibly inactivated enzyme complex (E-I*). Thus, clavulanic acid may behave like a susceptible substrate, reversible inhibitor, or irreversible inhibitor depending upon the relative ratios of E + P, E-T, and E-I* formed (18).

Sulbactam is considered to be 2–5 times less potent a β-lactamase inhibitor than clavulanic acid on a weight-to-weight basis, although this can be compensated for by increasing the sulbactam concentration (19). With clavulanate, cephalosporinases are inhibited less effectively than penicillinases or broad-spectrum β-lactamases. In vitro, sulbactam may have a slightly broader spectrum of inhibition than clavulanic acid and has been shown to be an effective inhibitor of β-lactamases of the Richmond types II, III, IV, and V, which are either plasmid or chromosomally mediated. Sulbactam has poor inhibitory activity against chromosomally mediated, inducible, or constitutive β-lactamases found in *Proteus*, *Citrobacter*, and *Enterobacter* (20). Sulbactam is also reported to inhibit type VI β-lactamases from *B. fragilis* (14). Although the primary mechanism of protection appears to be its ability to inhibit hydrolysis by β-lactamase enzymes, sulbactam also exhibits high-affinity binding to penicillin-binding proteins (PBP), such as PBP Ia of *Escherichia coli*.

Tazobactam, like clavulanic acid and sulbactam, is an irreversible inhibitor of Richmond types II, III, IV, and V β-lactamases (21,22). Comparative activity against β-lactamase–producing anaerobes has been reported to be relatively equal among the three inhibitors (23). Against chromosomally mediated Richmond type I β-lactamases, however, tazobactam has been reported to demonstrate the best activity of the three β-lactamase inhibitors (22,24).

IV. ANTIMICROBIAL SPECTRUM

Bacteria can develop resistance to the actions of β-lactam antibiotics through several different means, including alterations in receptor sites on penicillin-binding proteins or alterations in porin proteins on the outer membranes, that can limit the penetration of β-lactam antibiotics into the periplasmic space (25,26). The production of β-lactamase enzymes, however, remains the primary mechanism by which bacteria resist the actions of β-lactam antibiotics (4). As one would therefore expect, the combination of a β-lactamase inhibitor with selected β-lactam antibiotics has been shown to expand the antimicrobial spectrum of those β-lactam antibiotics to many otherwise resistant organisms. The susceptibility patterns given below are generalizations only and are not substitutes for the actual susceptibility patterns of individual institutions. This is particularly true for tertiary care hospitals in which antimicrobial resistance is a major problem.

Ampicillin as a single agent has activity against most gram-positive bacteria including *Streptococcus pneumoniae*, *Enterococcus faecalis*, non–penicillinase-producing staphylococci, *Listeria monocytogenes*, gram-negative bacteria including *Salmonella*, *Shigella*, and non–β-lactamase–producing strains of *Neisseria gonorrhoeae*, *Haemophilus influenzae*, *E. coli*, and *Proteus mirabilis*, as well as most anaerobic bacteria. The addition of sulbactam has been shown to expand ampicillin's spectrum of activity to include β-lactamase–producing *Staphylococcus*, *Klebsiella*, *Enterobacter*, *Serratia*, *Citrobacter*, and *Bacteroides* spp. Of relevance to the elderly population, this combination has no activity against methicillin-resistant *Staphylococcus aureus* and certain hospital-acquired aerobic gram-negative bacilli such as *Pseudomonas* spp. and *Acinetobacter* spp. These bacteria are capable of developing resistance through mechanisms not attributable to β-lactamase production.

Amoxicillin, as an oral analog of ampicillin, has a spectrum of activity identical to that of ampicillin. However, as an oral agent, antimicrobial activity is primarily limited by achievable plasma concentrations. Just as sulbactam expands ampicillin's antimicrobial spectrum, clavulanic acid expands the activity of amoxicillin to include β-lactamase–producing aerobic gram-positive, gram-negative, and anaerobic bacteria that would otherwise be resistant.

Ticarcillin alone is a broad-spectrum antibiotic that has good activity against most aerobic gram-positive, gram-negative (including *Enterobacter* and *Pseudomonas aeruginosa*), and anaerobic bacteria. Ticarcillin, as is the case with ampicillin, is susceptible to degradation by β-lactamases. The addition of clavulanic acid to ticarcillin expands activity to many otherwise resistant organisms including β-lactamase–producing strains of *H. influenzae*, *N. gonorrhoeae*, *Staphylococcus* spp., and many species of *Enterobacteriaceae*, especially *Klebsiella pneumoniae*, *Citrobacter diversus*, and *Proteus vulgaris* (27,28). In a study of 51 clinical isolates of ticarcillin-resistant, gram-negative bacilli, the addition of clavulanic acid to ticarcillin was shown to lower minimal inhibitory concentrations (MICs) at least threefold in the vast majority of isolates. Of note, against 8 strains of ticarcillin-resistant *P. aeruginosa*, only 1 strain was inhibited by the addition of clavulanic acid (29). In an in vitro test against 32 strains of ticarcillin-resistant *B. fragilis*, the combination of ticarcillin plus clavulanic acid was shown to inhibit all 32 strains (30).

Cefoperazone, like ticarcillin, has a broad spectrum of activity against gram-positive, gram-negative (including some strains of *P. aeruginosa*), and anaerobic bacteria. Cefoperazone is stable against plasmid-mediated, chromosomally mediated inducible β-lactamases in the *Enterobacteriaceae* and *Pseudomonas* families (31). It has been reported that cefoperazone in combination with sulbactam is synergistic against virtually all cefoperazone-resistant isolates of *E. coli*, *K. pneumoniae*, *Citrobacter* spp., *Providencia* spp., and *Enterobacter* spp.; however, no synergistic activity was evident against cefoperazone-resistant *Pseudomonas* strains (32). However, in another study, 27 of 40 (67%) *Pseudomonas* spp. that were originally resistant to cefoperazone (MIC $\geq$ 64 μg/ml) had at least a twofold reduction in MICs to the 2:1 combination of cefoperazone and sulbactam (33).

Piperacillin is also a broad-spectrum antibiotic with good activity against gram-positive, gram-negative, and anaerobic bacteria. The in vitro activity of piperacillin combined with tazobactam at a ratio of 8:1 was compared to that of ticarcillin/clavulanic acid against 5889 aerobic isolates and 60 strains from the *B. fragilis* group (34). Piperacillin/tazobactam was consistently equal to or slightly more active than ticarcillin/clavulanic acid against all staphylococci, *Streptococcus* spp., and enterococci. Against nonenteric gram-negative bacilli, piperacillin/tazobactam inhibited 86% of strains tested compared with 33% for ticarcillin/clavulanic acid. Against anaerobes, piperacillin/tazobactam inhibited all 60 strains tested (34).

V. CLINICAL PHARMACOLOGY

A. Amoxicillin/Clavulanate Potassium

Both amoxicillin trihydrate and clavulanate potassium are stable in the presence of gastric acid and are well absorbed following oral administration. Serum concentrations of amoxicillin and clavulanic acid do not differ significantly whether they are coadministered or given separately. Peak serum concentrations usually occur 1–2.5 h following oral administration for both amoxicillin and clavulanic acid. No accumulation of either drug appears to occur even after multiple dosing in healthy adult subjects (35,36). Amoxicillin/clavulanic acid absorption does not appear to be influenced by coadministration with food (35,37–40), milk (39), antacids (39,40), or ranitidine (40). Coadministration with cimetidine, however, has been reported to result in statistically significant increases in maximum serum concentration (C_{max}) and area under the plasma concentration-time curve (AUC) values (approximately 15–30%) for both amoxicillin and clavulanic acid (39). Although this has not been demonstrated with antacids or ranitidine, the authors postulate that cimetidine may increase intraluminal pH and therefore the solubility of amoxicillin and clavulanic acid.

Clavulanic acid and amoxicillin both distribute extensively into body tissues and fluids such as blister fluids (36), synovial fluid (41), noninfected ascites (42), and peritoneal fluid (43). Less than 10% of peak serum concentrations, however, distribute to bone (41), sputum (44), and saliva (45). Neither clavulanic acid nor amoxicillin penetrate sufficiently into the cerebrospinal fluid (CSF) for clinical use in the treatment of bacterial meningitis (46). Both clavulanic acid and amoxicillin cross the placenta and achieve approximately 50% of their respective serum concentrations in amniotic fluids (47,48). At concentrations of 1–100 μg/ml, clavulanic acid is approximately 22–30% bound to human serum proteins, while amoxicillin is approximately 17–20% bound to serum proteins (49).

Serum concentrations of amoxicillin and clavulanic acid both decline in a biphasic manner. The mean elimination half-lives of amoxicillin and clavulanic acid are 1.3 h and 1 h, respectively (35,36,50,51,52). Mean total clearances for both amoxicillin and clavulanic acid are approximately 25 L/h (35). After oral administration, amoxicillin is excreted largely unchanged in urine with about 60–80% of drug recovered intact after 6 h. Clavulanic acid is more extensively metabolized with the major metabolite being 1-amino-4-hydrooxy-butan-2-one. Thirty to fifty percent of the administered dose is recovered intact in urine after 6 h (35,36,50–52).

Studies that have examined the effect of age on the pharmacokinetics of amoxicillin/clavulanic acid have been conducted primarily in pediatric subjects, with little change reported in their pharmacokinetic profiles. Formal studies examining the pharmacokinetics of the combination drugs as a function of old age have not been reported. However, several studies have indicated that the pharmacokinetics of amoxicillin/clavulanic acid are associated with the degree of renal impairment (51,53,54). The total body and renal clearances of both amoxicillin and clavulanic acid decline with diminishing renal function. As renal function has been shown to be significantly influenced by the aging process (55), dosage adjustments for impaired renal function should be carefully considered when dosing elderly patients.

B. Ticarcillin Disodium/Clavulanate Potassium

The pharmacokinetics of intravenously administered clavulanic acid and ticarcillin disodium have also been studied as separate drugs and in combination. No significant effect on any pharmacokinetic value for either drug is in evidence when the two drugs are coadministered. Immediately upon completion of a 30-min intravenous infusion of 3 g of ticarcillin and 0.1 g of clavulanic acid, peak serum concentrations have been reported to range from 293 to 388 μg/ml for ticarcillin (mean 324 μg/ml) and 5.3–10.3 μg/ml for clavulanic acid (mean 8.0 μg/ml) (56).

As is the case with amoxicillin/clavulanic acid, ticarcillin/clavulanic acid distributes readily into many tissues and fluids. Clavulanic acid has a higher volume of distribution than does ticarcillin, with steady-state values at 16.3 and 8.98 L, respectively (56). The tissue penetration of ticarcillin/clavulanic acid was examined, and it was found that both agents penetrated blister fluid rapidly with peak blister fluid to serum level ratios of 58% and 77% for ticarcillin and clavulanic acid, respectively, at 1 h (57).

The elimination half-lives for both ticarcillin and sulbactam are approximately 1 h. Clavulanic acid is more extensively metabolized than is ticarcillin with renal clearance accounting for only 43% of total plasma clearance. Renal clearance for ticarcillin is approximately 70% of total plasma clearance (56). Seventy-five percent of the administered dose of ticarcillin and 52% of the clavulanic acid dose can be recovered unchanged in urine after 6 h (58).

Studies specifically evaluating the effect of age on the pharmacokinetics of ticarcillin/clavulanic acid are not available. However, as is the case with amoxicillin/clavulanic acid, studies regarding the behavior of ticarcillin/clavulanic acid in patients with renal impairment should provide a reasonable guideline for prescribing this drug in elderly patients. The influence of abnormal renal function on the pharmacokinetics of ticarcillin has been examined. The normal half-life of ticarcillin rises from 71 min in individuals with normal renal function to 3.7 h in patients with creatinine clearances of <10 ml/min. Therefore, it has been suggested that the dosage interval be increased as renal function declines (60).

C. Ampicillin Sodium/Sulbactam

Sulbactam is not well absorbed by humans when administered orally and must be administered parenterally. Certain ester formulations of sulbactam, such as sultamicillin, the tosylate salt of the double ester of sulbactam and ampicillin, demonstrate 80% bioavailability in clinical trials; however, they have yet to reach the commercial market (60–62).

Immediately following a 15-min, single-dose, intravenous infusion of ampicillin 2 g and sulbactam 1 g, mean peak serum concentrations of 120 and 60 μg/ml are reached, respectively. When given in multiple doses, generally no accumulation of either ampicillin or sulbactam occurs in healthy adults. After intramuscular injection, both ampicillin and sulbactam reach 100% of bioavailability, with peak concentrations occurring within 30 min (63).

The apparent volume of distributions for ampicillin and sulbactam at steady state are similar, with both drugs being detectable at significant levels in intraperitoneal fluid (64), blister fluid (65), appendix (66), bile and biliary tissue (67), intestinal mucosa (68), and female genital tissue (69). Penetration into CSF occurs primarily in the presence of inflamed meninges (70–72). Appreciable concentrations of ampicillin and sulbactam have also been found in samples of prostate and appendiceal tissue (73). Both sulbactam and ampicillin readily cross the placental barrier (74), and excretion into human milk has also been reported (75).

The mean elimination half-lives for ampicillin and sulbactam are almost identical at approximately 1 h in healthy subjects. Sulbactam is primarily eliminated by renal excretion with renal clearance (mean 12.2 L/h) accounting for 77% of total clearance (15.7 L/h). More than 75% of an administered dose can be recovered unchanged in urine within the first 8–12 h (63,65).

The pharmacokinetic values after administration of ampicillin/sulbactam reveal distinct pharmacokinetic differences for young and old healthy subjects. As would be expected from two drugs that are dependent on renal excretion as their primary means of elimination, age-related declines in renal function correspond closely with a decline in total drug clearance for both drugs. Elimination half-lives about 1.5 times longer for both ampicillin and sulbactam after a single dose administration and significantly increased area under the concentration-time curves (AUC) in healthy elderly subjects compared to young subjects have been reported. Neither ampicillin nor sulbactam was shown to be at risk for achieving toxic levels in elderly subjects despite the reduction in clearance (76).

D. Cefoperazone/Sulbactam

The pharmacokinetics of cefoperazone and sulbactam have been investigated individually and in combination (77–82). After a 2-g cefoperazone/ 1-g sulbactam intravenous infusion over 15 min, peak serum concentrations have been reported at 208 and 29 μg/ml, respectively, in patients with normal renal function (81). Following 2-g intramuscular injections of cefoperazone, peak serum concentrations range from 97 to 111 μg/ml within 1–2 h.

Serum protein binding of cefoperazone is approximately 90% (78) but only 38% for sulbactam (83). Both cefoperazone and sulbactam are extensively distributed throughout body tissues and fluids. Cefoperazone penetration into CSF during bacterial meningitis has been reported; however, penetration is considered unreliable, and therefore the drug should be used with caution for the treatment of meningitis (84). Biliary concentrations of cefoperazone reach levels 8–18 times that of blood, suggesting the biliary tract is an important pathway for elimination (82). Cefoperazone crosses the placenta readily, but breast milk concentrations are extremely low (85,86).

The elimination half-life of sulbactam is approximately 1 h, while that of cefoperazone ranges from 1.6–2.6 h. Cefoperazone is extensively metabolized and eliminated through bile, while sulbactam is primarily renally cleared. As expected, cefoperazone clearance is less likely to be affected by diminished renal function (80,81).

The pairing of cefoperazone and sulbactam represents the first β-lactamase inhibitor/β-lactam antibiotic combination with dissimilar pharmacokinetic profiles. Differences in protein binding and elimination pathways would suggest that certain physiological conditions such as aging, renal disease, and hepatic disease could alter the pharmacokinetic balance between these two drugs. Cefoperazone pharmacokinetics has been studied in ambulatory elderly volunteers in comparison to young adults (87). Elderly subjects were found to have a slightly higher elimination half-life (2.2 vs. 2.0 h) in comparison to the young subjects and a reduction in total clearance (60 vs. 85 ml/min/1.73 m^2) (87). The multidose pharmacokinetics of intravenously administered cefoperazone and sulbactam has also been evaluated in six infected, seriously ill elderly patients. Both drugs were reported to have slower elimination and greater pharmacokinetic variability in these patients as compared with values previously reported for normal, healthy volunteers (88). This is not unexpected, as the function of organs involved in drug elimination are generally compromised during acute illness.

E. Piperacillin/Tazobactam

Tazobactam has been combined with piperacillin in a combination of 1:8 in investigational studies. Unlike other combinations of β-lactamase inhibitors and β-lactam antibiotics, the pharmacokinetic behavior of tazobactam has been shown to be influenced by the presence of piperacillin. Higher peak levels of tazobactam and reduced plasma and renal clearances of tazobactam have been observed. One possible explanation cited by the authors is interference of the tubular secretion of tazobactam by piperacillin (89).

Apart from the interaction between tazobactam and piperacillin, the two drugs are well matched pharmacokinetically. Peak plasma concentrations are achieved 30 min after a 4-g piperacillin plus 0.5-g tazobactam infusion in healthy adult subjects with tazobactam levels reported to range between 13.7 and 37.1 μg/ml (mean of 24.3 μg/ml) and peak piperacillin levels ranging from 136 to 290.4 μg/ml (mean of 223.7 μg/ml). Tazobactam has an apparent volume of distribution of 14.6 l at steady-state. Tazobactam has been shown to penetrate inflammatory exudate rapidly, achieving approximately 67% of plasma concentrations compared with piperacillin's 50% penetration ability. Elimination half-lives for both tazobactam and piperacillin are approximately 1 h with renal clearance the primary means of elimination. Percent urinary recovery of intact tazobactam and piperacillin after 24 h have been reported as 56.8 and 49.8%, respectively (89).

VI. CLINICAL INDICATIONS

A. Amoxicillin/Clavulanic Acid

The efficacy of this oral antibiotic combination for a broad number of types of infections has been extensively reviewed, and it is clear that this is a very useful drug in general outpatient practice (11,17). It has been most extensively studied in the treatment of urinary tract infections (UTI) and is effective for UTI due to susceptible pathogens (90,91). Based on the literature, which includes both young and old patients, the drug may be used in older patients as empiric therapy for the potentially anaerobic infections of the head and neck including chronic sinusitis and periodontal infection. Also, the drug could be used for mild to moderate community- and nursing home–acquired pneumonia and bronchitis in cases in which an oral drug is appropriate. Moreover, the drug could be prescribed to treat complicated urinary tract infection due to susceptible pathogens and most soft tissue infections. Mild to moderate diabetic foot infections, even when complicated by osteomyelitis, may also be treated with this drug. Amoxicillin/clavulanic acid may also be used to complete an antimicrobial course of therapy initiated with a parenteral combination drug.

B. Ampicillin/Sulbactam and Ticarcillin/Clavulanic Acid

These two drug combinations have spectra similar to most third-generation cephalosporins, with an added advantage that both have anaerobic activity comparable to the second-generation cephalosporins (e.g., cefoxitin and cefotetan). Moreover, ampicillin/sulbactam will effectively treat infections in which enterococci or *Listeria monocytogenes* are potential pathogens, which is not true for any of the cephalosporins. Ampicillin/sulbactam has been used effectively to treat a wide variety of infections and is associated with minimal side effects (92–94). In a study of 754 patients with a variety of infections, an efficacy rate of about 80% was observed (93). Considering that the majority of patients were over 60 years of age and 80% suffered from moderate to severe infections, this was an unexpectedly high clinical efficacy rate (93). When ampicillin/sulbactam was used to treat severe mixed infections in which aerobic gram-negative bacilli were present, the use of ampicillin/sulbactam did not obviate the use of an aminoglycoside (94). Additional studies have confirmed the effectiveness of ampicillin/sulbactam to treat moderate to severe respiratory infection (95,96), allowing its use in place of cefoxitin. (97).

Like ampicillin/sulbactam, ticarcillin/clavulanic acid has been used to treat a variety of infections (14). It has been used successfully in oncology patients in combination with vancomycin (98) and cases of community-acquired pneumonia in which the mean age was 55 years (99). It compared well with piperacillin alone in the treatment of hospitalized patients with urinary tract infection (UTI), achieving a clinical efficacy rate of 97% (100), but was disappointing with only 5 of 18 bacteriological and clinical cures for adult women with pyelonephritis (101). However, 29 of 34 patients (86%) with serious, complicated UTI showed clinical improvement when treated with ticarcillin/clavulanic acid (102). Ticarcillin/clavulanic acid compared well with cefazolin in the treatment of skin and soft tissue infection, with a good clinical response of approximately 80% (103). Similarly, the drug combination has been used successfully in the treatment of bone and joint infections (104,105). Additionally, the drug combination has been used in the prophylaxis of penetrating abdominal trauma and has compared well as far as efficacy with the potentially nephrotoxic combination of clindamycin plus gentamicin (106). Moreover, in a predominantly geriatric population of patients with serious intraabdominal infection, ticarcillin/

clavulanic acid had reasonable efficacy in comparison to the community standard of clindamycin plus gentamicin (107,108). Finally, ticarcillin/clavulanic acid can be used to treat a variety of infections in patients with poor renal function when dosages are adjusted accordingly (109).

The role of ampicillin/sulbactam and ticarcillin/clavulanic acid in the treatment of infections in elderly patients has not been clearly delineated. However, it can be expected that these two drugs would be effective in the treatment of most head and neck infections and in cases of community- and nursing home–acquired pneumonia. In hospital-acquired pneumonia, which is usually caused by mixed anaerobic pathogens, methicillin-susceptible *S. aureus*, and aerobic gram-negative bacilli, these two drugs could be used for empiric therapy when *P. aeruginosa* and other potentially resistant gram-negative bacilli are not suspected. Moreover, either combination could be used as "single-agent" therapy for intraabdominal infection, with the caution that ticarcillin/clavulanic acid has limited activity against enterococci. Both drugs could also be prescribed to treat complicated urinary tract infections due to susceptible pathogens and soft tissue infections including diabetic foot infection.

C. Cefoperazone/Sulbactam

This drug combination has improved activity over cefoperazone alone against anaerobes and methicillin-susceptible *S. aureus*. Therefore, it could be used to treat pneumonia and intraabdominal infection, with the caution that the drug is not effective against enterococci and has limited activity against *P. aeruginosa*. In fact, cefoperazone/sulbactam was superior to clindamycin plus gentamicin (87% cures vs. 62% cures) in the treatment of intraabdominal infection in a large group of patients. Not surprisingly, failures in both groups were partially attributable to undrained abscesses and the presence of enterococci and *Pseudomonas* spp. (110). This drug shows promise in the treatment of severe intraabdominal infection in elderly patients.

D. Piperacillin/Tazobactam

Since the addition of tazobactam to piperacillin increases the antimicrobial spectrum of piperacillin to include β-lactamase–producing methicillin-susceptible *S. aureus*, *H. influenzae*, and *B. fragilis*, this drug combination could be used as a single agent for the treatment of pneumonia, intraabdominal infection, and complicated UTIs. Given the activity of piperacillin, even those UTI caused by *P. aeruginosa* could potentially be treated with piperacillin/tazobactam. Recently, piperacillin/tazobactam was used successfully to treat severe community-acquired soft tissue infections, with 22 of 25 patients showing clinical response (111). Delineation of the role of this drug in the treatment of infections in older patients will require further investigation.

VII. ADMINISTRATION OF DRUG

Amoxicillin/clavulanic acid potassium (Augmentin®) is available in orally administered tablets, chewable tablets, and powder for suspension. Each '250' or '500' tablet contains 250 mg or 500 mg of amoxicillin, respectively, and 125 mg clavulanic acid as the potassium salt. Because the ratio of amoxicillin to clavulanate potassium differs for the '250' (2:1) and '500' (4:1) tablets, two '250' tablets are not equivalent to a '500' tablet and should not be substituted. Chewable tablets and powder for oral suspensions are available in

'125' and '250' strengths (indicating mg of amoxicillin) in a 2:1 ratio of amoxicillin to clavulanate potassium. Amoxicillin/clavulanate potassium is dosed similarly to amoxicillin alone. The usual adult oral dose of amoxicillin and clavulanate potassium is one '250' tablet every 8 h. A '500' tablet every 8 h may be given for more severe infections and respiratory tract infections. In patients with a creatinine clearance (Crcl) of less than 30 ml/min, the dose and/or dosing interval of amoxicillin/clavulanate potassium should be adjusted in response to the degree of renal impairment. Patients with Crcl of 15–30 ml/min should receive the usual dose every 12–18 h; adults with Crcl of 5–15 ml/min should receive the usual dose every 20–36 h, and adults with Crcl less than 5 ml/min should receive the usual dose every 48 h. Adults undergoing hemodialysis can be given one '500' tablet after each dialysis and halfway through each dialysis period.

Ticarcillin disodium/clavulanate potassium (Timentin®) is administered parenterally and is currently available in two different ratios: 30:1 (3 g of ticarcillin and 100 mg of clavulanate) and 15:1 (3 g of ticarcillin and 200 mg of clavulanate). Ticarcillin disodium/clavulanate potassium is dosed similarly to ticarcillin alone. The usual dosage for treatment of systemic and urinary tract infections for average adults weighing 60 kg or more is 3.1 g of the 30:1 combination every 4–6 h. The usual dosage in moderate infections is 200 mg of ticarcillin per kg daily given in divided doses every 4–6 h. In severe infections the dose should be increased to 300 mg/kg daily given in divided doses every 4 h. In urinary tract infections, a dosage of 3.2 g (15:1 for ticarcillin/clavulanate) every 6–8 h should be sufficient. In patients with renal impairment, an initial loading dose of 3.1 g of the combined drug is recommended with the following maintenance dose modifications based on creatinine clearance determinations: patients with Crcl of 30–60 ml/min should receive 2 g (based on the ticarcillin component) every 4 h; patients with Crcl of 10–30 ml/min should receive 2 g every 8 h; patients with Crcl less than 10 ml/min should receive 2 g every 12 h; and those with hepatic dysfunction and a Crcl under 10 ml/min should receive 2 g every 24 h. Patients on peritoneal dialysis should receive 3.1 g of the combined drug every 12 h. Patients on hemodialysis should receive 3.1 g of the combined drug after each dialysis and 2 g (based on the ticarcillin component) every 12 h between dialysis.

Ampicillin sodium/sulbactam sodium (Unasyn®) is administered parenterally and available in two dosage strengths: 1.5 g (1 g ampicillin and 0.5 g sulbactam) and 3 g (2 g ampicillin and 1 g sulbactam). The recommended adult dose is 1.5–3.0 g of ampicillin/sulbactam every 6–12 h, depending on severity of infection. The total dose of sulbactam should not exceed 4 g per day; therefore, if more than 8 g of ampicillin is required, it should be supplemented by ampicillin alone. Dosage adjustment is necessary in renal impairment. Patients with Crcl of 15–30 ml/min should receive 1.5–3.0 g of ampicillin/sulbactam every 12 h, and those with Crcl of 5–14 ml/min should receive 1.5–3.0 g every 24 h.

No special dosage adjustments for these β-lactam antibiotic/inhibitor combinations have been specifically recommended for elderly patients. However, due to the association between advancing age and diminished renal function, the Cockcroft equation, which takes age into consideration, should be used when estimating creatinine clearance values:

For males

$$\text{Clcr} = (140 - \text{age})(\text{wt in kg})/72 \times \text{Scr (mg/dl)}$$

For females

$$\text{Clcr} = [140 - \text{age})(\text{wt in kg})/72 \times \text{Scr (mg/dl)}] \times 0.85$$

where:

wt = lean body weight
kg = kilograms
Scr = serum creatinine

VIII. DRUG MONITORING AND ADVERSE EFFECTS

The major adverse effects reported with ampicillin and amoxicillin are hypersensitivity reactions, rash, and gastrointestinal (GI) symptoms. Hematological, renal, hepatic, and nervous system side effects, as well as local reactions, may also occur. Reported hypersensitivity reactions are similar to those reported with other penicillins and include eosinophilia or rash, angioedema, exfoliative dermatitis or erythema multiforme, and rarely Stevens-Johnson syndrome. Serum sickness–like reactions have also been reported. Although all penicillins may cause urticarial hypersensitivity rash, ampicillin and amoxicillin can also cause a generalized erythematous maculopapular rash. GI side effects appear to be dose related, are associated with oral administration, and include nausea, vomiting, anorexia, epigastric distress, diarrhea, and gastritis. Black hairy tongue, glossitis, and stomatitis have also been reported. While the frequency and severity of adverse effects from these aminopenicillins are similar, diarrhea occurs more frequently with ampicillin.

The safety profile of amoxicillin/clavulanate potassium that can be summarized from clinical trials involving 9700 patients worldwide indicates that, with the exception of more frequent GI effects, adverse effects associated with amoxicillin/clavulanate potassium are similar to those reported with amoxicillin alone. Adverse drug reactions to amoxicillin/clavulanate potassium occurred in 13.1% of patients and included diarrhea (4.1%), nausea (3.0%), vomiting (1.8%), indigestion (1.6%), rash (1.1%), stomatitis (1%), candida vaginitis (1%), nine cases of urticaria, and one case of anaphylaxis. In general, adverse effects were dose related, mild, and transient. Treatment was discontinued in less than 3% of patients (17).

Ampicillin/sulbactam also appears to be well tolerated according to data gathered by the manufacturer from 1764 patients in the United States and Europe. Less than 10% of patients reported side effects, and only 0.7% of patients discontinued drug treatment secondary to adverse effects. The most commonly reported side effect was related to ampicillin/sulbactam's parenteral route of administration: injection site pain, particularly when administered intramuscularly (3.6%). Other adverse effects occurring in more than 1% of patients included diarrhea (2.2% of U.S. patients, 1.9% overall), phlebitis (1.2%), and nausea (1.2% in European patients, but only 0.1% in U.S. patients) (92).

Adverse reactions from extended-spectrum penicillins such as ticarcillin most frequently include hypersensitivity reactions, GI side effects, and local reactions. In addition, patients receiving high doses of ticarcillin may develop hemorrhagic manifestations associated with abnormalities of coagulation tests, such as bleeding time and platelet aggregation. As with the aminopenicillins, the addition of a β-lactamase inhibitor to ticarcillin does little to alter the antibiotic's side effect profile; adverse effects reported with ticarcillin/clavulanate potassium are similar to those reported with ticarcillin alone.

Transient elevations in liver function enzymes have been reported for the entire β-lactam class, including the inhibitors, but the clinical significance is unclear.

REFERENCES

1. Abraham EP, Chain E. An enzyme from bacteria able to destroy penicillin. Nature 1940; 146:837.
2. Kirby WMM. Extraction of a highly potent penicillin inactivator from penicillin-resistant staphylococci. Science 1944; 99:452–3.
3. Wise R. Beta-lactamase inhibitors. J Antimicrob Chemother 1982; 9(suppl B):31–40.
4. Tipper DJ. Mode of action of β-lactam antibiotics. Rev Infect Dis 1979; 1:39–54.
5. Dever LA, Dermody TS. Mechanisms of bacterial resistance to antibiotics. Arch Intern Med 1991; 151:886–95.
6. Neu HC, Fu KP. Clavulanic acid, a novel inhibitor of β-lactamases. Antimicrob Agents Chemother 1978; 14:650–5.
7. Neu HC. Contribution of β-lactamases to bacterial resistance and mechanisms to inhibit β-lactamases. Am J Med 1985; 79(suppl 5B):2–12.
8. Nord CE. Mechanisms of β-lactam resistance in anaerobic bacteria. Rev Infect Dis 1986; 8(suppl 5):543–8.
9. Maadux MS. Effects of β-lactamase-mediated antimicrobial resistance: the role of β-lactamase inhibitors. Pharmacotherapy 1991; 11(suppl 2):40S–50S.
10. Bauernfeind A. Classification of β-lactamases. Rev Infect Dis 1986; 8(suppl 5):470–81.
11. Bush K. Recent developments in β-lactamase research and their implications for the future. Rev Infect Dis 1988; 10:681–90.
12. Sawai T, Mitsuhashi S, Yamagishi S. Drug resistance of enteric bacteria. XIV. Comparison of β-lactamases in gram-negative rod bacteria resistant to α-aminobenzylpenicillin. Jpn J Microbiol 1968; 12:423–34.
13. Richmond MH, Sykes RB. The β-lactamases of gram-negative bacteria and their possible physiologic role. In: Rose AH, Tempest DW, eds. Advances in microbial physiology. New York: Academic Press, 1973:31–88.
14. Neu HC. Beta-lactamase inhibition: therapeutic advances. Am J Med 1985; 79(suppl 5B):194–6.
15. Ambler RP. The structure of β-lactamases. Philos Trans R Soc Lond [biol] 1980; 289:321–31.
16. Jaurin B, Grundström T. *amp*C cephalosporinase of *Escherichia coli* K-12 has a different evolutionary origin from that of β-lactamases of the penicillinase type. Proc Natl Acad Sci USA 1981; 78:4897–901.
17. Todd PA, Benfield P. Amoxicillin/clavulanic acid an update of its antibacterial activity, pharmacokinetic properties and therapeutic use. Drugs 1990; 39:264–307.
18. Bush K. Beta lactamase inhibitors from laboratory to clinic. Clin Microbiol Rev 1988; 1:109–23.
19. Arisawa M, Then RL. 6-Acetylmethylenepenicillanic acid: a potent β-lactamase inhibitor. I. Inhibition of chromosomally and R-factor-mediated β-lactamases. J Antibiot 1982; 35:1578–83.
20. Fu K, Neu HC. Comparative inhibition of β-lactamases by novel β-lactam compounds. Antimicrob Agents Chemother 1979; 15:171–6.
21. Gutmann L, Kitzis MD, Yamabe S, et al. Comparative evaluation of a new β-lactamase inhibitor, YTR 830, combined with different β-lactam antibiotics against bacteria harboring known β-lactamases. Antimicrob Agents Chemother 1986; 29:955–95.
22. Jacobs MR, Aronoff SC, Johenning S, et al. Comparative activities of the β-lactamase inhibitors YTR 830, clavulanate, and sulbactam combined with ampicillin and broad-spectrum penicillins against defined β-lactamase-producing aerobic gram-negative bacilli. Antimicrob Agents Chemother 1986; 29:980–8.

23. Appelbaum PC, Jacobs MR, Spangler SK, et al. Comparative activity of β-lactamase inhibitors YTR 830, clavulanate, and sulbactam combined with β-lactams against β-lactamase-producing anaerobes. Antimicrob Agents Chemother 1986; 30:789–91.
24. Knapp CC, Sierra-Madero J, Washington JA. Activity of ticarcillin/clavulanate and piperacillin/tazobactam (YTR 830; CL-298, 741) against clinical isolates and against mutants derepressed for class I β-lactamase. Diagn Microbiol Infect Dis 1989; 12:511–15.
25. Nikaido H, Rosenberg EY, Foulds J. Porin channels in *Escherichia coli*. J Bacteriol 1983; 153:232–40.
26. Nikaido H. Bacterial resistance to antibiotics as a function of outer membrane permeability. J Antimicrob Chemother 1988; 22(suppl A):1–22.
27. Fuchs PC, Barry AL, Jones RN. In vitro activity and disk susceptibility of timentin: current status. Am J Med 1985; 79(suppl 5B):25–32.
28. Sutherland R, Beale AS, Boon RJ, et al. Antibacterial activity of ticarcillin in the presence of clavulanate potassium. Am J Med 1985; 79(suppl 5B):13–24.
29. Paisley JW, Washington II JA. Combined activity of clavulanic acid and ticarcillin against ticarcillin-resistant, gram-negative bacilli. Antimicrob Agents Chemother 1978; 14:224–7.
30. Bansal MB, Chuah SK, Thadepalli H. In vitro activity and in vivo evaluation of ticarcillin plus clavulanic acid against aerobic and anaerobic bacteria. Am J Med 1985; 9(suppl 5B):33–8.
31. Neu HC, Fu KP, Aswapokee N, Aswapokee P, Kung K. Comparative activity and β-lactamase stability of cefoperazone, a piperazine cephalosporin. Antimicrob Agents Chemother 1979; 16:150–7.
32. Fu K, Neu HC. Synergistic activity of cefoperazone in combination with β-lactamase inhibitors. J Antimicrob Chemother 1980; 7:287–92.
33. Knapp CC, Sierra-Madero, Washington JA. Comparative in vitro activity of cefoperazone and various combinations of cefoperazone/sulbactam. Diagn Microbiol Infect Dis 1990; 13:45–9.
34. Jones RN, Pfaller MA, Fuchs PC, et al. Piperacillin/tazobactam (YTR 830) combination comparative antimicrobial activity against 5889 recent aerobic clinical isolates and 60 *Bacteroides fragilis* group strains. Diagn Microbiol Infect Dis 1989; 12:489–94.
35. Nakagawa K, Watanabe K, Hattori N, et al. Phase I study of BRL25000 (clavulanic acid-amoxicillin). Chemotherapy (Tokyo) 1982; 30(suppl 2):98–110.
36. Wise R, Bennett SA, Dent J. The pharmacokinetics of orally absorbed cefuroxime compared with amoxicillin/clavulanic acid. J Antimicrob Chemother 1984; 13:603–10.
37. Eshelman FN, Spyker DA. Pharmacokinetics of amoxicillin and ampicillin: crossover study of the effect of food. Antimicrob Agents Chemother 1987; 14:539–43.
38. Staniforth DH, Lillystone RJ, Jackson D. Effect of food on the bioavailability and tolerance of clavulanic acid/amoxicillin combination. J Antimicrob Chemother 1982; 10:131–9.
39. Staniforth DH, Clarke HL, Horton R, et al. Augmentin bioavailability following cimetidine, aluminum hydroxide and milk. Int J Clin Pharmacol Ther Toxicol 1985; 23:154–7.
40. Deppermann KM, Lode H, Höffken G, et al. Influence of ranitidine, pipenzepine, and aluminum magnesium hydroxide on the bioavailability of various antibiotics, including amoxicillin, cephalexin, doxycycline, and amoxicillin-clavulanic acid. Antimicrob Agents Chemother 1989; 33:1901–7.
41. Grimer RJ, Karpinski MRRK, Andrews JM, et al. Penetration of amoxicillin and clavulanic acid into bone. Chemotherapy (Basel) 1986; 32:185–91.
42. Grange JD, Gouyette A, Gutmann L, et al. Pharmacokinetics of amoxycillin/clavulanic acid in serum and ascitic fluid in cirrhotic patients. J Antimicrob Chemother 1989; 23:605–11.
43. Wise R, Donovan IA, Drumm J, et al. The penetration of amoxicillin/clavulanic acid into peritoneal fluid. J Antimicrob Chemother 1983; 11:57–60.
44. Gould IM, Reid TMS, Legge JS. Amoxycillin/clavulanic acid levels in lower respiratory secretions. J Antimicrob Chemother 1988; 22:88–90.
45. Havard CWH, Fernando A, Brumfitt W, et al. A pilot study of 'Augmentin' in lower respiratory infections: pharmacokinetic and clinical results. Br J Dis Chest 1982; 6:255–60.

46. Decazes JM, Bure A, Wolff M, et al. Bactericidal activity against *Haemophilus influenzae* of cerebrospinal fluid of patients given amoxicillin-clavulanic acid. Antimicrob Agents Chemother 1987; 31:2018–19.
47. Matsuda S, Tanno M, Kashiwagura T, et al. Fundamental and clinical studies on BRL25000 (clavulanic acid-amoxicillin) in the field of obstetrics and gynecology. Chemotherapy (Tokyo) 1982; 30(suppl S2):38–44.
48. Takase Z, Shirafuji H, Uchida M. Clinical and laboratory studies on BRL 25000 (clavulanic acid-amoxicillin) in the field of obstetrics and gynecology. Chemotherapy (Tokyo) 1982; 30(suppl 2):579–86.
49. Hunter PA, Coleman K, Fisher J, et al. In vitro synergistic properties of clavulanic acid, with ampicillin, amoxicillin and ticarcillin. J Antimicrob Chemother 1980; 6:455–70.
50. Adam D, De Visser I, Koeppe P. Pharmacokinetics of amoxicillin and clavulanic acid administered alone and in combination. Antimicrob Agents Chemother 1982; 22:353–7.
51. Jackson D, Cooper DL, Filer CW, et al. Augmentin: absorption, excretion and pharmacokinetic studies in man. Postgrad Med 1984; 76(suppl):51–70.
52. Nilsson-Ehle I, Fellner H, Hedström S-A, et al. Pharmacokinetics of clavulanic acid, given in combination with amoxicillin, in volunteers. J Antimicrob Chemother 1985; 16:491–8.
53. Horber FF, Frey FJ, Descoeudres C, et al. Differential effect of impaired renal function on the kinetics of clavulanic acid and amoxicillin. Antimicrob Agents Chemother 1986; 29:614–19.
54. Usuda Y, Tajiri M, Yusa Y, et al. Serum and urine levels of amoxicillin and clavulanic acid following BRL 2500 (clavulanic acid-amoxicillin) administration to patients with various degrees of renal function. Chemotherapy (Tokyo) 1982; 30(suppl 2):91–7.
55. Papper S. The effects of age in reducing renal function. Geriatrics 1973; 28:83–7.
56. Scully, BE, Chin N-X, Neu HC. Pharmacology of ticarcillin combined with clavulanic acid in humans. Am J Med 1985; 79(suppl 5B):39–43.
57. Bennett S, Wise R, Weston D, et al. Pharmacokinetics and tissue penetration of ticarcillin combined with clavulanic acid. Antimicrob Agents Chemother 1983; 23:831–4.
58. Jackson D, Cockburn A, Cooper DL, et al. Clinical pharmacology and safety evaluation of timentin. Am J Med 1985; 79(suppl 5B):44–55.
59. Parry MF, Neu HC. Pharmacokinetics of ticarcillin in patients with abnormal renal function. J Infect Dis 1976; 133:46–8.
60. Ginsburg CM, McCracken Jr GH, Olsen K, et al. Pharmacokinetics and bactericidal activity of sultamicillin in infants and children. J Antimicrob Chemother 1985; 15:345–51.
61. Pressler T, Pedersen SS, Christiansen L, et al. Sultamicillin—a new antibiotic in the treatment of persistent lower respiratory tract infections caused by *Haemophilus influenzae*. J Antimicrob Chemother 1986; 17:529–33.
62. Rogers HJ, Bradbrook ID, Morrison PJ, et al. Pharmacokinetics and bioavailability of sultamicillin estimated by high performance liquid chromatography. J Animicrob Chemother 1983; 147:227–35.
63. Foulds G, Knirsch AK, Stankewich JP, et al. The parenteral kinetics of ampicillin/sulbactam in man. Int J Clin Pharmacol Res 1985; 5:79–86.
64. Houang ET, Colley N, Chapman M. Penetration of sulbactam-ampicillin and clavulanic acid-amoxicillin into the pelvic peritoneum. Antimicrob Agents Chemother 1985; 28:165–6.
65. Brown RM, Wise R, Andrews JM, et al. Comparative pharmacokinetics and tissue penetration of sulbactam and ampicillin after concurrent intravenous administration. Antimicrob Agents Chemother 1982; 21:565–7.
66. Foster MC, Kapila L, Morris DL, et al. A randomized comparative study of sulbactam plus ampicillin vs. metronidazole plus cefotaxime in the management of acute appendicitis in children. Rev Infect Dis 1986; 8(suppl 8):634–8.
67. Morris DL, Ubhi CS, Robertson CS, et al. Biliary pharmacokinetics of sulbactam plus ampicillin in humans. Rev Infect Dis 1986; 8(suppl 5):589–92.

68. Kager L, Malmborg AS, Nord CE, et al. Effects of ampicillin plus sulbactam on bowel flora in patients undergoing colorectal surgery. Antimicrob Agents Chemother 1982; 22:208–12.
69. Schwiersch U, Lang N, Wildfeuer DA. Concentrations of sulbactam and ampicillin in serum and the myometrium. Drugs 1986;(suppl 2):18–21.
70. Hanninen P, Rossi T. Penetration of sulbactam into cerebrospinal fluid of patients with bacterial meningitis receiving ampicillin therapy. Rev Infect Dis 1986; 8(suppl 5):620–9.
71. Sanders CV, Marier RL. Penetration of sulbactam into human cerebrospinal fluid. Abstract presented at the 13th International Congress of Chemotherapy, Vienna. Aug 28–Sep 2, 1983.
72. Stahl J-P, Bur J-P, Fredj G, et al. Penetration of sulbactam into the cerebrospinal fluid of patients with bacterial meningitis receiving ampicillin therapy. Rev Infect Dis 1986; 8(suppl 5):612–16.
73. Dørflinger T, Madsen PO. Antibiotic prophylaxis in transurethral surgery: a comparison of sulbactam-ampicillin and cefoxitin. Infection 1985; 13:66–9.
74. Dubois M, Coibion M, Deco J, et al. The transplacental transfer of sulbactam sodium co-administered with ampicillin to healthy pregnant women in labor. In: Spitzy KH, Karrer, eds. Proceedings of the 13th Congress of Chemotherapy. Vol 1. Vienna: Verlag H Egermann, 1983:23.
75. Foulds G, Miller RD, Knirsch Ak, et al. Sulbactam kinetics and excretion into breast milk in post-partum women. Clin Pharmacol Ther 1985; 38:692–6.
76. Rho JP, Jones A, Woo M, et al. Single-dose pharmacokinetics of intravenously ampicillin plus sulbactam in healthy elderly and young adult subjects. J Antimicrob Chemother 1989; 24:573–80.
77. Bolton WK, Scheld WM, Spyker DA, et al. Pharmacokinetics of cefoperazone in normal volunteers and subjects with renal insufficiency. Antimicrob Agents Chemother 1981; 19:821–5.
78. Craig WA. Single-dose pharmacokinetics of cefoperazone following intravenous administration. Clin Ther 1980; 3(special issue):46–9.
79. Lode H, Kemmerich B, Koeppe P, et al. Comparative pharmacokinetics of cefoperazone and cefotaxime. Clin Ther 1980; 3(special issue):80–8.
80. Reitberg DP, Marble DA, Schultz RW, et al. Pharmacokinetics of cefoperazone (2.0 g) and sulbactam (1.0 g) coadministered to subjects with normal renal function, patients with decreased renal function, and patients with end-stage renal disease on hemodialysis. Antimicrob Agents Chemother 1988; 32:503–9.
81. Rho JP, Castle S, Smith K, et al. Effect of impaired renal function on the pharmacokinetics of coadministered cefoperazone and sulbactam. J Antimicrob Chemother 1992; 29:701–9.
82. Shimizu K. Cefoperazone: absorption, excretion, distribution, and metabolism. Clin Ther 1980; 3(special issue):60–79.
83. Foulds G. Pharmacokinetics of sulbactam/ampicillin in humans: a review. Rev Infect Dis 1986; 8(suppl 5):503–11.
84. Cable D, Overturf G, Edralin G. Concentrations of cefoperazone in cerebrospinal fluid during bacterial meningitis. Antimicrob Agents Chemother 1983; 23:688–91.
85. Takase Z, Shirafuji H, Uchida M. Fundamental and clinical studies of cefoperazone (T-1551) in the field of obstetrics and gynecology. Chemotherapy (Tokyo) 1980; 28(suppl 6):825–36.
86. Matsuda S, Furuya H. Fundamental and clinical studies on cefoperazone (T-1551) in the field of obstetrics and gynecology. Chemotherapy (Tokyo) 1980; 28(suppl 6):774–88.
87. Meyer BR, Mendelson MH, Deeter RG, et al. Pharmacokinetics of cefoperazone in ambulatory elderly volunteers compared with young adults. Antimicrob Agents Chemother 1987; 31:925–9.
88. Schwartz JI, Jauregui LE, Bachmann KA, et al. Multiple-dose pharmacokinetics of intravenously administered cefoperazone and sulbactam when given in combination and to infected, seriously ill, elderly patients. Antimicrob Agents Chemother 1988; 32:730–5.
89. Wise R, Logan M, Cooper M, et al. Pharmacokinetics and tissue penetration of tazobactam administered alone and with piperacillin. Antimicrob Agents Chemother 1991; 35:1081–4.

90. Raz R, Rottensterich E, Boger S, et al. Comparison of single-dose administration and three-day course of amoxicillin with those of clavulanic acid for treatment of uncomplicated urinary tract infection in women. Antimicrob Agents Chemother 1991; 35:1688–90.
91. Brumfitt W, Hamilton-Miller JMT. Comparative study of cephradine and amoxicillin-clavulanate in the treatment of recurrent urinary tract infections. Antimicrob Agents Chemother 1990; 34:1803–5.
92. Campoli-Richards DM, Brogden RN. Sulbactam/ampicillin a review of its antibacterial activity, pharmacokinetic properties, and therapeutic use. Drugs 1987; 33:577–609.
93. Shimada K. Clinical evaluation of sulbactam/ampicillin in Japan. Diagn Microbiol Infect Dis 1989; 12:1715–1745.
94. Reinhardt JF, Johnston L, Ruane P, et al. A randomized, double-blind comparison of sulbactam/ampicillin and clindamycin for the treatment of aerobic and aerobic-anaerobic infections. Rev Infect Dis 1986; 8(suppl 5):569–75.
95. Oviasu VO, Obasohan AO. Effectiveness of sulbactam/ampicillin in the treatment of lobar pneumonia. Curr Ther Res 1987; 41:99–104.
96. Castellano MA. Sulbactam/ampicillin in the treatment of lower respiratory infections. Drugs 1988; 35(suppl):53–56.
97. Lawrenz CA, Cole P, Theodorou A, et al. Therapeutic interchange of ampicillin-sulbactam for cefoxitin. Am J Hosp Pharm 1991; 48:2150–3.
98. Fainstein V, Elting L, Pitlik S, et al. Ticarcillin plus clavulanic acid in the treatment of patients with cancer. Am J Med 1985; 79(suppl 5B):62–6.
99. Mostow SR, O'Brien RF. Safety and effectiveness of ticarcillin plus clavulanate potassium in treatment of lower respiratory tract infections. Am J Med 1985; 79(suppl 5B):78–80.
100. Cox CE. Comparative study of ticarcillin plus clavulanate potassium versus piperacillin in the treatment of hospitalized patients with urinary tract infections. Am J Med 1985; 79(suppl 5B):88–90.
101. Sanders CV, Marier RL, Aldridge KE, et al. Safety and effectiveness of ticarcillin plus clavulanic acid in the treatment of community-acquired acute pyelonephritis in adult women. Am J Med 1985; 79(suppl 5B):96–100.
102. Gebhart RJ, Duma RJ, Patterson PM. Timentin in the treatment of symptomatic complicated urinary tract infection in adult patients. Am J Med 1985; 79(suppl 5B):101–5.
103. Pankey GA, Katner HP, Valainis GT, et al. Overview of bacterial infections of the skin and soft tissue and clinical experience with ticarcillin plus clavulanate potassium in their treatment. Am J Med 1985; 79(suppl 5B):106–15.
104. Gentry LO, Macko V, Lind R, et al. Ticarcillin plus clavulanic acid (timentin) therapy for osteomyelitis. Am J Med 1985; 79(suppl 5B):116–21.
105. Johnson CC, Reinhardt JF, Wallace SL, et al. Safety and efficacy of ticarcillin plus clavulanic acid in the treatment of infections of soft tissue, bone, and joint. Am J Med 1985; 79(suppl 5B):136–40.
106. Fabian TC, Boldreghini SJ. Antibiotics in penetrating abdominal trauma: comparison of ticarcillin plus clavulanic acid with gentamicin plus clindamycin. Am J Med 1985; 79(suppl 5B):157–60.
107. Fink MP, Helsmoortel CM, Arous EJ, et al. Comparison of the safety and efficacy of parenteral ticarcillin/clavulanate and clindamycin/gentamicin in serious intra-abdominal infections. J Antimicrob Chemother 1989; 24(suppl B):147–56.
108. Fink MP. Antibiotic therapy of intra-abdominal sepsis in the elderly: experience with ticarcillin and clavulanic acid. Surg Gynecol Obstet 1991; 172(suppl):36–41.
109. Dalet F, del Rio G, Torrellas A. Ticarcillin/clavulanate in severe infections in patients with varying renal function. J Antimicrob Chemother 1989; 24(suppl B):131–9.
110. Jauregui LE, Appelbaum PC, Fabian TC, et al. A randomized clinical study of cefoperazone and sulbactam versus gentamicin and clindamycin in the treatment of intraabdominal infections. J Antimicrob Chemother 1990; 25:423–33.
111. Gould IM, Ansari A, Harvey G, et al. Piperacillin/tazobactam in the treatment of serious acute soft tissue infection. Drugs Exp Clin Res 1991; 17:187–90.

12

Trimethoprim-Sulfamethoxazole

Leonard Williams
Veterans Affairs Medical Center and University of Florida College of Medicine, Gainesville, Florida

Bradley S. Bender
Veterans Affairs Medical Center, Gainesville, Florida

I. INTRODUCTION

Trimethoprim-sulfamethoxazole (TMP-SMX), also known as co-trimoxazole, remains an important, clinically effective antimicrobial agent. This drug combination exploits biochemical differences between humans and bacteria in order to selectively damage the parasite. It is an example of the practical application of a theoretical consideration, that is, if two drugs act on successive steps in the pathway of an essential enzymatic reaction in bacteria, the use of these drugs in combination will be synergistic (1,2). Since its introduction in 1968, the therapeutic effectiveness of TMP-SMX for numerous infections has contributed to the widespread use of the drug (3).

II. CHEMISTRY

Trimethoprim (2,4-diamino-5-[3,4,5-trimethoxybenzyl] pyrimidine), like pyrimethamine, the antimalarial agent, is one of the many 2,4-diamino-pyrimidines synthesized and tested for antimicrobial activity. Its structure is shown in Figure 1. Sulfamethoxazole is one of the sulfonamide drugs, which were the first effective antibiotics to be used systematically for the treatment of bacterial infections in man. *Sulfonamide* is the generic name for derivatives of para-aminobenzenesulfonamide (sulfanilamide) (Fig. 2). The minimal structural requirements for antibacterial activity are all contained in the sulfonamide itself, the essential portion being the para-NH_2 group. Sulfamethoxazole (3-[*p*-aminophenylsulfonamido]-5-methylisoxazole) is shown next to para-aminobenzoic acid in Figure 2. The $-SO_2NH_2$ group in this compound is not essential as such, but the important component is that the sulfur is directly linked to the benzene ring (1,4). In TMP-SMX the two drugs are combined in a ratio of 1:5 (TMP to SMX).

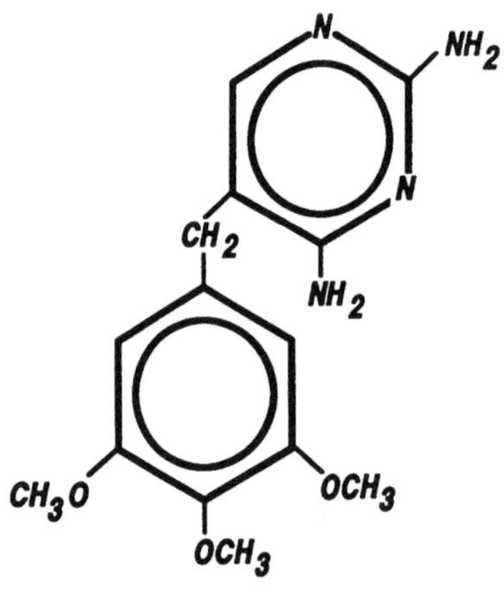

Figure 1 Structural formula of trimethoprim.

III. MECHANISM OF ACTION

The antimicrobial activity of the combination of TMP-SMX is due to its actions on two steps of the enzymatic pathway responsible for the synthesis of tetrahydrofolic acid. Sulfonamides are structural analogs and competitive antagonists of para-aminobenzoic acid (PABA) (Fig. 3). These compounds, therefore, prevent normal bacterial utilization of PABA for the synthesis of folic acid. Specifically, sulfonamides are competitive inhibitors of the bacterial enzyme responsible for the incorporation of PABA into dihydropteric acid, the immediate precursor of folic acid (Fig. 4). Bacteria that must synthesize their own folic acid are sensitive to the actions of sulfonamides; those that can utilize preformed folic acid are not affected. The bacteriostatic effect of sulfonamides can be counteracted by PABA. Mammalian cells are not affected by this mechanism because they cannot synthesize folic acid and require preformed folic acid in their diet. Some bacteria are also sulfonamide-insensitive because they, like mammalian cells, utilize preformed folate. Folic acid (dihydrofolate) is converted to tetrahydrofolate, which is required for the biosynthesis

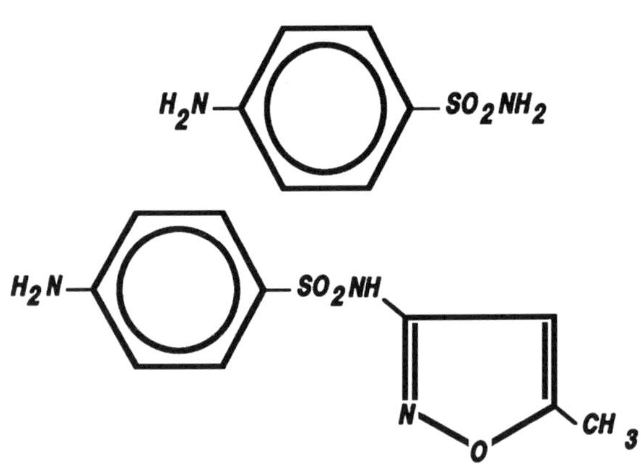

Figure 2 Structural formulas of sulfanilamide and sulfamethoxazole.

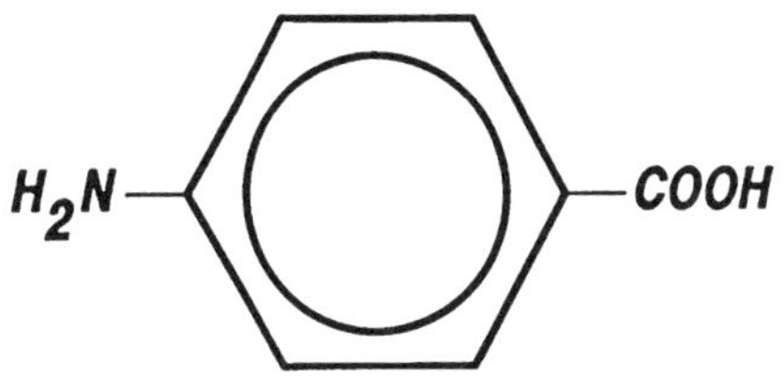

Figure 3 Structural formula of para-aminobenzoic acid.

of purines, pyrimidines, and certain amino acids. Trimethoprim prevents the reduction of dihydrofolate to tetrahydrofolate by inhibiting the activity of bacterial dehydrofolate reductase and interferes with the production of bacterial DNA (Fig. 4) (2,3,5).

The synergistic interaction between trimethoprim and sulfamethoxazole can be predicted by reason of their respective mechanisms. The optimal ratio of the concentrations of the two drugs for synergism is equal to the ratio of the minimal inhibitory concentrations of the agents acting independently. The most effective ratio for the largest number of bacteria is 20 parts of sulfamethoxazole per 1 part of trimethoprim (1,2,5). To achieve serum concentrations of 20:1, the drugs are combined in a ratio of 5:1.

IV. ANTIMICROBIAL SPECTRUM

TMP-SMX has a broad antimicrobial spectrum. It is effective against many of the important pathogens that infect elderly patients, such as *Escherichia coli*, *Proteus* spp., *Haemophilus influenzae*, *Neisseria* spp, *Streptococcus pneumoniae*, and *Listeria monocytogenes*. TMP-SMX has moderate activity against *Staphylococcus aureus*, *Klebsiella* spp., and *Enterococcus* spp. It has no activity against anaerobes (4,6). Other microorganisms susceptible to TMP-SMX include *Brucella* spp., *Branhamella catarrhalis*, *Haemophilus ducreyi*, *Chlamydia trachomatis*, *Salmonella typhi*, *Nocardia asteroides*, *Mycobacterium kansasii*,

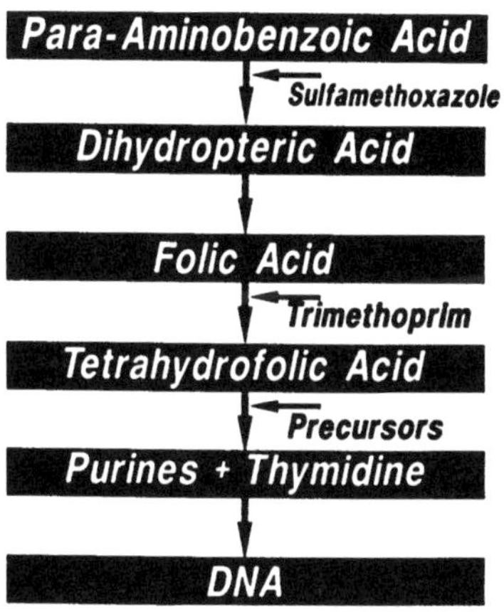

Figure 4 Mechanism of action of trimethoprim-sulfamethoxazole.

Table 1 Susceptibility of Organisms to Trimethoprim Alone and to Trimethoprim-Sulfamethoxazole (TMP-SMX), Expressed as Cumulative Percentage of Isolates Inhibited—Mayo Clinic 1989.

Organism	Trimethoprim (≤8 μg/ml)	TMP-SMX (≤0.5 and 9.5 μg/ml)
Acinetobacter calcoacericus var. *anitrasus*	37	78
Citrobacter diversus	100	100
C. freundii	67	67
Enterobacter aerogenes	99	98
E. agglomerans	100	100
E. cloacae	96	95
Escherichia coli	89	88
Klebsiella oxytocia	96	96
K. pneumoniae	100	87
Morganella morganii	85	89
Proteus mirabilis	82	82
P. vulgaris	60	74
Providencia rettgeri	81	69
P. stuartii	71	43
Pseudomonas aeruginosa	1	1
P. cepacia	94	100
P. fluorescens	2	7
Serratia liquefaciens	92	100
S. marcescens	86	83
Staphylococcus saprophyticus	ND	83
Xanthomonas maltophilia	1	22

Results are for isolates from all sources. Breakpoints for susceptibility used in this summary represent clinical practices at the Mayo Clinic. Some of the breakpoints differ from those defined by the National Committee for Clinical Laboratory Standards (NCCLS). These differences are minor, and the percentage of strains susceptible would not be affected substantially by application of the NCCLS guidelines. ND = insufficient data (results from fewer than 10 isolates). The following microorganisms have been shown to be susceptible to trimethoprim-sulfamethoxazole: *Brucella* species, *Chlamydia trachomatis, Haemophilus ducreyi, H. influenzae, Moraxella catarrhalis, Mycobacterium balnei (marinum), M. kansasii, M. scrofulaceum, Neisseria gonorrhoeae, Nocardia asteroides, Pneumocystis carinii, Pseudomonas pseudomallei, Salmonella typhi, Shigella* spp., and *Streptococcus pneumoniae.*

Reproduced with permission from Cockerill FR III, Edson RS: Trimethoprim-sulfamethoxazole. Mayo Clin Proc 66:1260–1269, 1991.

and *Mycobacterium scrofulaceum.* TMP-SMX is also effective in treating pneumonia caused by *Pneumocystis carinii* in patients who are immunocompromised (3,7). TMP-SMX is usually inactive against *Pseudomonas aeruginosa, Mycoplasma, Mycobacterium tuberculosis,* and *Treponema pallidum* (4). Table 1 summarizes the organisms that are susceptible to trimethoprim alone and to trimethoprim-sulfamethoxazole, which are expressed as cumulative percentages of isolates inhibited.

V. CLINICAL PHARMACOLOGY

A. Pharmacokinetics

1. Absorption

After oral administration, TMP and SMX are both efficiently absorbed whether administered alone or in combination. There are, however, some individual variations in absorption rates (8), but these seem to have no clinical significance. Trimethoprim is usually absorbed more rapidly than sulfamethoxazole after a single oral dose of the combined preparation. It appears that concurrent oral administration of these drugs retards the absorption of sulfamethoxazole (1). Trimethoprim usually reaches peak blood concentrations by 2 h, while peak concentrations of sulfamethoxazole occur by 4 h. The half-life of trimethoprim is approximately 11 h, while that of sulfamethoxazole is about 10 h (1). These drugs are well absorbed after oral administration even in the presence of acute gastroenteritis, and with concomitant administration of cimetidine or metoclopromide. Peak blood levels following a single oral dose of 160 mg of trimethoprim and 800 mg of sulfamethoxazole are 1–2 μg/ml for trimethoprim, 40–60 μg/ml for total sulfamethoxazole, and 30–50 μg/ml for unbound sulfamethoxazole. When the usual dose of 160 mg TMP and 800 mg SMX is given twice daily, a steady-state is reached in adults after 2–3 days and the steady-state peak serum concentrations are approximately 50% greater than the peak levels after a single dose (9). No noticeable changes in absorption occur in elderly patients with TMP-SMX in combination after oral administration (10).

Peak blood concentrations of TMP and SMX occur more rapidly after intravenous administration in comparison to the oral route. Because of some variability in oral absorption, peak concentrations of both drugs are often higher and more predictable after intravenous administration. After intravenous infusion of 160 mg of TMP and 800 mg of SMX over a period of 1 h, mean peak serum concentrations are 3.4 ± 0.3 μg/ml for TMP and 46.3 ± 2.7 μg/ml for SMX. When intravenous doses are given at 8-h intervals, the mean plasma peak and trough levels of TMP are 8.8 ± 0.9 μg/ml and 5.6 ± 0.6 μg/ml, respectively, and the mean peak and trough levels of SMX are 105.6 ± 10.9 μg/ml and 70.7 ± 7.3 μg/ml, respectively (3,11). Data on the impact of aging on the pharmacokinetics of intravenously administered TMP-SMX are not available.

2. Distribution

Because of its greater lipid solubility, trimethoprim is able to cross biological membranes and penetrate into extravascular and fatty tissues to a greater extent than sulfamethoxazole. In fact, the apparent volume of distribution of TMP is 100–120 L, compared to a volume of distribution of 12–18 L for sulfamethoxazole (8). Naber et al. showed that the volumes of distribution for these drugs did not differ in elderly patients whose mean age was 73.1 ± 2.9 years. In this study, the volume of distribution for TMP was 101.23 ± 29.52 L and 18.36 ± 5.23 L for SMX (10).

Because of unequal distribution, there is a wide range of concentration ratios of these two drugs in other body tissues and fluids. TMP is 45% bound to plasma protein, while SMX is 66% protein bound. The concentration of TMP is equal to or greater than the simultaneous plasma level in saliva, intracellular fluid, breast milk, prostatic tissue, sputum, lung tissue, vaginal secretions, bile, and urine. In contrast, the concentrations of SMX in all tissues and fluids except urine are considerably lower than those of the concomitant plasma concentrations (9). Of particular importance for older men is that the concentrations of TMP in prostatic fluid have been noted to be approximately 200% that of serum concentrations (12,13). Both TMP and SMX cross the human placenta (14). There are different reports for penetration of TMP and SMX into the cerebrospinal fluid (CSF) in patients, but in all cases the reported concentrations for both drugs in the CSF were ≤50% of the serum concentrations for both patients with inflamed or noninflamed meninges (3,8,15).

3. Metabolism

TMP-SMX is metabolized by the liver. Five to thirty percent of TMP is metabolized to oxide and hydroxylated metabolites, and about 20% of SMX is metabolized, predominantly by *N*-acetylation, although glucuronidation also occurs. The metabolites of both drugs have basically no antibacterial activity (3,8,11). The effect of age on liver metabolism of TMP-SMX is unknown.

4. Excretion

In patients with normal renal function, the plasma half-life of TMP is approximately 11 h, while that of SMX is about 9 h (16). Both TMP and SMX and their metabolites are excreted into the urine via glomerular filtration and tubular secretion, but only the parent compounds of both drugs are excreted into the bile (3). Naber et al. examined plasma and urine concentrations with time after a single dose of TMP-SMX in fixed combinations in six elderly subjects whose mean age was 73.1 ± 2.9 years (10). The mean plasma terminal phase half-lives for the study group were 10.31 ± 1.81 h for TMP and 11.79 ± 2.69 h for SMX, which were comparable to the half-lives (10–12 h) in young patients with normal function reported in the literature. While the total excretion of unchanged drug for TMP and SMZ in geriatric patients was comparable to that in younger people, the renal clearance value of 2.42 ml/min for SMZ was about 50% less than the corresponding renal clearance values for younger patients.

After an oral dose of TMP-SMX in adults with normal renal function, approximately 45–70% of SMX and 50–60% of TMP are excreted in the urine within 24 h; 20% of SMX and 80% of TMP are recovered in the urine in unchanged form (9). The elimination rate of neither TMP nor SMX is significantly affected by impaired renal function for creatinine clearances that are greater than 30 ml/min. When the creatinine clearance falls below this value, however, the elimination half-lives of both drugs can increase up to 45–60 h and the quantity of drug cleared by the kidney decreases (8).

Varoquaux et al. (17) showed that following a single-dose oral administration of TMP-SMX in six young and six elderly subjects, the urinary excretion of TMP and SMX was reduced by about 50% in the elderly group compared to young subjects; the renal clearance of TMP was significantly lower in the elderly group. Renal clearance of SMX, however, was not significantly different between the two groups.

Serum concentrations of SMX have been reported to be slightly lower in uremic patients than in normal subjects after a single dose, while serum concentrations of TMP were similar in both groups but tended to be higher in uremic subjects 5 h after dosing. The distribution of unbound SMX in tissues increased in renal insufficiency when there was little change in distribution into tissues of TMP with impaired renal function (16).

B. Drug Interactions

TMP-SMX may prolong the prothrombin time in patients receiving concomitant warfarin therapy. Although TMP-SMX displaces a small amount of warfarin from its binding sites to plasma proteins, the primary mechanism for the potentiation of anticoagulation is through selective inhibition of the metabolic clearance of the more potent S-enantiomorph form of warfarin (18). Also by means of inhibition of metabolic clearance, TMP-SMX may prolong the elimination half-life of phenytoin (19).

Sulfonamide-containing drugs potentiate the effect of oral sulfonylurea hypoglycemic agents (20). Sulfonamides augment the hypoglycemic effects of chlorpropamide in elderly persons as well as tolbutamide (21); recently, a symptomatic hypoglycemic episode has been reported in an elderly patient secondary to a TMP-SMX-glipizide drug interaction (22). Cases of thrombocytopenia in elderly patients receiving thiazide diuretics or furosemide chronically along with TMP-SMX have been reported (23).

The serum digoxin concentrations increased by 22% during trimethoprim therapy in nine elderly patients (median age 78 years) receiving chronic oral digoxin. The authors suggested that the increase in serum digoxin concentrations was due to decreased renal tubular secretion of digoxin (24).

There have been a number of reports concerning methotrexate toxicity in patients receiving TMP-SMX (25,26), with fatal results occurring in elderly patients (27). TMP-SMX should be used with caution in patients who receive methotrexate because sulfonamides may displace methotrexate from its plasma protein-binding sites resulting in increased free methotrexate concentrations. Toxic delirium due to an amantadine and TMP-SMX drug interaction has also been noted (28).

It should be noted, finally, that because TMP-SMX possesses antifolate properties, this drug could theoretically increase the incidence of folate deficiencies induced by other concomitantly used drugs such as pyrimethamine and phenytoin.

VI. CLINICAL INDICATIONS

TMP-SMX is currently approved by the Food and Drug Administration for treatment of a relatively limited number of infections: urinary tract infections (including complicated infections), acute exacerbations of chronic obstructive pulmonary disease (COPD), *Pneumocystis carinii* pneumonia, traveler's diarrhea, shigellosis, and otitis media. Otitis media is rarely seen in geriatric patients and will not be discussed further. Treatment for most of the other infections has not been evaluated extensively in older persons, but the lessons learned from studies in younger adults should be applicable.

A. Urinary Tract Infections (UTIs)

Probably the most common use of TMP-SMX in elderly persons is the treatment of UTIs. This is based on its activity against Enterobacteriaceae (the family of gram-negative bacilli that accounts for most urinary tract pathogens), proven efficacy and safety, and relatively low cost. Most studies on short-course antibiotic therapy of young women with uncomplicated UTIs report excellent results with either two double-strength tablets taken as a single dose (29) or one double-strength tablet taken twice daily for 3 days (30). In one study, however, single-dose TMP-SMX resolved catheter-induced UTI in 31 of 33 (94%) of women aged less than 65 years old compared to 10 of 18 (56%) women aged 65 years and older ($p = 0.002$). Ten days of therapy resolved the infection in 27/32 (84%) and 12 of 17 (71%) ($p = 0.17$) young and elderly women, respectively (31). Thus, elderly women should received at least 10 days of TMP-SMX for UTI.

Single-dose therapy with TMP-SMX is clearly ineffective in elderly men (32), and most clinicians would treat all men with at least 2 weeks of therapy. Prostatitis is a frequent concurrent problem of UTI. Because TMP penetrates well into the inflamed prostate, TMP-SMX is commonly prescribed for prostatitis. The duration of therapy is 2–6 weeks for acute prostatitis and up to 12 weeks for chronic bacterial prostatitis (3). Carbenicillin and more recently the quinolones are now more commonly used than TMP-SMX for treatment of prostatitis, particularly chronic bacterial prostatitis.

B. Respiratory Tract Infections

Sputum cultures from patients with exacerbations of COPD usually reveal nonencapsulated *H. influenzae*, *S. pneumoniae*, and other normal flora. TMP-SMX is probably as equally efficacious as doxycycline or ampicillin in the treatment of these exacerbations (33). The duration of treatment is 7–10 days. In patients with frequent exacerbations during the winter, several strategies are used: prescribing prophylactic use of daily or every-other-day antibiotics or giving the patient a prescription for a week's supply of drug with instructions to use it at the first sign of a flare-up (34).

Moraxella (Branhamella) catarrhalis is a gram-negative diplococcus that is a common cause of pneumonia in elderly patients (35). Most patients also have COPD or another serious underlying disease (35). Due to the increasing occurrence of beta-lactamase production by *M. catarrhalis*, TMP-SMX is currently the authors' initial antibiotic of choice for treating a respiratory infection caused by these organisms, but final therapy should be guided by in vitro susceptibility tests.

Pneumocystis carinii pneumonia (PCP) is the most frequently reported opportunistic infection in patients with the acquired immunodeficiency syndrome (AIDS), occurring in up to 80–90% of all AIDS patients (36,37). About 3% of AIDS cases occur in persons over 60 years old (38). Either TMP-SMX or pentamidine are the drugs of choice for treatment of PCP. TMP-SMX is given at dosage of 15–20 mg/kg/day (of TMP component) in three or four divided doses for 21 days (37,39). Side effects, such as rash, fever, and anemia, are more common in patients receiving such doses of TMP-SMX than in patients who receive lower doses of the drug. These adverse effects are rarely life-threatening and can be managed by reducing the TMP-SMX dose (39). Prophylaxis against PCP is also recommended for all patients who are infected with the human immunodeficiency virus and have CD4 cell counts less than 200/mm^3 (primary prophylaxis) or for any AIDS patient who has had a previous episode of PCP (secondary prophylaxis) (40,41).

C. Gastrointestinal Infections

About one-half of all travelers from industrialized countries visiting underdeveloped areas acquire traveler's diarrhea. The illness is usually mild (4–5 stools a day) and short-lived (3–4 days) (42,43). Enterotoxigenic *E. coli* is the most frequently implicated pathogen, but *Salmonella*, *Shigella*, parasites, and viruses are also encountered (43). Traveler's diarrhea responds well to 5 days of TMP-SMX (double-strength, twice daily) (43,44). TMP-SMX can also be used for prophylaxis at a dosage of one double-strength tablet daily (43,45). Because of increasing occurrence of resistance to TMP-SMX, quinolones are now more commonly prescribed for traveler's diarrhea (44).

TMP-SMX is also effective for treating *Salmonella* and *Shigella* infections, two of the more common causes of bacterial diarrhea (3,46). Treatment of mild cases of gastrointestinal salmonellosis is not recommended in younger patients because therapy results in prolonged fecal excretion of the organism (46). Because elderly persons in general have higher rates of bacteremia of all types and because *Salmonella* is known to invade the endothelium of major arteries (and cause mycotic aneurysm), many clinicians would treat all elders with salmonellosis (46). All patients with shigellosis should also be treated with antimicrobials (46).

D. Miscellaneous

TMP-SMX may be used for treating several other types of infections that are relatively more common in older adults. These include nocardiosis (47), *Listeria monocytogenes* meningitis (48), and serious gram-negative infections, including bacteremias (49).

VII. DRUG ADMINISTRATION

A. Preparations

TMP-SMX comes in oral suspension, tablets, and parenteral preparations. These preparations are packaged and marketed as the following:

Oral suspension: TMP 40 mg/5 ml and SMX 200 mg/5 ml
Tablets: TMP 80 mg and SMX 400 mg (single strength)
TMP 160 mg and SMX 800 mg (double strength)
Parenteral preparation for intravenous use: TMP 160 mg/ml and SMX 800 mg/ml

B. Dose and Routes of Administration

The usual dosage for adults is 800 mg of SMX plus 160 mg of TMP every 12 h for 10–14 days for most infections. Larger doses may be given in special circumstances, such as in patients with very serious or life-threatening disease (1). TMP-SMX therapy should be continued for 10–14 days for chronic or recurrent urinary tract infections, 1–4 months in men with chronic bacterial prostatitis, 7 days for enteritis, and 7–10 days for bronchitis. The treatment of traveler's diarrhea is 160 mg TMP and 800 mg SMX taken twice a day for 5 days. For prophylaxis against traveler's diarrhea, 160 mg TMP and 800 mg SMX is prescribed once daily during the period of risk up to a maximum of 2 weeks.

In older persons with feeding tubes or who have difficulty swallowing, the oral suspension may be preferable.

For severe infections, such as a gram-negative bacillary bacteremia, the intravenous dose is 8–10 mg/kg of TMP (as TMP-SMX) daily, given in two to four equally divided doses for up to 14 days. The maximum recommended dosage for TMP-SMX (as TMP) is 960 mg daily. *P. carinii* pneumonia is treated with TMP-SMX 15–20 mg/kg/day (of TMP component) in three or four divided doses for 21 days.

Significant dose adjustments of TMP-SMX are not necessary for most elderly patients with relatively normal renal functions. In patients who have moderately severe renal impairments (a creatinine clearance between 15 and 30 ml/min), the usual adult daily dose should be reduced by 50% (6). The drug should not be given when the creatinine clearance is less than 15 ml/min (1).

VIII. DRUG MONITORING AND ADVERSE REACTIONS

Serum levels of TMP-SMX are usually not measured in clinical practice.

A. Hematological Reactions

When TMP-SMX is given in recommended doses, it does not induce folate deficiency in normal persons (1). Patients who are reported to have megaloblastosis with TMP-SMX are many times found to have predisposing factors such as dietary folate deficiency (particularly among elderly persons), malabsorption, or alcoholism. There have been some reports of leukopenia, agranulocytosis, aplastic anemia, and thrombocytopenia with TMP-SMX usage (2,3,50).

Elderly persons, however, have been shown to be overrepresented among the serious reactions concerning TMP-SMX–associated blood dyscrasias (51).

B. Skin Reactions

About 75% of untoward reactions due to TMP-SMX involve the skin. These skin reactions include those known to occur with sulfonamide therapy, i.e., urticarial, erythematous, maculopapular, morbilliform, purpuric, and photosensitivity reactions. Rare exfoliative reactions including Stevens-Johnson syndrome and toxic epidermal necrolysis (Lyell's syndrome) have occurred in elderly patients (23).

C. Gastrointestinal Reactions

These reactions consist mainly of nausea and vomiting, while diarrhea is rare (3). Glossitis and stomatitis are common reactions (1). Mild and transient jaundice has been known to occur in patients taking TMP-SMX; this seems to be due to an allergic cholestatic hepatitis (1), and many patients had a previous history of hepatitis (50).

D. Central Nervous System Reactions

Reactions known to occur with sulfonamide therapy are seen, such as headache, hallucinations, and depression (50). Aseptic meningitis has been reported in a few cases in relation to TMP (52). In elderly patients with dementia, TMP-SMX has been reported to cause psychotic reactions (53).

E. Renal Reactions

A permanent deterioration in renal function may follow the use of TMP-SMX in patients with preexisting renal disease (54). A reversible decline in creatinine clearance has been noted in patients with normal renal function (55). Kastrup et al. have shown that the increase in serum creatinine may be due to an age-dependent reversible TMP-induced inhibition of the tubular secretion of creatinine rather than to a decrease in glomerular filtration rate (56). TMP-SMX is also associated with acute interstitial nephritis (57).

F. Cardiac Reactions

QT prolongation with paroxysmal ventricular tachycardia (58) and QT prolongation with torsades de pointes (59) have also been reported in relation to TMP-SMX administration.

REFERENCES

1. Mandell GL, Sande MA. Antimicrobial agents. Sulfonamides, trimethoprim-sulfamethoxazole, quinolones, and agents for urinary tract infections. In: Gilman AG, Rall TW, Nies AS, et al., eds. The pharmacological basis of therapeutics. 8th ed. New York: Pergamon Press, 1990:1047–64.
2. Hitchings GH. Mechanism of action of trimethoprim-sulfamethoxazole-I. J Infect Dis 1973; 128(suppl):433–6.
3. Cockerill FR, Edson RS. Trimethoprim-sulfamethoxazole. Mayo Clin Proc 1991; 66:1260–9.
4. Salter, AJ. Trimethoprim-sulfamethoxazole. An assessment of more than 12 years of use. Rev Infect Dis 1982; 4:196–236.
5. Burchall JJ. Mechanism of action of trimethoprim-sulfamethoxazole II. J Infect Dis 1973; 128(suppl):437–606.
6. Yoshikawa TT. Antimicrobial therapy for the elderly patient. J Am Geriatr Soc 1990; 38:1353–72.
7. Reeves DS. Sulfamethoxazole/trimethoprim: the first two years. J Clin Path 1971; 24:430–7.
8. Patel RB, Welling PG. Clinical pharmacokinetics of co-trimoxazole (trimethoprim-sulfamethoxazole). Clin Pharmacokinet 1980; 5:405–23.
9. Wormser GP, Keusch GT, Heel RC. Co-trimoxazole (trimethoprim-sulfamethoxazole): An updated review of its antibacterial activity and clinical efficacy. Drugs 1982; 24:459–518.
10. Naber K, Vergin H, Weigand W. Pharmacokinetics of co-trimoxazole and co-tetroxazine in geriatric patients. Infection 1981; 9:239–43.
11. Grose WE, Bodey GP, Loo TL. Clinical pharmacology of intravenously administered trimethoprim-sulfamethoxazole. Antimicrob Agents Chemother 1979; 15:447–51.
12. Winningham DG, Nemoy NJ, Stamey TA. Diffusion of antibiotics from plasma to prostatic fluid. Nature 1968; 219:139–43.
13. Meares EM. Long-term therapy of chronic bacterial prostatitis with trimethoprim-sulfamethoxazole. Can Med Assoc J 1975; 112(suppl):22–5.
14. Reid DWJ, Caille G, Kaufmann NR. Maternal and transplacental kinetics of trimethoprim and sulfamethoxazole, separately and in combination. Can Med Assoc J 1975; 112(suppl):67–72.
15. Dudley MN, Levitz RE, Quintiliani R, et al. Pharmacokinetics of trimethoprim and sulfamethoxazole in serum and cerebrospinal fluid of adult patients with normal meninges. Antimicrob Agents Chemother 1984; 26:811–14.
16. Welling PG, Craig WA, Amidon GL, et al. Pharmacokinetics of trimethoprim and sulfamethoxazole in normal subjects and patients with renal failure. J Infect Dis 1973; 128(suppl):556–66.
17. Varoquaux O, Lajoie D, Gobert C, et al. Pharmacokinetics of the trimethoprim-sulfamethoxazole combination in the elderly. Br J Clin Pharmacol 1985; 20:575–81.
18. O'Reilly RA. Stereoselective interaction of trimethoprim-sulfamethoxazole with the separated enantiomorphs of racemic warfarin in man. N Engl J Med 1980; 302:33–5.
19. Hansen JM, Kampmann JP, Siersbaek-Nielsen K, et al. The effect of different sulfonamides on phenytoin metabolism in man. Acta Med Scand 1979; 624(suppl):106–10.
20. Mihic M. Mautner LS, Leness JZ, et al. Effect of trimethoprim-sulfamethoxazole on blood insulin and glucose concentrations of diabetes. Can Med Assoc J 1975; 112(suppl):80–2.
21. Baciewicz AM, Swafford WB. Hypoglycemia induced by the interaction of chlorpropamide and co-trimoxazole. Drug Intel Clin Pharm 1984; 18:309–10.
22. Johnson JF, Dobmeier ME. Symptomatic hypoglycemia secondary to a glipizide–trimethoprim-sulfamethoxazole drug interaction. Drug Intel Clin Pharm 1990; 24:250–1.
23. Frisch JM. Clinical experience with adverse reactions to trimethoprim-sulfamethoxazole. J Infect Dis 1973; 128(suppl):607–11.
24. Petersen P, Kastrup J, Bartram R, et al. Digoxin-trimethoprim interaction. Acta Med Scand 1985; 217:423–7.
25. Frain, JB. Methotrexate toxicity in a patient receiving trimethoprim-sulfamethoxazole (Letter). J Rheumatol 1987; 14:176–77.

26. Jeurissen ME, Boerbooms AM, van de Putte LB. Pancytopenia and methotrexate with trimethoprim-sulfamethoxazole (Letter; Comment). Ann Intern Med 1989; 111:261.
27. Groenendal H, Rampen FH. Methotrexate and trimethoprim-sulfamethoxazole—a potentially hazardous combination. Clin Exp Dermatol 1990; 15:350–60.
28. Speeg KV, Leighton JA, Maldonado AL. Toxic delirium in a patient taking amantadine and trimethoprim-sulfamethoxazole. Am J Med Sci 1989; 298:410–12.
29. Fihn SD, Johnson C, Roberts PL, et al. Trimethoprim-sulfamethoxazole for acute dysuria in women: A single-dose or 10-day course; a double-blind, randomized trial. Ann Intern Med 1988; 108:350–7.
30. Trienekens TAM, Stobberingh EE, Winkens RAG, et al. Different lengths of treatment with co-trimoxazole for acute uncomplicated urinary tract infections in women. Br Med J 1989; 299:1319–22.
31. Harding GKM, Nicolle LE, Ronald AR, et al. How long should catheter-acquired urinary tract infection in women be treated? Ann Intern Med 1991; 114:713–19.
32. Nicolle LE, Bjornson J, Harding GKM, et al. Bacteriuria in elderly institutionalized men. N Engl J Med 1983; 309:1420–5.
33. Chodosh S, Eichel B, Ellis C, et al. Comparison of trimethoprim-sulfamethoxazole with ampicillin in acute infectious exacerbation's of chronic bronchitis: A double-blind crossover study. Rev Infect Dis 1982; 4:517–27.
34. Reynolds HY. Chronic bronchitis and acute infectious exacerbations. In: Mandell GL, Douglas RG, Bennett JE, eds. Principles and Practice of Infectious Diseases. New York: Churchill Livingstone, 1990: 531–5.
35. Wright PW, Wallace RJ, Shepherd JR. A descriptive study of 42 cases of *Branhamella catarrhalis* pneumonia. Am J Med 1990; 88(suppl 5A):2–8.
36. Phair J, Munoz A, Detels R, et al. and the Multicenter AIDS Cohort Study Group. The risk of *Pneumocystis carinii* pneumonia among men infected with human immunodeficiency virus type I. N Engl J Med 1990; 322:161–5.
37. Kovacs JA, Masur H. *Pneumocystis carinii* pneumonia: Therapy and prophylaxis. J Infect Dis 1988; 158:254–9.
38. Centers for Disease Control. Update: acquired immunodeficiency syndrome—United States, 1991. MMWR 1992; 41:463–8.
39. Sattler FR, Cowan R, Nielsen DM, et al. Trimethoprim-sulfamethoxazole compared with pentamidine for treatment of *Pneumocystis carinii* pneumonia in the acquired immunodeficiency syndrome. Ann Intern Med 1988; 109:280–7.
40. Bender BS. Inhaled pentamidine and prevention of pneumocystis pneumonia. N Engl J Med 1991; 325:736.
41. Bender BS. Outpatient management of patients infected with human immuno-deficiency virus. J Fam Prac 1992; 34:464–82.
42. Steffen R, van der Linde F, Gyr K, et al. Epidemiology of diarrhea in travelers. JAMA 1983; 249:1176–80.
43. Quinn TC, Bender BS, Bartlett JG. New developments in infectious diarrhea. Disease-A-Month 1986; 32:165–244.
44. Ericsson CD, Johnson PC, DuPont HL, et al. Ciprofloxacin or trimethoprim-sulfamethoxazole as initial therapy for travelers' diarrhea. Ann Intern Med 1987; 106:216–20.
45. DuPont HL, Galindo E, Evans DG, et al. Prevention of travelers' diarrhea with trimethoprim-sulfamethoxazole and trimethoprim alone. Gastroenterology 1083; 84:75–80.
46. Blacklow NR. Infectious diarrhea. In: Gleckman RA, Gante NM, eds. Infections in the elderly. Boston: Little, Brown and Company, 1983:159–75.
47. Smego RA, Moeller MB, Gallis HA. Trimethoprim-sulfamethoxazole therapy in *Nocardia* infections. Arch Intern Med 1983; 143:711–18.

48. Spitzer PG, Hammer SM, Karchmer AW. Treatment of *Listeria monocytogenes* infection with trimethoprim-sulfamethoxazole: Case report and review of the literature. Rev Infect Dis 1986; 8:427–30.
49. Quintilliani R, Levitz RE, Nightingale CH. Potential role of trimethoprim-sulfamethoxazole in the treatment of serious hospital-acquired bacterial infections. Rev Infect Dis 1987; 9:S160–S165.
50. Lawson DH, Paice BJ. Adverse reactions to trimethoprim-sulfamethoxazole. Rev Infect Dis 1982; 4:429–33.
51. Keisu M, Wiholm BE, Palmblad J. Trimethoprim-sulfamethoxazole-associated blood dyscrasias. Ten years' experience of the Swedish spontaneous reporting system. J Intern Med 1990; 228:353–60.
52. Carlson J, Wiholm BE. Trimethoprim associated aseptic meningitis. Scand J Infect Dis 1987; 19:687–91.
53. McCue JD, Zandt JR. Acute psychoses associated with the use of ciprofloxacin and trimethoprim-sulfamethoxazole. Am J Med 1991; 90:528–9.
54. Kalowski S, Nanra RS, Matthew T, et al. Deterioration in renal function is associated with co-trimoxazole therapy. Lancet 1973; 2:394–7.
55. Shouval D. Ligumsky M, Ben-Ishay D. Effect of co-trimoxazole on normal creatinine clearance. Lancet 1978; 1:244–5.
56. Kastrup J, Petersen P, Bartram R, et al. The effect of trimethoprim on serum creatinine. Br J Urol 1985; 57:265–8.
57. Kleinknect D, Vanhille P, Morel-Maroger L, et al. Acute interstitial nephritis due to drug hypersensitivity. An up-to-date review with a report of 19 cases. Adv Nephrol 1983; 12:377–408.
58. Wiener I, Rubin DA, Martinez E, et al. QT prolongation and paroxysmal ventricular tachycardia occurring during fever following trimethoprim-sulfamethoxazole administration. Mt Sinai J Med 1981; 48:53–5.
59. Lopez JA, Harold JG, Rosenthal MC. QT prolongation and torsades de pointes after administration of trimethoprim-sulfamethoxazole. Am J Cardiol 1987; 59:376–7.

13

Aminoglycosides

Darwin E. Zaske
University of Minnesota, Minneapolis, and St. Paul-Ramsey Medical Center, St. Paul, Minnesota

The aminoglycosides are the mainstay in the treatment of serious, often life-threatening, gram-negative bacillary infections afflicting the elderly patient. Although the aminoglycosides exhibit differences in their antibacterial spectrum and clinical applications, they have similar pharmacological activities, pharmacokinetic properties, and risks of toxicity. Their inherent risks of nephrotoxicity and ototoxicity are a major disadvantage of the aminoglycoside antibiotics and reduce their clinical utility. The following discussion summarizes the chemical, pharmacological, and pharmacokinetic properties of these agents with a specific emphasis on the geriatric patient.

I. CHEMISTRY

A. History and Source

The aminoglycoside antibiotics are an older class of broad-spectrum antibiotics with activity against aerobic and facultative gram-negative bacilli, staphylococci, and some *Mycobacterium* species. Streptomycin was the first isolated aminoglycoside from *Streptomyces griseus* in 1944 by Schatz, Bugie, and Waksman. Neomycin was later (1949) isolated from *Streptomyces fradiae* by Waksman and Lechevalier. Kanamycin was isolated in 1957 by Umezawa and coworkers at the Japanese National Institutes of Health. Gentamicin was derived from the actinomycete *Micromonspora purpurea* in 1963 by Weinstein and coworkers. Tobramycin (from *Streptomyces tenebrarius*), amikacin (semisynthetic derivative of kanamycin A), and netilmicin (semisynthetic derivative of sisomicin) are more recent additions to the group and are less susceptible to the common methods of enzyme-mediated resistance.

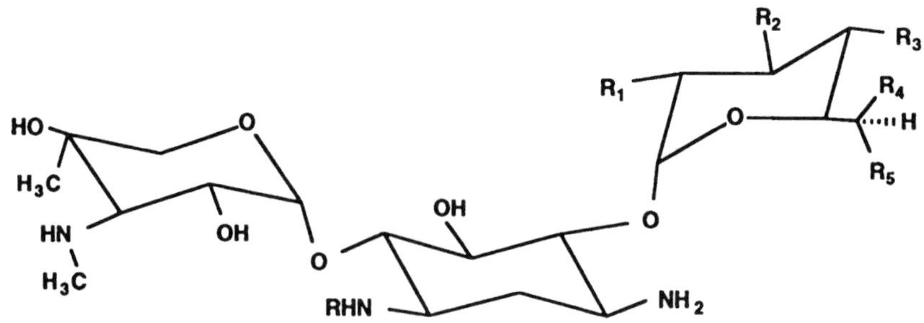

Antibiotic	R	R1	R2	R3	R4	R5
Gentamicin B	H	OH	OH	OH	H	NH_2
Gentamicin C_{1a}	H	NH_2	H	H	H	NH_2
Gentamicin C_1	H	NH_2	H	H	CH_3	$NHCH_3$
Gentamicin C_2	H	NH_2	H	H	CH_3	NH_2

Figure 1 The gentamicin family of aminoglycosides: The side chains of the different gentamicin-related molecules, and the basic nucleus of gentamicin are illustrated. The marketed formulation of gentamicin is a combination of gentamicin C_{1a}, C_1, and C_2.

B. Structure

The aminoglycosides consist of two or more amino sugars joined by a glycosidic linkage to a hexose nucleus. The hexose nucleus is either streptidine (for streptomycin) or 2-deoxystreptamine (for other aminoglycosides). The compounds containing three amino sugars are the neomycin family, and the gentamicin (Fig. 1) and kanamycin families (Fig. 2) contain two amino sugars. These two families, gentamicin and kanamycin, contain the currently used aminoglycosides. The commercially available gentamicin is a combination of gentamicin C_1, C_{1a}, and C_2, which are a different methylation of the amino sugar. Sisomicin and netilmicin (Fig. 3) contain a different 3-amino sugar (garosamine). The kanamycin family includes kanamycin A and B, tobramycin, and amikacin.

II. MECHANISM OF ACTION

The antibacterial mechanism of action (1,2) of aminoglycosides is rapidly bactericidal for sensitive organisms, especially those in the growing phase. This rapid lethal effect is apparently not explained by their capacity to inhibit protein synthesis or their effect on the translation of mRNA at the ribosome. The transport of aminoglycosides across the cell is an active process requiring oxygen. These compounds are thus not active in an anaerobic environment. The transport is also enhanced by an alkaline environment where less of the drug is ionized and more of the unionized drug is available for transportation across the cell membrane. Conversely, the transport of aminoglycosides in a more acidic environment is lessened, and, therefore, these agents are less active in an acidic or anaerobic environment. These agents are more active in reproducing cells, but are still lethal with resting cells. Their activity with resting cells differentiates the aminoglycosides from the β-lactams and may be important clinically.

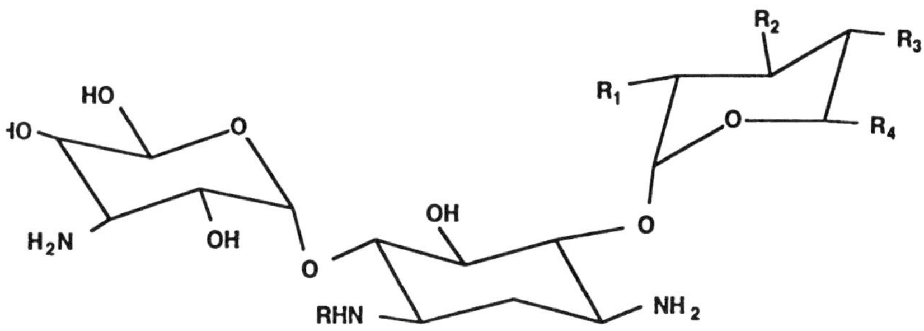

Antibiotic	R	R_1	R_2	R_3	R_4
Kanamycin A	H	OH	OH	OH	H
Kanamycin B	H	NH_2	OH	OH	H
Tobramycin	H	NH_2	H	OH	NH_2
Amikacin	HABA	OH	OH	OH	NH_2

Figure 2 The kanamycin family of aminoglycosides: The basic nucleus for kanamycin and the side chains for different kanamycin-related molecules are illustrated. The HABA (hydroxy-amino butyric acid) chain for amikacin is S-4-amino-2-hydroxylbutyryl, which prevents the nucleotidylation and phosphorylation at the 2″ position.

The aminoglycosides diffuse through the aqueous channels formed by porin proteins in the outer membrane of the gram-negative bacteria and enter the periplasmic space. They are further transported across the cytoplasmic membrane, which is an oxygen-dependent process that is reliant upon electron transport. This energy-dependent phase can be rate limiting and can be blocked or inhibited by divalent cations (i.e., calcium or

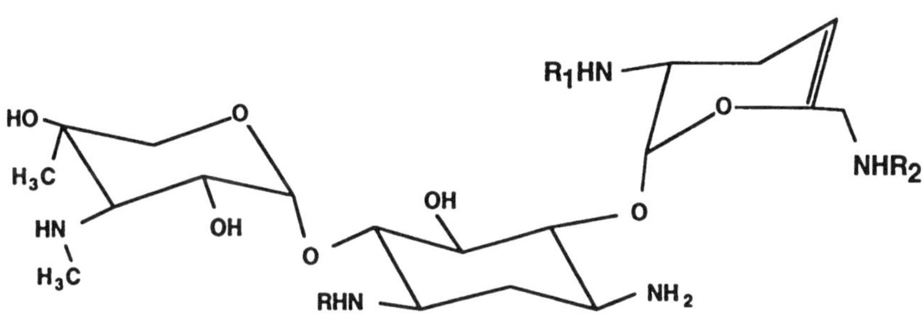

Antibiotic	R	R_1	R_2
Sisomicin	H	H	H
Netilmicin	CH_3CH_2	H	H

Figure 3 The sisomicin and netilmicin molecules are related to the gentamicin family as illustrated.

magnesium), hyperosmolarity, an acidic environment, and/or an anaerobic environment (i.e., an abscess). After transport across the cytoplasmic membrane, aminoglycosides bind to polysomes and inhibit synthesis of proteins, which further accelerates the transport of additional antibiotic. The binding to polysomes and inhibiting protein synthesis has been suggested to be linked to the disruption of the structure of the cytoplasmic membrane. This concept is consistent with the observation of leakage from the bacterial cell of small ions initially followed by larger molecules and then proteins immediately preceding death of the cell. The progressive disruption of the cellular envelope may explain the rapid lethal action of the aminoglycosides that occurs in resting cells.

Once transported across the bacterial cell membrane, the aminoglycosides attach to 30S and 50S ribosomal subunits. They cause misreading of genetic codes and formation of defective protein synthesis. A number of other steps in protein synthesis can also be affected. The aminoglycosides vary in their affinity for the ribosome and their capacity to cause misreading of mRNA. There appears to be a strong correlation between the agent's bactericidal activity and the ability to induce the misreading of the genetic code, but it remains to be proven whether this is the primary mechanism of action for the aminoglycosides.

A. Mechanisms of Resistance

Three major mechanisms of bacterial resistance are known to occur with aminoglycosides: (1) the production of inactivating enzymes, (2) the decrease in membrane permeability, and (3) a change in the 30S ribosomal binding protein.

Penetration of aminoglycosides through the pores in the outer membrane into the periplasmic space may be retarded in a few bacterial isolates, but is not an important mechanism of resistance that is encountered or acquired clinically. This mechanism may, however, explain the naturally occurring resistance found in anaerobic bacteria or facultative bacteria (e.g., *Pseudomonas maltophilia*) growing under anaerobic conditions. Such a mechanism of resistance can frequently be interrupted by the combination of β-lactam antibiotics which alter the structure of the cell wall and markedly improve the penetration of aminoglycosides into the bacteria.

Alterations in the ribosomal binding protein are less relevant clinically for most bacterial isolates. Isolates of *Escherichia coli*, *Pseudomonas aeruginosa*, and enterococci have been reported to have a change in amino acid content of ribosomal binding protein that also selectively alters the binding of aminoglycoside antibiotics. These strains or mutants occur infrequently, and therefore are not an important mechanism of resistance.

Inactivation of aminoglycosides by different enzymatic mechanisms is the most frequently occurring method of resistance clinically and is especially true for the nosocomial organisms causing hospital-acquired infections. After the drug has reached the periplasmic space, aminoglycosides may be altered by phosphorylation, adenylation, or acetylation of specific hydroxyl or amino groups on the molecule. Each of these enzymatic methods can affect different sites on the aminoglycoside molecule (Fig. 4). The genetic information for these enzymes is acquired by conjugation and the transfer of DNA as plasmids. This mechanism of resistance may also involve several antibiotics simultaneously. The different enzymes have markedly reduced the clinical usefulness of the older aminoglycosides, e.g., kanamycin, and have impacted the effectiveness of the more recent agents, e.g., gentamicin and tobramycin. Amikacin and netilmicin were engineered to be less susceptible to these enzyme mechanisms of resistance, but enzymatic mechanisms of resistance have

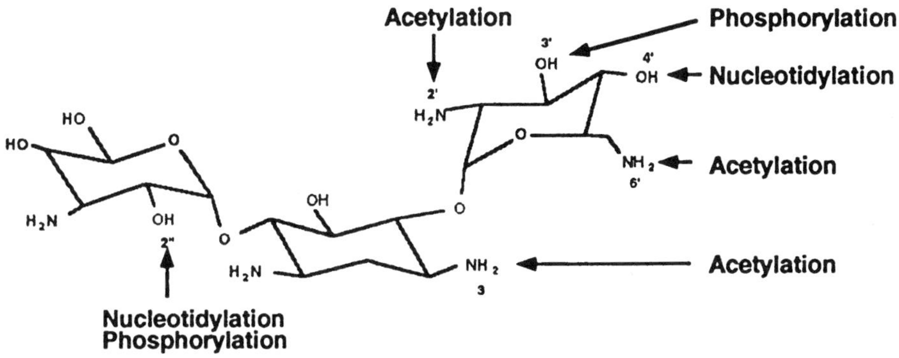

Figure 4 The most frequent methods of aminoglycoside resistance are enzymatic mechanisms involving acetylation, phosphorylation, and nucleotidylation at the indicated positions on the aminoglycoside nucleus.

been identified for these two agents (Fig. 4), and outbreaks of multiantibiotic resistant isolates (including amikacin and netilmicin) have been observed.

B. Structure-Activity Relationships

Structural modifications of the aminoglycosides have generally been conducted to develop molecules that would be more active against resistant strains. The understanding of different mechanisms of resistance at a molecular level has led scientists in a systematic manner to engineer new aminoglycosides that would be less susceptible to these identified mechanisms of resistance. Four general approaches have been undertaken to enhance the activity of the aminoglycosides: (1) removal of the functional group involved in the enzymatic inactivation (i.e., tobramycin), (2) steric shielding of the group involved in the enzymatic alteration (i.e., netilmicin), (3) steric shielding of a functional group remote to the site of chemical modification (i.e., amikacin), and (4) altering the glycoside conformation of the molecule to prevent enzymatic inactivation at several sites (i.e., 5-epi-sisomicin). New compounds combining several of these approaches have been identified, which are highly active against organisms resistant to amikacin. Designing compounds that can overcome mechanisms of permeability-resistance or that have fewer inherent risks of ototoxicity or nephrotoxicity (i.e., netilmicin) could receive future attention.

III. ANTIMICROBIAL SPECTRUM

The antibacterial activity of gentamicin, tobramycin, netilmicin, and amikacin is primarily directed against aerobic or facultative gram-negative bacilli (3–13). These organisms include many genera and species of Enterobacteriaceae including *E. coli*, *Klebsiella*, *Enterobacter*, *Serratia*, *Proteus*, and *Providencia* as well as *P. aeruginosa*. These aminoglycosides also have considerable activity against *Staphylococcus aureus* and *S. epidermidis*, but resistance to these agents, especially by staphylococci, can develop quickly.

The relative intrinsic activity of different aminoglycosides can vary substantially among different aerobic and facultative gram-negative bacilli. The older aminoglycosides, including kanamycin and streptomycin, are highly susceptible to different mechanisms of enzymatic inactivation and are not clinically useful for the treatment of infections caused by gram-negative bacilli. Tobramycin is generally more active against isolates of *P. aeruginosa* and *Proteus* species. Isolates of *Serratia marcescens* are generally more sensitive to gentamicin. Gentamicin-resistant gram-negative bacilli have mechanisms that are plasmid mediated and are frequently resistant to tobramycin except *Pseudomonas* species. Amikacin and netilmicin are less susceptible to the more frequent mechanisms of enzymatic inactivation. However, the nosocomial flora of many institutions have recently demonstrated resistance to many antibiotics including the aminoglycosides, and outbreaks of multiantibiotic resistance have been reported.

The aminoglycosides have little or no activity against the anaerobic bacteria. They have minimal activity against gram-positive bacteria except *Staphylococci*, and isolates of *Streptococcus pneumoniae* and *Streptococcus pyogenes* are highly resistant. Combinations of streptomycin or gentamicin with one of the penicillins are frequently synergistic or highly active. Gentamicin and tobramycin demonstrate considerable activity against isolates of *S. aureus* and *S. epidermidis*.

The activity of streptomycin against *Mycobacterium tuberculosis* was recognized in the late 1940s, and it became one of the first drugs available for the treatment of tuberculosis. Other species of *Mycobacterium* are generally resistant. The toxicity and the development of resistance to streptomycin has limited its current usage.

IV. CLINICAL PHARMACOLOGY

Large variations in serum concentrations are attained after a standardized dose of aminoglycoside. These variations are noted between patients and within an individual patient. Numerous physiological changes occur in patients who have sepsis, which explain the large interpatient and intrapatient variations in aminoglycoside elimination and distribution. These variations in serum concentrations may influence treatment outcomes since a relationship exists between concentrations and efficacy/safety.

A. Pharmacodynamics

1. Serum Concentration Versus Toxicity

The margin between therapeutic peak concentrations of aminoglycosides and those values associated with a higher risk of toxicity is relatively narrow. The peak serum concentration is defined as the value occurring immediately after the intravenous infusion. Peak serum concentrations for amikacin and kanamycin >32–34 μg/ml are associated with a higher risk of ototoxicity and nephrotoxicity (14). Sustained peak concentrations >12–15 μg/ml are associated with increased risk of developing nephrotoxicity and ototoxicity for gentamicin, tobramycin, and sisomicin. For netilmicin, increased risks of toxicity are associated with sustained peak concentrations >16 μg/ml. Peak serum concentrations of streptomycin should not exceed 30 μg/ml (15–17).

There is also a relationship between toxicity and the trough serum concentration of aminoglycosides (18–20). The trough concentration is the value immediately prior to a dose under steady-state conditions. A significant relationship between the trough concentration of streptomycin and the occurrence of vestibular toxicity was noted in patients receiving 0.75 g of streptomycin intramuscularly daily for treatment of tuberculosis (21). Patients with 24-h serum concentrations of streptomycin >3 μg/ml were significantly more likely to have vestibular toxicity than those who had 24-h serum concentrations <3 μg/ml. Higher risk of toxicity has also been associated with amikacin or kanamycin trough

Table 1 Serum Concentrations and Patient Response

Serum concentration	Response rate (%)	Comments	Ref.
Peaks of >5 μg/ml within first 72 h of treatment	84	Similar patient populations in both groups	24
"Therapeutic" serum concentrations not achieved	23		
Peaks of >8 μg/ml	89	Patients with gram-negative pneumonia	
"Therapeutic" serum concentrations not achieved	43		
1-h postinfusion serum concentrations of >5 μg/ml	Survival rate, 97.6	Patients with gram-negative bacteremia	26
Serum concentrations of <5 μg/ml	Survival rate, 79.1		
Mean peaks of 7.9 ± 1.8 μg/ml and mean troughs of 1.1 ± 0.6 μg/ml	88	Patients with gram-negative pneumonia involving *P. aeruginosa* or *Acinetobacter calcoaceticus*; multiple antibiotic-resistant pathogens, and grave prognosis	29
Postintramuscular administration: peaks of 6–8 μg/ml; Postintravenous bolus injection: 1-h postadministration concentrations of 8 μg/ml; All trough concentrations <2.0 μg/ml	94	Patients with complicated urinary tract infections (85% response rate with infections involving *Pseudomonas*)	29a
Individualized therapy: desired peaks of 8–12 μg/ml and troughs of 0.5–2 μg/ml	Survival rate, 64	Both treatment groups included patients with severe gram-negative sepsis	31
Conventionally dosed group, 3–5 mg/kg/day	Survival rate, 33		

concentrations >10 μg/ml (14). For gentamicin, tobramycin, and sisomicin, sustained trough concentrations >2 μg/ml are associated with increased risk of toxicity. For netilmicin, trough values >4 μg/ml are associated with a higher risk of toxicity.

2. *Serum Concentration Versus Efficacy*

Various investigators have reported a relationship between therapeutic serum aminoglycoside concentrations (defined below) and improved patient response (Table 1). Peak serum concentrations are associated with improved therapeutic success (22,23). Noone et al. (24) examined gentamicin concentrations and compared them with treatment response in 68 episodes of gram-negative sepsis during the first 72 h of treatment. Therapeutic concentrations were defined as peak concentrations >5 μg/ml for patients with soft-tissue infections, gram-negative septicemias, or urinary tract infections. For patients with a gram-negative pneumonia, peak concentrations of gentamicin >8 μg/ml were considered therapeutic. Treatment response was found to vary for these two groups of patients, with

84% of the patients who had therapeutic serum concentrations responding to treatment and only 23% of the patients who had inadequate serum concentrations responding to treatment.

Increased survival rates were also reported in patients with gram-negative bacteremia when treated with gentamicin (25). The 1-h post-infusion serum concentrations associated with increased survival were >5 μg/ml(26). A peak concentration of 20 μg/ml or greater for amikacin is considered therapeutic. Favorable patient response at this concentration was reported by Tally et al. (27). Klastersky et al. (28) showed that high serum bactericidal activity with amikacin was associated with increased response. Moore et al. (26) reported increased survival rates in patients with gram-negative sepsis when amikacin 1-h postinfusion serum concentrations were >20 μg/ml early in the course of therapy.

A higher incidence of breakthrough bacteremia is related to long periods of subinhibitory concentrations (25). Anderson et al. (23) reported a higher failure rate in patients who had excessively long periods of aminoglycoside serum concentrations below the inhibitory concentrations for the isolated pathogen. Of 42 patients being treated with antibiotics for gram-negative bacteremia, 20 cases (48%) ended in a second breakthrough or death due to the septic episode. Many patients receiving aminoglycosides demonstrate an extremely rapid half-life (1–2 h) of the drug, resulting in serum concentrations below the minimal inhibitory concentration (MIC) of the offending pathogen early in the dosing interval. For amikacin, the period of subinhibitory concentrations may be as much as 9–10 h of the conventional 12-h dosing interval. For gentamicin, tobramycin, and netilmicin, the period of subinhibitory concentrations may be as much as 4–6 h of a recommended 8-h dosing interval. Long periods of subinhibitory serum concentrations could be prevented by adjusting the dosing interval according to the elimination rate.

Improvement in morbidity and mortality of gram-negative infections might be achieved if the drug concentrations of patients were more carefully controlled to the upper concentrations of the therapeutic window for aminoglycosides. Cipolle et al. (29) reported a response rate of 88% for gram-negative pneumonia in patients whose doses were carefully monitored and adjusted using the Sawchuk-Zaske (30) method of aminoglycoside individualization. Burn patients with severe gram-negative sepsis whose dosing regimens were individualized had increased survival rates compared to a group that was dosed conventionally (31). Patient survival rates for the entire hospital course were 33% and 64% for the conventionally dosed and individually dosed groups, respectively. Survival rates for the first septic episode were 51.3% and 86.4%, respectively. Increased patient survival was also noted in burn patients treated with amikacin whose dosage regimens were individualized (32).

Interestingly, increasing patient age was also interactive with individualized methods in improving patient survival. Individualized dosing methods had a greater impact on the survival of geriatric patients. Thus, the geriatric patient benefited the most from individualized approaches to more quickly attain therapeutic serum concentrations. This observation would seem to be explained by the susceptibility of elderly patients to undertreated gram-negative sepsis and their limited reserve to withstand sepsis.

3. Therapeutic Serum Concentration

Gram-negative sepsis continues to have a high mortality rate with approximately one half of all fatalities occurring within the first 24 h (33). Survival has been related to the extent of the underlying disease, neutrophil count, and early use of appropriate antibiotics (34). Variations in half-life and distribution volume expose some patients to subtherapeutic concentrations and others to toxicity. The most direct and quantitative way of ensuring adequate as well as safe therapy within the first 72 h of treatment is to measure serum concentrations and adjust the patient's dosage regimen.

Guidelines for peak and trough serum concentrations can be established that minimize the risk of toxicity and maximize the likelihood of favorable treatment response. Within these guidelines, specific target peak and trough concentrations need to be selected for the patient being treated. These should be based on the patient's clinical condition, the type of infection, and the relative minimum inhibitory concentration of the suspected/isolated pathogen. Higher peak and trough serum concentrations are selected in patients who have more severe infections or who have a higher risk of treatment failure.

B. Pharmacokinetics

1. Absorption

Aminoglycoside antibiotics are poorly absorbed from the gastrointestinal tract except in patients who have extensive erosion of the gastrointestinal mucosa. Less than 1% of a dose of the drug is absorbed following either oral or rectal administration. After an oral dose of an aminoglycoside, resulting serum concentrations are very low in patients who have normal renal function (35,36), but systemic concentrations can approach or exceed toxic values in patients who have abnormal renal function.

The aminoglycosides must be given intravenously or intramuscularly to treat systemic infections. Absorption following intramuscular injection is reportedly consistent, rapid, and complete in normal volunteers. However, in severely ill patients, intramuscular absorption rates can vary considerably. This could be due in part to differences in regional blood flow that occur primarily in patients who are bedridden, obese, or hypotensive, or who have severely compromised cardiovascular function.

Peak serum aminoglycoside concentrations generally occur 20–60 min following intramuscular administration in patients who have normal renal functions and normal distribution volumes (25% of body weight). In patients who have abnormal renal functions or large distribution volumes, peak serum concentrations may not occur until 3–6 h after intramuscular administration. Peak serum concentrations following intravenous administration are attained immediately postinfusion.

Peritoneal administration may lead to high and potentially toxic serum concentrations. Systemic concentrations of kanamycin, after a 2- or 5-min intraperitoneal lavage, approach 15–25 μg/ml within 15–75 min (37). Substantial absorption may also occur when aminoglycosides are applied topically to wounds and burns, especially in continuous wound irrigations and with large surface area burns.

2. Distribution

Aminoglycosides distribute into bile, soft tissue, peritoneal, pleural, pericardial, and synovial fluids in adequate concentrations to treat most infections. These agents are less than 40% protein bound. Penetration of aminoglycosides into the eye is poor following systemic administration (38). To treat local ophthalmic infections, it may be necessary to administer the aminoglycoside either topically or by direct periocular injections. Aminoglycosides enter cerebrospinal fluid in subtherapeutic concentrations, even in the presence of inflamed meninges. Intrathecal or intraventricular administration of the drug is necessary to ensure optimal therapeutic concentrations.

Penetration of aminoglycosides into bile is variable (39,40). With biliary obstruction, aminoglycosides usually do not attain therapeutic concentrations in biliary fluid. Serious biliary infections such as cholecystitis can influence the pattern of biliary elimination. Inability to detect gentamicin and streptomycin in gallbladder and bile has been noted in patients with cholecystitis due to cystic obstruction (41,42). For patients without obstruc-

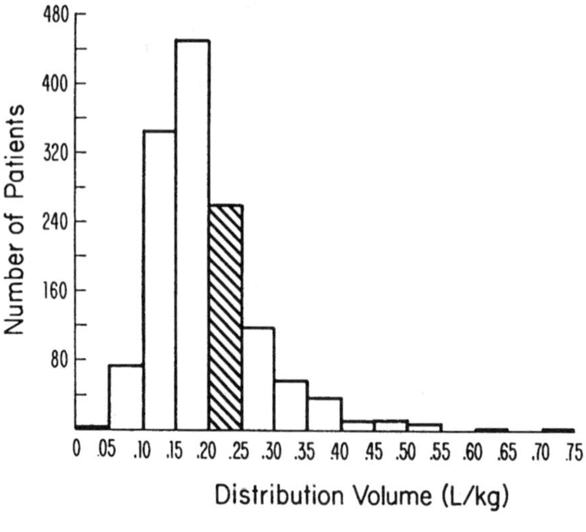

Figure 5 The distribution volume for gentamicin demonstrates substantial interpatient variability in a large group of patients initially treated for sepsis. This variation is similar for all aminoglycosides. During treatment, the variation is generally reduced because patients who are initially dehydrated have their fluid deficits replaced and patients who are initially fluid overloaded diuresis and their fluid volumes return to normal values.

tion, specimens of bile collected from gallbladder T-tube drainage contained 25–75% of the simultaneous concentrations of aminoglycoside in serum.

Aminoglycoside concentrations in bronchial secretions have been unpredictable (43,44). However, concentrations of 40% or more of corresponding serum concentrations of aminoglycosides have been found in bronchial secretions. Bronchial concentrations of the drug increased in parallel with those in serum (45). For this reason, it has been suggested that higher systemic concentrations will increase the efficacy of the antibiotic regimen for patients with pneumonia.

3. Volume of Distribution

The distribution volume is defined as the dose administered via an instantaneous infusion divided by the change in serum concentration. This pharmacokinetic parameter is usually expressed in liters or standardized to body weight (liters per kilogram). If, for example, 80 mg of aminoglycoside was administered to a patient as an instantaneous infusion and the change in serum concentration was 8 mg/L, the distribution volume would be 10 L.

The distribution volume of the highly water-soluble aminoglycoside closely resembles the volume of the extracellular fluid compartment. This compartment is 0.18–0.25 L/kg in normal individuals. However, wide variations occur both within and among individuals. In severely septic patients, the fluid and electrolyte status may vary considerably and further change the extracellular fluid volume and the aminoglycoside distribution volume. Expanded distribution volumes frequently occur in elderly patients who have congestive heart failure; contracted distribution volumes are frequently observed in elderly patients who are clinically dehydrated.

The distribution volume for gentamicin, tobramycin, amikacin, and netilmicin demonstrated a wide interpatient variation (Fig. 5). A 6- to 12-fold range was reported in

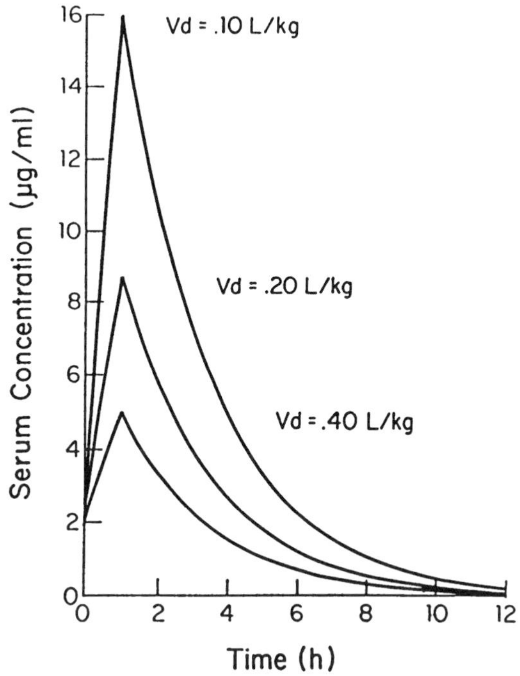

Figure 6 The interpatient variation in distribution volume can have an important effect on the serum concentration time profile for all aminoglycosides. Patients who are initially dehydrated and who have a small distribution volume will attain potentially toxic concentrations. If the same dose is administered to a patient who is fluid overloaded and has a large distribution volume, the patient may not attain therapeutic serum concentrations.

amikacin, netilmicin, tobramycin, and gentamicin (46,47) distribution volumes, respectively, in patients treated for gram-negative infection. This interpatient variation is similar for all aminoglycosides. The apparent volume of distribution for aminoglycosides varies from 0.13 to 0.48 L/kg with an average of 0.20 L/kg in adults (48–51). Evidence suggests that the pharmacokinetic data for streptomycin and kanamycin are similar to values determined for amikacin (15).

These interpatient differences in distribution volume can have a profound effect on the serum concentration-time profile (Fig. 6). The substantial variation in reported distribution volumes emphasizes the importance of calculating an individual patient's distribution volume to determine individual dosage requirements. An individual's distribution volume may be affected by several pathophysiological changes. Hydration status, congestive heart failure, peritonitis, gender, and renal failure are several factors that may influence aminoglycoside distribution volume. Clinically, dehydrated patients exhibit reduced distribution volumes for aminoglycosides. Patients who have congestive heart failure have increased extravascular fluid volumes and exhibit an increased aminoglycoside distribution volume. Patients with smaller distribution volumes require lower initial doses to attain therapeutic concentrations, while patients with larger distribution volumes require higher doses to attain the same values.

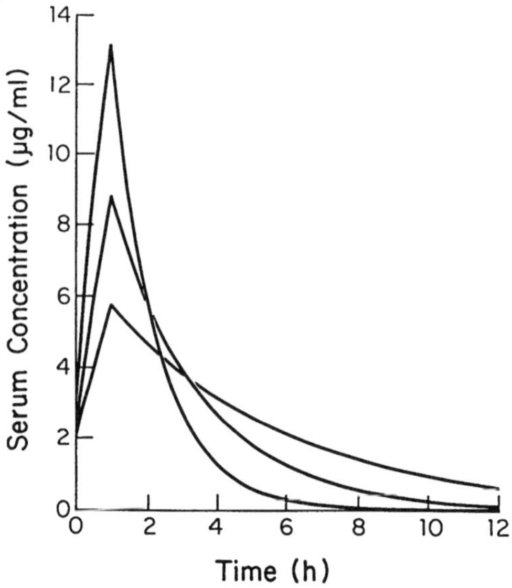

Figure 7 The intrapatient variation in distribution volume can have an important effect on the serum concentration time profile for all aminoglycosides. The clearance of aminoglycosides will remain constant in many patients, but the distribution can change within a patient and will cause changes in the drug's distribution volume. This change is totally independent of a change in serum creatinine and is frequently observed clinically. A change in both dose and dosing interval may be necessary to achieve desired serum concentrations.

Variations in aminoglycoside distribution volume can occur within an individual patient (52). Extracellular fluid volume, and thus, the aminoglycoside distribution volume, return toward normal values as a patient's underlying disease or infection resolves. For example, an elderly patient may have congestive heart failure secondary to their infection or sepsis. These patients who have congestive heart failure have a large distribution volume initially, but will return to normal values as the excess fluid is diuresed with diuretics/inotropes or the underlying infection resolves. Those patients who are clinically dehydrated generally receive intravenous fluids and as the fluid deficit is replaced, the distribution volume will increase.

These changes in distribution volume can affect elimination of the drug. As distribution volume decreases, half-life will decrease proportionately within the same patient and the drug's clearance will generally remain constant. This will also affect the serum concentration-time profile (Fig. 7). Such a change in half-life is independent of any change in renal function. These intrapatient variations in aminoglycoside distribution volume and half-life often necessitate adjustments in dosage regimens during a patient's treatment course.

In patients who have normal renal functions, a change in the extracellular fluid compartment, as estimated by distribution volume, is the second most important variable in explaining variance (r^2) in elimination rate and half-life (Fig. 8) (53). Changes in distribution volume affect aminoglycoside elimination rate by the following relationship:

$$\text{Elimination Rate} = \frac{\text{Clearance}}{\text{Volume of Distribution}}$$

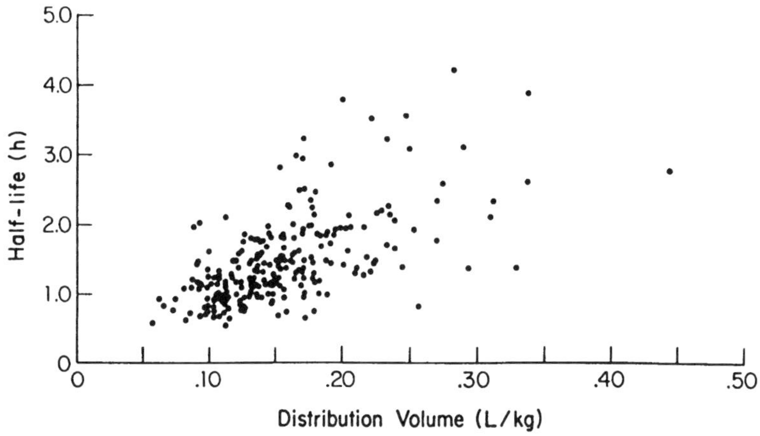

Figure 8 The relationship of gentamicin half-life and distribution volume is illustrated in 249 patients who had normal renal function (53). The larger the distribution volume caused a longer half-life of aminoglycoside. Alterations from normal values in the patient's aminoglycoside distribution volume and half-life are frequently observed in patients who have sepsis.

Aminoglycoside elimination rate and half-life are related in the following manner:

$$\text{Half-Life} = \frac{0.693}{\text{Elimination Rate}}$$

The half-life is thus directly related to the distribution volume and inversely related to clearance of the drug. Patients who have a large distribution volume will have a markedly prolonged half-life compared to patients who have similar renal function and a normal distribution volume. In contrast, patients who have a small distribution volume will have a shorter half-life.

4. Elimination

The major route of elimination of aminoglycosides is by the kidney via glomerular filtration. In general, 85–95% of the administered dose may be recovered unchanged in the urine. Additionally, active secretion has been suggested, but it accounts for only a small amount of drug elimination. Some tubular reabsorption may also occur. In patients with adequate renal function, urine concentrations of gentamicin, tobramycin, and netilmicin frequently exceed 300 μg/ml. Amikacin urine concentrations frequently exceed 1000 μg/ml. Urinary concentrations of aminoglycosides may be considerably less in patients with renal insufficiency, especially when renal function is less than 10% of normal. All of the aminoglycosides have similar pharmacokinetic properties within the same patient.

5. Half-Life

The half-life of a drug describes the time required for the serum concentration to decrease by 50% of the original concentration. It is a pharmacokinetic parameter describing the elimination rate of the drug. In volunteers with normal renal function, the half-life of aminoglycosides ranges from 2.5–4 h. However, wide variations in aminoglycoside elimi-

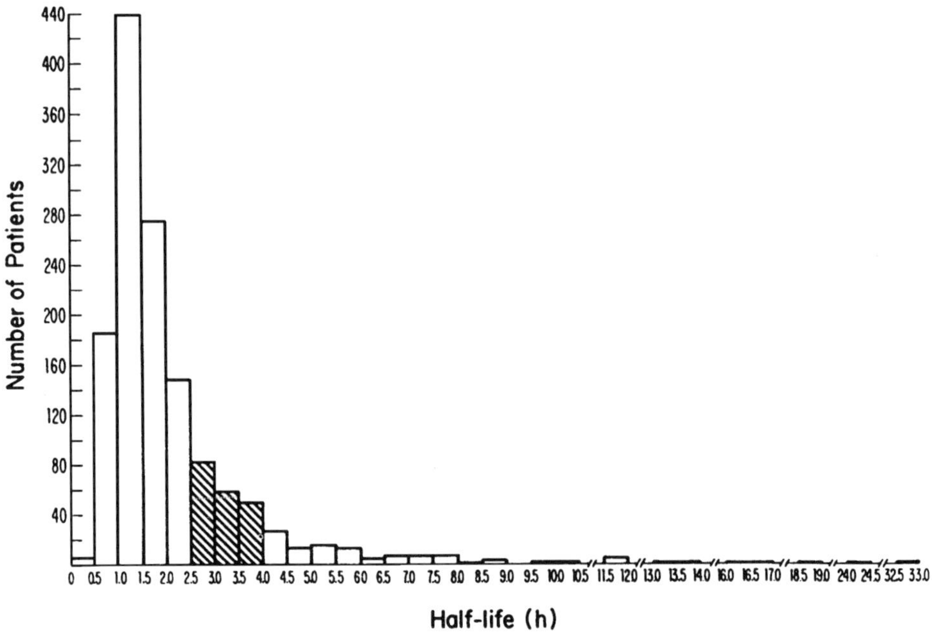

Figure 9 The half-life of gentamicin and other aminoglycosides demonstrate substantial variation in a group of patients treated for sepsis. This variation occurs in patients who have normal renal function as determined by serum creatinine (≤1.5 mg/dl) or creatinine clearance (>100 ml/min).

nation have been determined in seriously ill patients being treated with aminoglycosides.

Many physiological changes occur in patients who are treated with aminoglycosides due to underlying medical conditions or secondary to sepsis. Changes in factors such as cardiac output, renal blood flow, glomerular filtration, kidney perfusion, and the state of hydration will affect the disposition of aminoglycosides. This is of particular importance in the initial treatment of gram-negative sepsis when these physiological factors vary the most from patient to patient or within the same patient.

Substantial variation in aminoglycoside half-life exists among patients, even in those who have normal renal function (Fig. 9). All aminoglycoside agents have a similar degree of variation. The half-life of amikacin may range from 0.68–14.4 h in patients who have normal serum creatinine (≤1.5 mg/dl) and 0.68–7.2 h in patients with normal creatinine clearances (≥100 ml/h) in 67 subjects who are being treated for gram-negative sepsis. These variations have marked effects on serum aminoglycoside concentrations. The large number of patients who have a short half-life attain lower peak serum concentrations and can reach subinhibitory concentrations within the first 2 h of the dosing interval (Fig. 10).

6. Geriatric Populations

In general, elderly patients have progressively decreasing renal function with increasing age; glomerular filtration rate and aminoglycoside clearance are also decreased with increasing age (Table 2). These patients frequently require prolonged dosing intervals and lower daily dosages. Many geriatric patients who present to the hospital are clinically dehydrated and will require lower aminoglycoside doses to achieve desired peak serum concentrations. In contrast, elderly bedridden patients tend to have larger distribution

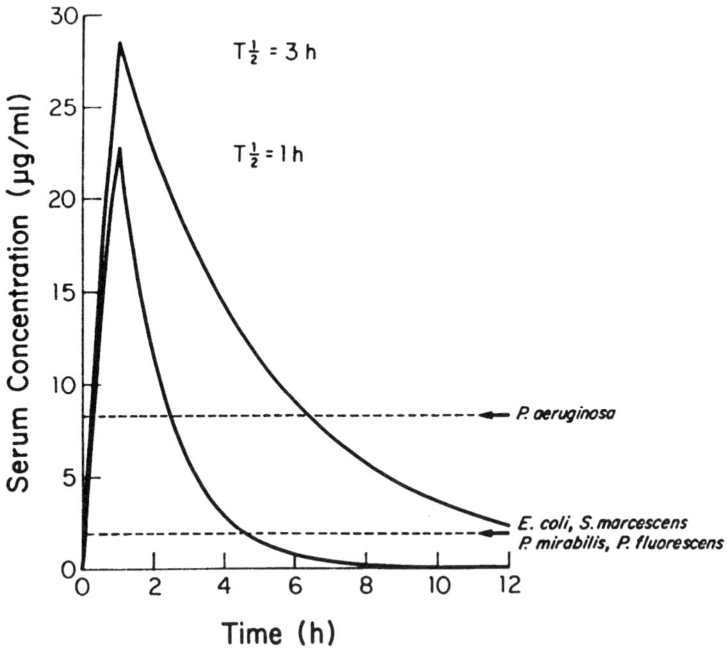

Figure 10 The short half-life of an aminoglycoside will result in subinhibitory serum concentrations within the first 1–2 h of the dosing interval. This further defines the need of shorter dosing intervals in select patients who are hyperdynamic.

Table 2 Clinical and Pharmacokinetic Data of Gentamicin in Geriatric Patients

Renal function	All patients (N = 417)	Normal SCr, ≤1.5 mg/dl (N = 302)	Abnormal SCr, >1.5 mg/dl (N = 115)	Abnormal CrCl, <100 ml/min (N = 410)	Normal CrCl, ≥100 ml/min (N = 7)
Age, y	76.56 ± 7.87	76.46 ± 7.92	76.83 ± 7.79	76.68 ± 86	69.71 ± 5.50
Weight, kg	65.62 ± 15.31	64.30 ± 14.59	69.07 ± 16.65	65.22 ± 14.99	88.91 ± 17.10
Serum creatinine, mg/dl	1.99 ± 1.77	1.05 ± 0.24	3.34 ± 2.09	2.01 ± 1.78	0.88 ± 0.29
Creatinine clearance, ml/min	42.36 ± 22.87	48.53 ± 22.59	27.64 ± 15.75	40.98 ± 20.72	114.85 ± 10.75
Hematocrit, %	35.15 ± 5.80	35.19 ± 5.73	35.06 ± 5.97	35.18 ± 5.79	—
Half-life, h	5.69 ± 6.55	4.43 ± 3.78	8.99 ± 10.19	5.75 ± 6.59	2.52 ± 0.88
Distribution volume, L/kg	0.23 ± 0.11	0.23 ± 0.12	0.22 ± 0.09	0.23 ± 0.11	0.20 ± 0.04
Elimination rate constant, h^{-1}	0.22 ± 0.18	0.25 ± 0.19	0.14 ± 0.11	0.22 ± 0.18	0.31 ± 0.14
Clearance, mg/h/kg	44.18 ± 30.24	49.67 ± 30.35	29.77 ± 24.88	43.86 ± 30.20	63.16 ± 28.10
Daily dose, mg/kg	3.53 ± 2.09	3.89 ± 2.13	2.60 ± 1.65	3.53 ± 2.09	4.04 ± 1.69

SCr = serum creatinine; CrCl = creatinine clearance.
Source: Ref. 81.

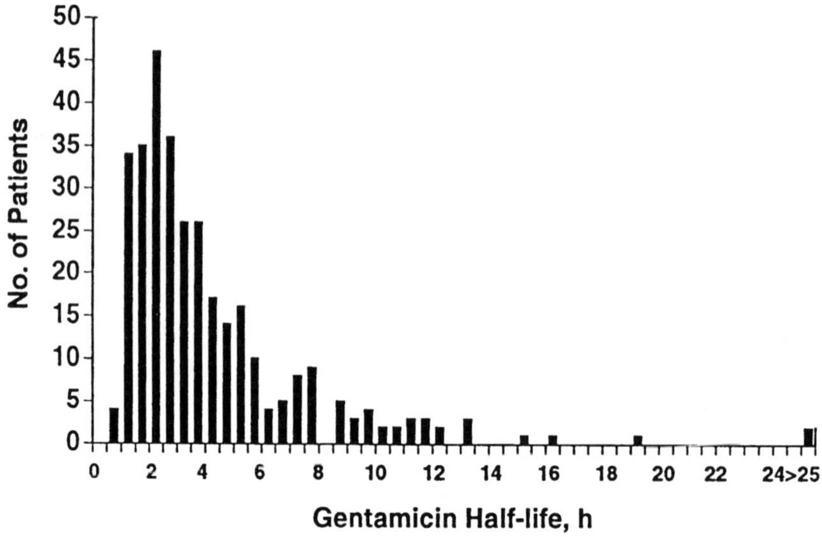

Figure 11 The half-life of gentamicin and other aminoglycosides are quite variable in geriatric patients who are treated for sepsis and who have a normal serum creatinine. Approximately 75% of these geriatric patients had half-lives shorter or longer than the reported normal range of 2.5–4.0 h in patients who had normal renal function.

volumes because many of these patients may have clinical signs or early signs of congestive failure (54). These patients frequently have underlying pathophysiological processes that alter aminoglycoside disposition. The elderly patient who develops severe gram-negative sepsis may develop congestive heart failure at the same time. These patients will probably have an expanded distribution volume and substantially prolonged half-life secondary to increased extracellular fluid and edema. These patients may also be at higher risks to toxicity or treatment failure.

The pharmacokinetic parameters of the aminoglycoside antibiotics demonstrate substantial interpatient variation. The half-life (Fig. 11) and distribution volume (Fig. 12) are more variable for all of the aminoglycosides in the elderly infected patients as compared to younger infected patients. The elderly patients' pharmacokinetic parameters are quite dynamic and are influenced by the same physiological changes that occur in other patients. Intrapatient changes in their pharmacokinetic parameters also frequently occur with all aminoglycosides, and many of these changes are not related to changes in renal function or serum creatinine.

7. *Patient Factors Affecting Pharmacokinetic Parameters*

Several patient factors/conditions have been identified that affect aminoglycoside disposition. The clinician can make better clinical judgments if he or she understands these physiological and pharmacokinetic relationships and the effect of different disease states on the patient's physiological parameters and thereafter on the drug's pharmacokinetic parameters. These factors are discussed in the following sections.

Renal Function. Patients who have compromised renal function have lower aminoglycoside elimination rates and more prolonged half-lives than patients who have normal

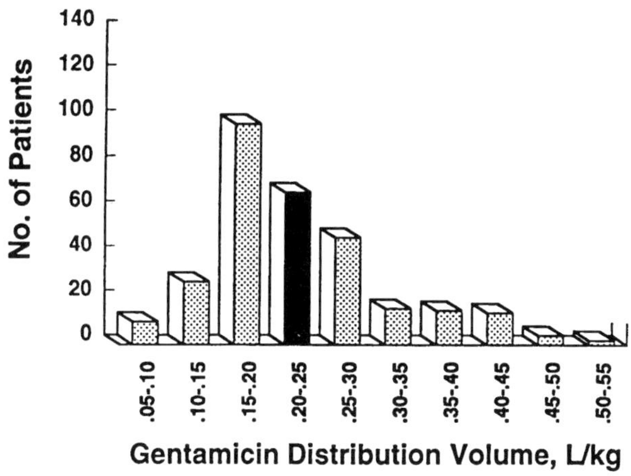

Figure 12 The distribution volume of gentamicin and other aminoglycosides are quite variable in geriatric patients who are treated for sepsis. Many of the geriatric patients are initially dehydrated and therefore have a smaller distribution volume as compared to a normal state. In contrast, some elderly patients have congestive heart failure concurrently with sepsis and will have a larger distribution volume until the excess fluid is diuresed.

renal function. The relationship between aminoglycoside elimination and estimates of renal function was originally established in healthy individuals. The variables of creatinine clearance (estimates) and aminoglycoside clearance were reported to be highly correlated (55,56). In patients with gram-negative sepsis, however, there is a marked decrease in the association of these variables (Fig. 13). The half-life and elimination rate of these agents vary considerably for specific estimates of renal function. Only 35% of the variance (r^2) in gentamicin elimination rate was explained by changes in creatinine clearance (31,57). In one report, about 56% of the variance in gentamicin half-life could be explained by changes in serum creatinine (58). Similar relationships are also reported with tobramycin (59), sisomicin (60), netilmicin (61,62) and amikacin (63–65). Additionally, the association with measured creatinine clearance via a 24-h urine collection, and predicted creatinine clearance was found to be very low in the septic patient for the four commonly used methods (Fig. 14).

Patients with Ascites. Patients who have ascites can have markedly increased extracellular fluid compartments (66). These patients exhibit large aminoglycoside distribution volumes and prolonged half-lives. The distribution volume of gentamicin was determined in one study of eight patients who had ascites (67). The distribution volumes in these patients were markedly increased, indicating the drug distributed into ascitic fluid. The large distribution volumes reported in this study were further substantiated in another study in which tobramycin pharmacokinetics were determined in eight patients who had ascites secondary to alcoholic liver cirrhosis (68). The maximum concentration of tobramycin in ascitic fluid occurred at 4.4 ± 1.7 h after administration.

In dosing patients who have severe hepatic disease, this third spacing phenomenon should be considered in estimating dosage requirements. A larger aminoglycoside dose must be given to these patients to ensure that desired peak concentrations will be achieved. These patients frequently require prolonged dosing intervals to prevent high trough concen-

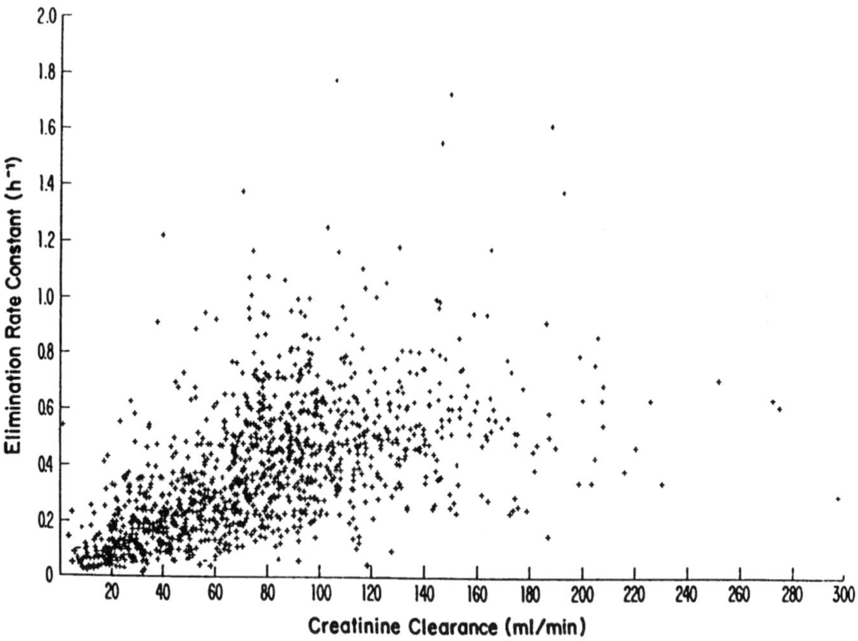

Figure 13 The relationship of gentamicin elimination rate and creatinine clearance demonstrates a moderate association ($r^2 = 0.30$). The relationship of gentamicin clearance and creatinine clearance is slightly improved ($r^2 = 0.38$).

trations. The prolonged half-life occurs even in those patients who have normal renal function. Additionally, the extracellular fluid compartment can change rapidly in these patients if effective diuretic therapy is instituted that is combined with fluid restriction. Similarly, aminoglycoside distribution volume and half-life can also change rapidly in these patients during aminoglycoside therapy, and serum aminoglycoside concentrations must be carefully monitored to determine the necessary dosage adjustments.

Dialysis Patients. Clearance of all aminoglycoside agents during dialysis is similar. The amount of aminoglycoside removed during dialysis can vary considerably between and within patients (69–71). Blood and dialysate flow rates, duration of dialysis treatment, and type of dialyzer membrane are major factors that determine the amount of drug removed during hemodialysis. Clearance of the aminoglycoside is directly proportional to the flow rate. Septic patients may exhibit fluctuating flow rates because of hypotension and other changes occurring hemodynamically. The amount of drug dialyzed may also be influenced by the type of membrane in the dialyzer machine. Different membrane types can have different extraction efficiencies. Recently, three different hemodialyzers were evaluated and it was found that the performance of each markedly differed with respect to elimination and clearance characteristics of gentamicin and tobramycin (72). The amount of drug that is removed is directly proportional to the duration of dialysis. The longer the dialysis period, the greater the amount of drug that is removed.

A rebound phenomenon appears to occur with serum concentrations of patients after hemodialysis, which may influence the calculated replacement dosages for these patients.

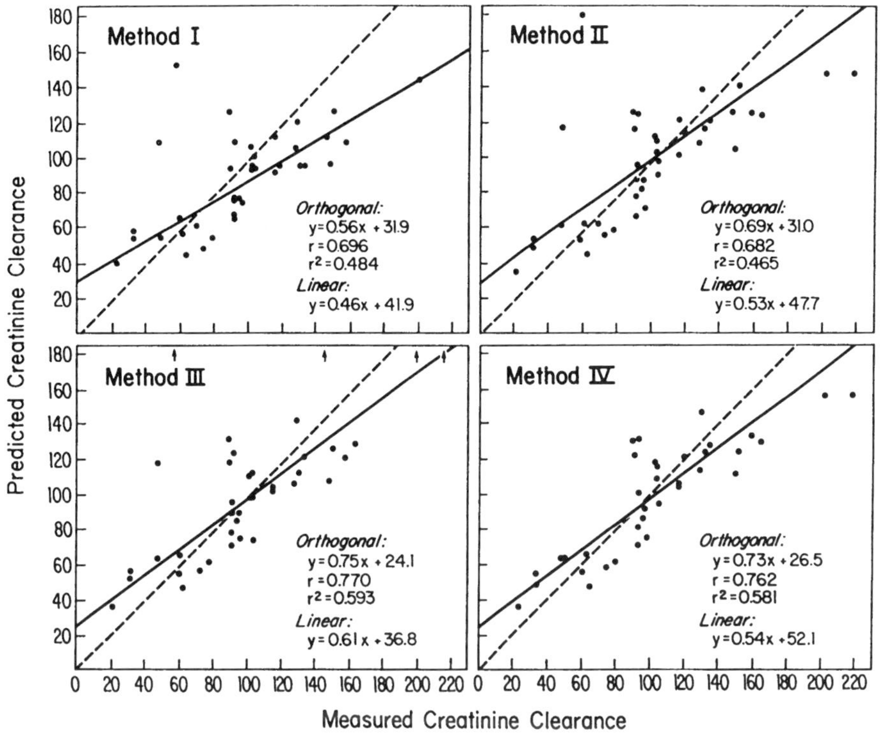

Figure 14 The association of measured creatinine clearance (from a 24-h urine collection) and predicted creatinine clearance from four commonly used methods were surprisingly low in theseptic patients. This is an important source of error in estimating aminoglycoside clearance and thereby dosage requirements.

This phenomenon was reported in seven acute renal failure patients receiving gentamicin (73). The blood samples from these patients were collected immediately postdialysis and 1-h postdialysis. In all seven cases, the 1-h postdialysis gentamicin concentration was higher than the concentration determined for the sample collected immediately postdialysis. The mean increase in gentamicin serum concentration was 25.7%, which could be due to release of the drug from tissues back into the blood. Such a finding may be clinically important since serum aminoglycoside samples are commonly obtained immediately postdialysis, and the drug concentrations in these samples are used to calculate replacement doses.

For hemodialysis patients, after an initial dose of 2.0 mg/kg of gentamicin the maintenance dosage regimens are 1.0 mg/kg or half of the loading dose, administered after each dialysis period (55). Suggested initial amikacin dosage regimen for hemodialysis patients is 7.5 mg/kg, and subsequent doses are 3.75 mg/kg after each dialysis (69). The clinician must consider those factors that can influence aminoglycoside therapy: time of dialysis in relation to the last administered dose, length of dialysis treatment, type of dialyzer used, amount of ultrafiltration, amount of intrinsic aminoglycoside clearance, flow rates, and time of serum sampling.

The factors governing aminoglycoside exchange across the peritoneal membrane are less well understood. Peritoneal dialysis is less efficient than hemodialysis in removing systemically administered aminoglycosides. Studies show that peritoneal dialysis accounted for only 15–20% of the total body clearance of tobramycin (74). For amikacin, the mean half-life and clearance are 19.9 ($\pm$ 3.2) h and 6.4 ($\pm$2.0) ml/min/m^2, respectively (69). In one study, the half-life of kanamycin decreased from 84 to 12 h after a 22-h peritoneal dialysis, and the peritoneal clearance was 8.3 mg/min (75). Dwell time, duration of peritoneal dialysis, and volume of fluid are important variables affecting the elimination of aminoglycosides by peritoneal dialysis.

Peritoneal dialysate has been mixed with aminoglycosides to reduce the risk of intraperitoneal infections. Absorption of aminoglycosides from the peritoneal dialysate can result in therapeutic serum concentrations. Aminoglycoside absorption from the peritoneal cavity is rapid in patients undergoing continuous ambulatory peritoneal dialysis. Equal gentamicin concentrations occur in serum and dialysate at 24 h following administration of a single intraperitoneal dose of 7.5 mg/L (76). Absorption of approximately half of the administered dose of gentamicin over a 6-h peritoneal dialysis period has been reported (77). Similar findings have been shown for tobramycin in which absorption of 52% of the administered dose of 1.5 mg/kg occurred during a 4-h dialysate dwelling period (74).

Febrile States. Serum concentrations of gentamicin in humans and in animals are affected by elevations in body temperature. Febrile subjects demonstrated lower gentamicin serum concentrations than did afebrile patients (78). Lower aminoglycoside serum concentrations in febrile patients may result from increased drug clearance. In febrile patients, the body's increased metabolic requirements can result in increased cardiac output, renal blood flow, and glomerular filtration. Thus, with increased renal perfusion and glomerular filtration, aminoglycoside clearance increases, resulting in lower serum concentrations.

Altered Hematocrits. A linear relationship between the reciprocal of the hematocrit and gentamicin half-life appears to be present (58). As the hematocrit increased, the gentamicin half-life decreased. The reciprocal of the hematocrit explains 43% of the variance in the half-life. Gentamicin distribution volume has also been reported to relate statistically to hematocrit (30). Changing the extracellular fluid volume and intravascular volume has a direct effect on the hematocrit and explains the basis for the relationship between hematocrit and distribution volume. Changes in half-life are probably affected by the distribution volume and explain the relationship between hematocrit and half-life. These findings may be clinically important in estimating dosage and dosing intervals.

Age. Although not confirmed by some investigators (79), age appears to be an important variable affecting aminoglycoside disposition, even when one accounts for the variation caused by renal function. There is a gradual decrease in elimination rate as the population ages, which continues after the patient reaches 60 years (80,81). The elimination rate and clearance of aminoglycosides continue to decrease within the geriatric population as age increases.

A number of physiological processes change as the population ages, which may account for the substantial variation in aminoglycoside kinetic parameters among different age groups. With increasing age, there is a decreasing proportion of total body water and/or muscle mass to the total body weight. Thus, aminoglycoside distribution volume will change, paralleling these changes in body water content. Additionally, aminoglycoside half-life may be a function of renal maturity (Fig. 15). Elderly patients have prolonged aminoglycoside half-lives secondary to reduced kidney function (81). Age explains additional variance in elimination rate of aminoglycosides and appears to also affect other

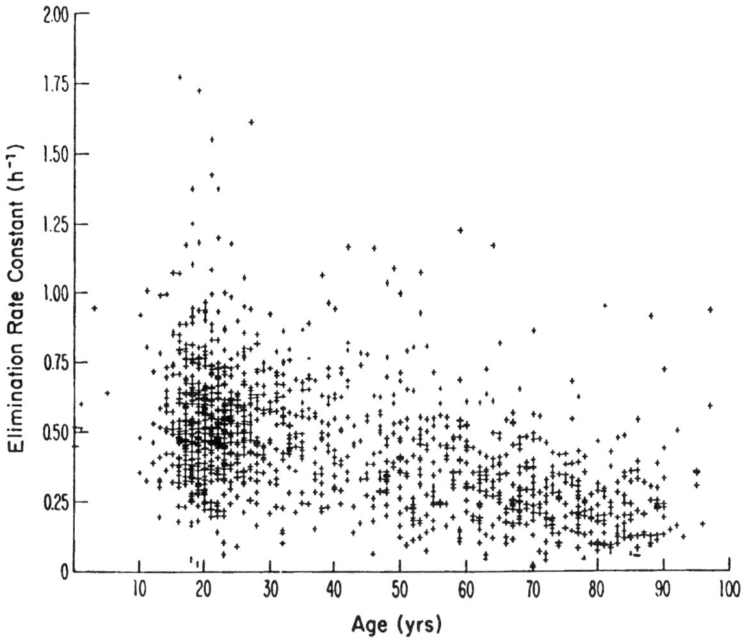

Figure 15 Aminoglycoside (gentamicin) elimination rate continually decreases with increasing age. This trend continues after the patient population reaches 60 years.

physiological functions related to aminoglycoside disposition (i.e., cardiovascular function).

Obesity. Lean body weight has a higher ratio of extracellular fluid to body mass as compared to adipose tissue. The aminoglycoside distribution volume on a per weight basis is less in adipose tissue than muscle mass. Originally, it was thought that aminoglycosides distribute into lean body mass only and not into excess weight or adipose tissue. However, pharmacokinetic studies indicate that aminoglycosides distribute into 5 or 6% of estimated excess weight (82–84). This closely approximates the extracellular fluid compartment of 8–10% that occurs in adipose tissue. Dosage estimates based on lean body weight could easily underestimate the dosage requirement of an obese patient. It is difficult to predict aminoglycoside requirements in obese patients without the benefit of serum concentration determinations.

Gender. Differences in aminoglycoside disposition have been associated with gender. Females reportedly have more rapid aminoglycoside half-lives and elimination rates than do males (30,58), which may be due to their smaller distribution volume in comparison to males. Females tend to have a lower proportion of muscle mass per kilogram body weight than do males. This significant relationship between elimination rate and gender was reported in 1640 patients who received individualized gentamicin therapy (30). The relationship was significant even after the influence of age and weight were used as covariants.

Burn Patients and Other Hypermetabolic Patients. Burn patients have two distinct postresuscitation phases in which aminoglycoside pharmacokinetic parameters can be substantially different. A wide variation in elimination rate, half-life, and distribution volume will occur in both phases (85). Aminoglycoside distribution volume is elevated during the initial phase of burn resuscitation and prior to the postburn diuresis phase. This is especially true in those who develop gram-negative sepsis and in the elderly patients who may not diurese the expanded fluid. The distribution volume in this phase frequently ranges from 0.3 to 0.5 L/kg or higher, and the half-life is excessively prolonged (5–7 h). These patients require larger doses and extended dosing intervals during this initial phase (79,85,86). After the diuretic phase, the distribution volume approaches the normal values of 0.15–0.2 L/kg, and the half-life decreases abruptly (32). These changes occur without parallel changes in creatinine clearance (87).

V. CLINICAL INDICATIONS

The aminoglycosides are prescribed for the treatment of life-threatening infections involving aerobic and facultative gram-negative bacilli that are aminoglycoside-sensitive. In combination with another antibiotic having a different spectrum of antimicrobial activity, they are agents of choice in the treatment of suspected or documented gram-negative sepsis. Aminoglycosides are commonly used to treat pneumonia, as well as urinary tract, pelvic, peritoneal, skeletal, and soft-tissue infections caused by gram-negative bacilli.

Aminoglycosides are indicated for the treatment of gram-negative bacillary meningitis or ventriculitis even though these agents penetrate poorly into cerebrospinal fluid in the presence of inflamed meninges. Therefore, they must be administered intrathecally or intraventricularly in addition to systemic therapy (88). Administration by the intrathecal lumbar route, however, often does not achieve therapeutic concentrations in the ventricle. It has been reported that direct administration of 5 mg of gentamicin or tobramycin into the ventricle resulted in adequate concentrations for up to 18–24 h in the lumbar and ventricular space (89). An Ommaya or Rickham reservoir can be used for repeated ventricular administration. However, if the ventricular infection is related to the catheter placement, the foreign body must generally be removed to ensure optimal response (90).

Aminoglycosides may be indicated for the treatment of select ophthalmic infections. Because these agents penetrate poorly into the eye following systemic administration, they must be administered by direct periocular injections or topically. Retrobulbar, subconjunctival, and topical administration result in marked regional variations in aminoglycoside concentrations (91). The method of administration should be carefully selected according to the infection site to ensure a favorable response (91).

Streptomycin and kanamycin are prescribed relatively infrequently in comparison to the newer aminoglycosides. Nevertheless, the combination of streptomycin and penicillin G are recommended in the treatment of enterococcal endocarditis (92). Streptomycin is also used in the treatment of tularemia and plague and is used in combination with tetracycline for the treatment of brucellosis (93–95). Additionally, it may be used in combination with antituberculous drugs for therapy of mycobacterial diseases. Amikacin and kanamycin are also occasionally used in the treatment of mycobacterial infections (96). Although it is not commonly used today, oral kanamycin has been prescribed for patients to reduce bacterial growth in the bowel prior to colorectal surgery (97–99).

VI. ADMINISTRATION

Aminoglycosides can be administered by either bolus injection, 30- to 60-min intermittent infusion, or continuous intravenous infusion. The use of bolus and continuous infusions has been discouraged because of a high risk of toxicity associated with these methods of administration (100,101). Intermittent infusions of 30–60 min give the drug time to equilibrate with the tissue compartment.

When determining dosage requirements, the adequacy of drug delivery should be considered. Residual solution in the intravenous container or in the administration set can lead to erroneous assumptions regarding the actual dose delivered to the patient. Patients in intensive care units may have additional intravenous fluids administered through the same administration set, which can increase the intraline fluid substantially to 20–25 ml. This volume may contain 20–50% of the actual aminoglycoside dose depending upon the original volume. Therefore, the administration set should be flushed after the drug has been administered to ensure that the patient has received all of the drug.

Infiltration of the infusion outside of the venipuncture site can considerably affect the actual amount of drug the patient receives. The infusion of other medications at the time of administering aminoglycosides should be avoided unless they are known to be compatible with the aminoglycoside. It is important to record the times of initiation and completion of the infusion because serum sampling strategies are performed in reference to these parameters. Trough concentrations that are drawn after the beginning of the next infusion may result in elevated assay determinations. Peak concentrations drawn before the end of the infusion may result in low determinations. The exact sampling times need to be recorded for ideal clinical use.

The parenteral preparations of aminoglycosides are generally marketed with preservatives to maintain stability. These preservatives can be irritating to tissues upon direct contact. Preservative-free preparations are available for intrathecal administration or periocular injections to prevent the irritation to tissue sites.

However, intramuscular injections of aminoglycosides are well tolerated and are absorbed well. In patients who are septic and hypotensive, intramuscular injections of aminoglycosides are discouraged because absorption may be altered or substantially delayed. Elderly patients' muscle mass may be decreased and perfusion may be further impaired.

A. Therapeutic Drug Monitoring

1. General Guidelines

The safe and effective use of aminoglycosides requires careful monitoring of serum concentrations and adjustment of doses and dosing intervals. Since approximately one-half of all fatalities due to gram-negative sepsis occur within the first 24 h, optimum serum concentrations should be attained as early as possible in the course of therapy. This may be especially true for the geriatric patients, where these patients may be more susceptible to mortality from gram-negative sepsis and may thus benefit more from early dosage adjustments to attain therapeutic serum concentrations (31).

During the past few years, highly accurate, rapid, and relatively inexpensive aminoglycoside assay procedures have become available to clinicians. Despite having these valuable assay methods available, many clinical aminoglycoside samples that are tested are inappropriately collected and erroneously interpreted. Several reports have defined some of the problems in interpreting serum gentamicin concentrations (102,103). Less than 50% of samples that were requested in their institutions were collected appropriately; drug administration times were poorly documented, and samples were collected at inappropriate times. In addition, only one of every five serum aminoglycoside determinations was appropriately interpreted relative to making therapeutic decisions. These problems may lead to suboptimal therapeutic outcomes and increased costs to both patients and their institutions.

A systematic approach for monitoring serum aminoglycoside concentrations is necessary. The laboratory and medical staff and the pharmacokinetic consultant must communicate effectively to optimize patient therapy. Carefully recorded drug administration and sample collection times are required. Both peak and trough concentrations at steady state should be maintained within the recommended therapeutic range. Serum aminoglycoside determinations are indicated to ensure adequate therapy based on therapeutic guidelines for a specific infection site, clinical condition, and/or pathogen. Serum aminoglycoside determinations are also necessary to prevent excessively high serum peak and trough concentrations that predispose the patient to toxicity. Serum aminoglycoside concentrations should be reassessed periodically in patients on prolonged therapy and in patients with changing renal function and distribution volume.

Although serum aminoglycoside determinations are necessary for optimizing patient response, several other more important parameters must be monitored. The clinician must monitor the patient's clinical response to aminoglycoside therapy both in terms of resolution of infection and preventing adverse effects.

2. *Sample Collection*

For dosage adjustments, serum specimens must be collected at ideal times and correctly interpreted to ensure optimal usage of each serum concentration determination. The serum samples should be collected in unheparinized tubes to avoid an interaction with the anticoagulant. Specimens that contain interacting substances such as β-lactams should be stored frozen if the sample cannot be rapidly assayed.

Several factors that can influence the aminoglycoside serum concentration determinations and/or subsequent dose and dosing interval adjustments should be considered. The clinician should be familiar with the assay methodology employed by the institution. Additionally, various substances have been reported to interact with the aminoglycosides (104–112) and/or interfere with the assay technique used (Table 3) (110,113,114). When interpreting serum concentration determinations and making dosage adjustments based on the results, these and several other factors should be considered.

3. *Assay Methodology*

Increased use of serum aminoglycoside concentration determinations has resulted in the development of several different assay techniques. The assay methods most commonly employed include microbiological assays (bioassays), immunoassays (radioimmunoassay), enzyme immunoassay (fluorescent immunoassay), and gas-liquid and high-pressure liquid chromatography (115). These methods can have interfering substances, which can lead to erroneous assay results (Table 3).

Bioassays were used extensively in early aminoglycoside investigations. A disadvantage of this method was the requirement of 24–48 h to achieve accurate results. The incubation time required has recently been reduced to less than 6 h. Another disadvantage is that numerous factors may influence the results including the reliability of the method in determining serum aminoglycoside concentrations. Temperature, pH, agar ion concentration, test strain, incubation time, and the presence of other antibiotics in the test sample can affect the results. Additionally, these assays lack reproducibility below 2 μg/ml.

Immunoassay techniques are available for several aminoglycoside antibiotics. These methods include the radioimmunoassay (RIA), fluorescent immunoassay (FIA), and enzyme multiplied immunoassay technique (EMIT). Radioactivity counting equipment, a scintillation counter (RIA), a spectrophotometer (EMIT), or a fluorometer (FIA) is

Table 3 Substances Interfering with Assays

Interfering substance	Assay method	Mechanism/Effect	Ref.
Sodium phosphate buffer, serum glucose concentration	Luciferase	Mechanism unknown; in the absence of phosphate buffer, sensitivity of the method may increase; high serum glucose affects bacterial growth, thus affecting MICs	110a
Serum bilirubin	Agar diffusion	Mechanism unknown; many inhibit aminoglycoside concentration measurements	110a
Serum uric acid, serum creatinine, alkaline phosphatase	Bioassay	Mechanism unknown; elevated levels of these substances may result in erroneously low aminoglycoside determinations	111
Heparin (>50 to 100 units/ml)	Agar diffusion RIA	Questionable reversible complex formation; may result in falsely low aminoglycoside serum concentrations	112

MICs = minimal inhibitory concentrations; RIA-radioimmunoassay.

required by these assays. Immunoassays are rapid; results are available within minutes to a few hours. These sensitive, specific, and rapid assays are extremely useful for dosage adjustment in the clinical setting.

Gas-liquid chromatography (GLC) and high-pressure liquid chromatography (HPLC) assays are chemical techniques. They are highly specific for the compounds tested; the HPLC method can separate the three major components of the gentamicin complex. A disadvantage, however, is the high cost of the equipment and the labor-intensive nature of this methodology. These are used primarily in a research environment and are not extensively used by clinical laboratories.

Serum aminoglycoside concentrations when measured by different assay methods can vary considerably. In a study that evaluated 35 serum gentamicin samples by three assay techniques, the serum gentamicin concentrations as determined by the EMIT, RIA, and radiometric assay (BACTEC) differed significantly (116). The BACTEC assay markedly underestimated serum gentamicin concentrations that were > 72 μg/ml, relative to the EMIT and RIA values. Falsely low peak serum concentrations can predispose a patient to toxicity. The coefficients of determination (r^2) were 0.73 and 0.83 for EMIT versus BACTEC and for RIA versus BACTEC, respectively. BACTEC overestimated concentrations below 1.5–2.0 μg/ml. Falsely elevated trough serum concentrations can expose the patient to subinhibitory serum concentrations. The coefficients of determination (r^2) were 0.65 and 0.68 for EMIT versus BACTEC and for RIA versus BACTEC, respectively. The EMIT technique was reportedly the most accurate method for serum gentamicin concentration determinations.

Such assay-dependent differences in serum aminoglycoside concentrations can result in substantial variations in calculated pharmacokinetic parameters. Subsequently, these

Table 4 Initial Dosage Regimens in Geriatric Patients with Normal Renal Function

	Total Daily Dose (mg/kg/day)[a]			
Age	Gentamicin	Tobramycin	Amikacin	Netilmicin
60–80 y	≤3 q8h	≤3 q8h	≤7.5 q8h	≤3 q8h
>80 y	≤2 q12h	≤2 q12h	≤5 q12h	≤2 q12h

[a]Measure serum concentrations within first 72 h of treatment (preferably first 24 h) and adjust dosages to attain therapeutic values.

kinetic parameters will influence dose and dosing interval calculations. The clinician should be aware of the differences in determinations by the various assay methods employed in their institution. Significant differences in aminoglycoside measurements from RIA and EMIT assays do occur. Gentamicin serum concentration data resulting from EMIT gave higher mean values for the distribution volume, half-life, and total body clearance; the mean percentage differences for these parameters were 25, 11, and 15% higher, respectively, for EMIT as compared to RIA determinations (116a). In another study, significant differences were found in distribution volume, total body clearance, and dosage calculations resulting from RIA and FIA methods (117). The mean percent differences between the RIA and FIA values for these calculations were 10.3, 9.8, and 9.8%, respectively, with RIA having smaller values. Estimates of the elimination rate constant and half-life were reportedly identical.

B. Individualizing Dosing Regimens

1. Initial Therapy

Generally, similar initial dosage regimens are recommended for gentamicin, tobramycin, and netilmicin. The recommended initial dose for adult and geriatric patients is 1–2 mg/kg administered at 8- or 12-h intervals (Table 4). Lower dosages (i.e., 1 mg/kg) should be prescribed for the elderly patients who appear to be clinically dehydrated. In contrast, higher initial dosages (i.e., 2 mg/kg), but longer dosing intervals should be prescribed for patients who have expanded extracellular fluid compartments such as the patient with congestive heart failure. Suggested initial dosage regimens for patients who have impaired renal function or hemodialysis patients are 1–2 mg/kg (55–57).

Similar initial dosage regimens are recommended for amikacin, kanamycin, and streptomycin. The recommended initial dose for adults are 5–7.5 mg/kg, regardless of the patient's renal function (118). In the treatment of urinary tract infections, a total dose of 10 mg/kg/day of amikacin given in two or three divided doses is usually effective (119). Suggested initial dosage regimens of amikacin for hemodialysis patients is 7.5 mg/kg, and subsequent doses are 3.75 mg/kg after each dialysis (69). In selecting the initial aminoglycoside dose, the clinician should consider those factors reported to affect the aminoglycoside distribution volume. Two of these factors include the patient's hydration status and the presence of edema. Overhydrated patients and those who have edema will have larger distribution volumes and require higher doses to achieve a desired peak concentration. For patients who are moderately to morbidly obese, lean body weight should be calculated to estimate the distribution volume of the drug. The severity of the infection should also be considered.

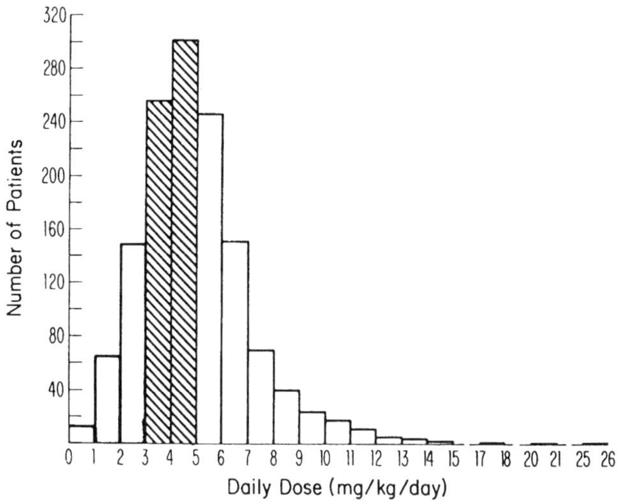

Figure 16 The dosage requirements of gentamicin are illustrated for 1369 patients who had a normal serum creatinine. These requirements varied substantially in these patients.

These considerations will aid the clinician in selecting an initial dose at the upper or lower end of the dosing range.

Various dosing charts and nomograms have been proposed and are available to assist the clinician in estimating dosage requirements in patients who have normal or compromised renal function. Such dosing regimens are based on statistical correlations between aminoglycoside elimination rate and estimates of renal function (usually serum creatinine or creatinine clearance). However, these relationships can have substantial error in predicting dosage requirements. Aminoglycoside dosage requirements can vary substantially from patient to patient, even in those who have normal renal function (Fig. 16) (see also previous section on Pharmacokinetics). Additionally, although patients who have abnormal renal function generally have reduced daily dosage requirements because of reduced aminoglycoside clearance, there is considerable overlap in dose and dosing interval requirements between patient groups. Aminoglycoside dosing charts and nomograms are useful as initial guidelines only.

2. *Nomograms*

Various dosage regimens can produce substantial variations in serum aminoglycoside concentrations, and the drug doses should be subsequently adjusted based on serum concentration determinations and clinical response. Several dosing methods for aminoglycosides have been published for patients who have normal or compromised renal function. These include the Sarubbi-Hull, "Rule of Eights," Dettli, Siersbaek-Nielsen, and Chan methods. The predictability of these methods is low (Fig. 17) (120) and is due to a low association between drug elimination and renal function, a wide variation in distribution volume, and recently identified factors not previously considered in such nomograms (see discussion below).

The method of Sarubbi-Hull utilizes serum creatinine, lean body weight, age, and sex to predict creatinine clearance (118). For certain ranges of creatinine clearance, low, medium, and high dosage regimens are selected (121). The clinician has the option to select different doses and dosing intervals for varying degrees of renal function and severity of infection. Of the several dosing methods available, this method considers more patient variables, which may improve estimates of glomerular filtration rate and aminoglycoside elimination.

The "Rule of Eights" method suggests a dose be administered at variable intervals depending on the patient's serum creatinine (56,122). Doses are given every 8 h for patients with normal serum creatinine. For patients who have abnormal renal function, the dosing interval is calculated by multiplying the patient's serum creatinine by a factor of eight and rounding the value to convenient intervals of 12, 18, 24, 36, or 48 h. This approach can result in prolonged subinhibitory serum concentrations, especially in patients who have severely compromised renal function. Additionally, this approach does not consider other factors recognized to influence aminoglycoside disposition.

The Dettli method utilizes estimates of lean body weight to determine the aminoglycoside distribution volume (123). The elimination rate constant is estimated from the patient's creatinine clearance. The following equation has been proposed:

$$\text{Kd} = \text{CCr(cal)} \times 0.0024 + 0.01$$

where Kd is the overall elimination rate constant, 0.0024 is the slope of the line, 0.01 is the y-intercept, and CCr(cal) is the patient's calculated creatinine clearance. The individual dosage regimen is then calculated from the estimated elimination rate constant. The clinician selects desired peak and trough serum concentrations and calculates a dosage regimen to achieve these. The clinician has the advantage of being able to select each patient's therapeutic endpoint.

The method of Siersbaek-Nielsen utilizes serum creatinine, lean body weight, and sex to estimate each patient's creatinine clearance (124). The distribution volume for all patients is assumed to be 0.26 L/kg of lean body weight. The lean body weight is estimated from *Geigy's Scientific Tables*, which utilizes the patient's age, sex, and height (125). This method suggests loading doses of 1.0–2.0 mg/kg of lean body weight, and the maintenance doses are determined as a percentage of the loading dose. The dosing intervals are determined for specific creatinine clearances. The aminoglycoside is administered every 8, 12, or 24 h.

The dosing nomogram of Chan et al. (126) utilizes a standard loading dose followed by a maintenance dose derived from a published nomogram. These maintenance doses are adjusted according to creatinine clearance estimates, and the dosing interval is 8 h. Utilization of fixed dosing intervals can lead to substantial drug accumulation in patients who have compromised renal function.

Dosing methods derived from nomograms have several sources of errors and limitations. In general, these nomograms assume a constant distribution volume throughout the patient population and do not take into account the wide intrapatient and interpatient variation that has been reported. Nomograms use calculated clearance rather than measured estimates of creatinine clearance, which can represent an important source of error (87). In addition, several factors known to affect aminoglycoside disposition other than renal function, such as lean body weight, hemodynamic changes, and underlying disease states, are not considered in dosage nomograms.

Lesar et al. (120) clinically evaluated four commonly used predictive dosing methods for gentamicin dosing. They compared the Sarubbi-Hull, Dettli, "Rule of Eights" and Chan methods with an individualized method in 96 consecutive septic patients. These four

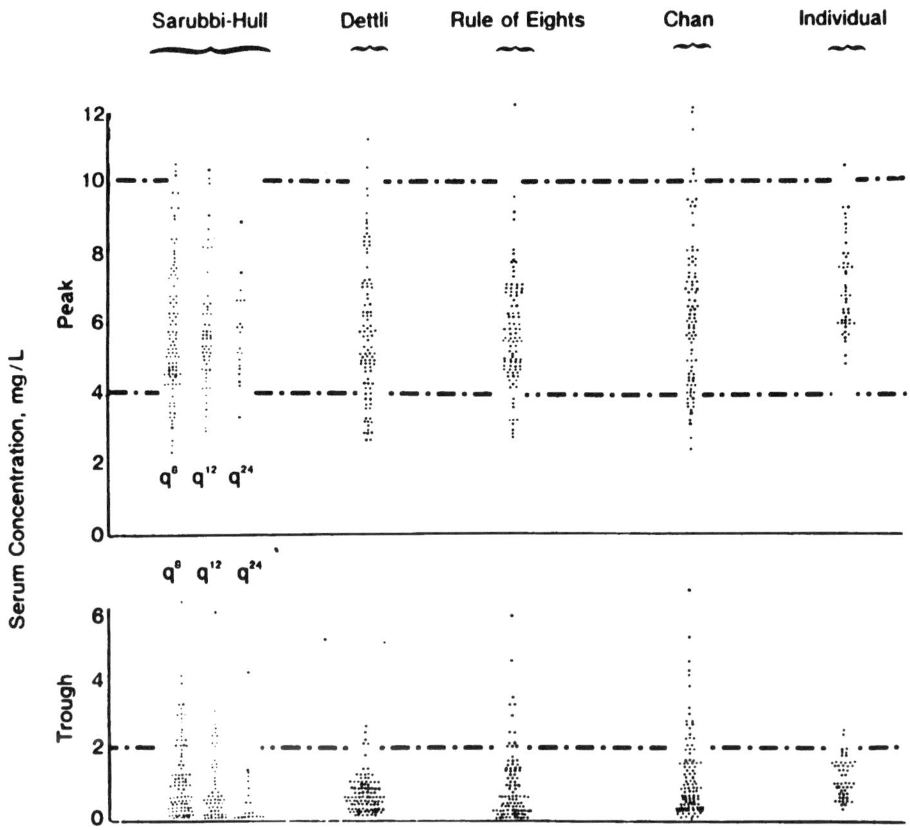

Figure 17 The four commonly used nomograms of Sarubbi-Hull, "Rule of Eights," Dettli, and Chan methods have substantial error and should only be used as initial dosage estimates until serum concentrations can be measured and an appropriate dosage regimen can be determined.

dosing methods were found to result in a large proportion of patients with subtherapeutic or potentially toxic serum concentrations (Fig. 17). At times, toxic peak serum concentrations may occur concurrently with subtherapeutic trough values, or vice versa. Therapeutic serum concentrations (peaks of 6 to 10 μg/ml, troughs of ≤2 μg/ml) were achieved in 78%, 43%, 28% and 39% of patients who were dosed according to the four methods, respectively (Fig. 17). A large number of these patients had long periods of subtherapeutic serum concentrations. The individualized method produced therapeutic serum concentrations in 90% of patients.

C. Maintenance Therapy

1. Trial and Error Method

Many institutions have had the capacity for routine laboratory assay of aminoglycosides for several years. However, necessary elements for quality assurance have not been initiated, and consequently many inadvertent errors in aminoglycoside administration have occurred in these institutions. Clinical serum samples are often obtained in an uncontrolled

Table 5 Suggested Alterations in Dose or Dosing Interval Using Measured Peak and Trough Serum Concentrations

Measured serum concentrations compared to desired values		Suggested change in dosage regimens	
Trough	Peak	Dose[a]	Dosing interval[a]
Same	Same	No change	No change
Higher	Higher	Decrease or no change	Increase
Higher	Lower	Increase	Increase
Lower	Lower	Increase or no change	Decrease
Lower	Higher	Decrease	Decrease
Same	Higher	Decrease	No change
Same	Lower	Increase	No change
Higher	Same	No change or increase	Increase
Lower	Same	No change or decrease	Decrease

[a]The dose and dosing intervals must bc in practical increments that the nursing staff can administer. Intervals of 4, 6, 8, 12, 24, or 48 h are routinely used in our institution.

manner. The aminoglycoside dose, sampling, and infusion times are important data that are frequently disregarded or not accurately recorded. Omitting these can lead to incorrect interpretation of serum concentration determinations and incorrect dosage adjustments (102,103).

Many clinicians collect peak and/or trough serum samples and make dosage adjustments empirically (Table 5). Empirical dosage adjustments introduce a trial-and-error approach to attaining desired serum concentrations. Obtaining these concentrations is useful only if the samples are collected under controlled conditions and if steady-state conditions (at four to five drug half-lives) are present. Many of these conditions are difficult to control clinically. Prior aminoglycoside doses and infusion times must be accurately recorded, and the distribution volume should remain constant if use of this method is to be optimal. A quantitative, individualized method avoids the added time of trial-and-error approaches and reduces the risk of patients being exposed to either subtherapeutic or toxic serum concentrations. Quantitative approaches to dosage adjustment may become especially important during the advent of prospective reimbursement.

2. *The Bayesian Approach*

Sheiner et al. (127,128) have proposed the application of Bayesian techniques to pharmacokinetics and thereby estimating dosage requirements. This approach considers not only population-derived pharmacokinetic parameters but also previous serum concentration values obtained in a specific patient, and thus is designed to emphasize individual data when available. When individual data are unavailable, population values are used. The decrease in the number of serum determinations combined with the use of population averages may result in a less precise dosage estimate for a specific patient. The clinical utility of this approach awaits further validation in the elderly patient who demonstrates considerable variability.

3. *Individualized Method*

Dosage regimens necessary to achieve therapeutic aminoglycoside serum concentrations can be quantitatively determined by using simple pharmacokinetic principles (30). Individ-

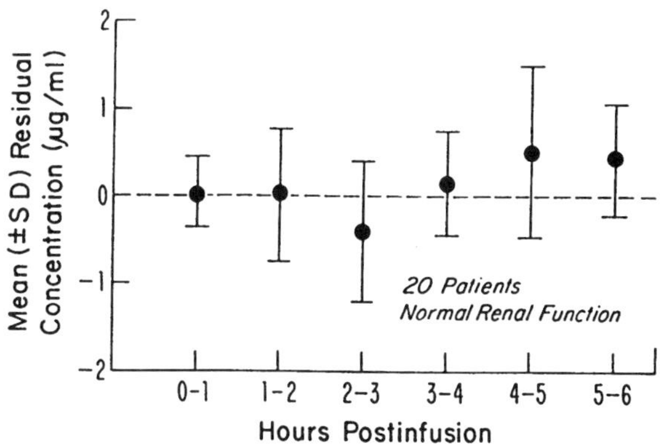

Figure 18 The biases observed in using a one-compartment model is illustrated over the initial 6 h after a 1-h infusion. The error in using a one-compartment model is minimal as indicated by a low mean residual concentration found each hour over the 6-h period.

ualized pharmacokinetic parameters are determined from the patient's serum concentration versus time data. Such pharmacokinetic parameters are then used to calculate an optimal dosage regimen for a specific patient. Individualized dosing regimens have been successfully applied in the clinical setting and found to achieve desired peak and trough serum concentrations. The dosing regimens can be rapidly calculated within 12–24 h of initiation of therapy. This is important in severely ill (i.e., septic) patients who require therapeutic serum concentrations early in therapy. In addition, this method can help avoid potentially toxic serum concentrations.

One-Compartment Versus Two-Compartment Model. Aminoglycoside antibiotics have been found to exhibit multicompartmental pharmacokinetics in some patients. This phenomenon is especially true in elderly patients who generally have decreased renal functions. Following a rapid intravenous bolus dose of aminoglycoside, an early distribution phase may occur, resulting in a biexponential decline in serum concentration. This distribution phase is very rapid and generally does not occur with 1-h infusions except in patients who have abnormal renal function (e.g., elderly persons) and a large distribution volume. A third phase has been reported, which may reflect drug redistribution from the tissue compartment back into the blood. This phase has been proposed to explain drug accumulation and to be related to nephrotoxicity (129,130).

A one-compartment model adequately characterizes the aminoglycoside disposition with minimal bias and provides information to rapidly estimate dosage requirements (Fig. 18). This is especially true with concentrations encountered clinically. Following a 1-h infusion, the serum concentration of aminoglycosides decline in a monoexponential manner so that a linear relationship is observed between the log of the serum concentration and time. Aminoglycosides also follow linear pharmacokinetic principles. A change in dose will produce a proportional change in the area under the concentration versus time curve (AUC).

Serum Sampling Strategy. Serum samples must be collected at ideal times and correctly interpreted to ensure optimal use of each serum concentration determination. Sampling times are influenced by factors that affect drug distribution and elimination; thus, the serum sampling strategy should be determined for each patient to provide the most reliable information (131).

The serum concentration versus time data in most patients receiving 1-h infusions of aminoglycosides can be characterized by a one-compartment model. When assuming this model, there are two points on the postinfusion concentration versus time curve that provide the largest amount of information describing the pharmacokinetic behavior of the drug. The first point, the zero-time postinfusion point, is necessary to estimate the distribution volume of the drug. The second point, at 1.5 half-lives of the drug postinfusion, is important in estimating the elimination rate constant. Each patient's serum sampling strategy should be scheduled to obtain serum samples according to these criteria.

Choosing three postinfusion specimens for aminoglycoside determinations may be especially important in critically ill patients where the margin of acceptable error may be less (131). In other patients, two postinfusion specimens obtained under well-controlled conditions will provide clinically adequate estimates of pharmacokinetic parameters and dosage requirements. Additional data points will add more information describing the concentration versus time curve up to a critical number; thereafter, the amount of information gained diminishes markedly after three or four specimens (assuming a one-compartment model). A predose sample is required only if the patient has received a previous dose.

In adults who have normal renal function, the first serum sample should be collected after a 1-h infusion of aminoglycoside is complete. The sample should be obtained at 15–30 min rather than immediately postinfusion to reduce the potential for error. For example, if a sample is collected at 2 min postinfusion and is incorrectly recorded by 1 min, the error in time is 50%. If, however, the same error is made for a 20-min postinfusion sample, the error is only 5%. These errors can substantially affect pharmacokinetic parameter estimates, especially in patients who have rapid elimination rates.

The second and third serum samples should be collected to characterize two to three half-lives of the drug. In those who have normal renal function, the timing of samples depends primarily on the patient's age and estimated renal function. In older patients who have normal function, samples should be obtained 3–6 h postinfusion. For patients who have abnormal renal function, the sampling interval can be calculated by estimating the half-life of the drug by multiplying the serum creatinine by a factor of four. Sampling times should be obtained over at least two estimated half-lives.

Linear Versus Nonlinear Fitting of Concentration Versus Time Data. The serum concentration versus time data can be fitted either by linear or nonlinear regression analysis assuming a one-compartment model. Linear regression analysis fits the log of the serum concentration with time. A semilog graph paper or a programmable hand-held calculator can be used for this purpose (Fig. 19). The line of best fit is determined by the smallest vertical difference in the log of the serum concentration. In nonlinear regression analysis, the absolute serum concentration versus time are fit using more sophisticated computer resources. The line of best fit is determined by the smallest vertical difference in the absolute serum concentration. In nonlinear regression analysis, the serum concentration and time are fitted in a linear manner that will allow for equal weighting of all data points. In linear regression analysis, the data points at the lower concentration values are weighted and can add bias to the data fitting. In general, the patient's estimated pharmacokinetic parameters determined by either method are similar if the data fit well.

Dosage Calculation. From the serum concentration versus time data, a patient's kinetic parameters can be determined (i.e., elimination rate constant, half-life, and distribution volume). Two or three serum samples obtained over two to three estimated half-lives of the drug (as discussed above) are sufficient for these parameter estimates (30). Serum samples are preferably collected within the first dosing interval to avoid requiring a

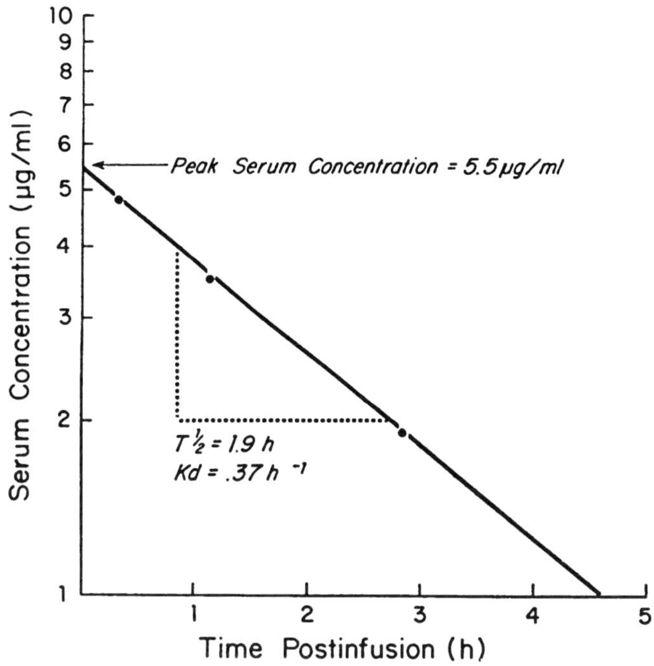

Figure 19 The fitting of log of serum concentration and time are illustrated. The actual serum concentration time data are indicated. The estimated peak serum concentration (at zero time postinfusion) and the estimated half-life are illustrated.

predose sample. The clinician selects desired peak and trough concentrations according to the patient's clinical status, type of infection, and pathogen (Table 6). These desired concentrations and the patient's pharmacokinetic parameters are then used to calculate the patient's dosage requirements. The serum concentration versus time data are fitted using least-squares regression analysis. A one-compartment model is assumed for the aminoglycoside disposition. As mentioned earlier, the fitting of data points can be either a linear or nonlinear regression analysis.

Table 6 Serum Concentration Guidelines

	Gentamicin	Tobramycin	Netilmicin[a]	Amikacin
Peak (µg/ml)				
Moderate to severe	6–8	6–8	6–8	20–25
Life-threatening	8–10	8–10	8–10	25–28
Trough (µg/ml)				
Moderate to severe	<1	<1	<1	<4
Life-threatening	<2	<2	<2	<8

[a]Higher peak and trough serum concentrations may be safely utilized if clinical or bacteriological data demonstrate the need.

The elimination rate constant (Kd), half-life ($t^{1/2}$), and zero-time postinfusion serum concentration (Cp_{max}) can be estimated by fitting the concentration versus time data. The distribution volume (Vd) of the drug is then calculated using these estimates and the following equation, which considers the amount of drug eliminated during the infusion period:

$$Vd = \frac{Ko}{Kd} \frac{1 - e^{-Kdt'}}{Cp_{max} - (Cp_{min}{}^{-Kdt'})}$$

where Ko is the rate of infusion (mg/h), t′ is the infusion period (h), Kd is the drug's elimination rate constant (h^{-1}), Cp_{min} is the predose serum concentration (μg/ml), and Cp_{max} is the peak concentration. The infusion rate (Ko) is the dose (mg) administered over time (h).

The patient's dosing interval (T) is calculated knowing the desired peak concentration ($Cp_{max\text{-}D}$), desired trough concentration ($Cp_{min\text{-}D}$), and infusion period (t′). The dosing interval can be calculated by:

$$T = \frac{1}{Kd} \ln \frac{Cp_{min\text{-}D}}{Cp_{max\text{-}D}} + 1.$$

The calculated dosing interval should be rounded off to a clinically convenient unit such as 4, 6, 8, or 12 h.

The aminoglycoside infusion rate (Ko) in mg/h is then calculated to achieve the desired serum concentrations. The following equation is used, which considers the amount of drug remaining from the previous dose and the amount eliminated during the infusion period:

$$Ko = Kd\ Vd\ Cp_{max\text{-}D} \frac{(1 - e^{-KdT})}{(1 - e^{-Kdt'})}$$

The infusion rate (mg/h) is then calculated. The aminoglycoside dose is equal to the rate of infusion (Ko) times the length of infusion (t′). The dose is rounded off to increments that can be conveniently prepared by pharmacy and administered by nursing. Computer programs are widely available for these calculations, including small programmable calculators and microcomputers.

With the use of the individualized method, desired peak and trough serum concentrations have been consistently obtained with gentamicin, tobramycin, amikacin, and netilmicin. Substantial variability in dosage requirements (see Table 2) was noted in septic elderly patients who had normal renal function (Fig. 20). Some elderly patients required dosing intervals shorter than 8 or 12 h (Fig. 21), and several patients required dosing intervals beyond 8 or 12 h. Overall, between 35 and 45% of patients treated with aminoglycosides required dosage regimens higher than those commonly recommended. Between 10 and 15% of patients required dosages less than those commonly recommended, even though they had abnormal renal function. The incidence of ototoxicity and nephrotoxicity compared favorably to previous studies in which dosages were not individualized.

Cost Effectiveness/Cost-Benefit Rationale. Achieving therapeutic aminoglycoside serum concentrations early in the treatment course is important, especially in severely ill elderly patients. This goal may be achieved rapidly and safely in institutions that utilize a workable, systematic approach to dosing aminoglycoside antibiotics. Improved aminoglycoside therapy may result in reduced length of hospitalization and reduced patient

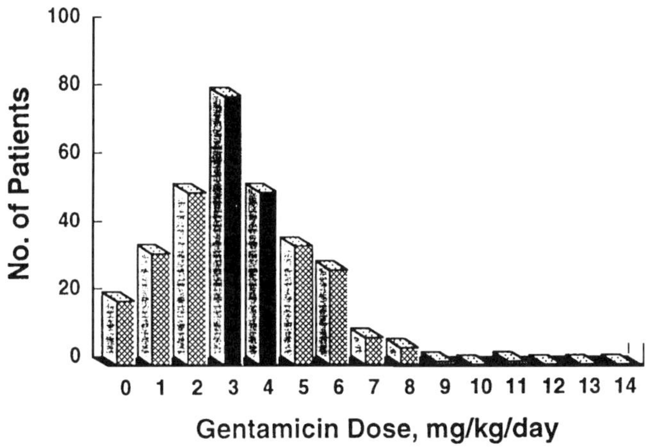

Figure 20 The dosage requirements of gentamicin are illustrated for 302 geriatric patients who had a normal serum creatinine. These requirements varied substantially in these patients who were treated for sepsis. (Reprinted with permission.)

morbidity and mortality. Institutional expenses may be reduced secondary to lower cost of pharmaceuticals (especially in the elderly patients) and less potential for medicolegal risks. A cost-benefit ratio of 8:1 has been reported in one study in which the cost-benefit of a pharmacokinetic service utilizing an individualized method of dosing aminoglycosides was evaluated (132). This means that for every dollar spent to monitor serum concentrations and to individualize dosage regimens, society had the potential to realize an $8 return. A

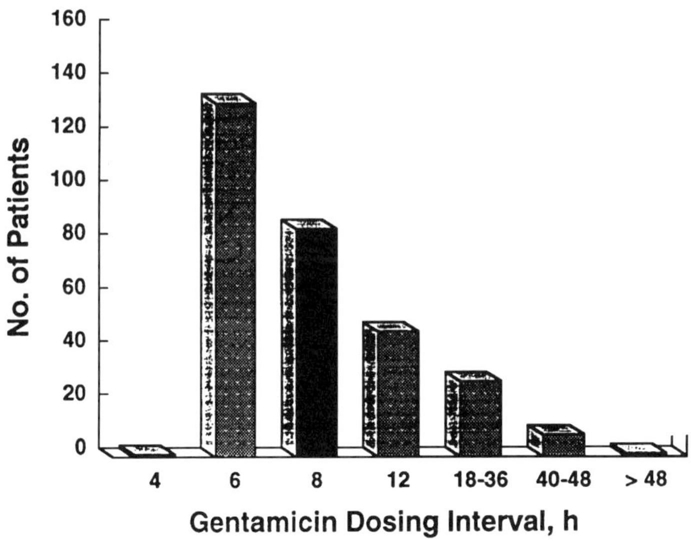

Figure 21 The dosage interval of gentamicin is illustrated for 302 geriatric patients who had a normal serum creatinine. (Reprinted with permission.)

Table 7 Risk Factors for Aminoglycoside Toxicity

Ototoxicity	Nephrotoxicity
Age	Age
Renal insufficiency	Renal insufficiency
Elevated trough serum concentrations	Elevated trough serum concentrations
Elevated peak serum concentrations	Elevated peak serum concentrations
Total daily dose	Total daily dose
Cumulative dose	Cumulative dose
Concurrent ototoxic drugs	Concurrent ototoxic drugs
Prior aminoglycoside exposure	Prior aminoglycoside exposure
Dialysis	Hypovolemia
Duration of treatment	Duration of treatment
Hypovolemia	Sepsis

broad view of improving drug therapy results in optimal patient care as well as many societal and institutional benefits.

VII. ADVERSE DRUG REACTIONS

Two of the most common adverse drug effects due to aminoglycosides are ototoxicity and nephrotoxicity. Several host factors contribute to the development of these adverse reactions (Table 7). Additional adverse reactions attributed to the aminoglycosides include neuromuscular blockade; hypersensitivity reactions; minor local, gastrointestinal, hematological, and central nervous system effects; and the potential for teratogenicity. The relative frequency of these reactions is low (Table 8).

A. Ototoxicity

Eighth cranial nerve toxicity causing cochlear and/or vestibular dysfunction has been observed with the use of aminoglycosides. Such abnormalities and deficits are especially devastating for older adults because of the common occurrences of age-associated hearing loss, gait disturbances, and falls. Eighth cranial nerve injury results from destruction of hair cells in the cochlear and/or vestibular apparatus. Toxicity can be bilateral or unilateral and may occur at a variable length of time after initiation or discontinuation of aminoglycoside therapy. The cochlear dysfunction presents as a perceptive hearing loss that may be preceded by a feeling of fullness in the ears or tinnitus. It usually affects those frequencies above 4000 Hertz (Hz) and generally does not include frequencies utilized in the conversational range. Cochlear toxicity is often irreversible, and it is not compensated for by physiological processes. The clinical symptoms of vestibular damage include dizziness, vertigo, ataxia, and/or nystagmus (133,134). The effects of vestibular toxicity can be overcome by physiological compensatory functions (i.e., vision), although the patient may have difficulty maintaining balance under poorly lit conditions. However, in elderly patients, compensatory mechanisms may not be adequate because of coexisting presence of poor vision and unsteady balance and gait. Histopathological examination of the inner ear has shown that neomycin, amikacin, and kanamycin are primarily associated with loss of hair cells in the organ of Corti (135,136). The changes that are seen in the cytoplasm

Table 8 Frequency of Aminoglycoside-Associated Reactions

Reaction	Incidence and clinical comments
Ototoxicity—cochlear and vestibular	0.5–3%; reported incidences vary considerably
Nephrotoxicity	2–10%; reports indicate a wide variation and these reactions are usually reversible
Neuromuscular blockade	Exact incidence unknown; patients at high risk should be monitored carefully due to the seriousness of the reaction
Hypersensitivity reactions—rash, eosinophilia, drug fever	1–3% overall; various reports indicate about 7%, 0.1 to 11%, and 6% for rash, eosinophilia, and drug fever, respectively
Reactions at site of injection—pain, tenderness, erythema, phlebitis	Exact incidence unknown; primarily associated with intramuscular injections
Superinfections	Incidence varies; depends on concurrent antibiotic therapy and patients' underlying disease
Headache and nausea	<1%; questionable association
Abnormal liver tests	Reported, but not definitely associated with aminoglycoside therapy

of the hair cells are an increase in lysosomes, swelling of the mitochondria, loss of ribosomes, and changes in the endoplasmic reticulum with eventual formation of vacuoles, myelin figures, and loss of the cytoplasmic architecture (136,137). The most susceptible cells are found in the basal end; these are responsible for high-frequency hearing function. As the lesion advances, it involves the hair cells toward the apex, and lower frequencies affecting conversational hearing function are affected (138,139). Gentamicin and streptomycin have had the greatest association with vestibular toxicity (140,141). Histopathological examination has demonstrated vestibular toxicity to be primarily associated with loss of hair cells in the macula of the utricle or saccule and the crest of the semicircular canal (27,88,89,142–145).

Damage to the hair cell appears to be correlated with high concentrations of aminoglycosides within the perilymph. Aminoglycosides readily diffuse into the perilymph of the inner ear where high concentrations are maintained. This is due to an electrochemical interaction between the positively charged, basic cationic aminoglycoside and the negatively charged, acid mucopolysaccharides in the inner ear. Animal studies have shown that the concentrations of amikacin in the perilymph are linearly related to the dose. The elimination half-life from perilymph is substantially longer compared to serum elimination half-life. Moreover, concentrations of the drug are higher in the inner ear than in serum (146). Maintaining optimal serum concentrations of an aminoglycoside will likely prevent excessive perilymph and endolymph concentrations and reduce the damage to hair cells. Various mechanisms have been proposed to explain the toxicity induced by aminoglycosides. Early investigations with kanamycin in animals revealed suppression of respiratory enzyme activity in outer hair cells, inhibition of the Emden-Meyerhof pathway, and impairment of adenine triphosphatase activity of the organ of Corti (147–149). These studies suggest that aminoglycosides induce toxic effects by interference with carbohydrate metabolism and energy utilization. Neomycin, tobramycin, gentamicin, and kanamycin

Table 9 Summary of Ototoxicity

Criteria	Incidence (%)[a]				Ref.
	Gentamicin	Tobramycin	Sisomicin	Netilmicin	
Auditory toxicity: decrease in perception of ≥ 15 dB in one or both ears at any frequency; symptoms of deafness, tinnitus, dizziness				15.8 (19)	154a
Vestibular toxicity: change in ice water caloric responses					
Auditory toxicity: decrease in acuity by >20 dB, presence of tinnitus	8 (40)		4 (39)		154b
Auditory toxicity: decrease in auditory acuity by >15 dB at ≥2 frequencies in one or both ears		12 (84)		3 (73)	154c
Auditory toxicity: mean decrease of >10 dB in auditory acuity and/or a decrease of ≥15 dB in ≥2 frequencies in either ear				4.8 (21)	154d
Auditory toxicity: decrease in auditory threshold of ≥15 dB at a single frequency	43[b] (3)	25[b] (2)			154e
Vestibular toxicity: abnormality in caloric nystagmus	33[c] (3)	100[c] (2)			
Auditory toxicity: not clearly defined	0[b] (20)	5[b] (20)			154f
Vestibular toxicity: vertigo, dizziness, headache	0[c] (21)	4[c] (25)			

[a]Number of subjects in parentheses.
[b]Cochlear or auditory toxicity.
[c]Vestibular toxicity.

competitively inhibit the binding of calcium to polyphosphoinositide-rich homogenates of cerebral tissue from guinea pigs (150,151). Since polyphosphoinositides are preferentially distributed in tissues that are sensitive to aminoglycosides, it has been proposed that active amino groups in the antibiotic bind to phosphate groups of polyphosphoinositides at high ionic strength and in competition with calcium (152). Formation of an aminoglycoside-polyphosphoinositide complex would have a strong influence on the integrity of the plasma membrane, e.g., excitability.

Studies differ in their reported incidence of aminoglycoside-induced ototoxicity. In general, the incidence of *overt clinical* ototoxicity has been found to range from 0.5–3% (135). Studies using audiometry or electronystagmography, which can determine subclinical changes in eighth cranial nerve function, have reported an incidence of toxicity as high as 20% to 25% (Table 9) (153–154f). However, these studies frequently involved patients with an increased number of risk factors associated with ototoxicity. Differences in the reported incidence of toxicity may be due to different patient populations, differences in administration of aminoglycosides, differences in dosage adjustment, lack of precise and uniform criteria in assessing ototoxicity, failure to obtain baseline studies of auditory and vestibular functions, inaccurate monitoring of drug dosage regimens, and failure to consider the coadministration of other potentially ototoxic agents. Additionally, reported

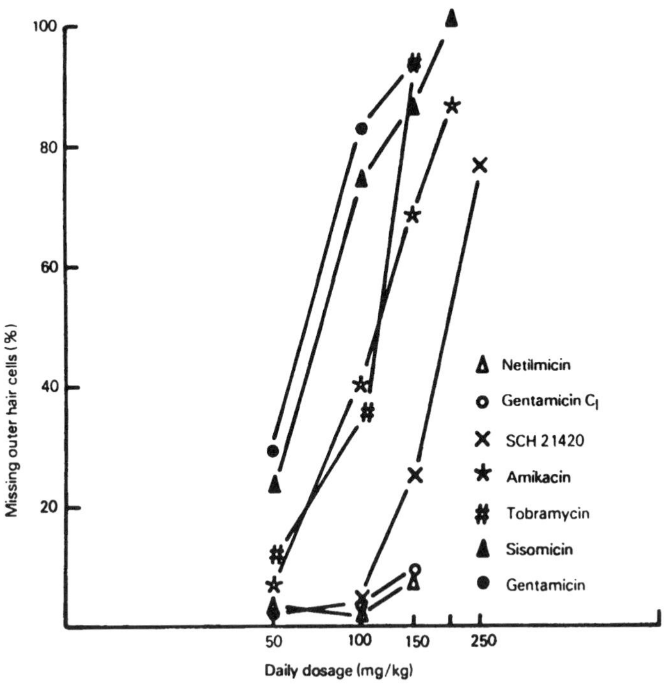

Figure 22 The relationship of dose and ototoxicity demonstrates substantial variability from one aminoglycoside to another in an animal model.

methods for evaluating eighth cranial nerve function have not been uniform for both audiometric and electronystagmographic evaluation.

In animal models, the ototoxic dose-response relationships of the four most commonly prescribed aminoglycosides are substantially different (Fig. 22). Netilmicin appears to have the least ototoxic potential, while gentamicin has the highest. In a guinea pig model, the ototoxic potentials of these four agents on a weight basis were found as follows (133): gentamicin = tobramycin > amikacin ≥ netilmicin. Since amikacin is used in higher dosages, the clinical risk of toxicity is similar to gentamicin and tobramycin. The intrinsic toxicity of netilmicin is similar to amikacin on a weight bases, but it is generally dosed similarly to gentamicin. Comparative clinical studies have found no significant differences in the incidence of ototoxicity of gentamicin, tobramycin, and amikacin. Lerner et al. found netilmicin to be significantly less ototoxic than tobramycin (3% vs. 12%) in a controlled study (155).

B. Nephrotoxicity

Aminoglycoside-induced nephrotoxicity is often difficult to distinguish from pathophysiological sequelae secondary to sepsis or to a patient's underlying disease. This is especially true in the elderly patient, who frequently has age-related decline in renal function, concurrent medical conditions, or drug therapy complicating the association of changing renal function with aminoglycoside therapy. Hypotension and shock, which often accompany gram-negative sepsis in elderly patients, may cause the kidney to develop acute tubular necrosis if the hypotensive state is not successfully treated. Changes in renal parenchyma caused by hypoperfusion cannot be differentiated clinically and histologically from toxic changes associated with aminoglycosides. Measuring serum concentrations of aminoglycosides and adjusting their dosage regimens may prevent the cellular damage from either sepsis or the aminoglycoside therapy.

Nephrotoxicity secondary to aminoglycosides classically occurs at least 5 days after initiating treatment, typically presenting as nonoliguric renal failure. Nephrotoxicity presents as a gradual rise in serum creatinine and blood urea nitrogen and impaired urinary concentrating ability. Tubular necrosis, lysosomal cytosegrosomes (autophage vacuoles), and myeloid bodies are found on histological examination of the kidneys. Proteinuria and aminoaciduria, glycosuria, and electrolyte disturbances may also occur. A decrease in glomerular filtration rate generally occurs as a later manifestation of nephrotoxicity and is generally rapidly reversible during therapy or shortly after discontinuing the drug (156,157). Patients with a rise in serum creatinine should be reassessed for the need for continued aminoglycoside therapy.

Maximum elevation of serum creatinine may occur up to 1 week after stopping therapy, followed by a gradual improvement of 50–100% of baseline values over several weeks (158,159). The recovery phase of renal toxicity may be prolonged and is often associated with high-output renal failure, resulting in large volumes of urine. Initially, in the high-output phase, aminoglycoside clearance does not substantially increase. Even if the aminoglycoside is continued, the patient's serum creatinine may return to normal values (160,161). However, serum concentrations of aminoglycosides should be monitored and dosages adjusted, if necessary, to prevent further insult to the kidney.

Many patients will excrete lysosomal enzymes including *N*-acetyl-glucosaminidase (NAG), β-galactosidase (GAL), alanine aminopeptidase, and alkaline phosphatase within a few days of initiation of aminoglycoside therapy (162–164). Increased excretion of β_2-microglobulin is also found at this time (165–167). Urinary casts, urinary enzymes, and β_2-microglobulin have been measured in an effort to detect early renal damage and prevent toxicity before glomerular filtration is reduced (165). These tests are expensive, time consuming, and limited in availability. In addition, markers of renal tubular function are not specific for aminoglycoside toxicity. Other disease states are also associated with elevated urinary excretion of the same enzymes.

The precise mechanism of nephrotoxicity is not well defined, and the pathogenetic observations are often conflicting. The fact that aminoglycosides accumulate in the renal cortex and persist there for days following a single dose of drug has been advocated as a mechanism for nephrotoxicity (156). Schentag et al. (129,130) and French et al. (169) found that the duration of renal cortical accumulation correlated with signs of renal tubular damage in humans. They advocated the use of a two-compartment pharmacokinetic model to measure the effect of the slow aminoglycoside elimination phase. However, other investigators have found no association of tissue accumulation with nephrotoxicity (170–173). Neomycin concentrates in renal cortex at a relatively low rate, yet it has the highest nephrotoxicity potential of aminoglycosides tested (174). Netilmicin accumulates in renal cortex to approximately the same extent as gentamicin, yet it is significantly less nephrotoxic than gentamicin (172,175). Streptomycin, which is relatively free of nephrotoxicity, displays a much weaker affinity for renal tissue. Many unmarketed aminoglycosides are not highly concentrated in cortical tissues but are nephrotoxic (176).

Nephrotoxicity has also been related to the propensity of the drug to cause damage to intracellular organelles. Ultrastructural studies in animals demonstrate the formation of membranous whorls within renal proximal tubule lysosomes (177). Since lysosomes concentrate basic cationic substances (e.g., aminoglycosides), it is possible that aminoglycosides interact with acidic lipoproteins in the lysosomal matrix, inducing these conformational changes. The number of free amino groups seems to correlate to some degree with renal toxicity (178).

Other observations suggest that the common mechanism of aminoglycoside ototoxicity and nephrotoxicity might be interference with membrane phospholipid metabolism (179). Alterations in the structure and function for the outer membrane may result in detrimental effects on intracellular processes and organelles and may ultimately lead to cell death. Nonlysosomal effects that have been related to nephrotoxicity include inhibition of sodium-potassium adenosine triphosphatase and inhibition of oxidative phosphorylation in the mitochondria (180,181). It is unknown whether the reported changes in mitochondrial function precede, follow, or occur independently of impaired lysosomal function.

In general, the comparative data indicate a similar risk of nephrotoxicity with gentamicin, tobramycin, and amikacin (182). Netilmicin appears to be the safest agent based on limited clinical studies (155). Reported differences in nephrotoxicity incidence could in part be due to differences in study design, as may be the case with reported incidence of ototoxicity. Some of these include comparing different patient populations, inconsistencies in defining nephrotoxicity, and imprecise monitoring of dosage regimens and aminoglycoside serum concentrations.

Earlier studies reported a higher incidence of nephrotoxicity with gentamicin therapy in comparison to tobramycin therapy (168,183–185). Several risk factors that are known to be associated with nephrotoxicity were not well controlled in these studies (Table 10). Gentamicin-treated patients often received cephalosporins concurrently. Aminoglycoside dosages were not carefully controlled, and serum concentrations were elevated (186). Peak serum concentrations were defined as 1-h postinfusion samples after a 20- to 30-min infusion. Dosages were adjusted to control the serum concentration between 5 and 10 μg/ml (183) for gentamicin and tobramycin, and 20–30 μg/ml for amikacin. But actual peak concentrations may have been much higher. For patients with an aminoglycoside half-life between 1.0 and 2.0 h, the true peak concentration immediately postinfusion would be between 10 and 20 μg/ml for tobramycin and gentamicin and 40–60 μg/ml for amikacin. Elevated peak concentrations are associated with increased potential for toxicity.

Several risk factors associated with nephrotoxicity are controversial. Preexisting renal insufficiency is thought to predispose a patient to development of nephrotoxicity. However, renal insufficiency may result in less aminoglycoside exposure to the kidney, thus less potential drug accumulation. Previous aminoglycoside therapy is also thought to be an increased risk factor. Patients previously exposed to aminoglycosides, however, may have immature proximal tubular cells that have replaced the mature cells destroyed by previous therapy. These immature cells are less susceptible to aminoglycoside destruction; thus previous aminoglycoside therapy may have a protective rather than destructive effect on the kidney (161).

C. Neuromuscular Blockade

Aminoglycoside-associated neuromuscular blockade was first thought to be rare (187). However, this potentially serious side effect may occur with greater frequency than previously thought (188). The mechanism of neuromuscular blockade involves interference with calcium and inhibition of the release of acetylcholine at the level of the presynaptic membrane (189–191). This reaction usually occurs in severely ill patients and has been

Table 10 Summary of Nephrotoxicity

Criteria	Incidence (%)[a]			Ref.
	Gentamicin	Tobramycin	Netilmicin	
SCr rise by ≥0.5 mg/dl			7 (28)	61
SCr rise by >0.4 mg/dl if baseline <3 mg/dl; >0.9 mg/dl if baseline >3 mg/dl			38 (34)	154
SCr rise by ≥0.5 mg/dl	1.2 (242)			47
SCr rise of 50% above baseline ≥1.3 mg/dl		4 (114)	1 (116)	155
SCr rise of 0.5 mg/dl above baseline of <1.5 mg/dl		7.6 (28)		197
SCr rise by ≥0.3 mg/dl or at least a doubling of SCr	a) 40 (25)	a) 28 (29)		154b
	b)20 (25)	b) 3.4 (29)		
SCr rise by >0.5 mg/dl rise in urine B_2-microglobulin levels and casts	37 (120)	22 (120)		198
SCr >110 μmol/l	27 (33)	10 (19)		152
SCr rise by ≥0.5 mg/dl after 6 days of therapy if baseline <2 mg/dl; 30% rise if baseline ≥2 mg/dl	10.2[b] (49)	18.4[b] (49)		18
	8[c] (50)	16.7[c] (48)		
SCr rise by >0.5 mg/dl above baseline	63	43		154e
SCr rise of ≥0.5 mg/dl if baseline <3; ≥1.0 mg/dl if baseline >3	26 (72)	12 (74)		183
SCr rise of ≥1/3 above baseline	55.2 (29)	15.1 (29)		184
SCr rise of ≥0.5 mg/dl if baseline <3; ≥1.0 mg/dl if baseline >3	9.8 (97)	7.8 (97)		199
Decrease clearance below 14% of baseline; rise in *N*-acetylglucosaminidase and alanine aminopeptidase levels	40 (13)	58 (12)		162
SCr rise above normal range (1.5 mg/dl) with ≥33% decrease in CrCl; SCr rise of 0.5 mg/dl in pts with abnormal SCr	24 (45)	9 (23)		185

SCr = serum creatinine; CrCl = creatinine clearance.
[a]Number of treatment courses in parentheses.
[b]McHenry dosing method.
[c]Individualized method.

associated with rapid administration, concurrent use of neuromuscular blocking agents (i.e., *d*-tubocurarine, succinylcholine, decamethonium), hypocalcemia, aminoglycoside accumulation or overdosage, and neuromuscular disease (i.e., myasthenia gravis, botulism). Due to the serious consequences of aminoglycoside neuromuscular blockade, all patients at increased risk should be monitored closely.

In milder cases of neuromuscular blockade, conservative treatment (including discontinuation of the aminoglycoside) usually suffices to reverse the toxicity. However, in the more severe cases involving postoperative respiratory depression, therapeutic intervention may be required. Supportive measures may include ventilator support and correction of any circulatory and/or metabolic abnormalities. Therapeutic measures may include administration of calcium salts or neostigmine (192–194). Dose and administration rate of calcium gluconate can vary, although 10–200 mg by slow intravenous infusion has been commonly used. Some patients may require up to 1 g of calcium gluconate for a

Table 11 Aminoglycoside Interactions

Interacting Drug(s)	Mechanism	Clinical Comments
Semisynthetic penicillins (carbenicillin, ticarcillin, piperacillin) and other beta-lactam antibiotics	Reversible complex formation	Aminoglycoside concentration determinations may be falsely low; may result in microbiologically inactive compounds; greatest effect may be seen with gentamicin and carbenicillin
Heparin (>5 to 10 units/ml)	Possible reversible complex formation	Aminoglycoside concentration determinations may be erroneously low
Amphotericin B	May exhibit synergistic nephrotoxicity	Patients receiving both agents concurrently should be closely monitored for renal function deterioration
Cephalosporins	May exhibit synergistic nephrotoxicity	May occur primarily with cephaloridine and cephalothin; closely monitor patient's renal function
Clindamycin	May enhance likelihood of aminoglycoside nephrotoxicity	Carefully monitor patient's renal function
Dimenhydrinate	May mask symptoms of aminoglycoside ototoxicity	Carefully monitor patient's cochlear and vestibular function
Ethacrynic acid	May potentiate aminoglycoside ototoxicity nephrotoxicity	Carefully monitor patient for nephrotoxicity and ototoxicity
Methoxyflurane	May have additive or synergistic nephrotoxicity	Closely monitor patient's renal function
Skeletal muscle relaxants and neuromuscular blocking agents	May be synergistic with aminoglycoside-induced neuromuscular blockade	Monitor patient closely for signs and symptoms of neuromuscular blockade

therapeutic response (195). For those patients who do not respond to calcium gluconate but show a positive response to edrophonium hydrochloride, administration of neostigmine (0.5–1.0 mg every 4 h intramuscularly) with 0.5 mg of atropine may be tried (192,193).

D. Hypersensitivity Reactions

Hypersensitivity reactions due to aminoglycosides have been reported rarely. Reactions may include rash, eosinophilia, anaphylaxis, and/or drug fever. Aminoglycoside antibiotics should be avoided in patients who have experienced signs and symptoms of aminoglycoside hypersensitivity in a previous treatment course. Alternative agents should be considered, as there may be cross-reactivity among the aminoglycosides. Occasional local reactions at the site of infusion have been reported, including pain, induration, and sterile abscesses. Hematological abnormalities including leukopenia, granulocytopenia, and thrombocytopenia are also extremely rare (196).

E. Interactions

Several chemical interactions can occur with the aminoglycosides (Table 11). These interactions are generally weak acids binding with weak bases, and the resulting complexes can be reversible when the complex is in equilibrium with the free acid and base. Generally, these chemical complexes are also devoid of antimicrobial activity, but may have added risks of toxicity.

The aminoglycosides can be inactivated in vitro when mixed with β-lactams in higher concentrations (104). These agents include the semisynthetic penicillins (i.e., carbenicillin, ticarcillin, piperacillin, and mezlocillin) and some cephalosporins. The aminoglycosides and the β-lactams form a water-soluble complex that is reversible (105). The complex formation is dependent on drug concentration, time, temperature, and pH. Higher concentrations of aminoglycoside and β-lactam, higher temperature of medium, longer time of incubation, and lower pH favor the formation of the complex. The aminoglycosides differ in their susceptibility to bind with β-lactams. Gentamicin and tobramycin are the least stable, and amikacin and netilmicin are the most stable (106–109). Therefore, β-lactams and aminoglycosides should not be mixed together in intravenous solutions. This interaction is not clinically important in vivo in patients who have renal function >10% of normal (108). Patients who have renal function <10% of normal will have substantial changes in measured serum concentrations and have less active drug measured in the vascular system (106). The toxic potential of the complex of aminoglycosides and β-lactams is not known. This chemical interaction can also be important in the processing and handling of serum samples that have both aminoglycoside and β-lactam present. This interaction can usually be halted by cooling or freezing the sample without excessive delays.

Heparin in higher concentrations (> 50–100 units/ml) can inactivate aminoglycosides (110,112). The resulting complex is reversible and is most likely a weak acid and weak base interaction. The antibacterial activity is apparently not affected, but lower concentrations of aminoglycosides are measured when utilizing the agar diffusion method (112). In vivo the interaction is most likely not significant when heparin is used in antithrombotic concentrations (5–10 units/ml). Serum samples obtained for aminoglycoside measurements should not be collected in heparinized tubes.

Other drugs have been reported to interact with aminoglycoside antibiotics. Many of these interactions can enhance the risk of toxicity (Table 11). Divalent cations such as calcium and magnesium and other endogenous substances can also bind aminoglycosides and reduce their antimicrobial activity (111).

VIII. SUMMARY

Aminoglycoside antibiotics remain the cornerstone of treatment for life-threatening gram-negative infections in elderly patients. The use of aminoglycosides has continued even with the introduction of newer beta-lactam antibiotics and parenteral quinolones. The major disadvantage of aminoglycosides is their association with ototoxicity and nephrotoxicity. These reactions have been reported for all aminoglycosides, although the risk may be less for netilmicin. Several factors may increase the risk of toxicity, including elevated serum concentrations. The disposition of aminoglycosides demonstrates substantial patient to patient variation. Measuring serum concentrations and dosage individualization are necessary to ensure optimal patient outcome and the most cost-effective treatment.

REFERENCES

1. Bryan LE, Van Den Elzen HM. Effects of membrane-energy mutations and cations on streptomycin and gentamicin accumulation by bacteria: a model for entry of streptomycin and gentamicin in susceptible and resistant bacteria. Antimicrob Agents Chemother 1977; 12:163–77.

2. Le Goffic, Capman ML, Tangy F, et al. Mechanisms of action of aminoglycoside antibiotics: binding studies of tobramycin and its 6′-N acetyl derivative to the bacterial ribosome and its subunits. Eur J Biochem 1979; 102:73–81.
3. Price KE, De Furia MD, Pursiano TA. Amikacin, an aminoglycoside with marked activity against antibiotic-resistant clinical isolates. J Infect Dis 1976; 134:S249–61.
4. Acar JF, Witchitz FL, Goldstein F, et al. Susceptibility of aminoglycoside-resistant gram-negative bacilli to amikacin: delineation of individual resistance patterns. J Infect Dis 1976; 134:S280–5.
5. Noone P. Use of antibiotics: aminoglycosides. Br Med J 1978; 8–19, 549–52.
6. Finland M, Gatner C, Wilcox C, et al. Susceptibility of recently isolated bacteria to amikacin in vitro: comparisons with four other aminoglycoside antibiotics. J Infect Dis 1976; 134:S297.
7. Hamada M, Homma Y, Kamamura I, et al. Antibacterial activity of dibekacin against gentamicin-resistant organisms. Jpn J Antibiot 1977; 30:203–5.
8. Farrell W, Wilks M, Drasae FA. Synergy between aminoglycosides and semisynthetic penicillins against gentamicin-resistant gram-negative rods. J Antimicrob Chemother 1979; 5:23–9.
9. Moellering Jr RC. Clinical microbiology and the in vitro activity of aminoglycosides. In: Welten A, Neu HC, eds. The aminoglycosides. microbiology, clinical use and toxicology. New York: Marcel Dekker, 1982:65.
10. Meyers BR, Hirschmann SZ. Antimicrobial activity in vitro of netilmicin and comparison with sisomicin, gentamicin, and tobramycin. Antimicrob Agents Chemother 1977; 11:118–21.
11. Dornbusch K, Hallander H. Gentamicin in gram-negative bacilli. Occurrence of modifying enzymes and their influence on susceptibility testing. Scand J Infect Dis 1980; 12:295–302.
12. Scheer M, Weinstein MJ, Waitz JA. Sisomicin: biochemical and microbiological profile. Infection 1979; 7(suppl 3):241–2.
13. Grimm H. Comparison of the antimicrobial effects of four aminoglycoside antibiotics. Infection 1979; 7(suppl 3):242–3.
14. Block RE, Lau WK, Weinstein RJ, et al. Ototoxicity of amikacin. Antimicrob Agents Chemother 1976; 9:956–61.
15. Erlanson P, Lundgren A. Ototoxic side effects following treatment with streptomycin, dihydrostreptomycin, and kanamycin. Acta Med Scand 1964; 176:147–63.
16. Luft FC, Randin LI, Sloan RS. Comparative low dose nephrotoxicities of dibekacin, gentamicin, and tobramycin. J Antimicrob Chemother 1982; 9:297–301.
17. Sato K, Yokota M, Doeda T. Evaluation of ototoxicity of aminoglycoside antibiotics in guinea pigs by scanning electromicroscopy. Current Chemotherapy Proceedings of the International Conference on Chemotherapy (ASM), 1980:609.
18. Matzke GR, Lucaroth PL, Shapiro HS. Controlled comparison of gentamicin and tobramycin nephrotoxicity. Am J Nephrol 1983; 3:11–18.
19. Dahlgren JG, Anderson ET, Hewitt WL. Gentamicin blood levels, a guide to nephrotoxicity. Antimicrob Agents Chemother 1975; 8:58–62.
20. Mawer GE, Ahmad R, Dobbs SM, et al. Prescribing aids for gentamicin. Br J Clin Pharmacol 1974; 1:45–50.
21. Line DH, Graham WP, Waterworth PM. Serum streptomycin levels and dizziness. Tubercle 1977; 51:76–81.
22. Jackson GG, Riff LJ. Pseudomonas bacteremia. Pharmacologic and other bases for failure of treatment with gentamicin. J Infect Dis 1971; 124:S185–91.
23. Anderson ET, Young LS, Hewitt WL. Simultaneous antibiotic levels in breakthrough gram-negative rod bacteremia. Am J Med 1976; 61:493–7.
24. Noone P, Parsons TMC, Pattison JR, et al. Experience in monitoring gentamicin therapy during treatment of serious gram-negative sepsis. Br Med J 1974; 1:477–81.
25. Bodey GP, Valdivieso M, Yap BS. The role of schedule in antibiotic therapy of the neutropenic patient. Infection 1980; 8(suppl 1):75–81.

26. Moore RD, Smith CR, Lietman PS. The association of aminoglycoside plasma levels with mortality in patients with gram-negative bacteremia. J Infect Dis 1984; 194(3):443–8.
27. Tally FP, Louie TJ, Weinstein WM, et al. Amikacin therapy for severe gram-negative sepsis: emphasis on infections with gentamicin-resistant organisms. Ann Intern Med 1975; 83:484–8.
28. Klastersky J, Meunier-Carpentier F, Prevost JM: Significance of antimicrobial synergism for the outcome of gram-negative sepsis. Am J Med Sci 1977; 273:157–67.
29. Cipolle RJ, Siefert RD, Zaske DE, et al. Hospital acquired gram-negative pneumonias: response rate and dosage requirements with individualized tobramycin therapy. Ther Drug Monit 1980; 2:273–82.
29a. Herting RL, Lane AZ, Lorber RR, et al. Netilmicin: chemical development and overview of clinical research. Scand J Infect Dis 1980; 23:S20–9.
30. Zaske DE, Cipolle RJ, Rotschafer JC, et al. Gentamicin pharmacokinetics in 1,640 patients: method for control of serum concentrations. Antimicrob Agents Chemother 1982; 21(3):407–11.
31. Zaske DE, Bootman JL, Solem LD, et al. Increased burn patient survival with individualized dosages of gentamicin. Surgery 1982; 91(2):142–9.
32. Zaske DE, Sawchuk RJ, Strate RG. The necessity of increased doses of amikacin in burn patients. Surgery 1978; 84:603–8.
33. Summer WR, Michael JR, Lipsky JJ. Initial aminoglycoside levels in the critically ill. Crit Care Med 1983; 11(12):948–50.
34. Kreger BE, Craven DE, McCabe WR. Gram-negative bacteremia: re-evaluation of clinical features and treatment in 612 patients. Am J Med 1980; 68:344.
35. Kunin CN. Absorption, distribution, excretion and fate of kanamycin. Ann NY Acad Sci 1966; 132:811–18.
36. Kunin DM, Chalmers TC, Leevy CN, et al. Absorption of orally administered neomycin and kanamycin. N Engl J Med 1960; 262:380–5.
37. Ericsson DC, Duke JH, Picking LK. Clinical pharmacology of intravenous and intraperitoneal aminoglycoside antibiotics in the prevention of wound infection. Am Surg 1978; 188:66–70.
38. Barza M, Kane A, Baum JL. Regional differences in ocular concentration of gentamicin after subconjunctival and retrobulbar injection in the rabbit. Am J Ophthamol 1977; 83:407–13.
39. Mendelson J, Portnoy J, Sigman H. Pharmacology of gentamicin in the biliary tract of humans. Antimicrob Agents Chemother 1973; 4:538.
40. Shiffmand DO. Evaluation of amikacin sulfate (Amikin). A new aminoglycoside antibiotic. JAMA 1977; 238:1547–50.
41. Pitt HA, Roberts RB, Johnson WB. Gentamicin levels in the human biliary tract. J Infect Dis 1973; 127:299.
42. Zazlow J, Counseller VS, Heilman FR. The excretion and concentration of penicillin and streptomycin in the abnormal human biliary tract. I: Gall bladder bile. Surg Gyn Obstet 1947; 84:16–20.
43. Riff JJ, Jackson GG. Pharmacology of gentamicin in man. J Infect Dis 1971; 124:598.
44. Odio W, Van Laer E, Klastersky J, et al. Concentrations of gentamicin in bronchial secretions after intramuscular and endotracheal administration. J Clin Pharmacol 1975; 15:518.
45. Wong GA, Pierce TH, Goldstein E, et al. Penetration of antimicrobial agents into bronchial secretions. Am J Med 1975; 59:219.
46. Zaske DE, Strate RG, Mossier NR. Amikacin pharmacokinetics: wide interpatient variation in 98 patients. J Clin Pharmacol 1991; 31:158–63.
47. Zaske DE, Cipolle RJ, Strate RG. Gentamicin dosage requirements: wide interpatient variations in 242 surgery patients with normal renal function. Surgery 1980; 87:164–9.
48. Cabana BE, Taggart JC. Comparative pharmacokinetics of BB-K8 and kanamycin in dogs and humans. Antimicrob Agents Chemother 1973; 3:478–83.
49. Lode H, Grunert K, Koeppe P, et al. Pharmacokinetic and clinical studies with amikacin, a new aminoglycoside antibiotic. J Infect Dis 1976; 134:S316–22.

50. Howard JB, McCracken GH. Pharmacological evaluation of amikacin in neonates. Antimicrob Agents Chemother 1975; 8:86–90.
51. Haughey DB, Hilligoss DM, Grassi A, et al. Two-compartment gentamicin pharmacokinetics in premature neonates: a comparison to adults with decreased glomerular filtration rates. J Pediatr 1980; 96(2):325–30.
52. Zaske DE, Cipolle RJ, Strate RG, et al. Rapid gentamicin elimination in obstetric patients. Obstet Gynecol 1980; 56:559–64.
53. Zaske DE, Cipolle RJ, Strate RG, et al. Increased gentamicin dosage requirements rapid elimination in 249 gynecology patients. Am J Obstet Gynecol 1981; 139:896.
54. Yasuhara H, Kobayashi S, Sakamoto K, et al. Pharmacokinetics of amikacin and cephalothin in bed-ridden elderly patients. J Clin Pharmacol 1982; 22:403–9.
55. Cutler RE, Gyselynck AM, Fleet P, et al. Correlation of serum creatinine concentration and gentamicin half-life. JAMA 1972; 219:1037–41.
56. McHenry MC, Gavan TL, Gifford RW, et al. Gentamicin dosage for renal insufficiency: adjustments based on endogenous creatinine clearance, and serum creatinine concentrations. Ann Intern Med 1971; 74:192–7.
57. Kaye D, Levison ME, Labovitz ED. The unpredictability of serum concentrations of gentamicin: pharmacokinetics of gentamicin in patients with normal and abnormal renal function. J Infect Dis 1974; 130:150–4.
58. Barza M, Brown RB, Shen D, et al. Predictability of blood levels of gentamicin in man. J Infect Dis 1975; 132:165–74.
59. Cipolle RJ, Seifert RD, Zaske DE, et al. Systematically individualizing tobramycin dosage regimens. J Clin Pharmacol 1980; 20:570–80.
60. Humbert G, Fillastre JP, Leroy A, et al. Pharmacokinetics of sisomicin in normal subjects and patients with renal failure. Infection 1979; 7(suppl 3):265–6.
61. Rotschafer JC, Crossley KB, Zaske DE, et al. Clinical use of a one compartment model for determining netilmicin pharmacokinetic parameters and dosage recommendations. Ther Drug Monit 1983; 5:263–7.
62. Kahlmeter G. Netilmicin: clinical pharmacokinetics and aspects on dosage schedules; an overview. Scand J Infect Dis 1980; 23:S74–81.
63. Plantier J, Forrey AW, O'Neill MA, et al. Pharmacokinetics of amikacin in patients with normal or impaired renal function: radioenzymatic acetylation assay. J Infect Dis 1976; 134:S323–30.
64. Pack J. Hallynck T, Soep H, et al. Pharmacokinetics of amikacin in patients with renal insufficiency: relation of half-life and creatinine clearance. J Infect Dis 1976; 134:S331–41.
65. McHenry MC, Wagner JG, Hall PM, et al. Pharmacokinetics of amikacin in patients with impaired renal function. J Infect Dis 1976; 134:S343–8.
66. Lanao JM, Dominguez-Gil A, Macias JG, et al. The influence of ascites on the pharmacokinetics of amikacin. Int J Clin Pharmacol Ther Toxicol 1980; 18(2):57–61.
67. Gill MA, Kern JW. Altered gentamicin distribution in ascitic patients. Am J Hosp Pharm 1979; 36:1704–6.
68. Sampliner R, Perrier D, Powell R, et al. Influence of ascites on tobramycin pharmacokinetics. J Clin Pharmacol 1984; 24(1):43–6.
69. Regeur L, Colding H, Jensen H, et al. Pharmacokinetics of amikacin during hemodialysis and peritoneal dialysis. Antimicrob Agents Chemother 1977; 11:214–18.
70. Danish M, Schultz R, Jusko WJ. Pharmacokinetics of gentamicin and kanamycin during hemodialysis. Antimicrob Agents Chemother 1974; 6:841–7.
71. Campillo JA, Lanao JM, Dominguez-Gil A, et al. Disposition of dibekacin in patients undergoing hemodialysis. Eur J Clin Pharmacol 1980; 18:347–50.
72. Matzke GR, Halstenson CE, Keane WF. Hemodialysis elimination rates and clearance of gentamicin and tobramycin. Antimicrob Agents Chemother 1984; 25(1):128–30.
73. Bauer LA. Rebound gentamicin levels after hemodialysis. Ther Drug Monit 1982; 4:99–101.

74. Bunke CM, Aronoff R, Brier ME, et al. Tobramycin kinetics during continuous ambulatory peritoneal dialysis. Clin Pharmacol Ther 1983; 34(1):110–16.
75. Atkins RC, Mion C, Despaux E, et al. Peritoneal transfer of kanamycin and its use in peritoneal dialysis. Kidney Int 1973; 3:391–6.
76. DePaepe M, Lameire N, Belpaire F, et al. Peritoneal pharmacokinetics of gentamicin in man. Clin Nephrol 1983; 19(3):107–9.
77. Pancorbo S, Comty C. Pharmacokinetics of gentamicin in patients undergoing continuous ambulatory peritoneal dialysis. Antimicrob Agents Chemother 1981; 19:605–7.
78. Pennington JE, Dale DC, Reynolds HW, et al. Gentamicin sulfate pharmacokinetics: lower levels of gentamicin in blood during fever. J Infect Dis 1975; 132:270–5.
79. Bauer LA, Blouin RA. Influence of age on tobramycin pharmacokinetics in patients with normal renal function. Antimicrob Agents Chemother 1981; 20:587–9.
80. Zaske DE, Sawchuk RJ, Gerding DN, et al. Increased dosage requirements of gentamicin in burn patients. J Trauma 1976; 16:824–8.
81. Zaske DE, Irvine P, Strand L, et al. Wide interpatient variations in gentamicin dosage requirements for geriatric patients. JAMA 1982; 248(23):3112–26.
82. Schwartz SN, Pazin GJ, Lyon JA, et al. A controlled investigation of the pharamcokinetics of gentamicin and tobramycin in obese patients. J Infect Dis 1978; 138:499–595.
83. Sketris I, Lesar TS, Zaske DE, et al. Effect of obesity on gentamicin pharmacokinetics. J Clin Pharmacol 1981; 21:288–93.
84. Bauer LA, Blovin RA, Griffen WU, et al. Amikacin pharmacokinetics in morbidly obese patients. Am J Hosp Pharm 1980; 37:519–22.
85. Zaske DE, Cipolle RJ, Solem LD, et al. Rapid individualization of gentamicin dosage regimens in 66 burn patients. Burns 1981; 7:215–20.
86. Zaske DE, Chin T, Kohls PR, et al. Initial dosage regimens of gentamicin in burn patients. J Burn Care Rehab 1991; 12:46–50.
87. Lott RS, Uden DL, Wargin WA, et al. Correlation of predicted versus measured creatinine clearance values in burn patients. Am J Hosp Pharm 1978; 35:717–20.
88. Wirt TC, McGee ZA, Oldfield EH, et al. Intraventricular administration of amikacin for complicated gram-negative meningitis and ventriculitis. J Neurosurg 1979; 50:95–9.
89. Kaiser AB, McGee ZA. Aminoglycoside therapy of gram-negative bacillary meningitis. N Engl J Med 1975; 293:1215–20.
90. Rotschafer JC. Central nervous system infections. In: Applied therapeutics—the clinical use of drugs. Vancouver, WA: Applied Therapeutics Inc., 1988:763–80.
91. Barza M. Factors affecting the intraocular penetration of antibiotics. The influence of route, inflammation, animal species and tissue pigmentation. Scand J Infect Dis 1978; SI4:151–9.
92. Jawetz E, Sonne M. Penicillin-streptomycin treatment of enterococcal endocarditis: a re-evaluation. N Engl J Med 1966; 274:710.
93. Sawyer WD, Dangerfield HG, Hogge AL, et al. Antibiotic prophylaxis and therapy of airborne tularemia. Bacteriol Rev 1966; 30:542.
94. Butler T, Mahmoud AAF, Warren KS. Algorithms in the diagnosis and management of exotic diseases. XXV Plague. J Infect Dis 1977; 136:317.
95. Buchanan TM, Faber LC, Feldman RA. Brucellosis in the United States, 1960–1972; an Abattoir-associated disease. Medicine 1974; 53:403.
96. Gangadharam PRJ, Candler ER, Ramakrishna PV. In vitro antimycobacterial activity of some new aminoglycoside antibiotics. J Antimicrob Chemother 1977; 3:285–6.
97. Wapnick S, Guinto R, Reizis E, et al. Reduction of post-operative infection in elective colon surgery with preoperative administration of kanamycin and erythromycin. Surgery 1979; 85:317–21.
98. Boyle R, Nelson JS, Stonestreet BS, et al. Alterations in stool flora resulting from oral kanamycin prophylaxis of necrotizing enterocolitis. J Pediatr 1978; 93:857–61.

99. Noone P. Sisomicin, netilmicin and dibekacin: a review of their antimicrobial activity and therapeutic use. Drugs 1984; 27:548–78.
100. Bergeron MG, Beauchamp D, Poirer A, et al. Continuous versus intermittent administration of antimicrobial agents; tissue penetration and efficacy in vivo. Rev Infect Dis 1981; 3:84–97.
101. Powell SH, Thompson WL, Luthe MA, et al. Once daily versus continuous aminoglycoside dosing: efficacy and toxicity in animal and clinical studies of gentamicin, netilmicin, and tobramycin. J Infect Dis 1983; (5):147:918–32.
102. Anderson AC, Hodges JR, Barnes WG. Determination of serum gentamicin sulfate levels. Arch Intern Med 1976; 136:785–7.
103. Glynn TW, Pevonka MP, Yost RL, et al. Use of serum gentamicin levels in hospitalized patients. Am J Hosp Pharm 1978; 35:806–8.
104. Noone P, Pattison JR. Therapeutic implications of interaction of gentamicin and penicillins. Lancet 1971; 2:575–8.
105. Waitz JA, Drube CG, Moss Jr EL, et al. Biological aspects of the interaction between gentamicin and carbenicillin. J Antibiot 1972; 25:219–25.
106. Pickering LK, Gearheart P: Effect of time and concentration upon interaction between gentamicin, tobramycin, netilmicin or amikacin and carbenicillin or ticarcillin. Antimicrob Agents Chemother 1979; 15:592–6.
107. Holt HA, Broughall JM, McCarthy M, et al. Interactions between aminoglycoside antibiotics and carbenicillin or ticarcillin. Infection 1976; 4:107–9.
108. Ervin FR, Bullock Jr WE, Nuttall CE. Inactivation of gentamicin by penicillins in patients with renal failure. Antimicrob Agents Chemother 1976; 9:1004–11.
109. Lau A, Lee M, Flascha S, et al. Effect of piperacillin on tobramycin pharmacokinetics in patients with normal renal function. Antimicrob Agents Chemother 1983; 24(4):533–7.
110. Yourassowsky E, de Broe ME, Wieme RJ. Effect of heparin on gentamicin concentration in blood. Clin Chem Acta 1972; 42:189–91.
110a. Nilsson I. Factors affecting gentamicin assay. Antimicrob Agents Chemother 1980; 17(6):918–21.
111. Flournoy DJ. Reduction of gentamicin bioassay values in sera with elevated inorganic phosphorous, uric acid, creatinine, and alkaline phosphatase levels. Ther Drug Monit 1982; 4(2):95–7.
112. Schmelter RF, Dirksen W, Stalp JT, et al. Effect of heparin on radioimmunoassay of gentamicin. Am J Hosp Pharm 1981; 38:534–7.
113. Sabath LD, Casey JI, Ruch PA, et al. Rapid microassay for circulating nephrotoxic antibiotics. Antimicrob Agents Chemother 1970; 10:83–90.
114. Zaske DE, Crossley K. A new aminoglycoside. Minn Med 1978; 61:125.
115. Maitra SK, Yoshikawa TT, Guze LB, et al. Determination of aminoglycoside antibiotics in biological fluids: a review. Clin Chem 1979; 25:1361–7.
116. Matzke GR, Gwizdala C, Wery J, et al. Evaluation of three gentamicin serum assay techniques. Ther Drug Monit 1982; 4(2):195–200.
116a. Rotschafer JC, Morlock C, Strand L, et al: Comparison of radioimmunoassay and enzyme immunoassay methods in determining gentamicin pharmacokinetic parameters and dosages. Antimicrob Agents Chemother 1982;22(4):748–651.
117. Rotschafer JC, Berg HG, Nelson RB, et al. Observed differences in gentamicin pharmacokinetic parameters and dosage recommendations determined by fluorescent polarization immunoassay methods. Ther Drug Monit 1983; 5:443–7.
118. Sarubbi FA, Hull JH. Amikacin serum concentrations: prediction of levels and dosage guidelines. Ann Intern Med 1978; 89:612–18.
119. Cox CE. Amikacin therapy of urinary tract infections. J Infect Dis 1976; 134:S362–8.
120. Lesar TS, Rotschafer JC, Strand LM, et al. Gentamicin dosing errors with four commonly used nomograms. JAMA 1982; 248(10):1190–3.

121. Hull JH, Sarubbi FA. Gentamicin serum concentrations: pharmacokinetic predictions. Ann Intern Med 1976; 85:183–9.
122. Garamycin sulfate. In: Physician's desk reference. Oradell, NJ: Medical Economics Company, 1981:1607.
123. Dettli LC: Drug dosage in patients with renal disease. Clin Pharmacol Ther 1974; 16:274.
124. Siersbaek-Nielsen K, Hansen JM, Kampmann J, et al. Rapid evaluation of creatinine clearance. Lancet 1971; 1:1133–4.
125. Diem K, Lentner C, eds. Geigy's scientific tables. Ardsley, NY: Geigy Pharmaceuticals, 1970.
126. Chan RA, Benner EJ, Hoeprich PO. Gentamicin therapy in renal failure: a nomogram for dosage. Ann Intern Med 1976; 76:773–8.
127. Sheiner LB, Beal SL. Bayesian individualization of pharmacokinetics: simple implementation and comparison with non-Bayesian methods. J Pharmacokin Sci 1982; 71(12):1344–8.
128. Sheiner LB, Beal SL, Rosenberg B, et al. Forecasting individual pharmacokinetics. Clin Pharmacol Ther 1979; 26(3):294–305.
129. Schentag JJ, Jusko WJ, Vance JW, et al. Gentamicin disposition and tissue accumulation on multiple dosing. J Pharmacokinet Biopharm 1977; 5:559–79.
130. Schentag JJ, Cumbo TJ, Jusko WJ, et al. Gentamicin tissue accumulation and nephrotoxic reactions. JAMA 1978; 240:2067–9.
131. D'Argenio DZ. Optimal sampling times for pharmacokinetic experiments. J Pharmacokinetic Biopharm 1981; 9:739–56.
132. Bootman JL, Wertheimer AI, Zaske DE, et al. Individualizing gentamicin dosage regimens in burn patients with gram-negative septicemia: a cost benefit analysis. J Pharm Sci 1979; 68:267–72.
133. Brummett RE. Drug-induced ototoxicity. Drugs 1980; 19:412–28.
134. Neu HC, Bendush CL. Ototoxicity of tobramycin: a clinical overview. J Infect Dis 1976; 134:S206–18.
135. Jackson GG, Arcieri G. Ototoxicity of gentamicin in man: a survey and controlled analysis of clinical experience in the United States. J Infect Dis 1971; 124:S130–7.
136. Ballantyne J. Ototoxic drugs. In: Hinchcliffe R, Harrison D, eds. Scientific foundations of otolaryngology. Chicago-Year Book Medical Publishers Inc., 1976:849–62.
137. Quick CA. Chemical and drug effects on inner ear. In: Paperella MM, Shumrick DA, eds. Otolaryngology, Vol. 2. Philadelphia: WB Saunders Co., 1973:391–406.
138. Brummett RE, Fox KE, Bendrick TW, et al. Ototoxicity of tobramycin, gentamicin, amikacin and sisomicin in the guinea pig. J Antimicrob Chemother 1978; 4(suppl A):73–83.
139. Ylikoski J. Correlation between pure tone audiogram and cochlear pathology in guinea-pigs intoxicated with ototoxic antibiotics. Acta Otolaryngol 1974; 326:S42–62.
140. Nordstrom L, Banck G, Belfrage S, et al. Prospective study of the ototoxicity of gentamicin. Acta Pathol Microbiol Scand 1973; (B)81(suppl 241):58–61.
141. Cawthorne T, Ranger D. Toxic effect of streptomycin upon balance and hearing. Br Med J 1957; 1:1444–6.
142. Spoenllin, H. Zur ototoxicitat des Streptomyzins. Pract Otorhinolarying (Basel) 1966; 28:305–22.
143. Weinstein MJ, Marquez JA, Testa PT, et al. Antibiotic 6640, a new micromonospora-produced aminoglycoside antibiotic. J Antibiot (Tokyo) 1970; 23:551–4.
144. Weinstein MJ, Wagman GH, Waitz JA: Discovery and isolation of sisomicin. Infection 1976; 4(suppl 4):285–8.
145. Daschner F, Langmaack H. Activity of dibekacin compared with other aminoglycoside antibiotics. Antimicrob Agents Chemother 1978; 4(suppl A):47.
146. Federspil P, Schatzle W, Tiesler E. Pharmacokinetics and ototoxicity of gentamicin, tobramycin, and amikacin. J Infect Dis 1976; 134:S200–5.
147. Kaku Y, Farmer Jr JC, Hudson WR. Ototoxic drug effects on cochlear histochemistry. Arch Otolaryngol 1973; 98:282–6.

148. Tachibaba M, Mizukoshi O, Kuriyama K. Inhibitory effects of kanamycin on glycolysis in cochlea and kidney—possible involvement in the formation of ototoxicities and nephrotoxicities. Biochem Pharmacol 1976; 25:2297–301.
149. Linuma T, Mizukoshi O, Daly JF. Possible effects of various ototoxic drugs upon the ATP-hydrolyzing system in the stria vascularis and spiral ligament of the guinea pig. Larynogoscope 1967; 77:159–70.
150. Orsulakova A, Stockhorst E, Schacht J. Effect of neomycin on phosphoinositide labeling and calcium binding in guinea-pig inner ear tissues in vivo and in vitro. J Neurochem 1976; 26:285–90.
151. Schacht J. Biochemistry of neomycin ototoxicity. J Acoust Soc Am 1976; 59:940–4.
152. Weintraub RG, Duggin GG, Horvath JS, et al. Comparative nephrotoxicity of two aminoglycosides: gentamicin and tobramycin. Med J Austr 1982; 2:129–32.
153. Meyer RD, Lewis RP, Carmait ED, et al. Amikacin therapy for serious gram-negative bacillary infections. Ann Intern Med 1975; 83:790–800.
154. Bock BV, Edelstein PH, Meyer RD. Prospective comparative study of efficacy and toxicity of netilmicin and amikacin. Antimicrob Agents Chemother 1980; 17(2):217–25.
154a. Barza M, Lauermann MW, Tally FP, et al. Prospective, randomized trial of netilmicin and amikacin with emphasis on eighth-nerve toxicity. Antimicrob Agents Chemother 1980; 17(4):707–14.
154b. Klastersky J, Hensgens C, Gerard M, et al. Comparison of sisomicin and gentamicin in bacteriuric patients with underlying diseases of the urinary tract. Antimicrob Agents Chemother 1975; 7:742–7.
154c. Panwalker AP, Malow JB, Zimelis VM, et al. Netilmicin: clinical efficacy, tolerance and toxicity. Antimicrob Agents Chemother 1978; 13(2):170–6.
154d. Tablan OC, Milagros PR, et al. Renal and auditory toxicity of high dose, prolonged therapy with gentamicin and tobramycin in *Pseudomonas* endocarditis. J Infect Dis 1984; 149(2):257–63.
154e. Feig PU, Mitchell PP, Abrutyn E, et al. Aminoglycoside nephrotoxicity: a double-blind prospective randomized study of gentamicin and tobramycin. J Antimicrob Chemother 1982; 10:217–26.
154f. Feig PU, Mitchell PP, Abrütyn E, et al. Aminoglycoside nephrotoxicity: a double-blind prospective randomized study of gentamicin and tobramycin. J Antimicrob Chemother 1982; 10:217–26.
155. Lerner AM, Reyes MP, Cone LA, et al. Randomized controlled trial of the comparative efficacy, auditory toxicity, and nephrotoxicity of tobramycin and netilmicin. Lancet I: 1983; 1123–6.
156. Edwards CQ, Smith CR, Baughman KL, et al. Concentrations of gentamicin and amikacin in human kidneys. Antimicrob Agents Chemother 1976; 9:925–7.
157. Appel GB, Neu HC. Gentamicin in 1978. Ann Intern Med 1978; 89:528–38.
158. Appel GB, Neu HC. The nephrotoxicity of antimicrobial agents. N Engl J Med 1977; 296:663–70,722–8.
159. Bennett WM, Luft F, Porter G. Pathogenesis of renal failure due to aminoglycosides and contrast media used in roentgenography. Am J Med 1980; 69:767–74.
160. Houghton DC, Hartnett M, Campbell-Bowell M, et al. A light and electron microscopic analysis of gentamicin nephrotoxicity in rats. Am J Pathol 1976; 82:589–612.
161. Luft FC, Randin LJ, Sloan RS, et al. Recovery from aminoglycoside nephrotoxicity with continued drug administration. Antimicrob Agents Chemother 1978; 14:284–7.
162. Keys TF, Kurtz SB, Jones JD, et al. Renal toxicity during therapy with gentamicin or tobramycin. Mayo Clin Proc 1981; 56:556–9.
163. Wellwood JM, Simpson PM, Tighe FR, et al. Evidence of gentamicin nephrotoxicity in patients with renal allografts. Br Med J 1975; 3:278.

164. Mondorf AW, Zegelman M, Kose J, et al. Comparative studies of the action of aminoglycosides and cephalosporins in the proximal tubule of the kidney. J Antimicrob Chemother 1978; 4S:53.
165. Trollfors B, Alestig K, Krantz I, et al. Quantitative nephrotoxicity of gentamicin in nontoxic doses. J Infect Dis 1980; 141(3):306–9.
166. Schentag JJ, Plaut ME. Patterns of urinary beta2-microglobulin excretion by patients treated with aminoglycosides. Kidney Int 1980; 17:654–61.
167. Kaye WA, Griffiths WC, Trebbin W, et al. Gentamicin induced B2-microglobinuria (abstract). Washington, DC: American Society of Nephrology, 1979:153A.
168. Schentag JJ, Plaut ME, Cerra FB, et al. Aminoglycoside nephrotoxicity in critically ill surgical patients. J Surg Res 1979; 26:270–9.
169. French MA, Cerra FB, Plaut ME, et al. Comparison of amikacin and gentamicin in critically ill patients. In: Nelson JD, Grassi C, eds. Current Chemotherapy and Infectious Disease. Washington, DC: American Society for Microbiology, 1980; 628.
170. Gilberg DN, Houghton DC, Bennett WM, et al. Reversibility of gentamicin nephrotoxicity in rats: recovery during continuous drug administration. Proc Soc Exp Biol Med 1979; 160:99–102.
171. Luft FC, Kleit SA. Renal parenchymal accumulation of aminoglycoside antibiotics in rats. J Infect Dis 1974; 130:656.
172. Soberon L, Bowman RL, Pastoriza-Munoz E, et al. Comparative nephrotoxicities of gentamicin, netilmicin and tobramycin in the rat. J Pharmacol Exp Ther 1979; 210:334–43.
173. Bowman RL, Silverblatt FJ, Kaloyanides GJ. Comparison of the nephrotoxicity of netilmicin and gentamicin in rats. Antimicrob Agents Chemother 1977; 12:474.
174. Kaloyanides GJ, Pastoriza-Munoz E. Aminoglycoside nephrotoxicity. Kidney Int 1980; 18:571–82.
175. Luft FC, Bloch R, Bloan RS, et al. Comparative nephrotoxicity of aminoglycoside antibiotics in rats. J Infect Dis 1978; 138:541–5.
176. Personal communication (letter) from the Schering Corporation: renal toxicity and antibiotic uptake in rats, March 27, 1985.
177. Silverblatt FJ. Antibiotic nephrotoxicity. Urol Clin North Am 1975; 2:557–67.
178. Cronin RE. Aminoglycoside nephrotoxicity: pathogenesis and prevention. Clin Nephrol 1979; 11:251–6.
179. Humes DH, Weinberg JM, Knauss TC. Clinical and pathophysiologic aspects of aminoglycoside nephrotoxicity. Am J Kidney Dis 1982; (1)2:5–29.
180. Leitman PS. Aminoglycoside inhibition of renal sodium-potassium ATPase: a possible model for nephrotoxicity. Antimicrob Agents Chemother 1978; 18:328.
181. Fillastre JP, Kuhn SM, Bendirdjian JP, et al. Prediction of antibiotic nephrotoxicity. Adv Nephrol 1976; 6:343–70.
182. Guay DRP. Netilmicin. Drug Int Clin Pharm 1983; 17:83–91.
183. Smith CR, Lipsky JJ, Laskin OL, et al. Double-blind comparison of the nephrotoxicity and auditory toxicity of gentamicin and tobramycin. N Engl J Med 1980; 302:1106–9.
184. Kumin GD. Clinical nephrotoxicity of tobramycin and gentamicin: a prospective study. JAMA 1980; 244(16):1808–10.
185. Fee Jr WE, Vierra V, Lathrop GR. Clinical evaluation of aminoglycoside toxicity: tobramycin versus gentamicin, a preliminary report. J Antimicrob Chemother 1978; 4(suppl A):31–6.
186. Zaske DE, Crossley KB, Strate RG. Tobramycin and gentamicin toxicity (letter). N Engl J Med 1980; 303(17):1102–3.
187. Warner A, Sanders E. Neuromuscular blockade associated with gentamicin therapy. JAMA 1971; 215:1153–4.
188. Pittinger CB, Eryasa Yi, Adamson R. Antibiotic-induced paralysis. Anesth. Analg. 1970; 49:487–501.
189. Finegold SM: Toxicity of kanamycin in adults. Ann NY Acad Sci 1966; 132:942–56.

190. L'Hommedieu CS, Nicholas D, Armes DA, et al. Potentiation of magnesium sulfate-induced neuromuscular weakness by gentamicin, tobramycin, and amikacin. J Pediatr 1983; 102(4):629–31.
191. Albiero L, Bomonte F, Ongini E, et al. Comparison of neuromuscular effects and acute toxicity of some aminoglycoside antibiotics. Arch Int Pharmacodyn 1978; 233:343–50.
192. Argov Z, Mastaglia FL. Disorders of neuromuscular transmission caused by drugs. N Engl J Med 1979; 301(8):409–13.
193. McQuillen MR, Cantor HE, O'Rourke JR. Myasthenic syndrome associated with antibiotics. Arch Neurol 1968; 18:402–15.
194. Elmquist D, Josefesson JO. The nature and neuromuscular block produced by neomycin. Acta Physiol Scand 1962; 54:105–10.
195. Meyer RD. Amikacin: diagnosis and treatment five years later. Ann Int Med 1981; 95:328–32.
196. Gooding PG, Berman E, Lane AZ, et al. A review of results of clinical trials with amikacin. J Infect Dis 1976; 134:S441–5.
197. Bergeron MG, Lessard C, Ronald A, et al. Three to eight weeks of therapy with netilmicin: toxicity in normal and diabetic patients. J Antimicrob Chemother 1983; 12:245–8.
198. Schentag JJ, Plaut ME, Cerra FB. Comparative nephrotoxicity of gentamicin and tobramycin: pharmacokinetic and clinical studies in 201 patients. Antimicrob Agents Chemother 1981; 19(5):859–66.
199. Fong IW, Fenton RS, Bird R. Comparative toxicity of gentamicin versus tobramycin: a randomized prospective study. J Antimicrob Chemother 1981; 7:81–8.

14

Quinolones

David R. P. Guay
University of Minnesota, Minneapolis, and St. Paul-Ramsey Medical Center, St. Paul, Minnesota

Modern antimicrobial chemotherapy has evolved at a rapid pace over the past six decades. Over this period of time, agents such as the sulfonamides, β-lactams (penicillins and cephalosporins), carbapenems, monobactams, macrolides, tetracyclines, chloramphenicol, clindamycin, nitroimidazoles, trimethoprim, β-lactam/β-lactamase inhibitor combinations, vancomycin, and aminoglycosides have been introduced. In addition, the fluoroquinolone class was introduced in the mid-1980s with the introduction of norfloxacin in 1986 and ciprofloxacin in 1987. In the 1990s, additional fluoroquinolone agents have emerged, including ofloxacin, enoxacin, and lomefloxacin in the United States as well as others such as pefloxacin that are only available outside the United States at present.

This chapter focuses on those fluoroquinolones currently available in the United States and reviews their role in modern antimicrobial chemotherapy in the elderly population. However, data for other fluoroquinolones will be supplied as well where geriatric-specific data exist.

I. CHEMISTRY

A. Development

The microbiological activity of nalidixic acid was first reported in 1962 (1). However, the clinical utility of this agent was limited by a narrow spectrum of activity (only against gram-negative aerobes), unfavorable pharmacokinetic properties (only useful for urinary tract infections), and a high propensity for the rapid development of bacterial resistance (2). During the 1960s and 1970s, chemical alterations to the quinolone nucleus resulted in the introduction of compounds such as oxolinic acid, cinoxacin, pipemidic acid, and flumequine. Although these compounds displayed improved activity and pharmacokinetic properties compared to nalidixic acid, the improvement was not sufficient to enable their use for systemic infections.

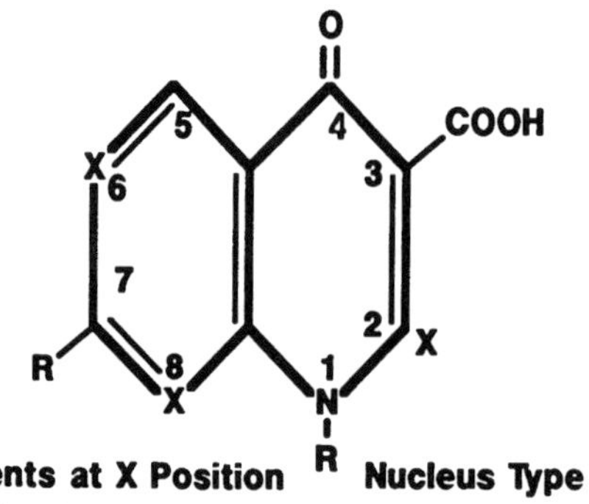

Substituents at X Position			Nucleus Type
2	6	8	
C	C	C	Quinolone
N	C	C	Cinnoline
C	N	N	Pyridopyrimidine
C	C	N	Naphthyridine

Figure 1

Despite the poor serum and tissue pharmacokinetic profiles of these early quinolones, as well as the problems with toxicity and the rapid development of bacterial resistance, interest in the quinolones remained high. Their apparent ability to disrupt bacterial DNA synthesis and replication by a unique mechanism of action had important potential, and cross-resistance with nonquinolone agents had not been found in clinical practice.

The introduction of ciprofloxacin during the mid-1980s heralded a major advance in the development of quinolone antimicrobial agents. Ciprofloxacin possessed potent broad-spectrum antimicrobial activity combined with a pharmacokinetic profile such that it was suitable for use in a wide range of systemic infections. Soon after its introduction, a number of other fluoroquinolones possessing similar properties became available in the United States, including ofloxacin, lomefloxacin, and temafloxacin. However, toxicity issues led to the withdrawal of temafloxacin in June 1992.

The development of quinolones, in general, has progressed along two paths, one leading to agents with improved pharmacokinetic profiles and the other leading to agents with improved antimicrobial activity. The path toward improved pharmacokinetic profiles is exemplified by ofloxacin, lomefloxacin, and enoxacin, which offered improved bioavailability and tissue penetration compared to previous agents. The other developmental path is exemplified by ciprofloxacin, which provided significant improvements in antimicrobial activity compared to previous agents (3).

B. Structure-Activity Relationships

The quinolones are a series of synthetic antimicrobial agents, each retaining a fundamental nuclear structure known as the "quinolone nucleus" (Fig. 1). These agents were developed from narrow-spectrum, less potent, pharmacokinetically inferior precursors exemplified by nalidixic acid, which was effective against a limited number of pathogens, as illustrated in Table 1. Nalidixic acid possessed a nitrogen substituent instead of a carbon atom at position 8 of the quinolone nucleus, giving rise to a naphthyridine nucleus (Fig. 1). Before the introduction of ciprofloxacin, nalidixic acid was often referred to as a "naphthyridine."

Substitutions of nitrogen atoms at other positions of the quinolone nucleus have in turn given rise to the "cinnoline" nucleus (nitrogen substituent at position 2) and the "pyridopyrimidine" nucleus (nitrogen substituents at positions 6 and 8).

Oxolinic acid was the next quinolone to enter clinical use (4). It differed from nalidixic acid by the possession of only one nitrogen substituent (at position 1), which produced a "quinolone" nucleus. Compared with the in vitro activity of nalidixic acid, oxolinic acid was 5–10 times more active against the Enterobacteriaceae, but not against *Pseudomonas aeruginosa*, and also possessed activity against *Staphylococcus aureus*.

During the 1970s, cinoxacin was developed (5). Structurally this agent differed from oxolinic acid by having cinnoline nucleus. Cinoxacin possessed less gram-positive activity compared to oxolinic acid and had similar in vitro activity compared to nalidixic acid; however, its pharmacokinetic properties were superior for the treatment of acute and chronic urinary tract infections. Both nalidixic acid and cinoxacin are rapidly absorbed, but hepatic metabolism results in urinary excretion of only 10–15% nalidixic acid as the parent compound compared to 60% for cinoxacin. This enabled treatment regimens of 1 g twice daily for cinoxacin compared to 1 g four times daily for nalidixic acid for the treatment of urinary tract infections.

Nalidixic acid, oxolinic acid, and cinoxacin all failed to achieve satisfactory serum or tissue concentrations to treat infections outside the urinary tract. Also, the rapid appearance of resistant mutants both in vitro and in vivo was reported (6). Organisms resistant to nalidixic acid were cross-resistant to oxolinic acid and cinoxacin and vice versa.

The next quinolones to enter clinical usage were pipemidic acid and flumequine (7,8). Pipemidic acid was synthesized using a pyridopyrimidine nucleus to which a piperazine substituent was attached at position 7. Importantly, this quinolone was the first to display substantial activity against *P. aeruginosa*, likely due to the piperazine substituent. However, pipemidic acid was only of use in the treatment of urinary tract infections due to its rapid urinary excretion. Flumequine was the first fluorinated quinolone carboxylic acid to be developed, and it had an antimicrobial spectrum and potency similar to that of oxolinic acid. As for pipemidic acid, flumequine was only of use in the treatment of urinary tract infections due to its rapid urinary excretion.

Norfloxacin was the first of the recently marketed fluoroquinolone class of agents (Fig. 2). Although the structure of these compounds differs, each has a fluorine atom at position 6 of the quinolone nucleus, giving rise to the name "fluoroquinolone." Chemically speaking, the label is imprecise. The alternative term "4-quinolone" has also been used to describe these compounds because the chemical name of the quinolone "nucleus" is 4-oxo-1,4-dihydroquinolone (9). However, in clinical practice most clinicians have reverted to the term "quinolone" in reference to the entire therapeutic class.

Norfloxacin was synthesized by attaching a fluorine atom at position 6 and a piperazine ring at position 7 of the quinolone nucleus. Subsequently, a large number of compounds based on this structure have been produced by chemists attempting to increase in vitro activity and/or improve the pharmacokinetic profile. These agents exhibit high intrinsic, broad-spectrum activity together with pharmacokinetic properties enabling their use for systemic as well as urinary tract infections.

As seen in Figure 2, the carboxylic acid group at position 3, the ketone group at position 4, and the fluorine substituent at position 6 are retained in the structures of these newer congeners. These groups at these positions optimize DNA gyrase binding, the primary site of action of the quinolones, and modification of these groups usually leads to substantial or total loss of activity.

Table 1 In Vitro Activity of Nalidixic Acid and Selected Fluoroquinolones

Bacterial species	MIC$_{50}$/MIC$_{90}$[a] (μg/ml)					
	Nalidixic acid	Norfloxacin	Ciprofloxacin	Ofloxacin	Lomefloxacin	Enoxacin
Gram-positive						
Staphylococcus aureus	50/100	0.8/6.3	0.5/1.0	0.4/0.4	1.0/2.0	0.08/3.1
Staphylococcus spp., coagulase negative	50/100	1.6/3.1	0.25/0.25	0.4/0.8	1.0/2.0	1.6/6.3
S. saprophyticus	>512/>512	2.0/4.0	0.5/0.5	1.0/1.0	2.0/2.0	2.0/2.0
Streptococcus pyogenes	>100/>100	1.6/6.3	0.5/2.0	1.6/3.1	3.1/8.0	6.3/12
S. agalactiae	>128/>128	2.0/4.0	0.5/1.0	2.0/2.0	16.0/16.0	4.0/8.0
Streptococcus spp., group C	>64/>64	4.0/8.0	0.5/2.0	1.0/2.0		
S. bovis		4.0/16	2.0/2.0	2.0/4.0		2.0/4.0
Streptococcus spp., group F	>64/>64	2.0/2.0	1.0/2.0			
Streptococcus spp., group G	>64/>64	2.0/4.0	0.25/1.0	1.0/2.0		8.0/16
Streptococcus, viridans group	128/>128	4.0/16	1.0/2.0	2.0/2.0	8.0/>12.5	16/32
S. pneumoniae	>128/>128	8.0/16	1.0/2.0	2.0/2.0	8.0/8.0	8.0/16
Enterococcus faecalis	>64/>64	4.0/8.0	2.0/4.0	2.0/4.0	8.0/12.5	8.0/16
E. faecium	>64/>64	4.0/8.0	1.0/2.0	3.1/6.2		
Listeria monocytogenes	>64/>64	2.0/4.0	0.5/0.5	0.5/1.0	2.0/8.0	8.0/16
Corynebacterium JK		1.0/4.0	0.25/1.0	0.25/1.0	3.2/>12.5	2.0/4.0
Corynebacterium D2		1.0/8.0	<0.3/1.0	0.5/0.5		
Enterobacteriaceae						
Escherichia coli	4.0/4.0	0.06/0.12	0.02/0.03	0.06/0.12	0.1/0.39	0.1/0.4
Klebsiella pneumoniae	2.0/16	0.12/0.5	0.03/0.06	0.1/0.2	0.25/1.0	0.2/0.8
K. oxytoca	2.0/8.0	0.12/0.25	0.03/0.13		0.2/0.5	0.2/0.8
Enterobacter aerogenes	2.0/8.0	0.1/0.4	0.03/0.06	0.1/0.8	0.25/0.50	0.2/0.8
E. cloacae	2.0/8.0	0.1/0.4	0.02/0.13	0.05/0.1	0.39/0.50	0.2/0.4
E. agglomerans	2.0/8.0	0.2/0.2	0.03/0.13	0.6/2.0		0.2/0.4
Citrobacter freundii	4.0/8.0	0.06/0.5	0.02/0.13	0.6/2.0	0.25/1.0	0.2/0.4

C. diversus	2.0/8.0	0.02/0.2	0.02/0.13	0.1/0.4	0.12/0.12	0.1/0.2
Proteus mirabilis	2.0/8.0	0.01/0.5	0.06/0.13	0.1/0.2	0.25/1.0	0.4/0.8
P. vulgaris	4.0/8.0	0.1/0.4	0.02/0.06	0.1/1.6	0.12/0.39	0.4/1.6
Providencia stuartii	16/32	0.12/1.0	0.03/0.5	0.4/1.6	0.50/1.0	0.8/16
P. rettgeri	8.0/16	0.5/1.0	0.13/0.25	0.4/1.6	0.50/4.0	0.8/16
Morganella morganii	4.0/8.0	0.02/0.06	0.02/0.03	0.01/0.02	0.12/0.40	0.1/0.4
Salmonella typhi	2.0/2.0	0.03/0.06	0.01/0.02	0.03/0.06		0.12/0.12
Salmonella spp.	2.0/4.0	0.06/0.06	0.01/0.02	0.06/0.06	0.12/0.25	0.12/0.12
Shigella spp.	4.0/8.0	0.03/0.06	0.01/0.02	0.06/0.12	0.12/0.25	0.12/0.12
Yersinia enterocolitica	2.0/2.0	0.06/0.06	0.02/0.02	0.06/0.12	0.03/0.25	0.12/0.12
Serratia marcescens	12/>100	0.8/3.1	<0.1/1.0	0.4/1.6	0.50/4.0	0.8/6.3
Other gram-negative						
Pseudomonas aeruginosa	16/16	1.0/2.0	0.12/0.5	1.0/2.0	2.0/8.0	1.0/4.0
P. maltophilia	8.0/16	1.0/4.0	1.0/2.0	0.8/3.1	8.0/12.5	4.0/8.0
P. cepacia	16/16	4.0/8.0	1.0/2.0	0.8/3.1	8.0/25.0	12/25
P. pseudomallei		4.0/8.0	2.0/8.0	8.0/32		8.0/32
Plesiomonas shigelloides	1.0/1.0	0.02/0.02	0.01/0.01	0.02/0.02		0.03/0.06
Aeromonas hydrophila	0.25/0.5	0.02/0.03	0.01/0.02	0.02/0.03	0.06/0.12	0.03/0.06
Acinetobacter calcoaceticus subsp. *anitratum*	32/256	8.0/64	0.13/0.25	1.0/4.0		1.0/2.0
A. calcoaceticus subsp. *lwoffi*	8.0/32	4.0/8.0	0.06/0.13	0.25/0.5		0.5/1.0
Hafnia alvei		0.12/0.12	0.03/0.03	0.06/0.06	0.12/1.0	0.06/0.12
Neisseria meningitidis	0.5/0.5	0.02/0.03	0.01/0.01	0.02/0.02	0.1/0.4	0.02/0.03
N. gonorrhoeae	1.0/1.0	0.03/0.06	0.01/0.01	0.02/0.06	0.05/0.10	0.1/0.25
Campylobacter jejuni	2.0/8.0	0.25/0.5	0.06/0.12	0.12/0.25	0.40/1.0	0.25/0.5
C. coli	4.0/4.0	0.4/0.8	0.2/0.4	0.4/0.8	0.25/0.25	1.0/2.0
Helicobacter pylori	32/64	2.0/2.0	0.25/0.25	1.0/1.0	2.0/4.0	8.0/8.0
Vibrio cholerae	0.5/1.0	0.01/0.02	0.005/0.01	0.01/0.01		0.03/0.03
V. parahaemolyticus	1.0/1.0	0.03/0.06	0.06/0.06	0.06/0.12		0.12/0.25
Haemophilus influenzae	0.5/1.0	0.06/0.06	0.01/0.01	0.03/0.03	0.10/0.10	0.12/0.12
H. parainfluenzae		0.03/0.13	0.02/0.03	0.06/0.25		0.25/0.25
H. ducrei	8.0/16	0.06/0.12	0.02/0.02	0.03/0.03		0.12/0.12
Gardnerella vaginalis	256/256	16/16	1.0/1.0	2.0/2.0		16/32

Table 1 Continued

Bacterial species	MIC$_{50}$/MIC$_{90}$[a] (μg/ml)					
	Nalidixic acid	Norfloxacin	Cipro-floxacin	Ofloxacin	Lomefloxacin	Enoxacin
Moraxella catarrhalis	1.0/2.0	0.5/0.4	0.02/0.03	0.05/0.1	0.10/0.10	0.06/0.06
Moraxella spp.		0.13/1.0	<0.3/0.5	0.5/1.0		
Legionella pneumophila	1.0/1.0	2.0/2.0	0.5/0.5	0.25/0.5	0.03/≤0.25	2.0/2.0
Legionella spp.		0.08/0.2	0.01/0.02	0.01/0.02	1.0/4.0	0.1/0.2
Pasteurella multocida		0.60/0.13	0.01/0.02	<0.06/0.06		0.12/0.5
Eikenella corrodens	1.0/2.0	0.03/0.06	0.01/0.02	0.02/0.03		0.06/0.13
Bordetella pertussis		0.25/0.25	<0.1/<0.1	0.12/0.12		0.5/0.5
Anaerobic						
Peptococci	128/256	8.0/64	0.25/2.0	0.5/4.0		0.25/2.0
Peptostreptococci	512/512	4.0/16	0.5/8.0	2.0/8.0	1.0/4.0	0.5/8.0
Clostridium perfringens	8.0/64	1.0/8.0	0.25/1.0	1.0/2.0	1.0/3.1	4.0/16
Clostridium spp.	64/256	1.0/2.0	1.0/4.0	1.0/16	2.0/16.0	4.0/32
C. difficile	>128/>128	64/128	8.0/16	8.0/16	25.0/50.0	64/128
Bacteroides fragilis	512/512	32/>128	4.0/8.0	4.0/8.0	12.5/32.0	16/32
Bacteroides spp., non–B. *fragilis*	128/256	8.0/128	1.0/4.0	1.0/2.0		4.0/16
Fusobacterium spp.	128/256	8.0/16	2.0/2.0	2.0/4.0		16/32
Eubacterium spp.	>128/>128	4.0/32	8.0/16	2.0/4.0		16/32

Capnocytophaga spp.	8.0/16	1.0/2.0	0.12/0.25	0.12/0.5		
Mobiluncus spp.	>64/>64	32/32	0.5/1.0			8.0/8.0
Other						
Mycobacterium tuberculosis		4.0/8.0	0.5/1.0	0.6/1.3		5.0/>5
M. avium complex		16/>16	2.0/16	2.5/10		
M. chelonei		16/>16	1.0/8.0	10/>20		
M. fortuitum		0.5/2.0	0.3/0.3	1.3/1.3		
M. kansasii		4.0/8.0	1.0/1.0	0.5/1.0		
M. xenopi		2.0/4.0	0.5/1.0	1.0/2.0		
Nocardia asteroides	>128/>128	32/64	4.0/8.0	4.0/16		8.0/32
Mycoplasma pneumoniae		6.3/12	2.0/2.0	1.0/2.0	2.0/8.0	1.0/8.0
M. hominis	>256/>256	4.0/16	1.0/1.0	0.4/0.8	4.0/8.0	4.0/8.0
Chlamydia trachomatis		25/25	1.6/1.6	0.8/0.8	2.0/4.0	6.3/6.3
Ureaplasma urealyticum		16/32	2.0/4.0	0.8/1.6	4.0/8.0	32/64
Candida albicans			>100/>100	>100/>100		

[a]MIC_{50}/MIC_{90} = concentrations of drug which inhibited 50 and 90%, respectively, of ≥10 isolates. Representative MIC_{50} and MIC_{90} values were chosen for species for which multiple values were available.

Source: Refs. 13,17–25.

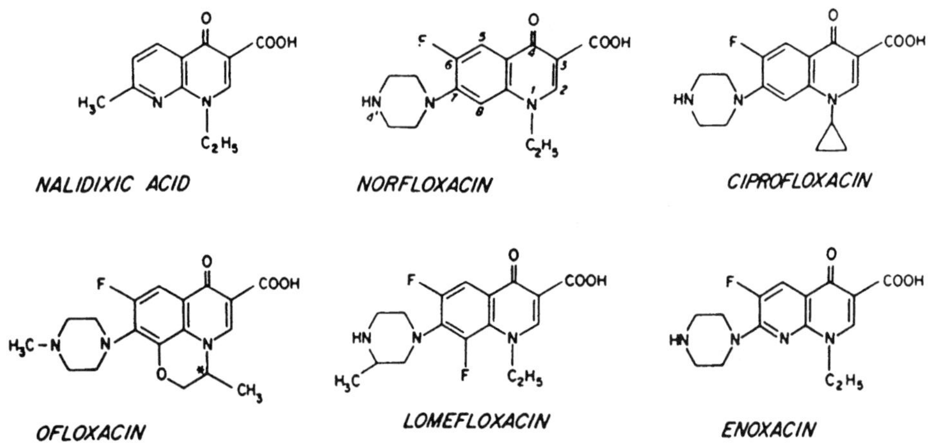

Figure 2

Similarly, ethyl groups are frequently found at position 1 and piperazinyl groups at position 7, although there is more scope for variation. For example, ciprofloxacin differs from norfloxacin by the presence of a cyclopropyl group instead of an ethyl group at position 1. This is responsible for the enhanced potency of ciprofloxacin. As seen for pipemidic acid, the piperazinyl group makes a substantial contribution to antimicrobial activity. Norfloxacin, ciprofloxacin, and enoxacin have a piperazin-1-yl substituent, and pefloxacin, ofloxacin, difloxacin, fleroxacin, and amifloxacin have a 4-methyl-piperazin-1-yl substituent. Attachment of a methyl group in the alpha position to the nitrogen of the piperazine substituent at position 7 (see 1 in Fig. 2) greatly improves the lipid solubility of lomefloxacin compared to norfloxacin, ofloxacin, and ciprofloxacin. The large size of the methyl group prevents binding to the nitrogen and thereby reduces the gamma-aminobutyric acid (GABA) receptor activity and prevents the formation of α-oxypiperazine metabolites, which are believed to be responsible for the interaction between the quinolones and hepatically metabolized drugs (vide infra).

In addition to chemical modifications, it has also been found that the activity of certain quinolones that are racemic mixtures (e.g., ofloxacin) is a consequence of the individual activity of their stereoisomers. For example, S-ofloxacin has been reported to be twice as active against a range of gram-positive and gram-negative bacteria as the S,R mixture of ofloxacin currently marketed (10). Although further details of quinolone structure-activity relationships are beyond the scope of this chapter, an excellent review is available in the recent literature (11).

In summary, differences among the quinolones currently marketed or approved are the result of differences among the chemical groups attached at position 1 of the basic quinolone nucleus. These chemical groups are in large measure responsible for the spectrum of activity and the pharmacokinetic profiles of specific quinolone agents.

As the quinolone class continues to be developed, key goals include improved reliability of coverage for gram-positive organisms and anaerobes, reduced propensity for the development of resistance, improved serum and tissue concentration profiles, and an improved side effect profile including a lower propensity for central nervous system (CNS) side effects.

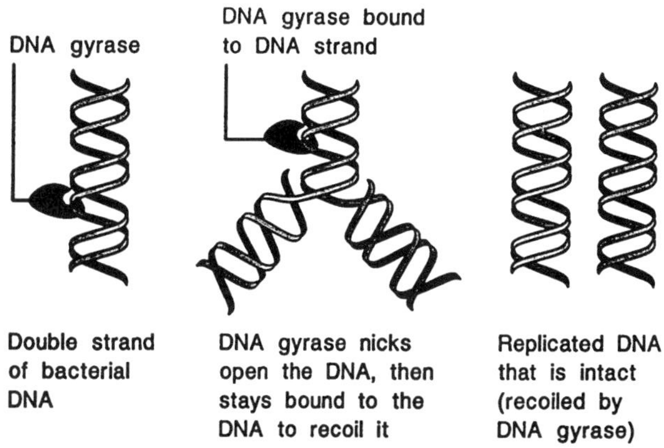

Figure 3

II. MECHANISM OF ACTION

The primary site of action of fluoroquinolones is bacterial DNA gyrase, the bacterial enzyme involved in the coiling and uncoiling of bacterial DNA. By inhibiting bacterial DNA gyrase, fluoroquinolones interfere with bacterial DNA replication, the segregation of bacterial chromosomes, and transcription (12,13).

As shown in Figure 3, DNA gyrase produces nicks in double-stranded DNA. These nicks provide sites for genetic replication or gene expression to start. After the chromosome has been duplicated or the gene expressed, DNA gyrase repairs the nicks, realigning the two strands of DNA into the proper orientation.

By interfering with this process, quinolones inhibit the repair process needed for the DNA to return to its normal coiled structure. The bacterial DNA is left with enraptured nicks, which inhibit proper gene expression. Importantly, the quinolones do not interfere with gene expression or chromosomal replication in humans because bacterial DNA gyrase is approximately 100 times more sensitive to quinolones than the comparable enzyme in human cells.

Quinolones have a primary bactericidal effect as demonstrated by their activity against both replicating and dormant microorganisms (14). Even though this antibacterial activity is correlated with their potency as DNA synthesis inhibitors, mechanisms involving RNA and protein synthesis may also be involved. In addition, overlap in the pathways of bactericidal activity of quinolones and β-lactams has been demonstrated in mutant strain studies (15).

III. ANTIMICROBIAL SPECTRUM

A. In Vitro Activity

Minimal bactericidal concentrations (MBCs) for currently available fluoroquinolones range from one to not more than four times higher than their minimal inhibitory concentrations (MICs). As a result, these agents are bactericidal at concentrations that are readily achievable in serum and most tissue sites (16). This bactericidal activity makes the quinolones potentially useful for immunocompromised patients as well as elderly patients whose immune systems are unable to combat infections effectively and for patients with especially serious infections such as gram-negative sepsis, gram-negative nosocomial pneumonia, and infective endocarditis.

In vitro antimicrobial activity of the fluoroquinolones, as exemplified by MIC values, is detailed in Table 1 (13,17–25). The fluoroquinolones exhibit substantial activity in vitro against the Enterobacteriaceae including *Escherichia coli*, *Klebsiella pneumoniae*, *Enterobacter* spp., *Citrobacter* spp., *Proteus* spp., *Salmonella* spp., *Shigella* spp., as well as other gram-negative aerobic bacteria including *Neisseria gonorrhoeae*, *N. meningitidis*, and the respiratory pathogens *Haemophilus* spp., *Legionella* spp., and *Moraxella catarrhalis*. In particular, the activity of these agents against *P. aeruginosa* makes them the first oral agents potentially effective in the treatment of systemic infections caused by this microorganism.

In general, activity against gram-positive aerobes is moderate for *Staphylococcus* spp. but generally less so against *Streptococcus* spp. Activity against both gram-negative anaerobes (e.g., *Bacteroides* spp.) and gram-positive anaerobes (e.g., *Peptococcus* spp.) is limited or poor. As a result, the broad-spectrum activity of the fluoroquinolones has important exceptions including *Streptococcus* spp., *Enterococcus* spp., *Pseudomonas* spp. (other than *P. aeruginosa*), most of the anaerobes, *Nocardia* spp., *Mycoplasma* spp., and slow-growing mycobacteria (13).

More recent studies with newer quinolones have documented improved antimicrobial activity or suggested novel applications compared to marketed or approved agents. WIN 57273, BMY 40062, PD 117558, PD 127391, sparfloxacin, temafloxacin, and tosufloxacin show enhanced activity against various staphylococci, streptococci, enterococci, *Corynebacterium* spp., *Listeria monocytogenes*, and *Bacillus* spp. These agents also possess increased activity against a variety of anaerobes, notably *Clostridium perfringens*, *C. difficile*, and the *Bacteroides fragilis* group. A number of the newer agents, notably those containing a cyclopropyl group, are more active than reference quinolones against *Mycobacterium leprae*. Improved antibacterial activity of the newer agents against *Mycoplasma hominis*, *Ureaplasma urealyticum*, *Acinetobacter* species, and *Xanthomonas maltophilia* has also been noted. Recent work with pefloxacin, ciprofloxacin, and ofloxacin has revealed useful in vitro activity against protozoa, including *Plasmodium* spp., *Trypanosoma cruzi*, and *Leishmania donovani*, but not against *Toxoplasma gondii* (26).

The fluoroquinolones also exhibit a significant postantibiotic effect. The ability of these agents to cause the rate of bacterial growth to remain depressed after exposure and subsequent removal of the drug in a manner similar to the aminoglycosides and imipenem/cilastatin has received considerable recent attention (27). This is of particular interest since it may allow for less frequent dosing with these agents (28).

B. Resistance

The unique mechanism of action of the new fluoroquinolones contributes to maintenance of antimicrobial activity. As mentioned above, these agents interfere with bacterial DNA replication, segregation of bacterial chromosomes, and transcription. They also bind DNA gyrase–DNA complexes. As a result, single-step mutation to resistance for these new fluoroquinolones is considerably less frequent than for the earlier quinolones and occurs at a very low level for many species of bacteria (29).

Microorganisms may produce enzymes that destroy or modify certain antimicrobials and hence confer resistance to these agents. Examples include β-lactamases, which cleave the β-lactam ring of penicillins and cephalosporins, and the adenylases, acetyltransferases,

Table 2 Mean Pharmacokinetic Parameters of Oral Quinolones in Healthy Young Volunteers

Quinolone[a]	C_{max} (mg/L)	T_{max} (h)	t1/2 (h)	AUC (mg/L · h)	V_D (L)	% renally unchanged (h)
Norfloxacin	1.5	1.5	3.3	5.4	—	27 (24)
Ciprofloxacin	1.5	1.1	3.3	5.8	348	29 (24)
Ofloxacin	4.0	1.4	5.0	29.0	102	73 (24)
Enoxacin	2.3	1.6	4.9	16.0	175	44 (72)
Lomefloxacin	3.8	2.0	6.4	37.0	103	57 (24)

[a]single oral 400 mg doses.
C_{max} = peak serum or plasma concentration; T_{max} = time to C_{max}; t 1/2 = terminal disposition half-life; AUC = area under the concentration-versus-time curve; V_D = apparent volume of distribution.
Source: Refs. 31, 33–35.

and phosphorylases, which add adenyl, acetyl, and phosphate groups to the aminoglycosides. Microorganisms may also inherit antimicrobial resistance genes through acquisition of plasmids from other bacteria. Plasmids are extrachromosomal fragments of DNA that carry resistance genes, usually to a multitude of antimicrobial agents. Fortunately, neither of these mechanisms of antimicrobial resistance have been noted with the fluoroquinolones to date.

The evolution of penicillin resistance and macrolide resistance in *S. pneumoniae* tends to correlate with the level of consumption of these agents. The increased activity of some as yet experimental fluoroquinolones against gram-positive organisms is encouraging as potential alternative treatments for resistant *S. pneumoniae* strains (30).

Widespread quinolone usage may carry a risk of pressure for selection of resistant strains, especially where the quinolone agents have modest or low activity against specific organisms. Since the introduction of norfloxacin and ofloxacin, for example, resistance among strains of *P. aeruginosa* has increased in Germany, and since the introduction of ciprofloxacin, some acute and long-term care institutions have reported an increased prevalence of quinolone-resistant strains of methicillin-resistant and methicillin-susceptible *S. aureus* (31). In addition, quinolone-resistant enterococci have been noted with increasing frequency in long-term care facility residents (32). To help prevent the spread of resistant pathogens, careful selection of antimicrobials is essential, especially in community acquired respiratory tract infections (30).

IV. CLINICAL PHARMACOLOGY

A. Pharmacokinetic Overview

The pharmacokinetic parameters of marketed or approved quinolones after oral administration to healthy young subjects are illustrated in Table 2 (31,33–35). Peak serum or plasma concentrations (C_{max}) vary from 1.5 mg/L for norfloxacin and ciprofloxacin to two- to threefold higher values for most other agents, as assessed from single 400-mg dose data, with time to C_{max} of 1–2 h. Terminal disposition half-lives (t1/2) vary as well, from 3.5 h for norfloxacin and ciprofloxacin to 5–8 h for ofloxacin, enoxacin, and lomefloxacin. The longer t1/2 of lomefloxacin has allowed approval of a once-daily dosing regimen for this agent. Area under the concentration-versus-time curve (AUC), a measure of exposure of the patient to drug, also varies substantially between agents, ranging from 5.5 mg/L · h for norfloxacin and ciprofloxacin to 30 mg/L · h for ofloxacin and lomefloxacin, as assessed from single 400-mg dose data. Oral bioavailability is generally good to excellent, but may not always be complete: norfloxacin (30–50%), ciprofloxacin (60–85%), ofloxacin (95%), enoxacin (89%), and lomefloxacin (>80%) (33,36–40). Food does not significantly alter quinolone oral bioavailability (13).

Unlike the β-lactams and aminoglycosides, the fluoroquinolones exhibit excellent tissue distribution characteristics. While β-lactams seldom achieve tissue to serum concentration ratios in excess of 0.4:1 (41,42) and aminoglycosides seldom achieve such ratios in excess of 0.5:1 (except in the kidney where high tissue binding predisposes to nephrotoxicity) (43,44), the quinolones usually achieve minimal tissue-to-serum concentration ratios of 2:1 (13,33,34).

Tissue distribution is facilitated by the minimal binding of the quinolones to serum proteins, being 14–25% for norfloxacin, ciprofloxacin, ofloxacin, and lomefloxacin and 18–54% for enoxacin. Large volumes of distribution of these agents, in the order of 1–3 L/kg body weight, reflect widespread tissue distribution as well. Quinolone bioavailability to interstitial fluid (as reflected by blister fluid studies) ranges from 90 to 125%. Concentration ratios of quinolones in selected body tissues and fluids to serum or plasma may be summarized as follows (13):

urine	25-to several hundredfold
renal tissue	2- to 10-fold
prostatic tissue	0.7- to 2.3-fold
prostatic fluid	0.1- to 0.3-fold
bile	2- to 10-fold
bronchial secretions	0.2- to 1-fold
lung tissue	1.6- to 4-fold
bone	0.3- to 0.8-fold
cerebrospinal fluid	0.4- to 0.9-fold

Unlike most β-lactams and aminoglycosides that undergo elimination primarily via the renal route in unchanged form, quinolones undergo a complex process of elimination from the body, including hepatic metabolism, renal and biliary elimination, and transintestinal secretion. Quinolones represent a range of complexity in elimination processes including those having balanced hepatic metabolism and renal elimination (norfloxacin, ciprofloxacin, enoxacin), those having primarily hepatic metabolism (pefloxacin), and those having primarily renal elimination (ofloxacin, lomefloxacin). As will be discussed in Sec. VI, various degrees of dosage regimen adjustment for renal impairment are needed with marketed and approved quinolones. Dosage adjustment to compensate for dialysis loss is unnecessary as these agents are poorly dialyzed by either hemo- or peritoneal dialysis (≤14% loss in dialysate).

B. Pharmacokinetics in Elderly Persons

In contrast to most antimicrobial classes, the pharmacokinetics of the quinolones have been assessed extensively in both healthy elderly volunteer and elderly patient populations. An exhaustive compilation of these data (with comparative data to younger populations, where available) is presented in Table 3 (45–80). Table 4 illustrates results of selected studies examining the body tissue and fluid penetration characteristics of quinolones in predominantly or exclusively elderly patient populations (54,75,80–117).

Several age-related factors may affect the rate and/or extent of drug absorption: gastric acidity, splanchnic blood flow, gastric motility, small bowel motility, and number of viable mucosal cells are reduced in elderly persons. However, studies evaluating the bioavailability of quinolones in elderly subjects have revealed that absolute oral bioavailability is maintained, if not enhanced, in this older age group, at least for ciprofloxacin (70,79). Despite this alteration in oral bioavailability, it was found that the effect of oral ciprofloxacin on intestinal microflora was not significantly different between healthy young and elderly volunteers receiving a 5-day therapy course of 500 mg twice daily (118). In addition, delivery of quinolones by nasogastric, nasoduodenal, or jejunostomy feeding tubes after crushing of the oral tablet formulations does not adversely affect oral bioavailability (119–123).

All of the quinolones exhibit low to modest binding to serum proteins (20–40%). Thus, the age-dependent decline in serum albumin, noted especially in the malnourished, chronically ill nursing home patient population, is unlikely to affect quinolone distribution. Another age-related factor of importance for drug distribution is the alteration in fat and lean body mass and water compartmentalization. Studies that have compared volume of distribution data between young and elderly subjects have revealed either no significant difference (70) or a significant reduction in the older age group (47,54,56,71,75). The one study revealing no difference between groups in volume of distribution utilized data derived after intravenous dosing (70), while those studies revealing a reduction in elderly persons utilized data derived after oral dosing (47,54,56,71,75). Although a true alteration in distribution of the quinolones may occur with aging, at least a portion of the differences noted in the oral dosing studies may be accounted for by the lack of correction of area under the curve for individual oral bioavailability. This latter point especially applies to those studies documenting a significant increase in peak plasma or serum concentration and no significant difference in terminal disposition half-life with aging (54,75). In addition, quinolones appear to be rapidly and efficiently distributed to peripheral compartments in elderly persons, as illustrated in Table 4. However, whether there is an alteration in quinolone tissue distribution as a function of age is unknown at present, as no comparative studies using body tissue or fluid sampling in patients of various ages have been performed.

Age-related reductions in hepatic and renal blood flow and glomerular filtration rate may be expected to alter the elimination of quinolones in elderly subjects. Reductions in total body and renal clearances and prolongations of terminal disposition half-life as a function of aging have been noted in comparative studies for amifloxacin (45), temafloxacin (47), lomefloxacin (54,56), ofloxacin (64), and ciprofloxacin (68,70–73,75). However, when clearance data are normalized for body weight (or body surface area) and level of renal function, these age-related changes virtually disappear. It thus appears that there are no age-specific alterations in quinolone metabolism and excretion, and dosing regimens should be chosen predominantly based upon the level of renal function (see Sec. VI).

C. Drug Interactions

Delineating the frequencies and types of pharmacokinetic and pharmacodynamic interactions of the quinolones with other drugs is important for several reasons. Since quinolones are often administered orally, absorptive interactions may compromise antimicrobial therapy. Because of their breadth of activity, agents of this class find substantial use in critically ill patients as well as geriatric patients, many of whom receive several medications (124). In addition, since older persons have an increased sensitivity to drug-induced toxicity and experience more adverse drug reactions, they may also exhibit an increased incidence

Table 3 Pharmacokinetics of Quinolones in Elderly Persons

Subjects	No./sex/age (y)	Drug	Dose (mg/route)	No. of doses	T_{max} (h)	C_{max} (mg/L)
Healthy volunteers	10/5M,5F/65–79	Amifloxacin	200/PO	1	1.65/1.60[a]	1.13/1.95[a]
Patients (LRTI)	12/10M,2F/63–80	Rufloxacin	400/PO	1 then		
			200/PO	6–9 q 24 h	4.3	6.46
Healthy volunteers	12/6M,6F/21–37	Temafloxacin	600/PO	1	1.17	3.54[c]
	12/6M,6F/73–80		600/PO	1	1.32	4.99[c]
Patients (UTI)	18/NS/70–100	Enoxacin	200/PO	1	1.40	1.90
Patients (UTI)	10/10M/57–88	Enoxacin	400/IV	≥5q12h then	NA	NA
			400/PO	≥5q12h	NA	NA
Healthy volunteers	15/NS/65–76	Fleroxacin	400/PO	7q24h	1.2	8.5
Patients (UTI)	12/4M,8F/63–88	Fleroxacin	800/PO	1	2.7	15.6
Patients (UTI)	8/8F/73–94	Norfloxacin	400/PO	1 then	2.0	1.36
			400/PO	15q12h	1.5	1.66
Patients (UTI)	8/3M,5F/74–88	Norfloxacin	400/PO	1 then	3.2	1.5
			400/PO	10q12h	3.0	2.2
Healthy volunteers	15/15M/20–28	Lomefloxacin	400/PO	1	1.25	2.00[c]
	17/17M/66–79		400/PO	1	1.63	2.61[c]
Healthy volunteers	12/3M,9F/65–80	Lomefloxacin	200/PO	1	0.96	2.40
			400/PO	1	1.31	4.48
Healthy volunteers	8/NA/18–30	Lomefloxacin	400/PO	1	1.25	4.15
	13/NA/60–75		400/PO	1	1.28	4.60
Patients (UTI)	11/3M,8F/75–90	Lomefloxacin	400/PO	1 then	2.60	4.81[c]
			400/PO	7q24h	1.98	6.33[c]
Healthy volunteers	12/6M,6F/66–86	Ofloxacin	200/PO	1	NA	3.6
Healthy volunteers	15/15M/66–81	Ofloxacin	400/PO	1	2.0	3.50
			400/PO	21q12h	1.9	6.04
Healthy volunteers	NA/allF/65–74	Ofloxacin	200/PO	1 then	1.3	3.34
			200/PO	"q12h to steady state"	1.9	4.74
			400/PO	1 then	1.4	7.77
			400/PO	"q12h to steady state"	1.3	9.71
Patients (ICU)	12/NA/69[g],59[h]	Ofloxacin	3 mg/kg/IV	1 then	NA	NA
			3 mg/kg/IV	13q12h	NA	NA
Patients (LRTI)	5/3M,2F/23–61	Ofloxacin	200/PO	9–13q12h	2.5[c]	2.86[c]
	11/8M,3F/67–86		200/PO	9–13q12h	3.0[c]	4.16[c]
Patients (NA)	12/NA/20	Ofloxacin	200/PO	1	0.8	2.64
	12/NA/20		400/PO	1	0.7	5.64
	12/NA/55		400/PO	1	1.25	5.08
	16/NA/>70		200/PO	1	2.0	3.60
Patients (UTI)	8/NA/20–32	Ofloxacin	200/PO	13q12h	NA	1.5[c]
	20/NA/67–82		200/PO	13q12h	NA	5.3[c]
Healthy volunteers	10/5M,5F/69–80	Pefloxacin	400/PO	1	NA	10.74[c]
			400/PO	15q12h	NA	23.63[c]
Patients (various diagnoses)	7/1M,6F/84[j]	Pefloxacin	400/IV	1	NA	11.5
	7/1M,6F/64[k]		400/PO	1	1.8	13.0
Patients (ICU)	10/5M,5F/55–79	Pefloxacin	6mg/kg/IV	1 then	NA	NA
			6mg/kg/IV	9q12h then	NA	13.1
			400/PO	19q12h	1.4	13.4

AUC (mg/L · h)	V_{ss}/f (L/kg)	Vd/f (L/kg)	Vb/f (L/kg)	t1/2 (h)	CL/f (L/h)	CL_r (L/h)	f (%)	Ref.
9.5/15.6[a]	NA	NA	2.05/1.28[a]	5.4/4.5[a]	0.259/0.199[a,b]	0.113/0.086[a,b]	NA	45
								46
154.9	NA	1.27	NA	28.7	2.1	NA	NA	
35.2[c]	NA	NA	3.28	8.7[c]	18.0[c]	7.08[c]	NA	47
60.3[c]	NA	NA	2.28[c]	10.3[c]	10.8[c]	4.26[c]	NA	
11.41[d]	NA	NA	NA	6.11	NA	NA	NA	48
47.59	1.52	NA	1.61	8.2	9.81	5.36	NA	49
41.02	NA	NA	NA	9.1	NA	NA	83.24	
NA	0.50	NA	NA	15.5	4.06	NA	NA	50
389	NA	0.9	NA	16	2.58	1.02	NA	51
9.37[d]	NA	NA	NA	5.18	NA	NA	NA	52
14.56	NA	NA	NA	5.43	NA	NA	NA	
9.47[d]	NA	NA	NA	5.0	NA	NA	NA	53
11.11	NA	NA	NA	5.3	NA	NA	NA	
17.27[c]	NA	3.70[c]	NA	6.65	27.12[c]	14.71	NA	54
23.55[c]	NA	2.31[c]	NA	7.07	17.76[a]	9.59	NA	
23.95	NA	NA	NA	8.54	NA	6.05	NA	55
49.23	NA	NA	NA	8.75	NA	5.06	NA	
NA	1.73[c]	NA	NA	7.3	12.12[c,e]	NA	NA	56
NA	1.50[c]	NA	NA	8.4	9.26[c,e]	NA	NA	
65.58[c,f]	NA	NA	NA	10.0	NA	NA	NA	57
73.30[c]	NA	NA	NA	10.3	NA	NA	NA	
22.9	1.42	NA	NA	8.5	10.14	8.28	NA	58
36.51	NA	NA	NA	6.42	NA	NA	NA	59
71.89	NA	NA	NA	7.36	NA	NA	NA	
31.28	NA	NA	NA	7.06	NA	NA	NA	60
54.43	NA	NA	NA	6.83	NA	NA	NA	
69.96	NA	NA	NA	6.54	NA	NA	NA	
123.7	NA	NA	NA	7.50	NA	NA	NA	
48[g],42[h]	NA	0.5[c,g],0.6[c,h]	NA	5.1[c,g],6.0[c,h]	4.29[c,g],4.42[c,h]	3.96[c,g]	NA	61
NA	NA	0.23[c,g],0.45[c,h]	NA	10.7[c,g],9.6[c,h]	1.56[c,g],2.81[c,h]	0.96[c,g]	NA	
13.25[c]	NA	NA	NA	7.03	NA	NA	NA	62
22.28[c]	NA	NA	NA	9.52	NA	NA	NA	
NA	NA	129.4[i]	NA	6.96	13.30	NA	NA	63
NA	NA	123.6[i]	NA	7.4	11.70	NA	NA	
NA	NA	139[i]	NA	9.5	10.26	NA	NA	
NA	NA	85.3[i]	NA	13.3	5.00	NA	NA	
12.1[c]	NA	NA	NA	5.7[c]	NA	NA	NA	64
14.2[c]	NA	NA	NA	17.8[c]	NA	NA	NA	
151.39[c]	NA	NA	NA	12.58[c]	2.88	NA	NA	65
197.87[c]	NA	NA	NA	17.32[c]	NA	NA	NA	
149.6[l]	NA	NA	NA	13.3	6.0[l]	NA	NA	66
208.2[l]	NA	NA	NA	12.4	4.3[l]	NA	NA	
87.5[c]	NA	1.3	NA	11.3[c]	5.45[c]	NA	NA	67
132.9[c]	NA	1.8	NA	19.4[c]	3.11[c]	NA	NA	
125.5[c]	NA	1.6	NA	21.1[c]	3.38[c]	NA	NA	

Table 3 Continued

Subjects	No./sex/age (y)	Drug	Dose (mg/route)	No. of doses	T_{max} (h)	C_{max} (mg/L)
Healthy volunteers	6/NA/<35	Ciprofloxacin	250/PO	1	2.08	1.29
	6/NA/>65		250/PO	1	1.75	2.44
	6/NA/<35		500/PO	1	1.08	2.57
	6/NA/>65		500/PO	1	1.28	1.94
Healthy volunteers	6/NA/69[m]	Ciprofloxacin	750/PO	3q12h	1.42	2.82
		Ciprofloxacin	750/PO	3q12h	1.17	2.34
		+ rifampin	600/PO	2q24h		
Healthy volunteers	8/8M/22–34	Ciprofloxacin	250/IV	1	NA	NA
			250/PO	1	1.2	1.24
			500/PO	1	1.0	2.35
			500/PO	9q12h	1.0	3.1
	8/8M/63–76		250/IV	1	NA	NA
			250/PO	1	1.1	1.47
			500/PO	1	1.4	2.83
			500/PO	9q12h	1.5	3.3
Healthy volunteers	12/12M/19–25	Ciprofloxacin	500/PO	1	1.33	2.26[c]
	12/12M/71–86		500/PO	1	1.08	3.24[c]
Healthy volunteers	10/10M/20–30	Ciprofloxacin	250/PO	1	1.3	1.2[c]
	10/6M,4F/60–73		250/PO	1	1.3	1.7[c]
Patients (no diagnoses stated)	12/NA/"young"	Ciprofloxacin	200/IV	1	NA	2.1[c]
	8/NA/"old"		200/IV	1	NA	3.7[c]
Patients (TURP)	11/11M/57–84	Ciprofloxacin	200/IV	1	NA	4.2
Healthy volunteers	12/12M/19–33	Ciprofloxacin	200/IV	1	NA	3.43[c]
Patients (TURP)	14/14M/57–84		200/IV	1	NA	4.15[c]
Healthy volunteers	6/NA/19[m]	Ciprofloxacin	100/PO	1	1.2	0.34[c]
Patients (UTI)	9/NA/74[m]		100/PO	1	1.3	0.86[c]
Patients (MRSA colonization)	6/NA/68–76	Ciprofloxacin	750/PO	1 then	2.2	5.9
			750/PO	13q12h then	1.5	6.2
			750/PO	to 28q12h total	2.0	6.2
	6/NA/67–95	Ciprofloxacin	750/PO	1 then	1.9	4.2
		+ rifampin	750/PO	13q12h then	2.0	7.5
			750/PO	to 28q12h total	2.3	6.9
Patients (LRTI)	20/12M,8F/64–92	Ciprofloxacin	750/PO	1 then	1.5	6.65
			750/PO	≥27q12h	1.3	8.83
Patients (LRTI)	9/7M,2F/67–90	Ciprofloxacin	200/IV	≥5q12h then	NA	3.6
			750/PO	≥5q12h	1.9	7.6
Patients (LRTI)	12/8M,4F/51–80	Ciprofloxacin	200/IV	9q12h	NA	NA

C_{max} = peak serum/plasma concentration; T_{max} = time to C_{max}; AUC = area under the serum/plasma concentration-versus-time curve (for single dose data represents AUC from time zero to infinity and for steady-state data represents AUC over the dosing interval, unless otherwise stated); V_{ss}/f = volume of distribution at steady-state normalized to bioavailability; Vd/f = volume of distribution normalized to bioavailability; Vb/f = volume of distribution at the terminal phase of the concentration-versus-time curve normalized to bioavailability; t1/2 = terminal disposition half-life; CL/f = total body clearance normalized to bioavailability; CL_R = renal clearance; f = absolute oral bioavailability; NA = not available or applicable; LRTI = lower respiratory tract infection; UTI = urinary tract infection; ICU = intensive care unit; TURP = transurethral resection of the prostate; MRSA = methicillin-resistant *Staphylococcus aureus*.

[a]Male/Female.

[b]l/h per kg.

AUC (mg/L · h)	V_{ss}/f (L/kg)	Vd/f (L/kg)	Vb/f (L/kg)	t1/2 (h)	CL/f (L/h)	CL_g (L/h)	f (%)	Ref.
8.22[f]	NA	NA	NA	NA	NA	22.4[c]	NA	68
13.30[f]	NA	NA	NA	NA	NA	9.9[c]	NA	
14.78[f]	NA	NA	NA	NA	NA	42.1[c]	NA	
16.09[f]	NA	NA	NA	NA	NA	13.2[c]	NA	
NA	NA	NA	NA	4.52	NA	NA	NA	69
NA	NA	NA	NA	4.72	NA	NA	NA	
8.1	132[n]	NA	NA	3.45	29.22	16.14[c,e]	NA	70
4.7[c]	NA	NA	NA	3.55	NA	17.28[c]	58[c]	
10.3[c]	NA	NA	NA	3.55	NA	15.54[c]	63[c]	
14.3[c]	NA	NA	NA	4.03	NA	15.12[c]	NA	
8.9	130[n]	NA	NA	3.79	26.04	12.96[c]	NA	
6.4[c]	NA	NA	NA	3.50	NA	13.02[c]	72[c]	
13.8[c]	NA	NA	NA	3.48	NA	12.66[c]	79[c]	
20.5	NA	NA	NA	4.28	NA	12.06	NA	
10.00[c]	3.76[c]	NA	NA	3.69[c]	54.48[c]	23.74[c]	NA	71
20.88[c]	2.47[c]	NA	NA	6.83[c]	23.64[c]	9.14[c]	NA	
5.55[cf]	NA	NA	NA	3.7	NA	19.09[c]	NA	72
7.43[c,f]	NA	NA	NA	4.3	NA	13.26[c]	NA	
NA	NA	NA	NA	5.8[c]	NA	NA	NA	73
NA	NA	NA	NA	6.3[c]	NA	NA	NA	
8.17	1.74	NA	NA	4.17	26.46	NA	NA	74
5.37[c]	1.94[c]	NA	2.52[c]	3.58	37.92[c]	19.68	NA	75
8.79[c]	1.69[c]	NA	2.09[c]	4.31	24.42[c]	NA	NA	
0.81[c,o]	NA	NA	NA	3.9	NA	NA	NA	76
1.95[c,o]	NA	NA	NA	4.0	NA	NA	NA	
35.1	NA	NA	NA	3.42	21.74	NA	NA	77
33.1	NA	NA	NA	3.82	25.46	NA	NA	
34.7	NA	NA	NA	4.26	23.60	NA	NA	
30.0	NA	NA	NA	3.98	34.72	NA	NA	
39.4	NA	NA	NA	3.32	20.96	NA	NA	
36.7	NA	NA	NA	3.76	23.58	NA	NA	
41.85	NA	NA	2.71[c]	4.92	22.18	6.66	NA	78
47.70	NA	NA	4.40[c]	4.87	19.05	8.90	NA	
14.6	1.5	NA	1.8	5.7	16.47	9.47	NA	79
39.9	NA	NA	NA	4.2	NA	NA	78	
9.99	NA	NA	2.59	4.95	23.3	NA	NA	80

[c] $p < 0.05$.
[d] $AUC_{0\text{-}12}$.
[e] l/h/1.73m².
[f] $AUC_{0\text{-}24}$.
[g] Mean for mechanically ventilated patients.
[h] Mean for non–mechanically ventilated patients.
[i] Liters.
[j] Mean for IV group
[k] Mean for PO group
[l] per 65 kg body weight
[m] Mean
[n] l/1.73m².

Table 4 Tissue Penetration of Quinolones in Elderly Persons

Drug	Body fluid/tissue	No. (sex)	Dose (mg) [frequency]	Route	Mean concentration (mg/l or g/kg)		C_t:C_s	Sampling time (h)		Ref.
					tissue	serum		tissue	serum	
Lomefloxacin	Blister fluid	17(17M)	400[1]	PO	2.50	2.61	0.96	3	3	54
					0.48	0.24	2.00	24	24	
					36.71[a]	23.55[a]	1.56			
Pefloxacin	Ascites	10(9M,1F)	400[1]	IV	1.53	2.21	0.69	24	24	81
					1.20			48	48	
Ciprofloxacin	Peritoneum	10(5M,5F)	750[1]	PO	0.29	1.3	0.22	4–8.5	4–8.5	82
Norfloxacin	Muscle	8(2M,6F)	400[1]	PO	0.87[b]	1.09	0.80	3–6	3–6	83
Ciprofloxacin		17(12M,5F)	200[1]	IV	3.82[c,d]	1.47	2.59			84
					2.91[c,e]	1.18	2.46			
					1.79[b,f]	0.82	2.17			
Ciprofloxacin		18(9M,9F)	400[1]	IV	31.6[c]			0–1		85
		18(14M,4F)	750[4q12h] then	PO						
			400[1]	IV	21.8[c]			0–1		
Ciprofloxacin	Mediastinal fat	17(12M,5F)	200[1]	IV	1.04[g]	1.51	0.69			84
Ciprofloxacin		18(9M,9F)	400[1]	IV	3.1			3–5		85
		18(14M,4F)	750[4q12h] then	PO						
			400[1]	IV	2.0			1–3		
Ciprofloxacin	Bone	20(8M,12F)	200[1]	IV	0.54	0.61	0.89	0.5–24	0.5–24	86
Pefloxacin		15(10M,5F)[i]	400[4q12h] then	IV						87
			400[q12h for 3–96 months]	PO	4.05			2[h]	2[h]	
Lomefloxacin		32(18M,14F)	400[1]	PO			0.7	1–12	1–12	88
Enoxacin		24	400[1]	PO	0.7	2.0	0.34	1.45–5.5	1.45–5.5	89
			400[2q12h]	PO	0.9	2.1	0.45	1.45–5.5	1.45–5.5	
			400[1]	IV	0.9	1.8	0.48	1.45–5.5	1.45–5.5	
			400[2q12h]	IV	1.1	3.1	0.35	1.45–5.5	1.45–5.5	
		7[i]	400[2–3q12h]	PO	1.3	2.8	0.39	1.45–5.5	1.45–5.5	

Ciprofloxacin	Aqueous humor	25	200[2q12h]	IV	0.21			1.0		90
Ciprofloxacin		30(22M,8F)	1000[1]	PO	0.73	2.20	0.33	1.5–8.0	1.5–8.0	91
Ciprofloxacin		40(22M,18F)	400[1]	IV	0.20	0.73	0.27	3	3	92
			750 [2q12h]	PO	0.33	0.82	0.40	12	12	
Pefloxacin		20(12M,8F)	400[1]	IV			0.75	24	24	93
Pefloxacin		38(21M,17F)	800[1] then	PO						94
			400[5q12h]	PO	4.21	5.24	0.89	24	24	
Ciprofloxacin	Vitreous	40(22M,18F)	400[1]	IV	0.14	0.54	0.26	6	6	92
Pefloxacin	Lens	38(21M,17F)	800[1] then	PO	4.59			12		94
			400[5q12h]	PO	1.68			48		
Ciprofloxacin	Sputum	8	200[1] then	IV	8.5[j]	11.7[j]	0.73			95
			200[5q12h]	IV	10.2[j]	12.8[j]	0.80			
Ciprofloxacin		8	3mg/kg[3q12h] then	IV	0.95[k]	2.95[k]	0.32(0.66)[l]			96
			3mg/kg[to total of 7q12h]	IV	0.76[k]	2.43[k]	0.33(0.55)[l]			
Enoxacin		20(13M,7F)	400[1]	PO	2.2	1.9	1.16	5	5	97
			600[1]	PO	4.0	3.4	1.18	5	5	
			400[4q12h]	PO	2.4	2.5	0.96	5	5	
Enoxacin		19(12M,7F)	400[1]	PO	3.0[k]	4.0[k]	0.75			98
			400[5q12h]	PO	2.7[k]	4.8[k]	0.56			
			600[1]	PO	5.6[k]	5.6[k]	1.00			
			600[5q12h]	PO	6.9[k]	7.4[k]	0.93			
Ofloxacin		52	400[1]	PO	2.0	2.1	0.83	1–2	1–2	99
					2.1	2.6	0.81	5–6	5–6	
					0.4	0.5	0.80	24	24	
Lomefloxacin		9	400[7–11q24h]	PO	4.1[k]	4.2[k]	0.98(1.26)[m]			100
Ciprofloxacin	Lung tissue	8	200[11–23q12h]	IV	21.7[n]	1.4[n]	16.9	2	2	80
Ciprofloxacin		29(21M,8F)	500[8q12h]	PO	4.40	3.01	1.47	2–7	2–7	101
		10(5M,5F)	200[1]	IV	3.94	1.62	2.31	0.33–2	0.33–2	
Ciprofloxacin		25(19M,6F)	200[1]	IV	4.53	0.99	4.58	0.83	0.83	102
					3.62	0.44	8.23	2.08	2.08	
					3.77	0.36	10.47	4.0	4.0	
Enoxacin		15(15M)	600[1]	PO	7.0	2.0	3.50	2.8	2.8	98

Table 4 Continued

Drug	Body fluid/tissue	No. (sex)	Dose (mg) [frequency]	Route	Mean concentration (mg/l or g/kg)		C_t:C_s	Sampling time (h)		Ref.
					tissue	serum		tissue	serum	
Ciprofloxacin	Pleural exudate	5(4M,1F)	200[1]	IV	1.4[k](17.0)[a]	2.0[k](8.1)[a]	0.70[k](2.10)[a]			103
Norfloxacin	Epididymis	10(10M)	400[5q12h]	PO	3.39	0.91	3.74	4.0	4.0	104
Pefloxacin		10(10M)	400[4q12h] then	PO						105
			400[1]	IV	14.02			2.7–11.3		
Rufloxacin	Prostatic tissue	16(16M)	400[1] then	PO						106
			200[1][o]	PO	6.68	3.53	1.89			
Ofloxacin		20(20M)	300[1] then	PO						107
			300[1][p]	PO	4.55	3.74	1.22			
			300[1] then	PO						
			300[1][q]	PO	3.12	3.43	0.91			
			300[1] then	PO						
			300[1][r]	PO	2.59	2.63	0.98			
			300[1] then	PO						
			300[1][s]	PO	2.09	1.97	1.06			
Ofloxacin		21(21M)	400[1]	PO	3.47	2.10	1.65	8.5–13.0	8.5–13.0	108
Ofloxacin		28(28M)	400[1]	PO			1.06	1.58–7.75	1.58–7.75	109
Lomefloxacin		20(20M)	400[3q24h]	PO	5.00	2.36	2.12	0.1–7.1	0.1–7.1	110
Lomefloxacin		12(12M)	400[1]	PO	6.46	4.63	1.53	1.6	1.6	111
Ciprofloxacin		17(17M)	200[1]	IV	1.87	0.81	2.45	1–2.5	1–2.5	75
					0.13	0.09	1.86	16–18	16–18	
Ciprofloxacin		15(15M)	750[1]	PO	2.07	4.86	0.43	1–4	1–4	112
Ciprofloxacin		25(25M)	500[3q12h]	PO	4.46	1.62	2.75	1.5–10.5	1.5–10.5	113
Enoxacin		20(20M)	200[2q12h]	PO	3.10	1.26	2.53			114
Enoxacin		14(14M)	400[1]	PO	2.20	1.57	1.40	0.92–8.0	0.92–8.0	115
Enoxacin		16(16M)	400[5q12h]	PO	5.15	2.07	2.49	2	2	116
					2.50	0.98	2.55	15	15	

Fleroxacin		10(10M)	400[1]	PO	4.35	3.95	1.10	1.5–4	1.5–4	117
Fleroxacin	Prostatic secretion	9(9M)	400[1]	PO	1.67	4.51	0.37	1–4	1–4	117
Ciprofloxacin		17(17M)	200[1]	IV	0.62	0.82	0.48	1–2.5	1–2.5	75
					0.06	0.09	0.86	16–18	16–18	
Rufloxacin		12(12M)	400[1] then	PO						106
			200[1][o]	PO	5.5	3.67	1.5			

C_t: C_s = ratio of tissue concentration to serum concentration

[a]AUC_{0-24}.

[b]Skeletal muscle.

[c]Cardiac muscle.

[d]Beginning of cardiopulmonary bypass.

[e]End of cardiopulmonary bypass.

[f]End of surgery.

[g]Before cardiopulmonary bypass.

[h]After last dose of at least 7 days' treatment.

[i]Osteomyelitis.

[j]Day 1 = $AUC_{0-\infty}$; day 3 = AUC_{0-12}.

[k]Peak concentration.

[l]Based on AUC_{0-12} ratio of sputum:serum.

[m]Based on AUC_{0-24} ratio of sputum:serum.

[n]2h post last drug administration.

[o]400 mg dose 16 h preop then 200 mg dose 5 h preop.

[p]Doses administered at 14 and 2 h preop.

[q]Doses administered at 16 and 4 h h preop.

[r]Doses administered at 19 and 7 h preop.

[s]Doses administered at 22 and 10 h preop.

and severity of drug–drug interactions. Finally, the quinolones are such a structurally diverse group that the extrapolation of drug-drug interactions from one to another of these agents may not be appropriate.

1. Absorption Interactions

The deleterious effect of multivalent cations on the oral bioavailability of quinolones was first reported in 1985 (125). Since this pivotal report, numerous investigations have duplicated and extended this observation (Table 5).

The concomitant oral administration of magnesium- or aluminum-containing antacids has been found to result in substantial 6- to 10-fold decreases in the absorption of oral quinolones. Even when dose administrations of the agents were separated by 2 or more hours, substantial reductions in quinolone absorption persisted (126–140). Studies of the oral co-administration of calcium-containing antacids with oral quinolones have produced conflicting results, with some reporting no significant effects (126–128) while others reported significant reductions in absorption (129,136,137,139). More recent studies documenting the significant reduction in norfloxacin and ciprofloxacin bioavailability with co-administration of milk and yogurt lend credence to the deleterious effect of calcium on quinolone bioavailability (141,142). Recent studies have documented substantial reductions in quinolone bioavailability when co-administered with sucralfate. Again, this interaction persisted even when dose administrations of the agents were spaced 2 or more hours apart (136,143–145). Further studies have documented substantial reductions in quinolone bioavailability when co-administered with iron preparations or multiple vitamins with minerals such as zinc, magnesium, copper, and manganese (133,138), although one study did not find a significant interaction with iron (126). It is hypothesized that the reduction in quinolone absorption is due to the formation of insoluble and hence unabsorbable drug-cation complexes or chelates in the gastrointestinal tract. This has been confirmed in ciprofloxacin-iron binding experiments (133). It appears that the complexation or chelation involves the 4-keto and 3-carboxyl groups of the quinolones. It is thus recommended not to use magnesium-, aluminum-, or calcium-containing antacids, sucralfate, or iron/vitamin-mineral preparations concomitantly with quinolones. Histamine H_2-receptor antagonists such as ranitidine and cimetidine have, in general, not been shown to alter quinolone absorption (132,146,147). Thus, these agents can be recommended as alternative noninteracting antiulcer therapy.

An important consideration in the therapy of infections in debilitated older nursing home residents is the effect of enteral feedings on quinolone bioavailability, especially when examining the cation content of these products. Studies in normal volunteers (120,121) and older nursing home residents (78,79) have revealed that the bioavailability of ciprofloxacin and temafloxacin is not significantly altered in the presence of such feedings administered by a nasogastric tube.

2. Distribution Interactions

The quinolones are plasma protein-bound to the extent of only 20–40%. Ciprofloxacin does not displace bilirubin from albumin, which suggests that interactions involving displacement of other drugs from their carrier proteins are unlikely to occur during co-administration of quinolones (148). The absence of such an interaction with the quinolones may be of particular importance to elderly, debilitated patients with hypoalbuminemia who receive multiple drugs.

Table 5 Effects of Multivalent Cations on Quinolone Absorption

Quinolone	Cation preparation/ Schedule	Mean % change in C_{max}	Mean % change in AUC	Ref.
Enox	Mg/Al antacid			131
	0.5 h prequinolone	−70*	−73*	
	2 h prequinolone	−38	−48*	
	8 h prequinolone	−9	−17	
Oflox	Mg/Al antacid			128
	2 h prequinolone	−30*	−21*	
	24 h prequinolone	−5	−5	
	2 h postquinolone	+3	+5	
	Ca carb antacid			
	2 h prequinolone	+3	−4	
	24 h prequinolone	+9	−4	
	2 h postquinolone	+3	−2	
Tema	Mg/Al antacid			140
	8 doses day prior to study and 5 doses on study day	−59*	−61*	
Cipro	Mg/Al antacid			125
	24 h prequinolone	−94*	—	
Cipro	Mg/Al antacid			127
	with meals (PO_4 binder)	−65	—	
	Ca carb antacid			
	with meals (PO_4 binder)	+13	—	
Norflox	Mg/Al antacid			137
	simultaneous with quinolone	−95*	—	
	2 h postquinolone	−24*	−20	
	Ca carb antacid			
	simultaneous with quinolone	−66*	−63*	
Oflox	Mg trisilicate			126
	simultaneous with quinolone	−2	+19	
	Al OH			
	simultaneous with quinolone	−29*	−19	
	Ca carb			
	simultaneous with quinolone	−18	+10	
	$FeSO_4$			
	simultaneous with quinolone	+9	+35	
Oflox	Mg/Al antacid			134
	simultaneous with quinolone	−24	—	
Cipro	$FeSO_4$			138
	325 mg tid × 7 days	−75*	−63*	
	Multivit with Zn			
	once daily × 7 days	−32*	−22*	
Cipro	$FeSO_4$			133
	300 mg simultaneous with quinolone	−33*	−42*	
	Fe gluc			
	600 mg simultaneous with quinolone	−57*	−64*	
	Multivit with Fe/Zn			
	once simultaneous with quinolone	−53*	−52*	

Table 5 Continued

Quinolone	Cation preparation/ Schedule	Mean % change in C_{max}	Mean % change in AUC	Ref.
Cipro	Sucralfate			144
	1 gm 6 and 2 h prequinolone	−30*	−30*	
Norflox	Sucralfate			145
	1 gm simultaneous with quinolone	−90*	−98*	
	1 gm 2 h prequinolone	−28	−43	
Cipro	Sucralfate			143
	1 g QID × 1 day	−90*	−88*	
	then simultaneous with quinolone			
Cipro	Ca carb			139
	simultaneous with quinolone	−38*	−41*	
Cipro	Mg/Al antacid			135
	5–10 min prequinolonc	−80*	−85*	
	2 h prequinolone	−74*	−77*	
	4 h prequinolone	−13	−30*	
	6 h prequinolone	0	+9	
	2 h postquinolone	+32*	+7	
Cipro	Ca carb antacid			129
	simultaneous with quinolone	−47*	−42*	
	Mg/Al antacid			
	simultaneous with quinolone	−81*	−84*	
Norflox	Mg/Al antacid			136
	simultaneous with quinolone	−95	−98	
	2 h post-quinolone	−24	−22	
	Ca carb antacid			
	simultaneous with quinolone	−66	−62	
	Sucralfate			
	simultaneous with quinolone	−90	−98	
	2 h pre-quinolone	−28	−42	

% change = change from baseline or placebo control; C_{max} = peak serum or plasma concentration; AUC = area under the plasma or serum concentration-versus-time curve; enox = enoxacin; oflox = ofloxacin; tema = temafloxacin; cipro = ciprofloxacin; norflox = norfloxacin; Mg = magnesium; Al = aluminum; OH = hydroxide; Ca = calcium; carb = carbonate; $FeSO_4$ = ferrous sulfate; Multivit = multiple vitamins; Zn = zinc; gluc = gluconate; * = statistically significant difference compared to baseline or placebo control.

3. Metabolism Interactions

A number of the quinolones have been found to reduce the hepatic metabolism of co-administered drugs such as the xanthines theophylline (149–168) and caffeine (169–174) (Table 6). In contrast to the absorption interactions with multivalent cations, which appear to be generalizable to the entire quinolone drug class, differences do exist between individual quinolones in their propensity to inhibit hepatic xanthine metabolism. A recent meta-analysis of quinolone-theophylline interaction studies revealed that enoxacin, ciprofloxacin, and norfloxacin (in descending order) are clinically significant inhibitors of theophylline metabolism while ofloxacin and lomefloxacin (and based on Ref. 162,

Table 6 Effect of Quinolones on Methylxanthine Pharmacokinetics

Quinolone	Mean % change in steady-state conc.	Mean % change in CL	Mean % change in $t_{\frac{1}{2}}$	Ref.
Theophylline				
Enox				159
400 bid	+109*	−55*	—	
Norflox				151
400 bid	—	−8*	+9*	
Norflox				150
400 bid	—	−10	+26	
Cipro				161
750 bid	—	−31*	—	
Oflox				152
400 bid	+9*	−15*	—	
Norflox				153
400 bid	—	−15*	+13*	
Lomeflox				156
400 qd	—	−7	+4*	
Enox				158
25 bid	—	−53*	+35*	
100 bid	—	−66*	+74*	
400 bid	—	−73*	+83*	
Enox				162
400 bid	+91*	−65*	+187	
Tema				
400 bid	−55	−10	+9	
Enox				166
400–600 bid	+155*	−42*	—	
Enox				163
200 tid	+118*	−65*	—	
Enox				167
400 bid	+163*	−64*	+159*	
Cipro				
500 bid	+66*	−30*	+42*	
Oflox				
400 bid	+2	−5	+2	
Oflox				160
200 tid	—	0	+6	
Norflox				
200 tid	—	−7	+15	
Enox				149
400 bid	+243*	−74*	—	
Lomeflox				168
400 bid	—	+7	+3	
Norflox				154
200 tid	—	−4	—	
Enox				
200 tid	—	−84*	—	

Table 6 Continued

Quinolone	Mean % change in steady-state conc.	Mean % change in CL	Mean % change in $t_{\frac{1}{2}}$	Ref.
Oflox				
200 tid	—	−11	—	
Cipro				
200 tid	—	−22*	—	
Enox				165
600 bid	+248*	—	—	
Cipro				157
750 bid	+87*	—	—	
Caffeine				
Norflox				169
800 bid	—	−35*	+23	
Cipro				172
750 bid	—	−45*	+58*	
Tema				174
600 bid	0	+1	−7	
Cipro				
750 bid	+877*	−145*	+116*	
Oflox				171
200 bid	—	+2	−3	
Norflox				
400 bid	—	−16	+16*	
Cipro				
100 bid	—	−17	+6	
250 bid	—	−57*	+15*	
500 bid	—	−58*	+26	
Enox				
100 bid	—	−138*	+103*	
200 bid	—	−176*	+126*	
400 bid	—	−346*	+258*	
Lomeflox				173
400 qd	−6	−3	0	

% change = change from baseline or placebo control; CL = total body clearance; t½ = terminal disposition half-life; enox = enoxacin; norflox = norfloxacin; cipro = ciprofloxacin; lomeflox = lomefloxacin; tema = temafloxacin; oflox = ofloxacin; * = statistically significant difference compared to baseline or placebo control.

temafloxacin) are clinically insignificant inhibitors (175). By using a simple pharmacokinetic model that allowed cross-comparison between quinolone-caffeine interaction studies, a relative potency index of quinolone interaction has been developed: enoxacin (100), ciprofloxacin (11), norfloxacin (9), and ofloxacin (0) (176).

Few other substrates have been examined. Enoxacin decreased the metabolism of the less active enantiomer of warfarin, R-warfarin, without potentiation of the anticoagulant effect (177). Temafloxacin was shown not to potentiate the anticoagulant effect of warfarin in healthy subjects (178). However, case reports have documented quinolone-associated increases in prothrombin time in patients receiving warfarin concurrently with ciprofloxacin, ofloxacin, and norfloxacin (179–183). Pending additional information, patients who are receiving long-term warfarin therapy in whom a quinolone is to be used should be monitored for changes in prothrombin time. Ciprofloxacin does not impair the elimination of diazepam (184). It has been demonstrated that elderly subjects are not more sensitive than young volunteers to the inhibitory effect of ciprofloxacin on hepatic metabolism of antipyrine (185). In addition, rifampin does not induce the metabolism of ciprofloxacin, suggesting that the two agents may be used concomitantly in standard clinical dosing regimens (69,77), an important finding when considering combination therapy of infection or eradication of the carrier state of methicillin-resistant *Staphylococcus aureus.*

The mechanism of these interactions is largely unexplored. It has been suggested that inhibition of metabolism may be related to the 4-oxo-metabolites of the quinolones, but more recent data suggest that the sequence N*-C=N-C-N-C (where N* = nitrogen on the piperazine ring) is the entity responsible for metabolic inhibition (171,186). It appears that metabolic inhibition is dose-related, at least for enoxacin and ciprofloxacin (158,171).

Clinically, caution is advised when using any quinolone in combination with a xanthine compound such as theophylline. Close monitoring of serum theophylline concentrations is recommended in any patient receiving these drugs. The clinical significance of inhibited metabolism of other drugs remains unclear at present. Until further data become available, clinicians should be aware of the possibility of reduced drug metabolism resulting in adverse effects whenever the quinolones are co-administered with drugs that depend on hepatic metabolism for their elimination.

4. *Pharmacodynamic Interactions*

Quinolones may rarely produce central nervous system adverse effects such as restlessness, headaches, tremors, hallucinations, and seizures (see Sec. VII). These agents have been demonstrated in animal models to inhibit in vitro the binding of the inhibitory neurotransmitter gamma-aminobutyric acid (GABA) to its receptors in mouse brain (187–191). In addition the nonsteroidal antiinflammatory drugs (NSAIDs) flurbiprofen, indomethacin, and fenbufen have been shown in vitro to potentiate this effect of the quinolones. Predicted interactions include an increase in the epileptogenic potential of theophylline, opiates, antidepressants, neuroleptics, and other agents when co-administered with quinolones, potentially with further enhancement during concomitant quinolone-NSAID therapy. Indeed, reports of seizures in Japan during concomitant enoxacin-fenbufen therapy resulted in a warning to physicians (191). Further studies will be necessary to demonstrate the clinical significance of this pharmacodynamic interaction.

V. CLINICAL INDICATIONS

Quinolones have been used to treat a broad range of bacterial infections including upper and lower respiratory tract infections, skin and skin structure infections, bone and joint infections, urinary tract infections, prostatitis, infectious diarrhea, and sepsis (12,13,31). Newer agents such as the quinolones have been promoted for their high potency and broad spectrum of activity, ease of administration, favorable adverse event profile, and lack of cross-reactivity with penicillin. However, there is the risk that these sophisticated and expensive agents may become first-line therapy, even where they may be unnecessary or insufficient treatment (192).

This section will critically evaluate the clinical indications for quinolone therapy of infections in the geriatric population. The selected references cited in Tables 7 through

Table 7 Open Trials of Quinolones in the Treatment of Urinary Tract Infections in Elderly Patients

Drug	Dosing regimen (mg/frequency/route)	Mean duration of therapy (days)[a]	No. patients	Clinical efficacy (% cure)	Bacteriological eradication (%)	Adverse events	Ref.
Norfloxacin	400/b.i.d./PO	6.8 (5–10)	19	NA	84	None reported	193
Norfloxacin	400/b.i.d./PO	NA (7–30)	95	NA	85	Dyspepsia, sluggishness, nausea, heartburn, dizziness, rash, ↑SGOT, ↑BUN, eosinophilia (11.6% overall incidence)	194
Ciprofloxacin	200–250/b.i.d./PO	5 (NA)	28	NA	89	Nausea, vomiting, depression (7.1% overall incidence)	195
Ciprofloxacin	250/b.i.d./PO	7 (NA)	38	NA	84	GI, neurological, skin rash (11% overall incidence)	196
	500/b.i.d./PO	7 (NA)	34	NA	87		
	750/b.i.d./PO	7 (NA)	38	NA	86		
Ciprofloxacin	500/b.i.d./PO	10.1 (9–11)	53	98	89	↑LDH, ↑serum creatinine, eosinophilia (7% overall incidence)	197
Ciprofloxacin	500/b.i.d./PO	NA (7–10)	30	NA	93	Nausea, fever, disorientation, vertigo, ↑SGOT (22.9% overall incidence, 2/7 withdrew due to adverse events)	198
Ciprofloxacin	500/b.i.d./PO	7 (NA)	25	NA	84	Eosinophilia, ↓WBC, crystalluria, granular casts, ↑serum creatinine, ↑BUN, nausea (28% overall incidence)	199

Ciprofloxacin	500–750/b.i.d./PO	10 (5–17)	57	100	84	Nausea, vomiting, headache, ↑hepatic enzymes (14% overall incidence)	200
Ciprofloxacin	750/b.i.d./PO	15 (NA)	14	100	100	None reported	201
Enoxacin	200/b.i.d./PO	7 (NA)	20	85	75	Nausea, anorexia, diarrhea, dizziness, lethargy, tinnitus, numbness (40% overall incidence)	202
Enoxacin	200/b.i.d./PO 400/b.i.d./PO	NA (4–14)[b]	11 56	81[b]	61[b]	Gastrointestinal, CNS, palpitations, candidal vaginitis (36% overall incidence)	203
Lomefloxacin	400/q.d./PO	NA (7–10)	63	92[c]	80	Diarrhea, ↑SGOT, ↑SGPT, others not specified (no quantitation of adverse events)	204
Pefloxacin	400/b.i.d./PO	NA (10–21)	88	77[c]	95	Gastrointestinal neurological, allergic, arthralgias, myalgias (33% overall incidence)	205
Fleroxacin	200/q.d./PO 400/q.d./PO 600/q.d./PO	8.9 (6–14) 9.0 (7–12) 8.0 (1–10)	20 21 21	86 77 71	64 59 36	Oliguria, psychosis, photosensitivity, nausea, vomiting, ↑hepatic enzymes, insomnia, nightmares, rash, eosinophilia, others not stated (43.3% overall incidence)	206

Table 7 Continued

Drug	Dosing regimen (mg/frequency/route)	Mean duration of therapy (days)[a]	No. patients	Clinical efficacy (% cure)	Bacteriological eradication (%)	Adverse events	Ref.
Fleroxacin	200/q.d./PO	10 (NA)	28	NA	86	Insomnia, abdominal discomfort, nausea, others not stated (3.6, 13.8, 42.9% overall incidences in 200, 400, 600 mg groups, respectively)	207
	400/q.d./PO	10 (NA)	29	NA	83		
	600/q.d./PO	10 (NA)	28	NA	89		

NA = not available; SGOT = serum aspartate aminotransaminase; BUN = blood urea nitrogen; GI = gastrointestinal; LDH = lactate dehydrogenase; WBC = white blood cell; CNS = central nervous system; SGPT = serum alanine aminotransferase.

[a]Range in parentheses.

[b]Pooled results for 200 and 400 mg recipients.

[c]Clinical success (cure or improvement).

17 were chosen based upon their predominantly or exclusively elderly (≥65 years old) patient populations. Space limitations prevent this listing from being exhaustive.

A. Urinary Tract Infections (UTIs)

Uncomplicated lower UTIs are treatable with a number of highly effective and well-established antimicrobial regimens such as ampicillin or amoxicillin, trimethoprim/sulfamethoxazole (TMP/SMX), and nitrofurantoin. Although effective, the quinolones do not appear to produce significantly better clinical or bacteriological cure rates (Tables 7 and 8 (193–226). However, for patients who are allergic to these older agents, quinolone therapy is a reasonable alternative.

Although single-dose quinolone therapy of uncomplicated UTIs with norfloxacin (800 or 1200 mg), ciprofloxacin (100 or 250 mg), ofloxacin (100 mg), fleroxacin (200,400, or 600 mg), and pefloxacin (800 mg) has been highly effective in treating younger women with infections caused by Enterobacteriaceae (31), similar data do not exist for such therapy in older women, and hence single-dose therapy is not recommended at present in elderly females. By definition, UTI in males is complicated in nature, and single-dose therapy is similarly not recommended.

Three-day therapy of uncomplicated lower UTIs with quinolones and traditional antimicrobials has been the subject of numerous studies, albeit most commonly in the young and middle-aged female patient population (31). Although some data documenting the efficacy of 3-day quinolone regimens in the elderly patient population exist (211,213), such regimens should be approached with caution until further confirmatory studies are performed.

In studies examining the therapy of complicated UTIs, quinolones have been documented to be similar or superior to traditional antimicrobials in their ability to eradicate bacteriuria. Traditional agents evaluated were TMP/SMX, amoxicillin, mezlocillin, other β-lactams, and a variety of other agents, including parenteral agents. Response rates for the quinolones ranged from 53 to 100% (mean 87%), while those for traditional agents ranged from 30 to 100% (mean 78%) (31). Similar findings have been noted in studies performed in predominantly or exclusively elderly patient populations (majority of studies cited in Tables 7 and 8). However, patients with complicated UTIs, particularly those caused by *P. aeruginosa*, may suffer relapse if the infecting strains develop resistance during quinolone therapy. In addition, superinfections with enterococci may be problematic due to the variable sensitivity of these organisms to available quinolones (12,13,32).

B. Prostatitis

Patients with prostatic inflammation are classified into those with nonbacterial prostatitis, bacterial prostatitis, prostatodynia, or pelvic pain (227). Patients diagnosed with bacterial prostatitis are further characterized as acute or chronic in onset and course. Such classification is important in antimicrobial selection, and cure rates differ between these two types of bacterial prostatitis.

In acute bacterial prostatitis, symptoms typically have a rapid onset and usually respond quickly to treatment with a wide variety of antimicrobials. The acute inflammatory state allows for the ready accessibility of most agents into the infected gland. One would thus expect that results of quinolone therapy of acute bacterial prostatitis would not be substantially different from those of other agents, provided that the pathogen(s) is/are susceptible. In contrast, patients with chronic bacterial prostatitis (typically men over the

Table 8 Comparative Trials of Quinolones in the Treatment of Urinary Tract Infections in Elderly Patients

Study design	Drug	Dosing regimen (mg/frequency/route)	Mean duration of therapy (days)[a]	No. patients	Clinical efficacy (% cure)	Bacteriological eradication (%)	Adverse events	Ref.
C,R	Norfloxacin	400/b.i.d/PO	10 (NA)	14	86	92	Norfloxacin—none reported	208
	TMP/SMX	160/800/b.i.d./PO	10 (NA)	13	100	73	TMP/SMX—vomiting in 1 patient (8% overall incidence)	
C,R	Norfloxacin	400/b.i.d./PO	7 (NA)	20	NA	95	None reported	209
	Amoxicillin	250/t.i.d./PO	7 (NA)	20	NA	75		
C,R	Norfloxacin	400/b.i.d./PO	NA (≥7)	95	85	85	Norfloxacin—nausea, ↑SGOT, ↑SGPT (2.1% overall incidence)	210
	Pipemidic acid	400/b.i.d./PO	NA (≥7)	40	45	45	Pipemidic acid—indigestion (2.5% overall incidence)	
C,NR/R (depending on organism susceptibility)	Norfloxacin	400/b.i.d./PO	3 (NA)	35	NA	80	No adverse events reported for any agent	211
	Cefadroxil	1000/t.i.d./PO	3 (NA)	13	NA	31		
	TMP/SMX	160/800/b.i.d./PO	3 (NA)	23	NA	78		
C,R	Norfloxacin	200/b.i.d./PO	7 (NA)	114	81	79	Norfloxacin—1.2% overall incidence	212
	Pivmecillinam	200/t.i.d./PO	7 (NA)	96	71	52	Pivmecillinam—3.5% overall incidence) No specific adverse events reported in either group	
C,R	Norfloxacin	400/b.i.d./PO	3 (NA)	49	NA	86	Norfloxacin—↑hepatic function test values (4.1% overall incidence)	213
	TMP	300/q.d./PO	3 (NA)	51	NA	69	TMP—↑hepatic function test values (5.9% overall incidence)	

C,NR/R (depending on TMP/SMX susceptibility)	Ciprofloxacin	100/b.i.d./PO	5 (NA)	33	NA	94	Ciprofloxacin—nausea and flatulence (3% overall incidence)	214
		250/b.i.d./PO	5 (NA)	26	NA	88		
	TMP/SMX	160/800/b.i.d./PO	5 (NA)	16	NA	87	TMP/SMX—nausea (6% overall incidence)	
C,R	Ciprofloxacin	100/b.i.d./PO	5 (NA)	16	NA	94	Ciprofloxacin—drowsiness, ↑SGOT (12% overall incidence)	215
	TMP	200/b.i.d./PO	5 (NA)	16	NA	75	TMP—↓platelets (6% overall incidence)	
C,R	Ciprofloxacin	250/b.i.d./PO	7 (NA)	22	NA	82	Ciprofloxacin—↑hepatic function test values (4.5% overall incidence)	216
	TMP/SMX	160/800/b.i.d./PO	7 (NA)	23	NA	52	TMP/SMX—nausea, vomiting, pruritus, ↑serum creatinine (26.1% overall incidence)	
C,R	Ciprofloxacin	200/b.i.d./IV →500/b.i.d./PO	10 (NA)	38	100	100	Ciprofloxacin—urticaria, ↑SGOT, ↑SGPT, ↑BUN, ↑serum creatinine (10% overall incidence)	217
	Ceftazidime	500/t.i.d./IV	9 (NA)	39	92	87	Ceftazidime—↑BUN, ↑serum creatinine, ↑SGOT, ↑SGPT, ↑alk. phos., ↑ESR (8% overall incidence)	
C,R	Ciprofloxacin	500/b.i.d./PO	NA (7–10)	37	81	63	Ciprofloxacin—nausea (2.7% overall incidence)	218
	Aminoglycosides	various/various/IV	NA (7–10)	28	82	15	Aminoglycosides—rash (3.6% overall incidence)	

Table 8 Continued

Study design	Drug	Dosing regimen (mg/frequency/route)	Mean duration of therapy (days)[a]	No. patients	Clinical efficacy (% cure)	Bacteriological eradication (%)	Adverse events	Ref.
C,R	Enoxacin	400/b.i.d./PO	14 (NA)	89	93	81	Enoxacin—nausea, vomiting, others not stated (24% overall incidence)	219
	TMP/SMX	160/800/b.i.d./PO	14 (NA)	90	87	81	TMP/SMX—headache, nausea, vomiting, amblyopia, others not stated (13% overall incidence)	
C,R	Pefloxacin	400/b.i.d/IV or PO	NA (10–15)	76	84	72	Pefloxacin—7.7% overall incidence	220
	Cefotaxime	1000/t.i.d./IV or IM	NA (10–15)	79	70	53	Cefotaxime—17.6% overall incidence	
							No specific adverse events reported in either group	
C,R	Ofloxacin	200/q.d./IV	7 (NA)	34	78	75	No specific adverse events or quantitation reported in either group	221
	Piperacillin	4000/t.i.d./IV	7 (NA)	16	73	73		
C,R	Lomefloxacin	400/q.d./PO	NA (10–14)	72	92	97	Lomefloxacin—nausea, nervousness, pruritus, others not stated (18.7% overall incidence)	222
	Ciprofloxacin	500/b.i.d./PO	NA (10–14)	70	87	96	Ciprofloxacin—nausea, pruritus, others not stated (21.3% overall)	
C,R	Lomefloxacin	400/q.d./PO	NA (10–14)	84	96[b]	93	No specific adverse events or quantitation reported in either group	223
	Ciprofloxacin	500/b.i.d./PO	NA (10–14)	80	99[b]	98		

C,R	Fleroxacin	400/q.d./PO	10 (NA)	42	NA	81	No specific adverse events or quantitation reported in either group	224
	Norfloxacin	400/b.i.d./PO	10 (NA)	40	NA	78		
C,R	Fleroxacin	400/q.d./PO	10 (NA)	40	87[b]	87	Fleroxacin—rash, insomnia, nausea, gastrointestinal disturbances (17.5% overall incidence)	225
	Norfloxacin	400/b.i.d./PO	10 (NA)	39	90[b]	90	Norfloxacin—gastric pain, rash (5.1% overall incidence)	
C,R	Ofloxacin	100/b.i.d./PO	7 (NA)	18	83	63	Ofloxacin—rash, meteorism (6.7% overall incidence)	226
	Ciprofloxacin	250/b.i.d./PO	7 (NA)	22	68	63	Ciprofloxacin—pruritus, drug fever (6.5% overall incidence)	

C = controlled; R = randomized; NR = nonrandomized; NA = not available; TMP/SMX = trimethoprim/sulfamethoxazole; SGOT = serum aspartate aminotransaminase; SGPT = serum alanine aminotransaminase; BUN = blood urea nitrogen; ESR = erythrocyte sedimentation rate.

[a]Range in parentheses.

[b]Clinical success (cure or improvement).

age of 50 years) experience extended periods of asymptomatic infection with periodic episodes of acute symptoms suggestive of recurrent UTI (228). Pathogens involved in chronic bacterial prostatitis include the Enterobacteriaceae as well as gram-positive cocci, primarily staphylococci and enterococci, the latter being especially problematic in the older population. Treatment of chronic bacterial prostatitis is made more difficult by the inability to attain and maintain adequate prostatic tissue/fluid concentrations for many antimicrobials since diffusion into these compartments is limited in the absence of acute inflammation (229).

Previous treatment regimens of chronic bacterial prostatitis using older agents such as TMP/SMX and carbenicillin indanyl have been less than satisfactory. In light of their excellent penetration into prostatic fluid and tissue (Table 4), the use of quinolones in this disease entity has been the subject of intense investigation. Unfortunately, not all investigators have analyzed their results by separating patients with acute bacterial from those with chronic bacterial prostatitis. Moreover, the daily drug dose, duration of treatment, length of the follow-up period, and definition of cure have also varied among investigators, most of whom have carried out open, noncomparative studies (31).

Notwithstanding these deficiencies, an examination of the details of these studies is worthwhile. In one group of studies, a total of 154 patients with chronic bacterial prostatitis were treated with oral ciprofloxacin in doses ranging from 100 mg three times daily to 500 mg twice daily for durations of 10–259 days; most were treated for approximately 4 weeks. Follow-up ranged from 1 to 12 months. Cure rates ranged from 60 to 100%, with a mean cure rate of 73% (230–236). In general, these cure rates appear to be comparable, if not superior, to cure rates obtained with TMP/SMX, tetracyclines, and carbenicillin indanyl in previous studies. Similar results have been obtained with oral ofloxacin, norfloxacin, and enoxacin (237–245). Although further data are required, especially with respect to the utility of quinolones in chronic bacterial prostatitis due to enterococci and resistance/relapse rates, the quinolones may be viewed as a significant addition to the antimicrobial armamentarium for treatment of chronic bacterial prostatitis.

C. Upper Respiratory Tract Infections

Few data exist regarding the potential utility of quinolones in the therapy of upper respiratory tract infections (otitis media, tonsillitis, pharyngitis, and sinusitis), probably due to their marginal to modest activity against the major pathogens of these infections, i.e., streptococci, anaerobes, and staphylococci. In general, quinolone therapy of such infections is not to be encouraged.

An exception to this principle may be found in the treatment of malignant or invasive external otitis. Encouraging results of quinolone therapy of this disease entity, predominantly caused by *P. aeruginosa* and found in elderly diabetics, have been noted (Table 9) (246–250). Cure rates with oral quinolone therapy have been similar to those noted in other studies utilizing traditional parenteral antipseudomonal therapy. The potential advantages of oral quinolone therapy in this disease state include reduced cost, reduced length of hospital stay, reduced drug toxicity, and enhanced convenience.

D. Lower Respiratory Tract Infections (LRTIs)

Lower respiratory tract infections in geriatric patients include bronchitis (acute and chronic) and pneumonia (community-acquired, nosocomial, and aspiration) (251,252). These infections may be treated with a wide variety of antimicrobials. Typically, patients in this age

Table 9 Open Trials of Quinolones in the Treatment of Malignant External Otitis in Elderly Patients

Drug	Dosing regimen (mg/frequency/route)	Mean duration of therapy (days)[a]	No. patients	Clinical efficacy (% cure)	Bacteriological eradication (%)	Adverse events	Ref.
Ciprofloxacin + Rifampin	750/b.i.d./PO 600/b.i.d./PO	56 (42–84)	11	91	91	Nausea, diarrhea (18.2% overall incidence)	246
Ciprofloxacin	750–1000/b.i.d.-t.i.d./PO	NA (42–57)	23	91	91	Restlessness, headache, constipation, nausea, vertigo (13% overall incidence)	247
Ofloxacin	400/b.i.d./PO	49 (21–94)	24	83	83	Rash, pruritus, nausea, arthralgia (20.8% overall incidence)	248
Ofloxacin	200/b.i.d./PO	24 (12–39)	17	94	94	Weakness (11.8% overall incidence)	249
Ciprofloxacin Ofloxacin Pefloxacin	200–1000/b.i.d./IV or PO 200/t.i.d./PO 400/t.i.d./IV or PO	109 (20–200)[b]	12[b]	67[b]	75[b]	None reported to any agent	250

[a]Range in parentheses.
[b]Pooled results over the three drug groups.

Table 10 Open Trials of Quinolones in the Treatment of Lower Respiratory Tract Infections in Elderly Patients

Drug	Dosing regimen (mg/frequency/route)	Mean duration of therapy (days)[a]	No. patients	Clinical efficacy (% cure)	Bacterio-logical eradication (%)	Adverse events	Ref.
Ofloxacin	400/q.d. or b.i.d./PO	10 (NA)	30	87	90	Skin rash (3% overall incidence)	253
Ofloxacin	200/b.i.d./PO	8.8 (NA)	667	91	78[b]	GI, neurological, others not specified (5% overall incidence)	254
	300/b.i.d./PO			93			
	400/b.i.d./PO			92			
Ofloxacin	400/b.i.d./PO	10 (NA)	98	71	NA	Insomnia, headache, dizziness, nausea, vomiting, diarrhea, pruritus, ↑serum creatinine, eosinophilia (35% overall incidence)	255
Ofloxacin	400/b.i.d./PO	10 (NA)	4	75	NA	None reported	256
Ofloxacin	100–200/b.i.d./PO	NA (NA)	36	67	67	Nausea (2.8% overall incidence)	257
Ofloxacin	800/b.i.d./PO	7 (NA)	40	58	58	Nausea (2.5% overall incidence)	258
Ofloxacin	400/q.d./PO	10 (NA)	15	93	90[b]	Rash, stomach pain (6.7% overall incidence)	259
	400/b.i.d./PO	10 (NA)	15	80			
Ofloxacin +	200/b.i.d./IV→PO +	19 (NA)	38	84	NA	Confusion, skin rashes (7.9% overall incidence)	260
Penicillin G	12 mU/day/IV	7 (NA)					
Ciprofloxacin	500/b.i.d./PO	10 (NA)	20	70 (50)[c]	80 (54)[b,c]	Vomiting, stomach pain, nausea, hallucinations, chest pain, rash (8% overall incidence, 5 patients withdrew due to adverse events)	261
	750/b.i.d. (Lot A)/PO	10 (NA)	20	75 (50)[c]			
	750/b.i.d. (Lot B)/PO	10 (NA)	20	90 (55)[c]			
	1000/b.i.d./PO	10 (NA)	20	90 (55)[c]			
Ciprofloxacin	500/b.i.d./PO	NA (5–NA)	32	100	97	None reported	262
Ciprofloxacin	500/b.i.d./PO	9 (4–17)	42	17	48	None reported	263
Ciprofloxacin	200–300/b.i.d./IV	9 (NA)	41	63	63	Phlebitis, drug fever, ↑BUN and serum creatinine (7.3% overall incidence)	264

Ciprofloxacin	500/b.i.d./PO	9 (7–13)	28	93	93	None reported	265
Ciprofloxacin	500/b.i.d./PO	10 (NA)	31	81	81	Seizures, nausea, visual disturbances, abnormal liver function tests (13.7% overall incidence)	266
	750/b.i.d./PO	10 (NA)	20	90	95		
Enoxacin	600/b.i.d./PO	10 (NA)	15	100 (67)[c]	83 (60)[c]	Nausea, vomiting, seizures, hallucinations, dizziness (80% overall incidence) due to theophylline intoxication. Nine patients withdrew.	267
Enoxacin	800/b.i.d./PO	10 (NA)	30	80	97	Gastric pain (3.3% overall incidence)	268
Pefloxacin	400/b.i.d.-t.i.d./IV or PO	9 (2–14)	59	63	81	Nausea, epigastric pain, vomiting, anorexia, rash (15.4% overall incidence)	269
Pefloxacin	400/b.i.d./IV	9 (NA)	15	73	67	None reported	270
Pefloxacin	400/b.i.d./PO or IV	9 (5–14)	101	43	91	Gastrointestinal disturbances, urticaria, CNS disturbance, dyspnea (16.7% overall incidence)	271
Temafloxacin	300–600/b.i.d./PO	10 (NA)	36	86	81	Nausea, waterbrash (5.6% overall incidence)	272

NA = not available; CNS = central nervous system; GI = gastrointestinal; BUN = blood urea nitrogen.
[a]Range in parentheses.
[b]Pooled results over all of the study groups.
[c]Results at 1 day (7 days) after therapy.

Table 11 Comparative Trials of Quinolones in the Treatment of Lower Respiratory Tract Infections in Elderly Patients

Study design	Drug	Dosing regimen (mg/frequency/route)	Mean duration of therapy (days)[a]	No. patients	Clinical efficacy (% cure)	Bacteriological eradication (%)	Adverse events	Ref.
C,R	Ciprofloxacin	500/b.i.d./PO	9.8 (5–10)	26	81	87	Ciprofloxacin—mild hallucinations (4% overall incidence)	273
	Amoxicillin	250/t.i.d./PO	9.4 (4–10)	22	82	64	Amoxicillin—confusion and nightmares (5% overall incidence)	
C,R	Ciprofloxacin	750/b.i.d./PO	14.4 (4–17.5)	30	76	NA	Ciprofloxacin—↑SGOT, eosinophilia, rash, ↑serum creatinine (13% overall incidence)	274
	Cefamandole	1000/q.i.d./IM	13.6 (5–14)	30	70	NA	Cefamandole—pain on IM injection, eosinophilia (20% overall incidence)	
C,R	Ciprofloxacin	200/b.i.d./IV →500/b.i.d./PO	6 (2–10)[b] 6 (1–11)[c]	23	100[d]	NA	Ciprofloxacin—seizures (4.3% overall incidence)	275
	Ceftazidime	2000/t.i.d./IV →suitable PO agent	7 (1–15)[b]	21	71[d]	NA	Ceftazidime—rash, ↓WBC, ↑SGOT, ↑SGPT (9.5% overall incidence)	
C,R	Ciprofloxacin	200/b.i.d./IV →500–750/b.i.d./PO	7 (NA)[b]	37	97[d]	63	Ciprofloxacin—headache, ↑hepatic function tests, nausea, ↑serum theophylline	276
	Ceftazidime	1000–2000/b.i.d.-t.i.d./IV	9 (NA)	34	97[d]	77	Ceftazidime—headache, candidiasis No quantitation of adverse events in either group	

C,R	Ciprofloxacin	500/b.i.d./PO	11 (10–12)	20	60[d]	NA	Ciprofloxacin—none reported	277
	Amoxicillin/ clavulanate	1000/250/t.i.d./PO	11 (5–12)	20	60[d]	NA	Amoxicillin/ clavulanate—gastrointestinal distress (5% overall incidence)	
C,R	Ciprofloxacin	500–750/b.i.d./PO	7 (NA)	73	22	68	Ciprofloxacin—nausea, headache (4% overall incidence)	278
	Amoxicillin	250–500/t.i.d./PO	7 (NA)	67	10	46	Amoxicillin—dizziness, gastrointestinal disturbance (3% overall incidence)	
C,R	Ciprofloxacin	200–400/b.i.d./IV →750/b.i.d./PO	3 (2–6)[b]	24	50[d]	NA	Ciprofloxacin—↑SGOT, ↑SGPT, ↑LDH, ↑alk phos, eosinophilia, candiduria (9 episodes)	279
	Ceftriaxone	2000/q.d./IV →1000/q.d./IM	4 (2–10)[b]	26	54[d]	NA	Ceftriaxone—↑SGPT, ↑alk phos, eosinophilia, diarrhea, drug fever, IM injection site pain, candiduria (10 episodes)	
C,R	Ciprofloxacin	250/b.i.d./PO	10 (NA)	29	56	NA	Ciprofloxacin—nausea, vomiting, ↑serum theophylline	280
	Ampicillin	500/q.i.d./PO	10 (NA)	28	71	NA	Ampicillin—facial flushing, itchy eyes, nausea, vomiting. No quantitation of adverse events in either group	
C,R	Ofloxacin	400/b.i.d./PO	8 (NA)	7	100	100	Ofloxacin—rash (14% overall incidence)	281
	TMP/SMX	160/800/b.i.d./PO	8 (NA)	10	80	80	TMP/SMX—none reported	

Table 11 Continued

Study design	Drug	Dosing regimen (mg/frequency/route)	Mean duration of therapy (days)[a]	No. patients	Clinical efficacy (% cure)	Bacteriological eradication (%)	Adverse events	Ref.
C,R	Ofloxacin	400/b.i.d./PO	11 (5–16)	69	81	100	Ofloxacin—anorexia, nausea, vomiting, dysphagia, candidiasis, insomnia, myoclonus (10.7% overall incidence)	282
	"Usual Care Regimen"	(parenteral, at least initially)	11 (7–18)	64	69	98	"Usual Care"—diarrhea, glossitis, tinnitus, pain, ↓platelets, ↓WBC (8.3% overall incidence)	
C,R	Ofloxacin	200/b.i.d./PO	14 (NA)	39	97	94	Ofloxacin—none reported	283
	Pivmecillinam	700/t.i.d./PO	14 (NA)	42	98	97	Pivmecillinam—diarrhea (2.3% overall incidence)	
C,R	Ofloxacin	400/q.d./PO	NA (10–14)	87	77	89	Ofloxacin—gastrointestinal, allergic, CNS (14% overall incidence)	284
	Doxycycline	200→100/q.d./PO	NA (10–14)	91	63	76	Doxycycline—as for ofloxacin (12% overall incidence)	
C,R	Ofloxacin	200/b.i.d.-t.i.d./IV or PO	7 (NA)	59	27	95	Ofloxacin—nausea, vomiting, rashes, hypotension, headache, phlebitis (10.2% overall incidence)	285
	Amoxicillin/ clavulanate	625–2200/ b.i.d.,t.i.d.,q.i.d./IV or PO	8 (NA)	33	30	82	Amoxicillin/ clavulanate—none reported	
C,R	Ofloxacin	200/b.i.d./PO	NA (5–10)	34	84[e]	83	Ofloxacin—hallucinations, nightmares, spasms, gastrointestinal disturbances, candidiasis, rash (11 episodes)	286

	Erythromycin	500/b.i.d./PO	NA (5–10)	34	82[e]	75	Erythromycin—headache, vertigo, gastrointestinal disturbances, candidiasis (9 episodes)	
C,R	Temafloxacin	600/b.i.d./PO	NA (10)	43	89	91	Temafloxacin—pyuria, rash, vasodilation, lab abnormality (18% overall incidence)	287
	Cefotaxime	2000/t.i.d./IV	NA (10)	42	92	96	Cefotaxime—diarrhea, fever, pruritus, rash, phlebitis, urticaria, lab abnormality (27% overall incidence)	
C,R	Temafloxacin	600/q.d./PO	7 (6–14)	116	98[d]	98	Temafloxacin—headache, pain, vertigo, diarrhea, nausea, vomiting, candidiasis, xerostomia (8.6% overall incidence)	288
	Ciprofloxacin	500/b.i.d./PO	7 (4–14)	121	97[d]	98	Ciprofloxacin—pain, dizziness, diarrhea, candidiasis, vaginitis, ptosis, balanitis (5.8% overall incidence)	
C,R	Temafloxacin	300–600/b.i.d./PO	NA (7–14)	127[f] 168[g]	94[d] 95[d]	99 98	Temafloxacin—nausea, dizziness, dyspepsia, others (34.8% overall incidence)	289
	Ciprofloxacin or Amoxicillin	500–750/b.i.d./PO 500/t.i.d./PO	NA (7–14) NA (7–14)	107[f] 121[g]	93[d] 89[d]	91 92	Ciprofloxacin/ Amoxicillin—nausea, diarrhea, dyspepsia, others (33.6% overall incicence)	
C,R	Lomefloxacin	400/q.d./PO	NA (7–10)	170	80[d]	82	Lomefloxacin—headache, dizziness, nausea, diarrhea, abdominal pain, flatulence, pruritus, rash (24% overall incidence)	290

Table 11 Continued

Study design	Drug	Dosing regimen (mg/frequency/route)	Mean duration of therapy (days)[a]	No. patients	Clinical efficacy (% cure)	Bacteriological eradication (%)	Adverse events	Ref.
	Cefaclor	250/t.i.d./PO	NA (7–10)	153	65[d]	63	Cefaclor—dizziness, nausea, diarrhea, candidiasis, pruritus, rash, urticaria, xerostomia, taste changes (20% overall incidence)	
C,R	Fleroxacin	400/q.d./IV	NA (4–21)	15	NA	100	None reported in either group	291
	Ceftazidime	500–2000/t.i.d./IV	NA (4–21)	6	NA	100		
C,R	Enoxacin	400/b.i.d./PO	NA (7–10)	24	88[d]	88	Enoxacin—nausea, vomiting, diarrhea (12.5% overall incidence)	292
	TMP/SMX	160/800/b.i.d./PO	NA (7–10)	26	96[d]	100	TMP/SMX—nausea, vomiting, abdominal pain, rash (15.4% overall incidence)	
C,R	Enoxacin	400/b.i.d./PO	8 (7–12)	23	52	76	Enoxacin—↑serum theophylline (15/16 patients)	293
	Amoxicillin	1000/t.i.d./PO	8 (7–12)	14	50	71	Amoxicillin—none reported	
C,R	Pefloxacin	400/b.i.d./PO	NA (>4)	69	74[d]	91	Pefloxacin—allergy, fatigue, phlebitis, digestive disorders (15.9% overall incidence)	294
	Ceftazidime	2000/b.i.d./IV	NA (>4)	70	81[d]	88	Ceftazidime—allergy, digestive disorders, CNS disorders, lab abnormalities (20.4% overall incidence)	

C,R	Temafloxacin	600/b.i.d./PO	NA (7–14)	21	100	100	Nausea, diarrhea, dizziness reported for both agents	295
	Ciprofloxacin	750/b.i.d./PO	NA (7–14)	20	100	100	No quantitation of overall incidence	

NA = not available; C = controlled; R = randomized; TMP/SMX = trimethoprim/sulfamethoxazole; SGOT = serum aspartate aminotransferase; SGPT = serum alanine aminotransferase; WBC = white blood cell; LDH = lactate dehydrogenase; alk phos = alkaline phosphatase; CNS = central nervous system; lab = laboratory.

[a]Range in parentheses.

[b]Intravenous.

[c]Oral.

[d]Clinical success (cure or improvement).

[e]Satisfactory response.

[f]Smokers.

[g]Elderly.

group are treated empirically with broad-spectrum agent(s) prior to the availability of culture results (if bronchopulmonary secretions are obtained at all) (see Chap. 26). With increases in the prevalence of β-lactam resistance among several common respiratory pathogens such as *H. influenzae* and *M. catarrhalis*, it has become common among clinicians to rely more heavily on agents that are β-lactamase stable.

The pharmacokinetic and microbiological properties of the quinolones have engendered much interest, as well as controversy, in their use in the treatment of LRTIs in elderly patients. Tables 10 and 11 illustrate the results of open and comparative LRTI trials of quinolones in elderly patients, respectively (253–295).

In general, the quinolones have been comparable to various comparator agents in terms of clinical cure and bacteriological eradication rates in LRTI therapy in predominantly or exclusive elderly patient populations. A limited number of studies of selected quinolones suggest their superior clinical efficacy over comparator agents, for example, ofloxacin versus cefaclor and amoxicillin and ciprofloxacin versus cefaclor, josamycin, and ceftazidime (reviewed in Ref. 31). Still other studies suggest greater bacteriological efficacy for quinolones as compared to other agents, for example, ofloxacin versus amoxicillin, ciprofloxacin versus ampicillin and cephalexin, and both of these quinolones versus cefaclor (reviewed in Ref. 31). Although comparisons of efficacy among quinolones can be complicated by disparities in clinical and bacteriological criteria for diagnosis and evaluation, in general, these agents are equally effective clinically and bacteriologically as determined from summary data analysis (31) and direct comparative studies (288,289,295).

The role of quinolones in the treatment of pneumococcal infections has not been fully established. Considering the unfavorable relationship between serum concentrations of these agents and the MICs for the pneumococcus, the clinical results to date have been surprising. The mean rate of clinical cure or improvement for ciprofloxacin and ofloxacin has been reported to be 91% for pneumococcal LRTIs (31). However, the mean bacteriological eradication rate for the two agents for *S. pneumoniae* has been reported to be only 73% (31). These reasonable results of quinolone therapy of pneumococcal LRTIs have probably been the result of excellent penetration into respiratory tissue/fluid (Table 4).

However, reservations have been expressed regarding the efficacy of quinolones in the treatment of known or suspected pneumococcal infections (192,279,296–298), based upon their less favorable bacteriological eradication rates. As such, if *S. pneumoniae* is suspected as a potential LRTI pathogen, empiric therapy with a quinolone augmented with penicillin or ampicillin has been recommended (297), at least until the presence of the pneumococcus has been excluded. Quinolones should not be viewed as first-line antipneumococcal agents. Moreover, should *S. pneumoniae* be isolated in pure culture, therapy should be changed to a β-lactam, if possible. Quinolone monotherapy of "mixed" *S. pneumoniae* infections may be justified provided that the patient can be carefully monitored.

E. Skin, Soft Tissue, and Bone Infections

Osteomyelitis and, to a lesser extent, septic arthritis are infectious conditions characterized by a high frequency of failures of therapy and recurrence of infection due to short-term treatment, inadequate choice of antimicrobial, formation of abscess and sequestrum, and other as yet unknown factors (299). These failures of therapy are also partially influenced by the use of orthopedic fixation devices and prosthetic implants of various types that perpetrate the infectious process. The organisms most encountered in adult cases of osteomyelitis and septic arthritis include *S. aureus*, coagulase-negative staphylococci, and gram-negative facultative and aerobic bacilli including *P. aeruginosa*. Gram-negative

Table 12 Open Trials of Quinolones in the Treatment of Soft Tissue and Bone Infections in Elderly Patients

Drug	Dosing regimen (mg/frequency/route)	Mean duration of therapy (days)[a]	No. patients	Clinical efficacy (% cure)	Bacteriological eradication (%)	Adverse events	Ref.
Ciprofloxacin	500–750/b.i.d./PO	19,85,115(NA)[b]	48	84	75	Rash, GI intolerance, ↑ hepatic enzymes (32% overall incidence)	303
Ciprofloxacin	500/b.i.d./PO 750/b.i.d./PO 300/b.i.d./IV	69 (17–189)[c]	13 13 1	74[c]	74[c]	Nausea (3.7% overall incidence)	304
Ciprofloxacin	500–1500/b.i.d./PO	139 (15–476)	40	65	69	Phototoxicity, vision perturbation, rash, abdominal pain, drug fever, malaise, paresthesias, eosinophilia (22.5% overall incidence)	305
Ciprofloxacin	250/t.i.d./PO 500/b.i.d./PO	7 (2–12)[c]	19 2	70[c]	50[c]	Nausea, vomiting, ↑ SGOT, ↑ LDH, eosinophilia, ↑ platelets (28.6% overall incidence)	306
Ciprofloxacin	750/b.i.d./PO	86 (30–120)	20	95	95	Nausea (5% overall incidence)	307
Pefloxacin	400/b.i.d./IV → 400/b.i.d./PO	170 (75–180)	13	69	69	Arthralgia, rash, pruritus, nausea, photosensitivity (76.9% overall incidence)	308
Ofloxacin	9.8 ± 2.5 mg/kg/day/PO	100 (NA)	20	95	95	Bone and muscle pain, rash (15% overall incidence)	309

NA = not available; GI = gastrointestinal; SGOT = serum aspartate aminotransferase; LDH = lactate dehydrogenase.
[a]Range in parentheses.
[b]Means for soft tissue infections, nondiabetic osteomyelitis, diabetes mellitus with chronic soft tissue involvement, and osteomyelitis, respectively.
[c]Pooled results over all study groups.

facultative and aerobic bacilli are especially important in hematogenous spinal osteomyelitis, while gram-positive aerobic cocci are important in contiguous osteomyelitis and septic arthritis (300–302). One should remember that osteomyelitis, especially that of the contiguous type, is rarely due to a single organism. In most cases, a mixed flora is obtained upon culture of the infection site, making antimicrobial selection a difficult task.

Tables 12 and 13 illustrate the results of open and comparative trials of quinolones in skin, soft tissue, and bone infections in geriatric patients, respectively (303–314). Although the quinolones appear to be reasonable alternatives in the treatment of such infections, their modest coverage of gram-positive pathogens coupled with their superior gram-negative coverage suggests that these agents should be reserved for the treatment of complicated soft tissue infections such as infected pressure ulcers or chronic osteomyelitis and used with caution, if at all, in the treatment of acute osteomyelitis and septic arthritis. Development of resistance with subsequent therapeutic failure has been noted in infections due to *P. aeruginosa*, *S. aureus*, and *Serratia marcescens*, especially in the presence of prosthetic devices (31). The need for additional antianaerobic coverage with metronidazole or clindamycin during quinolone treatment of deep soft tissue infections is unresolved.

F. Miscellaneous Infections

Tables 14 and 15 document the results of open and comparative trials of the quinolones in the treatment of sepsis in elderly patients, respectively (315–317), while Tables 16 and 17 document results of such trials in the treatment of a variety of infections in older patients (318–329).

G. Summary

Currently available quinolones are suboptimal therapy for streptococcal infections. Similarly, monotherapy with currently available quinolones for outpatient-acquired pneumonia should be viewed with caution due to their suboptimal coverage of three major pathogens of this disease entity: *S. pneumoniae*, *M. pneumoniae*, and oral anaerobes. A similar argument may be applicable to the treatment of sinusitis and otitis media. For outpatient-acquired cellulitis—often due to β-hemolytic streptococci, which exhibit variable sensitivity to marketed quinolones—first-generation cephalosporins or antistaphylococcal penicillins remain the drugs of choice.

Clearly, the quinolones have many proven and potential indications in the geriatric population including treatment of UTIs caused by susceptible organisms resistant to standard therapy, UTIs in patients allergic to other agents and prostatitis; curative or suppressive therapy for chronic osteomyelitis; eradication of Salmonella and meningococcal carrier states, bacterial infectious diarrhea including "traveler's diarrhea," and invasive external otitis; and perhaps treatment of sepsis. Data are insufficient at present to support their routine use in the treatment of acute septic arthritis and osteomyelitis, bacterial meningitis, gram-positive or anaerobic bacteremia, and infective endocarditis.

VI. DRUG ADMINISTRATION

Tables 18 and 19 illustrate the oral and parenteral dosage formulations and regimens of quinolones marketed in the United States as of the time of this writing. In addition, dosage regimen adjustment for impaired renal function is recommended as follows:

norfloxacin, ciprofloxacin, enoxacin: halve the dose *or* double the dosing interval when creatinine clearance (CrCl) < 30 ml/min
ofloxacin: double the dosing interval for CrCl 10–50 ml/min; halve the dose *and* double the dosing interval for CrCl < 10 ml/min
lomefloxacin: standard initial dose, then halve the subsequent doses for CrCl < 40 ml/min

Dosage adjustment for the presence of hepatic dysfunction appears to be unnecessary with these agents.

VII. ADVERSE EFFECTS

The quinolones appear to be relatively safe and effective antimicrobial agents. Although, in general, exposure rates in general practice have been insufficient to detect relatively rare untoward effects or permit determination of precise rate data, worldwide exposure to a few agents such as ciprofloxacin, enoxacin, norfloxacin, ofloxacin, and pefloxacin has been sufficient to generate a profile of more common reactions and their rates.

To date, overall rates appear to be low and comparable to or less than those observed with other antimicrobial classes. Rates have ranged from 2–25% with a mean of 4–8% in large trials or reviews of pooled data (330). Tables 7 through 17 illustrate incidence and specific type adverse event data from selected clinical trials conducted in exclusively or predominantly elderly patient populations. Obviously, many factors are responsible for the wide range of incidence data, including differences in criteria for assessment of relationship to therapy, methods of data analysis, and geographic location.

With the exception of temafloxacin, adverse reactions to the quinolones have been innocuous or of mild to moderate severity. Severe reactions necessitating discontinuation of therapy have been infrequent, with rates for individual drugs as shown in Table 20 (330). Rates for gastrointestinal (GI), central nervous system (CNS), cutaneous, and musculoskeletal (MS) adverse events of selected quinolones are illustrated in Table 21 (330). The most common GI adverse effects include nausea, diarrhea, vomiting, epigastric burning, abdominal cramps, anorexia, and flatulence (in descending order). Pseudomembranous colitis has been decidedly rare among quinolone recipients for unknown reasons, although the maintenance of normal anaerobic gut flora due to the poor activity of most quinolones against anaerobes may be a factor. The most common CNS adverse events are related to stimulation and include tremulousness, anxiety, nervousness, insomnia, euphoria, nightmares, hallucinations, mania, and psychosis. MS reactions such as myalgia or arthralgia and cutaneous reactions are rarely seen.

Although convulsive seizures are rare events with quinolones, it appears that elderly patients may constitute an "at-risk" population in this regard (331–336). This appears to be the case whether considering seizures due to quinolone monotherapy or quinolone-theophylline drug–drug interaction. In fact, of the 17 patients reported by Grasela and Dreis to have developed seizures as a result of the interaction of ciprofloxacin or norfloxacin with theophylline, 13 were over 60 years of age (331). In view of the central nervous system excitatory effects of the quinolones, the theoretical potentiation of these effects by NSAIDs, and the interaction potential with methylxanthines, elderly patients should be monitored carefully for manifestations such as tremors, insomnia, and restlessness as premonitory signs of seizure potential.

Table 13 Comparative Trials of Quinolones in the Treatment of Soft Tissue and Bone Infections in Elderly Patients

Study design	Drug	Dosing regimen (mg/frequency/route)	Mean duration of therapy (days)[a]	No. patients	Clinical efficacy (% cure)	Bacterio-logical eradication (%)	Adverse events	Ref.
C,R	Ciprofloxacin	750/b.i.d./PO	7–10 (5–21)	24	96	88	Ciprofloxacin—diarrhea, ↑ SGOT, ↑ SGPT, ↑ serum creatinine	310
	Cefotaxime	2000/t.i.d./IV	7–10 (5–21)	32	94	69	Cefotaxime—candidiasis, dehydration, diarrhea (adverse events not quantified)	
C,R	Ciprofloxacin + local treatment[b]	250–750/b.i.d./PO	90 (NA)	18	17(67)[c]	33	Ciprofloxacin—resistant flora overgrowth, nausea (83.3% overall incidence)	311
	Local treatment[b]		90 (NA)	8	0 (13)[c]	13		
C,R	Ciprofloxacin	200/b.i.d./IV → 750/b.i.d./PO	25 (2–50)	32	75	78	Ciprofloxacin—superinfection in 9 patients; nausea, dizziness, altered mental status, ↓ platelets, hepatic necrosis (21.9% overall incidence)	312

	Ceftazidime	2000/t.i.d./IV	19 (3–42)	19	58	72	Ceftazidime—superinfection in 3 patients; allergic reaction, fever, eosinophilia (21.1% overall incidence)	
C,R	Enoxacin	400/b.i.d./PO	10 (NA)	16	56	93	Enoxacin—superinfection in 3 patients, no quantitation of adverse events	313
	Ceftriaxone	2000/q.d./IV	9 (NA)	14	69	92	Ceftriaxone—no quantitation of adverse events	
C,R	Pefloxacin	400/t.i.d./PO or IV →400/b.i.d./PO or IV	13 (3–45)	34	47	68	Pefloxacin—nausea, vomiting, ↑ hepatic function tests (11.8% overall incidence)	314
	Ceftazidime	2000/t.i.d./IV	10 (3–17)	33	39	67	Ceftazidime—none reported	

NA = not available; C = controlled; R = randomized; SGOT = serum aspartate aminotransferase; SGPT = serum alanine aminotransferase.
[a]Range in parentheses.
[b]Local treatment = chlorhexidine or potassium permanganate bathes, mechanical and enzymatic debridement, dextranomer or Duoderm® coverings.
[c]Cure or decreased ulcer size in parentheses.

Table 14 Open Trials of Quinolones in the Treatment of Sepsis in Elderly Patients

Drug	Dosing regimen (mg/frequency/route)	Mean duration of therapy (days)[a]	No. patients	Clinical efficacy (% cure)	Bacteriological eradication (%)	Adverse events	Ref.
Pefloxacin	400/b.i.d./IV	12 (5–19)	30	76	96	Anaphylaxis (3.3% overall incidence)	315

[a]Range in parentheses.

Table 15 Comparative Trials of Quinolones in the Treatment of Sepsis in Elderly Patients

Study design	Drug	Dosing regimen (mg/frequency/route)	Mean duration of therapy (days)[a]	No. patients	Clinical efficacy (% cure)	Bacterio-logical eradication (%)	Adverse events	Ref.
C,R	Ciprofloxacin	200/b.i.d./IV	11.8 (NA)	36	92	94	Rash, ↓ or ↑ platelets, WBC, vomiting, altered hepatic function tests, others not specified (overall incidence IV group = 22.7%, IV→PO group = 22.2%)	316
	Ciprofloxacin	200/b.i.d./IV →750/b.i.d./PO	13.8 (NA)	29	93	96		
C,R	Ofloxacin	200/b.i.d./PO	12.4 (NA)	9	100	100	Ofloxacin—none reported	317
	Ceftriaxone	1000/q.d./IM or IV	11.6 (NA)	9	100	100	Ceftriaxone—rash (11.1% overall incidence)	

NA = not available; C = controlled; R = randomized; WBC = white blood cell.
[a]Range in parentheses.

Table 16 Open Trials of Quinolones in the Treatment of Various Infections in Elderly Patients

Drug	Dosing regimen (mg/frequency/route)	Mean duration of therapy (days)[a]	No. patients	Clinical efficacy (% cure)	Bacterio-logical eradication (%)	Adverse events	Ref.
Ciprofloxacin	750/b.i.d./PO	13 (5–23)	25 (19 STI, 6 RTI)	48	52	Diarrhea, nausea, headache, blurred vision, rash (40% overall incidence, 2 patients withdrew due to adverse events)	318
Ciprofloxacin	250/b.i.d./PO 500/q.d./PO 500/b.i.d./PO	8.8 (NA)[b]	19 13 26 (24 RTI, 28 UTI, 6 other)	79[b]	88[b]	Epigastric pain, diarrhea, nausea (5.2% overall incidence)	319
Ciprofloxacin	750/b.i.d./PO	10.5 (3–42)	58 (34 UTI, 13 RTI, 9 STI, 1 bone, 1 sepsis)	78	85	Candidal colonization, GI upset, rash, chest pain, renal failure, tremors, ↑ theophylline level (29% overall incidence)	320
Ciprofloxacin	200–400/b.i.d.-t.i.d./IV →500–1000/b.i.d./PO if appropriate	5 (2–19)[c] 17.5 (0–93)[d]	32 (15 STI, 10 bone, 5 RTI, 1 perit., 1 UTI)	44	44	Rash, crystalluria, phlebitis, nausea, anorexia (32.4% overall incidence)	321
Ciprofloxacin	250–500/q.d.-b.i.d./PO	8 (1–18)	212 (UTI, RTI, GTI, STI, J—not quantitated)	76	89	Rash, gastric discomfort, diarrhea, headache, ↑SGOT, ↑SGPT, ↑serum creatinine (6.1% overall incidence)	322

Ciprofloxacin	200–300/b.i.d./IV →500–750/b.i.d./PO	13 (5–18) (N = 9)[c] 6 (2–15) →8 (2–165) (N = 31)[e]	40 (8 sepsis, 8 RTI, 5 UTI, 15 STI, 2 GTI, 1 endo, 1 bone)	63	75	Diarrhea, ↑serum creatinine (5.0% overall incidence)	323
Fleroxacin	400/q.d./IV	NA (1–21)	47 (38 UTI, 3 RTI, 6 STI)	96	91	Nausea, vomiting diarrhea, hypotension, injection site reaction (9% overall incidence)	324
Ofloxacin	300/b.i.d./PO	NA (NA)	74 (distribution of infections not stated)	91[f]	73 (RTI) 93 (UTI)	Vomiting, dermatitis, rash (4% overall incidence)	325
Ofloxacin	200/b.i.d./IV →200–400/b.i.d./PO—if appropriate	NA (3–10)	87 (30 UTI, 11 BJ, 8 GTI, 3 STI, 35 RTI, 8 sepsis)	75	86	Nausea, rash, phlebitis, renal failure (4.6% overall incidence)	326

NA = not available; STI = soft tissue infection; RTI = respiratory tract infection; UTI = urinary tract infection; perit = peritoneal infection; GTI = gastrointestinal tract infection; J = joint; endo = endocarditis; BJ = bone and/or joint; GI = gastrointestinal; SGOT = serum aspartate aminotransferase; SGPT = serum alanine aminotransferase.

[a]Range in parentheses.

[b]Pooled results over all study groups.

[c]Intravenous.

[d]Oral.

[e]IV→oral group.

[f]Cure or improvement.

Table 17 Comparative Trials of Quinolones in the Treatment of Various Infections in Elderly Patients

Study design	Drug	Dosing regimen (mg/frequency/route)	Mean duration of therapy (days)[a]	No. patients	Clinical efficacy (% cure)	Bacterio-logical eradication (%)	Adverse events	Ref.
C,R	Ciprofloxacin	200/b.i.d./IV	NA (NA)	32	79	79	↑ or ↓ platelets (14.7% ciprofloxacin group, 5.6% ceftazidime group)	327
	Ceftazidime	2000/t.i.d./IV	NA (NA)	36 (7 sepsis, 34 UTI, 29 RTI, 1 IA, 1 STI)	89	89		
C,R	Ciprofloxacin	200–300/b.i.d./IV →500/b.i.d./PO	16(7–25)[b]	16	41	54	Ciprofloxacin—rash (no quantitation of adverse events)	328
	Ceftazidime	1000–1500/b.i.d.-t.i.d./IV		16 (2 sepsis, 3 bone, 2 IA, 13 RTI, 13 STI, 5 UTI)	48	56	Ceftazidime—interstitial nephritis, renal failure, phlebitis (no quantitation of adverse events)	
C,R	Pefloxacin	400/t.i.d./IV →400/b.i.d./IV	10.5 (5–33)	21	71	86	Pefloxacin—none reported	329
	Cefotaxime	1000–2000/t.i.d./IV	8.5 (6–14)	18 (9 IA, 6 sepsis, 16 RTI, 5 STI, 10 UTI, 1 GU)	72	67	Cefotaxime—none reported	

NA = not available; C = controlled; R = randomized; UTI = urinary tract infection; RTI = respiratory tract infection; IA = intraabdominal infection; STI = soft tissue infection; GU = genitourinary infection.

[a]Range in parentheses.

[b]Pooled results over both study groups.

Table 18 Oral Dosage Regimens and Formulations of Quinolones Marketed in the United States

Quinolone	Formulation	Infection type	Regimen[a]
Norfloxacin	400 mg tablets	UTI	400 mg b.i.d.
Ciprofloxacin	250 mg tablets	UTI	250–500 mg b.i.d.
	500 mg tablets	LRTI,B + J,SSSI	500–750 mg b.i.d.
	750 mg tablets	Diarrhea	500 mg b.i.d.
Ofloxacin	200 mg tablets	LRTI	400 mg b.i.d.
	300 mg tablets	SSSI	400 mg b.i.d.
	400 mg tablets	UTI	200 mg b.i.d.
		Prostatitis	300 mg b.i.d.
Lomefloxacin	400 mg tablets	LRTI	400 mg q.d.
		UTI	400 mg q.d.

UTI = urinary tract infection; LRTI = lower respiratory tract infection; B + J = bone + joint infection; SSSI = skin and skin structure infection.
[a]q.d. = once daily, b.i.d. = twice daily; unadjusted for impaired renal function (for latter, see text).

Several investigator groups have attempted to identify factors associated with an increased risk for adverse reactions, including advancing age. Although Shah and Frech have suggested that advancing age predisposes to toxicity (337), other investigators have been unable to identify any relationship between risk and age (338–344). In addition, preliminary data suggest that increasing dosage or serum drug concentrations may be associated with increased risk of toxicity, but further data are needed to corroborate these findings (207,336,345,346).

VIII. CONCLUSION

Systematic investigation of structure-activity relationships has led to the development of the fluoroquinolone class of antimicrobials over the past decade. These agents are

Table 19 Parenteral (Intravenous) Dosage Regimens and Formulations of Quinolones Marketed in the United States

Quinolone	Formulation	Infection type	Regimen[a]
Ciprofloxacin	200 mg/20 mL vial	UTI	200–400 mg b.i.d.
	400 mg/40 mL vial	LRTI,SSSI,B + J	400 mg b.i.d.
	200 mg/100 mL premixed bag		
	400 mg/200 mL premixed bag		
Ofloxacin	400 mg/10 or 20 mL vial	UTI	200 mg b.i.d.
	400 mg/100 mL premixed bottle	Prostatitis	300 mg b.i.d.
	200 mg/50 mL premixed bag	LRTI, SSSI	400 mg b.i.d.
	400 mg/100 mL premixed bag		

UTI = urinary tract infection; LRTI = lower respiratory tract infection; SSSI = skin and skin structure infection; B + J = bone + joint infection.
[a]b.i.d. = twice daily; unadjusted for impaired renal function (for latter, see text).

Table 20 Adverse Reactions to Quinolones Necessitating Discontinuation of Therapy

Quinolone	Rate (%)
Ciprofloxacin	1.2–2.9
Enoxacin	2.6–6.5
Norfloxacin	1.0–1.2
Ofloxacin	1.4–1.7
Pefloxacin	1.3–2.2

Source: Ref. 330.

Table 21 Rates of Gastrointestinal, Central Nervous System, Cutaneous, and Musculoskeletal Adverse Reactions to Quinolones

	Rate (%)			
Quinolone	GI	CNS	Cutaneous	MS
Ciprofloxacin	2.1–8.1	0.4–4.4	0.4–1.9	0.08–0.2
Enoxacin	3.4–3.8	1.1–1.2	0.7	0.04
Norfloxacin	2.1–4.5	0.8–1.7	0.4–0.7	0.1
Ofloxacin	2.6–3.0	0.9–1.0	0.4–0.6	<1.0
Pefloxacin	4.2–5.6	0.9–1.1	2.2–2.4	0.9

GI = gastrointestinal; CNS = central nervous system; MS = musculoskeletal.
Source: Ref. 330.

characterized by a broad antimicrobial spectrum of activity and favorable pharmacokinetic properties, both of which lend themselves to extensive use in many patient populations, including the geriatric population. Although these agents have proven to be valuable additions to our therapeutic armamentarium, problems have emerged with their widespread use, including significant pharmacokinetic drug interactions, development of resistance, and misuse for infections for which they are unnecessary or insufficient therapy. Only with judicious use of these agents will we preserve their utility in the years to come.

REFERENCES

1. Lesher GY, Froelich EJ, Gruett MD, et al. 1,8-Naphthyridine derivatives. A new class of chemotherapeutic agents. J Med Pharm Chem 1962; 5:1063–5.
2. Ronald AR, Turck M, Petersdorf RG. A critical evaluation of nalidixic acid in urinary tract infections. N Engl J Med 1966; 275:1081–9.
3. Percival A. Impact of chemical structure on quinolone potency, spectrum, and side effects. J Antimicrob Chemother 1991; 28(suppl C):1–8.
4. Gleckman R, Alvarez S, Joubert DW, et al. Drug therapy reviews: oxolinic acid. Am J Hosp Pharm 1979; 36:1077–9.
5. Guay DRP. Cinoxacin (Cinobac, Eli Lilly & Co.). Drug Intell Clin Pharm 1982; 16:916–21.
6. Cameron DW, Ronald AR. The older DNA-gyrase inhibitors. Res Clin For 1985; 7:81–7.

7. Shimizu M, Takase Y, Nakamura S, et al. Pipemidic acid, a new antibacterial agent active against Pseudomonas aeruginosa. in vitro properties. Antimicrob Agents Chemother 1975; 8:132–8.
8. Rohlfing SR, Gerster JF, Kvam DC. Bioevaluation of the antibacterial flumequine for urinary tract use. Antimicrob Agents Chemother 1976; 10:20–4.
9. Smith JT. Awakening the slumbering potential of the 4-quinolone antibacterials. Pharmaceut J 1984; 233:299–305.
10. Neu HC, Chin N-X. In vitro activity of S-ofloxacin. Antimicrob Agents Chemother 1989; 33:1105–7.
11. Chu DTW, Fernandes PB. Structure-activity relationships of the fluoroquinolones. Antimicrob Agents Chemother 1989; 33:131–5.
12. Hooper DC, Wolfson JS. Fluoroquinolone antimicrobial agents. N Engl J Med 1991; 324:384–94.
13. Wolfson JS, Hooper DC. Fluoroquinolone antimicrobial agents. Clin Microbiol Rev 1989; 2:378–424.
14. Vergin H, Metz R. Review of developments in fluoroquinolones. Drugs Today 1991; 27:177–92.
15. Hooper DC, Wolfson JS. Mode of action of the new quinolones: new data. Eur J Clin Microbiol Infect Dis 1991; 10:223–31.
16. Fitton A. The quinolones: an overview of their pharmacology. Clin Pharmacokinet 1992; 22(suppl 1):1–11.
17. Segreti J, Nelson JA, Goodman LJ, et al. In vitro activities of lomefloxacin and temafloxacin against pathogens causing diarrhea. Antimicrob Agents Chemother 1989; 33:1385–7.
18. Talbot H, Romanowski B. In vitro activities of lomefloxacin, tetracycline, penicillin, spectinomycin, and ceftriaxone against *Neisseria gonorrhoeae* and *Chlamydia trachomatis*. Antimicrob Agents Chemother 1989; 33:2049–51.
19. Venezia RA, Prymas LA, Shayegani A, et al. In vitro activities of amifloxacin and two of its metabolites. Antimicrob Agents Chemother 1989; 33:762–6.
20. Kenny GE, Cartwright FD. Susceptibility of *Mycoplasma pneumoniae* to several new quinolones, tetracycline, and erythromycin. Antimicrob Agents Chemother 1991; 35:587–9.
21. Hirose T, Okezaki E, Kato H, et al. In vitro and in vivo activity of NY-198, a new difluorinated quinolone. Antimicrob Agents Chemother 1987; 31:854–9.
22. Van der Auwera P, Grenier P, Glupczynski Y, et al. In vitro activity of lomefloxacin in comparison with pefloxacin and ofloxacin. J Antimicrob Chemother 1989; 23:209–19.
23. Wise R, Andrews JM, Ashby JP, et al. In vitro activity of lomefloxacin, a new quinolone antimicrobial agent, in comparison with those of other agents. Antimicrob Agents Chemother 1988; 32:617–22.
24. Chin N-X, Novelli A, Neu HC. In vitro activity of lomefloxacin (SC-47111; NY-198), a difluoroquinolone-3-carboxylic acid, compared with those of other quinolones. Antimicrob Agents Chemother 1988; 32:656–62.
25. Mayer KH, Ellal JA. Lomefloxacin: a microbiological assessment and unique properties. Am J Med 1992; 92(suppl 4A):58*S*–62*S*.
26. Furet YX, Pechere JC. Newly documented antimicrobial activity of quinolones. Eur J Clin Microbiol Infect Dis 1991; 10:249–54.
27. Craig WA, Gudmundsson S. The post-antibiotic effect. In: Lorian V, ed. Antibiotics in laboratory medicine. Baltimore, MD: Williams & Wilkins, 1986:515–36.
28. Craig WA, Ebert S. Killing and regrowth of bacteria in vitro: a review. Scand J Infect Dis 1991; 74(suppl):63–70.
29. Neu HC. The quinolones. Infect Dis Clin North Am 1989; 3:625–39.
30. Baquero F, Martinez-Beltram J, Loza E. A review of antibiotic resistance patterns of Streptococcus pneumoniae in Europe. J Antimicrob Chemother 1991; 28(suppl C):31–8.
31. Guay DRP. Current role of fluoroquinolones. Pharmacotherapy 1992; 12(6 Pt 2):71*S*–85*S*.
32. Guay DRP, Somani SK, Cooper SL, et al. Antimicrobial resistance patterns in long-term care facilities. J Geriatr Drug Ther 1991; 6(2):29–44.

33. Neumann M. Clinical pharmacokinetics of the newer antimicrobial 4-quinolones. Clin Pharmacokinet 1988; 14:96–121.
34. Drusano GL. Pharmacokinetics of the quinolone antimicrobial agents. In: Wolfson JS, Hooper DC, eds. Quinolone antimicrobial agents. Washington, DC: American Society for Microbiology, 1989:71–105.
35. Gros I, Carbon C. Pharmacokinetics of lomefloxacin in healthy volunteers: comparison of 400 milligrams once daily and 200 milligrams twice daily given orally for 5 days. Antimicrob Agents Chemother 1990; 34:150–2.
36. Adhami S, Wise R, Weston D, et al. The pharmacokinetics and tissue penetration of norfloxacin. J Antimicrob Chemother 1984; 13:87–92.
37. Vance-Bryan K, Guay DRP, Rotschafer JC. Clinical pharmacokinetics of ciprofloxacin. Clin Pharmacokinet 1990; 19:434–61.
38. Chang T, Block A, Dunky A, et al. Pharmacokinetics of intravenous and oral enoxacin in healthy volunteers. J Antimicrob Chemother 1988; 21(suppl B):49–56.
39. Stone JW, Andrews JM, Ashby JP, et al. Pharmacokinetics and tissue penetration of orally administered lomefloxacin. Antimicrob Agents Chemother 1988; 32:1508–10.
40. Lamp KC, Bailey EM, Rybak MJ. Ofloxacin clinical pharmacokinetics. Clin Pharmacokinet 1992; 22:32–46.
41. Schentag JJ, Gengo FM. Principles of antibiotic tissue penetration and guidelines for pharmacokinetic analysis. Med Clin North Am 1982; 66:39–49.
42. Schentag JJ, Swanson DJ, Smith IL. Dual individualization-antibiotic usage calculation from the integration of in vitro pharmacodynamics and in vivo pharmacokinetics. J Antimicrob Chemother 1985; 15(suppl A):47–57.
43. Schentag JJ, Cumbo TJ, Jusko WE, et al. Gentamicin tissue accumulation and nephrotoxic reactions. JAMA 1978; 240:2067–9.
44. Schentag JJ, Jusko WJ, Vance JW, et al. Gentamicin disposition and tissue accumulation on multiple dosing. J Pharmacokinet Biopharm 1977; 5:559–77.
45. Stroshane RM, Silverman MH, Sauerschell R, et al. Preliminary study of the pharmacokinetics of oral amifloxacin in elderly subjects. Antimicrob Agents Chemother 1990; 34:751–4.
46. Cogo R, Rimoldi R, Mattina R, et al. Steady-state pharmacokinetics of rufloxacin in elderly patients with lower respiratory tract infections. Ther Drug Monitor 1992; 14:36–41.
47. Granneman GR, Guay DRP. The influence of age on the pharmacokinetics of temafloxacin. Am J Med 1991; 91(suppl 6A):71*S*–75*S*.
48. Wise R, Baker SL, Misra M, et al. The pharmacokinetics of enoxacin in elderly patients. J Antimicrob Chemother 1987; 19:343–50.
49. Marchbanks CR, Mikolich DJ, Mayer KH, et al. Pharmacokinetics and bioavailability of intravenous-to-oral enoxacin in elderly patients with complicated urinary tract infections. Antimicrob Agents Chemother 1990; 34:1966–72.
50. Marcotte A, Parent M, Bergeron MG, et al. Pharmacokinetics of fleroxacin after multiple doses in elderly population. Clin Pharmacol Ther 1989; 45:164.
51. Taburet AM, Devillers A, Thomare P, et al. Disposition of fleroxacin, a new trifluoroquinolone, and its metabolites. Pharmacokinetics in elderly patients. Clin Pharmacokinet 1990; 19:80–8.
52. Kelly JG, Deaney NB, Lavan J, et al. Chronic dose urinary and serum pharmacokinetics of norfloxacin in the elderly. Br J Clin Pharmacol 1988; 26:787–90.
53. MacGowan AP, Greig MA, Clarke EA, et al. The pharmacokinetics of norfloxacin in the aged. J Antimicrob Chemother 1988; 22:721–7.
54. LeBel M, Vallee F, Marcotte N, et al. Tissue penetration of lomefloxacin in young and elderly healthy volunteers. Pharmacotherapy 1989; 9:185.
55. Crome P, Morrison PJ. Pharmacokinetics of a single oral dose of lomefloxacin in healthy elderly volunteers. Drug Invest 1991; 3:183–7.

56. Woodworth J, Fitzsimmons S. Lomefloxacin pharmacokinetics in young and elderly subjects. Proceedings of the Twenty-Ninth Interscience Conference on Antimicrobial Agents and Chemotherapy, Houston, TX, 1989, abstract 1268.
57. Cowling P, Rogers S, McMullin CM, et al. The pharmacokinetics of lomefloxacin in elderly patients with urinary tract infection following daily dosing with 400 mg. J Antimicrob Chemother 1991; 28:101–7.
58. Rademaker CMA, Jones RW, Notarianni LJ, et al. Pharmacokinetics of a single dose of ofloxacin in healthy elderly subjects using noncompartmental and compartmental models. Pharm Weekblad 1989; 11:224–8.
59. Flor S, Beals B, Tack K, et al. Pharmacokinetics of ofloxacin in healthy geriatric subjects after single oral dose and during multiple oral dose administration. Proceedings of the Twenty-Seventh Interscience Conference on Antimicrobial Agents and Chemotherapy, New York, 1987, abstract 1261.
60. Louie T, Loewen R, Rayner E, et al. Pharmacokinetics and metabolism of ofloxacin in elderly women after single dose and during multiple oral dose administration. Proceedings of the Twenty-Ninth Interscience Conference on Antimicrobial Agents and Chemotherapy, Houston, TX, 1989, abstract 203.
61. Martin C, Lambert D, Saux P, et al. Modification of ofloxacin pharmacokinetics in mechanically ventilated patients. Pathol Biol 1990; 38:508–12.
62. Freymann H, Stapel A, Ruge W. Pharmacokinetics and efficacy of ofloxacin in patients with exacerbation of chronic bronchitis. Rev Infect Dis 1989; 11(suppl 5):*S*1107.
63. Veyssier P, Humbert G, Modai J, et al. Pharmacokinetics of oral ofloxacin, single and repeated doses in 55 year old subjects (N = 12). Comparison with kinetics in 20 year olds (N = 24) and elderly patients ≥ 70 years old (N = 16). Proceedings of the Third International Symposium on New Quinolones, Vancouver, Canada, 1990, abstract 441.
64. Graber H, Ludwig E, Arr M, et al. Pharmacokinetics of ofloxacin in young and elderly patients. Rev Infect Dis 1988; 10(suppl 1):*S*106.
65. Dow J, Frydman AM, Djebbar F, et al. Single- and multiple-dose pharmacokinetics of pefloxacin in elderly patients. Rev Infect Dis 1988; 10(suppl 1):*S*107.
66. Schmit JL, Hary L, Devandeville A. Pefloxacin kinetics in elderly ill patients. Proceedings of the Third International Symposium on New Quinolones, Vancouver, Canada, 1990, abstract 445.
67. Sultan E, Richard C, Pezzano M, et al. Pharmacokinetics of pefloxacin and amikacin administered simultaneously to intensive care patients. Eur J Clin Pharmacol 1988; 34:637–43.
68. Urso R, Segre G, Cerretani D, et al. Plasma and urine pharmacokinetics of ciprofloxacin in man after single oral administration. Eur J Pharmacol 1990; 183:1860–1.
69. Deeter RG, Weinstein MP, Swanson KA, et al. Comparative pharmacokinetics (PKS) of oral ciprofloxacin (CIP) alone in combination with rifampin (RIF) in healthy elderly volunteers. Proceedings of the Twenty-Ninth Interscience Conference on Antimicrobial Agents and Chemotherapy, Houston, TX, 1989, abstract 201.
70. Ljungberg B, Nilsson-Ehle I. Pharmacokinetics of ciprofloxacin in the elderly: increased oral bioavailability and reduced renal clearance. Eur J Clin Microbiol Infect Dis 1989; 8:515–20.
71. LeBel M, Barbeau G, Bergeron MG, et al. Pharmacokinetics of ciprofloxacin in elderly subjects. Pharmacotherapy 1986; 6:87–91.
72. Bayer A, Gajewska A, Stephens M, et al. Pharmacokinetics of ciprofloxacin in the elderly. Respiration 1987; 51:292–5.
73. Kitzes-Cohen R, Gilon D, Shachar H, et al. Comparison of pharmacokinetic parameters in old and young patients after a single intravenous dose of ciprofloxacin. Proceedings of the Third International Symposium on New Quinolones, Vancouver, Canada, 1990, abstract 11.
74. Kees F, Naber KG, Meyer GP, et al. Pharmacokinetics of ciprofloxacin in elderly patients. Arzneim Forsch 1989; 39:523–7.

75. Naber KG, Sorgel F, Kees F, et al. Pharmacokinetics of ciprofloxacin in young (healthy volunteers) and elderly patients, and concentrations in prostatic fluid, seminal fluid, and prostatic adenoma tissue following intravenous administration. Am J Med 1989; 87(suppl 5A):57*S*–59*S*.
76. Ball AP, Fox C, Ball ME, et al. Pharmacokinetics of oral ciprofloxacin, 100 mg single dose, in volunteers and elderly patients. J Antimicrob Chemother 1986; 17:629–35.
77. Chandler MHH, Toler SM, Rapp RP, et al. Multiple-dose pharmacokinetics of concurrent oral ciprofloxacin and rifampin therapy in elderly patients. Antimicrob Agents Chemother 1990; 34:442–7.
78. Guay DRP, Awni WM, Peterson PK, et al. Single and multiple dose pharmacokinetics of oral ciprofloxacin in elderly patients. Int J Clin Pharmacol Ther Toxicol 1988; 26:279–84.
79. Hirata CAI, Guay DRP, Awni WM, et al. Steady-state pharmacokinetics of intravenous and oral ciprofloxacin in elderly patients. Antimicrob Agents Chemother 1989; 33:1927–31.
80. Fabre D, Bressolle F, Gomeni R, et al. Steady-state pharmacokinetics of ciprofloxacin in plasma from patients with nosocomial pneumonia: penetration of the bronchial mucosa. Antimicrob Agents Chemother 1991; 35:2521–5.
81. Ducroix JP, Smail A, Tondriaux A, et al. Clinical and pharmacokinetic evaluation of pefloxacin for the treatment of ascitic fluid infections. Rev Infect Dis 1989; 11(suppl 5):*S*1302.
82. Dan M, Serour F, Poch F, et al. Penetration of ciprofloxacin into human peritoneal tissue. Proceedings of the Third International Symposium on New Quinolones, Vancouver, Canada, 1990, abstract 138.
83. Dan M, Serour F, Gorea A, et al. Penetration of norfloxacin into muscle tissue of the abdominal wall. Rev Infect Dis 1989; 11(suppl 5):*S*1076.
84. Schmidt W, Eigel P, Zurcher J, et al. Ciprofloxacin as prophylaxis in open-heart surgery: distribution into serum, myocardium, skeletal muscle, and mediastinal fat. Rev Infect Dis 1989; 11(suppl 5):*S*1016.
85. Mertes PM, Voiriot P, Dopff C, et al. Penetration of ciprofloxacin into heart valves, myocardium, mediastinal fat, and sternal bone marrow in humans. Antimicrob Agents Chemother 1990; 34:398–401.
86. Wacha H, Wagner D, Schafer V, et al. Concentration of ciprofloxacin in bone tissue after single parenteral administration to patients older than 70 years. Infection 1990; 18:173–6.
87. Dellamonica P, Bernard E, Etesse H, et al. The diffusion of pefloxacin into bone and the treatment of osteomyelitis. J Antimicrob Chemother 1986; 17(suppl B):93–102.
88. On A, Nightingale CH, Quintiliani R, et al. Lomefloxacin concentrations in bone after a single oral dose. Am J Med 1992; 92(suppl 4A):15*S*–17*S*.
89. Fong IW, Rittenhouse BR, Simbul M, et al. Bone penetration of enoxacin in patients with and without osteomyelitis. Antimicrob Agents Chemother 1988; 32:834–7.
90. Skoutelis AT, Gartaganis SP, Chrysanthopoulos CJ, et al. Aqueous humor penetration of ciprofloxacin in the human eye. Arch Ophthalmol 1988; 106:404–5.
91. Bron A, Talon D, Cellier T, et al. The intraoccular penetration of ciprofloxacin in man. Pathol Biol 1989; 37:730–3.
92. Mounier A, Adenis JP, Denis F. Ciprofloxacin levels in human eye after intravenous and oral administration. Pathol Biol 1988; 36:724–7.
93. Salvanet A, Fisch A, Lafaix C, et al. Pefloxacin concentrations in human aqueous humour and lens. J Antimicrob Chemother 1986; 18:199–201.
94. Salvanet-Bouccara A, Montay G, Fisch A, et al. Ocular penetration of pefloxacin into aqueous humour and lens after multiple oral doses in man. J Fr Ophthalmol 1991; 14:260–4.
95. Leroy A, Bonmarchand G, Fourdrinier F, et al. Penetration of ciprofloxacin into bronchial secretions in patients with severe respiratory disease. Proceedings of the Twenty-Ninth Interscience Conference on Antimicrobial Agents and Chemotherapy, Houston, TX, 1989, abstract 207.
96. Saux P, Martin C, Portet C, et al. Penetration of ciprofloxacin into bronchial secretions in mechanically-ventilated patients. Pathol Biol 1991; 39:515–19.

97. Fong IW, Vandenbroucke A, Simbul M. Penetration of enoxacin into bronchial secretions. Antimicrob Agents Chemother 1987; 31:748–51.
98. Wijnands WJA, Vree TB, Baars AM, et al. Pharmacokinetics of enoxacin and its penetration into bronchial secretions and lung tissue. J Antimicrob Chemother 1988; 21(suppl B):67–77.
99. Symonds J, Javaid A, Bone M, et al. The penetration of ofloxacin into bronchial secretions. J Antimicrob Chemother 1988; 22(suppl C):91–5.
100. Kovarik JM, Smit J, Sips DJ, et al. Steady state pharmacokinetics and sputum penetration of lomefloxacin (LOM) in chronic bronchitis patients. Proceedings of the Thirtieth Interscience Conference on Antimicrobial Agents and Chemotherapy, Atlanta, GA, 1990, abstract 1005.
101. Honeybourne D, Andrews JM, Ashby JP, et al. Evaluation of the penetration of ciprofloxacin and amoxycillin into the bronchial mucosa. Thorax 1988; 43:715–19.
102. Forst H, Ruckdeschel G, Unertl K, et al. Lung tissue concentrations of ciprofloxacin following intravenous administration in patients. Arzneim Forsch 1989; 39:618–19.
103. Morgenroth A, Pfeuffer HP, Seelmann R, et al. Pleural penetration of ciprofloxacin in patients with empyema thoracis. Chest 1991; 100:406–9.
104. Blondin C, Costa P, Bressolle F, et al. Norfloxacin concentrations in plasma and human epididymal tissue after repeated dosage by oral route. Pathol Biol 1991; 39:520–3.
105. Galtier M, Costa P, Laurelli JM, et al. Pefloxacin penetration into the epididymis. Rev Infect Dis 1989; 11(suppl 5):*S*1361–*S*1362.
106. Boerema JBJ, Bach D, Jol C, et al. Penetration of rufloxacin into human prostatic tissue and fluid. J Antimicrob Chemother 1991; 28:547–54.
107. Aagaard J, Knes J, Madsen PO. Prostatic tissue levels of ofloxacin. Urology 1991; 38:380–2.
108. Aubert J, Lefebvre MA, Couet W, et al. Diffusion of ofloxacin into the prostate and kidney. Rev Infect Dis 1988; 10(suppl 1):*S*170.
109. Fujita K, Munakata A. Serum and prostatic tissue concentrations of ofloxacin. Clin Ther 1988; 10(spec):32–5.
110. Kovarik JM, deHond JAPM, Hoepelman IM, et al. Intraprostatic distribution of lomefloxacin following multiple-dose administration. Antimicrob Agents Chemother 1990; 34:2398–401.
111. Leroy A, Humbert G, Fillastre J-P, et al. Penetration of lomefloxacin into human prostatic tissue. Am J Med 1992; 92(suppl 4A):12*S*–14*S*.
112. Dan M, Golamb J, Gorea A, et al. Concentration of ciprofloxacin in human prostatic tissue after oral administration. Antimicrob Agents Chemother 1986; 30:88–9.
113. Gombert ME, duBouchet L, Aulicino TM, et al. Prostatic tissue concentrations of ciprofloxacin after oral administration. Am J Med 1987; 82(suppl 4A):130–2.
114. Desai KM, Abrams PH, White LO. A double-blind comparative trial of short-term orally administered enoxacin in the prevention of urinary infection after elective tansurethral prostatectomy: a clinical and pharmacokinetic study. J Urol 1988; 139:1232–4.
115. Bergeron MG, Roy R, Lessard C, et al. Enoxacin penetration into human prostatic tissue. Antimicrob Agents Chemother 1988; 32:1433–4.
116. Charton M, Timbal Y. In vivo diffusion of enoxacin in healthy renal and adenomatous prostate tissue in man. Eur Urol 1990; 17:252–6.
117. Naber KG, Sorgel F, Kees F, et al. In vitro activity of fleroxacin against isolates causing complicated urinary tract infections and concentrations in seminal and prostatic fluid and in prostatic adenoma tissue. J Antimicrob Chemother 1988; 22(suppl D):199–207.
118. Ljungberg B, Nilsson-Ehle I, Edlund C, et al. Impact of ciprofloxacin on the intestinal microflora in young and elderly persons: no effect of altered drug absorption. Proceedings of the Third International Symposium on New Quinolones, Vancouver, Canada, 1990, abstract 195.
119. Druckenbrod RW, Healy DP. In vitro delivery of crushed ciprofloxacin through a feeding tube. Ann Pharmacother 1992; 26:494–95.

120. Yuk JH, Nightingale CH, Sweeney KR, et al. Relative bioavailability in healthy volunteers of ciprofloxacin administered through a nasogastric tube with and without enteral feeding. Antimicrob Agents Chemother 1989; 33:1118–20.
121. Lubowski TJ, Nightingale CH, Sweeney K, et al. The relative bioavailability of temafloxacin administered through a nasogastric tube with and without enteral feeding. Clin Pharmacokinet 1992; 22(suppl 1):43–7.
122. Yuk JH, Nightingale CH, Quintiliani R, et al. Absorption of ciprofloxacin administered through a nasogastric or a nasoduodenal tube in volunteers and patients receiving enteral nutrition. Diagn Microbiol Infect Dis 1990; 13:99–102.
123. Sahai J, Memish Z, Conway B. Ciprofloxacin pharmacokinetics after administration via a jejunostomy tube. J Antimicrob Chemother 1991; 28:936–7.
124. Yuk JH, Williams TW Jr. Drug interaction with quinolone antibiotics in intensive care unit patients. Arch Intern Med 1991; 151:619.
125. Hoffken G, Borner K, Glatzel PD, et al. Reduced enteral absorption of ciprofloxacin in the presence of antacids. Eur J Clin Microbiol 1985; 4:345.
126. Akerele JO, Okhamafe AO. Influence of co-administered metallic drugs on ofloxacin pharmacokinetics. J Antimicrob Chemother 1991; 28:87–94.
127. Fleming LW, Moreland TA, Stewart WK, et al. Ciprofloxacin and antacids. Lancet 1986; 2:294.
128. Flor S, Guay DRP, Opsahl JA, et al. Effects of magnesium-aluminum hydroxide and calcium carbonate antacids on bioavailability of ofloxacin. Antimicrob Agents Chemother 1990; 34:2436–8.
129. Frost DW, Lettieri JT, Noe A, et al. Effect of aluminum hydroxide and calcium carbonate antacids on ciprofloxacin bioavailability. Clin Pharmacol Ther 1989; 45:165.
130. Golper T, Hartstein AI, Morthland VH, et al. Effects of antacids and dialysate dwell times on multiple dose pharmacokinetics of oral ciprofloxacin in patients on continuous ambulatory peritoneal dialysis. Antimicrob Agents Chemother 1987; 31:1787–90.
131. Grasela TH Jr., Schentag JJ, Sedman AJ, et al. Inhibition of enoxacin absorption by antacids or rantidine. Antimicrob Agents Chemother 1989; 33:615–17.
132. Hoffken G, Lode H, Wiley PD. Pharmacokinetics and interaction in the bioavailability of new quinolones. Proceedings of the International Symposium on the New Quinolones, Geneva, Switzerland, 1986, abstract 141.
133. Kara M, Hasinoff BB, McKay D, et al. Clinical and chemical interactions between iron preparations and ciprofloxacin. Br J Clin Pharmacol 1991; 31:257–61.
134. Maesen FPV, Davies BI, Geraedts WH, et al. Ofloxacin and antacids. J Antimicrob Chemother 1987; 19:848–9.
135. Nix DE, Watson WA, Lener ME, et al. Effects of aluminum and magnesium antacids and ranitidine on the absorption of ciprofloxacin. Clin Pharmacol Ther 1989; 46:700–5.
136. Nix DE, Wilton JH, Schentag JJ, et al. Inhibition of norfloxacin absorption by antacids and sucralfate. Rev Infect Dis 1989; 11(suppl 5):*S*1096.
137. Nix DE, Wilton JH, Ronald B, et al. Inhibition of norfloxacin absorption by antacids. Antimicrob Agents Chemother 1990; 34:432–5.
138. Polk RE, Healy DP, Sahai J, et al. Effect of ferrous sulfate and multivitamins with zinc on absorption of ciprofloxacin in normal volunteers. Antimicrob Agents Chemother 1989; 33:1841–4.
139. Sahai J, Healy D, Stotka J, et al. Influence of chronic administration of calcium on the bioavailability of oral ciprofloxacin. Proceedings of the Twenty-Ninth Interscience Conference on Antimicrobial Agents and Chemotherapy, Houston, TX, 1989, abstract 211.
140. Granneman GR, Stephan U, Birner B, et al. Effect of antacid medication on the pharmacokinetics of temafloxacin. Clin Pharmacokinet 1992; 22(suppl 1):83–9.
141. Kivisto KT, Ojala-Karlsson P, Neuvonen PJ. Inhibition of norfloxacin absorption by dairy products. Antimicrob Agents Chemother 1992; 36:489–91.

142. Neuvonen PJ, Kivisto KT, Lehto P. Interference of dairy products with the absorption of ciprofloxacin. Clin Pharmacol Ther 1991; 50:498–502.
143. Garrelts JC, Godley PJ, Peterie JD, et al. Sucralfate significantly reduces ciprofloxacin concentrations in serum. Antimicrob Agents Chemother 1990; 34:931–3.
144. Nix DE, Watson WA, Handy L, et al. The effect of sucralfate pretreatment on the pharmacokinetics of ciprofloxacin. Pharmacotherapy 1989; 9:377–80.
145. Parpia SH, Nix DE, Hejmanowski LG, et al. Sucralfate reduces the gastrointestinal absorption of norfloxacin. Antimicrob Agents Chemother 1989; 33:99–102.
146. Sorgel F, Granneman R, Stephan U, et al. Effect of cimetidine on the pharmacokinetics of temafloxacin. Clin Pharmacokinet 1992; 22(suppl 1):75–82.
147. Wingender W, Foerster D, Beerman D. Effect of gastric emptying time on rate and extent of the systemic availability of ciprofloxacin. Proceedings of the Fourteenth International Congress of Chemotherapy, Kyoto, Japan, 1985, abstract P-37-91.
148. Stutman HR, Parker KM, Marks MI. Potential of moxalactam and other new antimicrobial agents for bilirubin-albumin displacement in neonates. Pediatrics 1985; 75:294–8.
149. Beckman J, Elsasser W, Gundert-Remy U, et al. Enoxacin—a potent inhibitor of theophylline metabolism. Eur J Clin Pharmacol 1987; 33:227–30.
150. Bowles SK, Popovski Z, Rybak MJ, et al. Effect of norfloxacin on theophylline pharmacokinetics at steady state. Antimicrob Agents Chemother 1988; 32:510–12.
151. Davis RL, Kelly HW, Quenzer RW, et al. Effect of norfloxacin on theophylline metabolism. Antimicrob Agents Chemother 1989; 33:212–14.
152. Gregoire SL, Grasela TH Jr., Freer JP, et al. Inhibition of theophylline clearance by coadministered ofloxacin without alteration of theophylline effects. Antimicrob Agents Chemother 1987; 31:375–8.
153. Ho G, Tierney MG, Dales RE. Evaluation of the effect of norfloxacin on the pharmacokinetics of theophylline. Clin Pharmacol Ther 1988; 44:35–8.
154. Niki Y, Soejima R, Kawane H, et al. New synthetic quinolone antibacterial agents and serum concentration of theophylline. Chest 1987; 92:663–9.
155. Nix DE, DeVito JM, Whitebread MA, et al. Effect of multiple dose oral ciprofloxacin on the pharmacokinetics of theophylline and indocyanine green. Br J Clin Pharmacol 1987; 19:263–9.
156. Nix DE, Norman A, Schentag JJ. Effect of lomefloxacin on theophylline pharmacokinetics. Antimicrob Agents Chemother 1989; 33:1006–8.
157. Raoof S, Wollschlager C, Khan FA. Ciprofloxacin increases serum levels of theophylline. Am J Med 1987; 82(supp 4A):115–18.
158. Rogge MC, Solomon WR, Sedman AJ, et al. The theophylline-enoxacin interaction: I. effect of enoxacin dose size on theophylline disposition. Clin Pharmacol Ther 1988; 44:579–87.
159. Rogge MC, Solomon WR, Sedman AJ, et al. The theophylline-enoxacin interaction. II. changes in the disposition of theophylline and its metabolites during intermittent administration of enoxacin. Clin Pharmacol Ther 1989; 46:420–8.
160. Sano M, Yamamoto I, Ueda J, et al. Comparative pharmacokinetics of theophylline following two fluoroquinolones co-administration. Eur J Clin Pharmacol 1987; 32:431–2.
161. Schwartz J, Jauregui L, Lettieri J, et al. Impact of ciprofloxacin on theophylline clearance and steady-state concentrations in serum. Antimicrob Agents Chemother 1988; 32:75–7.
162. Sorgel F, Mahr G, Granneman GR, et al. Effects of 2 quinolone antibacterials, temafloxacin and enoxacin, on theophylline pharmacokinetics. Clin Pharmacokinet 1992; 22(suppl 1):65–74.
163. Takagi K, Hasegawa T, Ogura Y, et al. Comparative studies on interaction between theophylline and quinolones. J Asthma 1988; 25:63–71.
164. Thomson AH, Thomson GD, Hepburn M, et al. A clinically-significant interaction between ciprofloxacin and theophylline. Eur J Clin Pharmacol 1987; 33:435–6.
165. Wijnands WJA, van Herwaarden CLA, Vree TB. Enoxacin raises plasma theophylline concentrations. Lancet 1984; 2:108–9.

166. Wijnands WJA, Vree TB, van Herwaarden CLA. Enoxacin decreases the clearance of theophylline in man. Br J Clin Pharmacol 1985; 20:583–8.
167. Wijnands WJA, Vree TB, van Herwaarden CLA. The influence of quinolone derivatives on theophylline clearance. Br J Clin Pharmacol 1986; 22:677–83.
168. Wijnands WJA, Cornel JH, Martea M, et al. The effect of multiple-dose oral lomefloxacin on theophylline metabolism in man. Chest 1990; 98:1440–4.
169. Carbo M, Segura J, de la Torre R, et al. Effect of quinolones on caffeine disposition. Clin Pharmacol Ther 1989; 45:234–40.
170. Fuhr U, Wolff T, Harder S, et al. Quinolone inhibition of cytochrome P-450-dependent caffeine metabolism in human liver microsomes. Drug Metab Dispos 1990; 18:1005–10.
171. Harder S, Staib AH, Beer C, et al. 4-quinolones inhibit biotransformation of caffeine. Eur J Clin Pharmacol 1988; 35:651–6.
172. Healy DP, Polk RE, Kanawati L, et al. Interaction between oral ciprofloxacin and caffeine in normal volunteers. Antimicrob Agents Chemother 1989; 33:474–8.
173. Healy DP, Schoenle JR, Stotka J, et al. Lack of interaction between lomefloxacin and caffeine in normal volunteers. Antimicrob Agents Chemother 1991; 35:660–4.
174. Mahr G, Sorgel F, Granneman GR, et al. Effects of temafloxacin and ciprofloxacin on the pharmacokinetics of caffeine. Clin Pharmacokinet 1992; 22(suppl 1):90–7.
175. Parent M, LeBel M. Meta-analysis of quinolone-theophylline interactions. DICP Ann Pharmacother 1991; 25:191–4.
176. Barnett G, Segura J, de la Torre R, et al. Pharmacokinetic determination of relative potency of quinolone inhibition of caffeine disposition. Eur J Clin Pharmacol 1990; 39:63–9.
177. Toon S, Hopkins KJ, Garstang FM, et al. Enoxacin-warfarin interaction: pharmacokinetic and stereochemical aspects. Clin Pharmacol Ther 1987; 42:33–41.
178. Millar E, Coles S, Wyld P, et al. Temafloxacin does not potentiate the anticoagulant effect of warfarin in healthy subjects. Clin Pharmacokinet 1992; 22(suppl 1):102–6.
179. Jolson HM, Tanner LA, Green L, et al. Adverse reaction reporting of interaction between warfarin and fluoroquinolones. Arch Intern Med 1991; 151:1003–4.
180. Kamada A. Possible interaction between ciprofloxacin and warfarin. DICP Ann Pharmacother 1990; 24:27–8.
181. Leor J, Matetzki S. Ofloxacin and warfarin. Ann Intern Med 1988; 109:761.
182. Linville D, Emory C, Graves L. Ciprofloxacin and warfarin interaction. Am J Med 1991; 90:765.
183. Linville T, Matanin D. Norfloxacin and warfarin. Ann Intern Med 1989; 110:751.
184. Wijnands WJA, Trooster JFG, Teunissen PC, et al. Ciprofloxacin does not impair the elimination of diazepam in humans. Drug Metab Dispos 1990; 18:954–7.
185. Waite NM, Rybak MJ, Krakovsky DJ, et al. Influence of subject age on the inhibition of oxidative metabolism by ciprofloxacin. Antimicrob Agents Chemother 1991; 35:130–4.
186. Hasegawa T, Nadai M, Kuzuya T, et al. The possible mechanism of interaction between xanthines and quinolone. J Pharm Pharmacol 1990; 42:767–72.
187. Hori S, Shimada J, Saito A, et al. Inhibitory effect of quinolones on gamma aminobutyric acid receptor-binding. Proceedings of the Twenty-Sixth Interscience Conference on Antimicrobial Agents and Chemotherapy, New Orleans, LA, 1986, abstract 438.
188. Hori S, Shimada J, Saito A, et al. Effect of new quinolones on gamma-aminobutyric acid receptor binding. Proceedings of the Twenty-Fifth Interscience Conference on Antimicrobial Agents and Chemotherapy, Minneapolis, MN, 1985, abstract 396.
189. Hori S, Shimada J, Saito A, et al. A study of enhanced epileptogenicity of new quinolones in the presence of anti-inflammatory drugs. Proceedings of the Twenty-Seventh Interscience Conference on Antimicrobial Agents and Chemotherapy, New York, NY, 1987, abstract 30.
190. Segev S, Rehavi M, Rubinstein E. Quinolones, theophylline, and diclofenac interactions with the gamma-aminobutyric acid receptor. Antimicrob Agents Chemother 1988; 32:1624–6.

191. Morikawa K, Nagata O, Kubo S, et al. Unusual CNS toxic action of new quinolones. Proceedings of the Twenty-Seventh Interscience Conference on Antimicrobial Agents and Chemotherapy, New York, 1987, abstract 255.
192. Freiden TR, Mangi RJ. Inappropriate use of oral ciprofloxacin. JAMA 1990; 264:1438–40.
193. Leigh DA, Emmanuel FXS. The treatment of *Pseudomonas aeruginosa* urinary tract infections with norfloxacin. J Antimicrob Chemother 1984; 13(suppl B):85–8.
194. Corrado ML, Grad C, Sabbaj J. Norfloxacin in the treatment of urinary tract infections in men with and without identifiable urologic complications. Am J Med 1987; 82(suppl 6B):70–4.
195. Leigh DA, Emmanuel FXS, Petch VJ. Ciprofloxacin therapy in complicated urinary tract infections caused by *Pseudomonas aeruginosa* and other resistant bacteria. J Antimicrob Chemother 1986; 18(suppl D):117–21.
196. Gasser TC, Graversen PH, Madsen PO. Treatment of complicated urinary tract infections with ciprofloxacin. Am J Med 1987; 82(suppl 4A):278–9.
197. Cox C. Ciprofloxacin in the treatment of urinary tract infections caused by *Pseudomonas* species and organisms resistant to trimethoprim-sulfamethoxazole. Am J Med 1987; 82(suppl 4A):288–9.
198. Ryan JL, Berenson CS, Greco TP, et al. Oral ciprofloxacin in resistant urinary tract infections. Am J Med 1987; 82(suppl 4A):303–6.
199. Preheim LC, Cuevas TA, Roccaforte JS, et al. Oral ciprofloxacin in the treatment of elderly patients with complicated urinary tract infections due to trimethoprim-sulfamethoxazole-resistant bacteria. Am J Med 1987; 82(suppl 4A):295–300.
200. Fass RJ. Efficacy and safety of oral ciprofloxacin for treatment of serious urinary tract infections. Antimicrob Agents Chemother 1987; 31:148–50.
201. Berman SJ, Schwartz SM. Clinical evaluation of ciprofloxacin with moderately severe bacterial infections. Am J Med 1987; 82(suppl 4A):233–5.
202. Roe CJ, Becker GJ, Whitworth JA, et al. Enoxacin in the treatment of complicated urinary tract infections. Aust NZ J Med 1987; 17:81–2.
203. Huttunen M, Kunnas K, Saloranta P. Enoxacin treatment of urinary tract infections in elderly patients. J Antimicrob Chemother 1988; 21(suppl B):105–11.
204. Bischoff W. Evaluation of lomefloxacin in urinary tract infection: efficacy and safety of once daily dosing, preliminary report. Proceedings of the Third International Symposium on New Quinolones, Vancouver, Canada, 1990, abstract 272.
205. Boerema JBJ, Pauwels R, Scheepers J, et al. Efficacy and safety of pefloxacin in the treatment of patients with complicated urinary tract infections. J Antimicrob Chemother 1986; 17(suppl B):103–9.
206. Wolfhagen MJHM, Hoepelman AIM, Verhoef J. Double-blind, dose-range-finding study of fleroxacin (RO 23-6240, AM-833) for treatment of complicated urinary tract infections. Antimicrob Agents Chemother 1990; 34:409–12.
207. Bernstein-Hahn L, Barclay CA, Iribarren MA, et al. Treatment of complicated urinary tract infections with fleroxacin: a dose-finding study. Rev Infect Dis 1989; 11(suppl 5):*S*1359.
208. Bendall MJ. A review of urinary tract infection in the elderly. J Antimicrob Chemother 1984; 13(suppl B):69–78.
209. Leigh DA, Smith EC, Mariner J. Comparative study using norfloxacin and amoxicillin in the treatment of complicated urinary tract infections in geriatric patients. J Antimicrob Chemother 1984; 13(suppl B):79–83.
210. Spanish Multicenter Study Group. Clinical experience with norfloxacin for urinary tract infections in Spain. Rev Infect Dis 1988; 10(suppl 1):*S*172–*S*173.
211. Tzias V, Dontas AS, Petrikkos G, et al. Three-day antibiotic therapy in bacteriuria of old age. J Antimicrob Chemother 1990; 26:705–11.
212. Jonsson M, Englund G, Norgard K. Norfloxacin vs. pivmecillinam in the treatment of uncomplicated lower urinary tract infections in hospitalized elderly patients. Scand J Infect Dis 1990; 22:339–44.

213. Ewer TC, Bailey RR, Gilchrist NL, et al. Comparative study of norfloxacin and trimethoprim for the treatment of elderly patients with urinary tract infection. NZ Med J 1988; 101:537–9.
214. Williams AA, Gruneberg RN. Ciprofloxacin and co-trimoxazole in urinary tract infections. J Antimicrob Chemother 1986; 18(suppl D):107–10.
215. Newsom SWB, Murphy P, Matthews J. A comparative study of ciprofloxacin and trimethoprim in the treatment of urinary tract infections in geriatric patients. J Antimicrob Chemother 1986; 18(suppl D):111–15.
216. Allais JM, Preheim LC, Cuevas TA, et al. Randomized, double-blind comparison of ciprofloxacin and trimethoprim-sulfamethoxazole for complicated urinary tract infections. Antimicrob Agents Chemother 1988; 32:1327–30.
217. Cox CE. Sequential intravenous and oral ciprofloxacin versus intravenous ceftazidime in the treatment of complicated urinary tract infections. Am J Med 1989; 87(suppl 5A):157*S*–159*S*.
218. Faug G, Brennan C, Wagener M, et al. Use of ciprofloxacin versus use of aminoglycosides for therapy of complicated urinary tract infection: prospective, randomized clinical and pharmacokinetic study. Antimicrob Agents Chemother 1991; 35:1849–55.
219. Cox CE, Drylie DM, Klimberg I, et al. A multicenter, double-blind, trimethoprim-sulfamethoxazole controlled study of enoxacin in the treatment of patients with complicated urinary tract infections. J Urol 1989; 141:575–8.
220. Marini U. Pefloxacin versus cefotaxime in patients with complicated urinary tract infections (UTI). Proceedings of the Third International Symposium on New Quinolones, Vancouver, Canada, 1990, abstract 264.
221. Schalkhauser K. Comparison of iv ofloxacin and piperacillin in the treatment of complicated urinary tract infections. J Antimicrob Chemother 1990; 26(suppl D):93–7.
222. Cox CE. A comparison of the safety and efficacy of lomefloxacin and ciprofloxacin in the treatment of complicated or recurrent urinary tract infections. Am J Med 1992; 92(suppl 4A):82*S*–86*S*.
223. Westenfelder M. The safety and efficacy of lomefloxacin and ciprofloxacin in the treatment of complicated urinary tract infections. preliminary data. Proceedings of the Third International Symposium on New Quinolones, Vancouver, Canada, 1990, abstract 323.
224. Dubois J, St.-Pierre C, Germain M, et al. Fleroxacin in urinary tract infections, a randomized, multi-dose, double-blind study versus norfloxacin. Proceedings of the Third International Symposium on New Quinolones, Vancouver, Canada, 1990, abstract 259.
225. Pummer K, Taufer M, Presterl E, et al. Efficacy and tolerance of fleroxacin vs. norfloxacin in the treatment of complicated urinary tract infections. Proceedings of the Third International Symposium on New Quinolones, Vancouver, Canada, 1990, abstract 280.
226. Kromann-Andersen B, Sommer P, Pers C, et al. Ofloxacin compared with ciprofloxacin in the treatment of complicated lower urinary tract infections. J Antimicrob Chemother 1988; 22(suppl C):143–7.
227. Naber KG, Boerema JBJ, Bischoff W, et al. An assessment of temafloxacin in the treatment of chronic bacterial prostatitis. J Antimicrob Chemother 1991; 28(suppl C):87–96.
228. Stamey TA. Urinary tract infections in males. In: Pathogenesis and treatment of urinary tract infections. Vol. 1. Baltimore, MD: Williams & Wilkins, 1980; 342–429.
229. Stamey TA, Meares EM, Winningham DG. Chronic bacterial prostatitis and the diffusion of drugs into prostatic fluid. J Urol 1970; 103:187–94.
230. Guibert J, Destree D, Acar JF. Ciprofloxacin (Bay 09867): clinical evaluation in urinary tract infections due to *Pseudomonas aeruginosa*. Chemioterapia 1986; 6(suppl 2):524–5.
231. Guibert J, Destree D, Konopka C, et al. Ciprofloxacin in the treatment of urinary tract infection due to enterobacteria. Eur J Clin Microbiol 1986; 5:245–8.
232. Langemeyer TNM, Ferwerda WHH, Hooghamp-Korstanje JAA, et al. Treatment of chronic bacterial prostatitis with ciprofloxacin. Pharm Weekblad 1987; 9(suppl):78.
233. Childs SJ. Ciprofloxacin in treatment of chronic bacterial prostatitis. Urology 1990; 35(suppl):15–18.

234. Weidner W, Shiefer HG, Dalhoff A. Treatment of chronic bacterial prostatitis with ciprofloxacin. Am J Med 1987; 82(suppl 4A):280–3.
235. Bischoff W, Bischoff H. Bacterial prostatitis: efficacy of ciprofloxacin versus sulfonamin-trimethoprim therapy. Proceedings of the Sixteenth International Congress of Chemotherapy, Jerusalem, Israel, 1989, abstract 211.
236. Okada K. Clinical studies on Bay 09867 in the field of urology. Chemotherapy 1985; 33(suppl 7):601.
237. Desplaces N, Gutmann L, Carlet G, et al. The new quinolones and their combinations with other agents for therapy of severe infections. J Antimicrob Chemother 1986; 17(suppl A):25–39.
238. Sabbaj J, Hoagland VL, Cook T. Norfloxacin versus cotrimoxazole in the treatment of recurring urinary tract infections in man. Scand J Infect Dis 1986; 48(suppl):48–53.
239. Cox CE. Ofloxacin in the management of complicated urinary tract infections including prostatitis. Am J Med 1989; 87(suppl 6C):61–8.
240. Guibert J, Acar JF. Ofloxacin (RU 43280): evaluation clinique dans les infections urinaires et prostatiques. Pathol Biol 1986; 34:494–7.
241. Suzuki K, Tamai H, Naide Y, et al. Laboratory and clinical study of ofloxacin in the treatment of bacterial prostatitis. Hinyo Kiyo 1984; 30:1505–18.
242. Kumamoto Y, Sakai S, Tamate H, et al. Therapeutic studies on chronic prostatitis - use of AT-2266. Hinyo Kiyo 1986; 32:1213–23.
243. Bologna M, Vaggi L, Flammini D, et al. Norfloxacin in prostatitis: correlation between HPLC tissue concentrations and clinical results. Drugs Expt Clin Res 1985; 11:95–100.
244. Remy G, Rouger C, Chavanet P, et al. Use of ofloxacin for prostatitis. Rev Infect Dis 1988; 10(suppl 1):173–4.
245. Asbach HW, Melekios M. Zur Behandlung der Urethroadexitis des Mannes mit Gyrasehemmern. In: Adam D, Knothe H, Lode H, Stille W, eds. Ofloxacin. Fortschr Antimikrob antineoplastisch Chemother 1986; 5:857–9.
246. Rubin J, Stoehr G, Yu VL, et al. Efficacy of oral ciprofloxacin plus rifampin for treatment of malignant external otitis. Arch Otolaryngol Head Neck Surg 1989; 115:1063–9.
247. Lang R, Goshen S, Kitzes-Cohen R, et al. Successful treatment of malignant external otitis with oral ciprofloxacin: report of experience with 23 patients. J Infect Dis 1990; 161:537–40.
248. Zikk D, Rapaport Y, Redianu C, et al. Oral ofloxacin therapy for invasive external otitis. Ann Otol Rhinol Laryngol 1991; 100:632–7.
249. Lery R, Shpitzer T, Shvero J, et al. Oral ofloxacin as treatment of malignant external otitis: a study of 17 cases. Laryngoscope 1990; 100:548–51.
250. Giamarellou H, Galanakis N, Christidis K, et al. Malignant external otitis and the newer quinolones. Rev Infect Dis 1989; 11(suppl 5):*S*1109–*S*1110.
251. Ebright JR, Rytel MW. Bacterial pneumonia in the elderly. J Am Geriatr Soc 1980; 28:220–3.
252. Verghese A, Berk SL. Bacterial pneumonia in the elderly. Medicine 1983; 62:271–85.
253. Maesen FPV, Davies BI, Baur C, et al. Clinical, microbiological, and pharmacokinetic studies on ofloxacin in acute purulent exacerbations of chronic respiratory disease. J Antimicrob Chemother 1986; 18:629–34.
254. Grassi C, Grassi GG, Mangiarotti P. Clinical efficacy of ofloxacin in lower respiratory tract infections. a multicenter study. Drugs 1987; 34(suppl 1):80–2.
255. Gentry LO, Lipsky B, Farber MO, et al. Oral ofloxacin therapy for lower respiratory tract infection. South Med J 1992; 85:14–18.
256. Lipsky BA, Tack KJ, Kuo C, et al. Ofloxacin treatment of *Chlamydia pneumoniae* (strain TWAR) lower respiratory tract infections. Am J Med 1990; 89:722–4.
257. Krcmery V Jr, Kettner M, Gocar E, et al. Ofloxacin in treatment of RTI in elderly caused by polyresistant bacteria. Proceedings of the Third International Symposium on New Quinolones, Vancouver, Canada, 1990, abstract 225.

258. Meek JCE, Maesen FPV, Davies BI. A prospective study of ofloxacin in acute exacerbations of chronic respiratory disease associated with *Pseudomonas aeruginosa*. J Antimicrob Chemother 1989; 24:447–53.
259. Maesen FPV, Davies BI, Baur C, et al. Clinical, microbiological and pharmacokinetic studies on ofloxacin in acute purulent exacerbations of chronic respiratory disease. J Antimicrob Chemother 1986; 18:629–34.
260. Dopff Ch, Mertes PM, Nace L, et al. Penicillin G-ofloxacin in combination: a response to the empirical treatment of community-acquired pneumonia (CAP). Pathol Biol 1990; 38:526–9.
261. Davies BI, Maesen FPV, Baur C. Ciprofloxacin in the treatment of acute exacerbations of chronic bronchitis. Eur J Clin Microbiol 1986; 5:226–31.
262. Fraschini F, Braga PC, Cosentina R, et al. Ciprofloxacin: multiple-dose pharmacokinetics and clinical results in patients with hypercrinic bronchopulmonary diseases. Int J Clin Pharmacol Res 1987; 7:63–71.
263. Haverkorn MJ. Ciprofloxacin therapy of respiratory tract infection with *Pseudomonas aeruginosa*. Eur J Clin Microbiol Infect Dis 1988; 7:661–4.
264. Peloquin CA, Cumbo TJ, Nix DE, et al. Evaluation of intravenous ciprofloxacin in patients with nosocomial lower respiratory tract infections. Arch Intern Med 1989; 149:2269–73.
265. Salvati F, Zubiani M, Antilli A, et al. Ciprofloxacin in the oral treatment of severe respiratory tract infections. Rev Infect Dis 1988; 10(suppl 1):*S*220–*S*221.
266. Brutel de la Riviere T, Daniels-Bosman MSM, ten Velde GPM. Two different dosages of ciprofloxacin in patients with respiratory tract infections. Pharm Weekblad 1989; 11:121–3.
267. Davies BI, Maesen FPV, Teengs JP. Serum and sputum concentrations of enoxacin after single dosing in a clinical and bacteriological study. J Antimicrob Chemother 1984:14(suppl C):83–9.
268. Scarpazza G, Della Torre F, Scaglione F, et al. Efficacy and safety of enoxacin in the treatment of respiratory infections. Int J Clin Pharmacol Res 1989; 9:43–7.
269. Vanderdouckt J, Hellebrand A, Cordier R. Clinical evaluation of pefloxacin in community-acquired lower respiratory tract infections. Curr Ther Res 1988; 43:82–91.
270. Bagnulo H, Pedreira W, Bazet C, et al. Pefloxacin in the treatment of *Acinetobacter anitratus* pneumonia in ventilated patients. Proceedings of the Third International Symposium on New Quinolones. Vancouver, Canada, 1990, abstract 327.
271. Grassi C, Catena E, de Iola G, et al. Pefloxacin in lower respiratory tract infections. J Antimicrob Chemother 1990; 26(suppl B):103–10.
272. Davies BI, Maesen FPV, Gubbelmans HLL, et al. Temafloxacin in acute purulent exacerbations of chronic bronchitis. J Antimicrob Chemother 1990; 26:237–46.
273. Gledhill IC, Ferguson WP, Lowry RC. Efficacy and safety of ciprofloxacin in patients with respiratory infections in comparison with amoxicillin. J Antimicrob Chemother 1986; 18(suppl D):133–8.
274. Peterson PK, Stein D, Guay DRP, et al. Prospective study of lower respiratory tract infections in an extended care nursing home program: potential role of oral ciprofloxacin. Am J Med 1988; 85:164–71.
275. Trenholme GM, Schmitt BA, Spear J, et al. Randomized study of intravenous/oral ciprofloxacin versus ceftazidime in the treatment of hospital and nursing home patients with lower respiratory tract infections. Am J Med 1989; 87(suppl 5A):116*S*–118*S*.
276. Haddow A, Greene S, Heinz G, et al. Ciprofloxacin (intravenous/oral) versus ceftazidime in lower respiratory tract infections. Am J Med 1989; 87(suppl 5A):113*S*–115*S*.
277. Schmidt EW, Zimmerman I, Pitzerfeld W, et al. Controlled prospective study of oral amoxicillin/clavulanate vs. ciprofloxacin in acute exacerbations of chronic bronchitis. J Antimicrob Chemother 1989; 24(suppl B):185–93.
278. Basran GS, Joseph J, Abbas AMA, et al. Treatment of acute exacerbations of chronic obstructive airway disease—a comparison of amoxycillin and ciprofloxacin. J Antimicrob Chemother 1990; 26(suppl F):19–24.

279. Hirata-Dulas CAI, Stein DJ, Guay DRP, et al. A randomized study of ciprofloxacin versus ceftriaxone in the treatment of nursing home-acquired lower respiratory tract infections. J Am Geriatr Soc 1991; 39:979–85.
280. Chmel H, Emmanuel G, Lie T, et al. A prospective, double-blind, randomized study comparing the efficacy and safety of low-dose ciprofloxacin with ampicillin in the treatment of bronchitis. Diagn Microbiol Infect Dis 1990; 13:149–51.
281. Hanninen P. Ofloxacin in lower respiratory tract infections. Drugs 1987; 34(suppl 1):179–80.
282. Sanders WE Jr, Morris JF, Alessi P, et al. Oral ofloxacin for the treatment of acute bacterial pneumonia: use of a nontraditional protocol to compare experimental therapy with "usual care" in a multicenter clinical trial. Am J Med 1991; 91:261–6.
283. Egede F, Kristensen I. A comparative study of ofloxacin and pivmecillinam in acute exacerbations of chronic bronchitis. Scand J Infect Dis 1990; 68:46–9.
284. Punakivi L, Keistinen T, Backman R, et al. Oral ofloxacin once daily and doxycycline in the treatment of acute exacerbations of chronic bronchitis. Scand J Infect Dis 1990; Suppl 68:41–5.
285. Khajotia R, Drlicek M, Vetter N. A comparative study of ofloxacin and amoxycillin/clavulanate in hospitalized patients with lower respiratory tract infections. J Antimicrob Chemother 1990; 26(suppl D):83–91.
286. Forsberg P, Maller R, Nilsson L. Comparative study of oral ofloxacin and erythromycin in the treatment of pneumonia. Rev Infect Dis 1989; 11(suppl 5):*S*1229–*S*1230.
287. Vogel F, Lode H. The use of oral temafloxacin compared with a parenteral cephalosporin in hospitalized patients with pneumonia. J Antimicrob Chemother 1991; 28(suppl C):81–6.
288. Kosmidis J. A double-blind study of once-daily temafloxacin in the treatment of bacterial lower respiratory tract infections. J Antimicrob Chemother 1991; 28(suppl C):73–9.
289. Davey PG. Efficacy of temafloxacin versus ciprofloxacin or amoxicillin for lower respiratory tract infections in smokers and the elderly. Am J Med 1991; 91(suppl 6A):101*S*–105*S*.
290. Gottfried MH, Ellison WT. Safety and efficacy of lomefloxacin versus cefaclor in the treatment of acute exacerbations of chronic bronchitis. Am J Med 1992; 92(supp 4A):108*S*–113*S*.
291. Farkas S, Chokreff M, Casey P, et al. A comparative study of fleroxacin (FLX) versus ceftazidime (CTZ) in the intravenous (IV) therapy of lower respiratory tract infections (LRTI). Proceedings of the Thirtieth Interscience Conference on Antimicrobial Agents and Chemotherapy, Atlanta, GA, 1990, abstract 1297.
292. Maasilta P, Mattson K, Leinonen M, et al. Enoxacin compared with trimethoprim-sulfamethoxazole in the treatment of lower respiratory tract infections in patients with chronic obstructive pulmonary disease. Rev Infect Dis 1988; 10(suppl 1):*S*221–*S*222.
293. Prigogine T, Glupczynski Y, Carpiaux JP, et al. Enoxacin in acute exacerbations of chronic bronchitis: a comparison with amoxycillin. J Antimicrob Chemother 1988; 21(suppl B):131–6.
294. Vanderdonckt J. Comparison of pefloxacin with ceftazidime in severe bronchopulmonary infections. J Antimicrob Chemother 1990; 26(suppl B):111–16.
295. Chaudhry A. Treatment of lower respiratory tract infections: a comparison of temafloxacin vs. ciprofloxacin. Proceedings of the Third International Symposium on New Quinolones, Vancouver, Canada, 1990, abstract 314.
296. Gordon JJ, Kauffman CA. Superinfection with *Streptococcus pneumoniae* during therapy with ciprofloxacin. Am J Med 1990; 89:383–4.
297. Yoshikawa TT. Treatment of nursing home-acquired pneumonia. J Am Geriatr Soc 1991; 39:1040–1.
298. Lee BC, Padula AM, Kimbrough RC, et al. Infectious complications with respiratory pathogens despite ciprofloxacin therapy. N Engl J Med 1991; 325:520–1.
299. Waldvogel FA, Vasey H. Osteomyelitis: the past decade. N Engl J Med 1980; 303:360–70.
300. Norden CW. Osteomyelitis. In: Mandell GL, Douglas RG Jr, Bennett JE, eds. Principles and practice of infectious diseases, 3rd ed. Churchill Livingstone, New York 1990:922–30.

301. Smith JW. Infectious arthritis. In: Mandell GL, Douglas RG Jr, Bennett JE, eds. Principles and practice of infectious diseases, 3rd ed. Churchill Livingstone, New York 1990:911–18.
302. Septimus EJ, Musher DM. Osteomyelitis: recent clinical and laboratory aspects. Orthoped Clin North Am 1979; 10:347–59.
303. Nix DE, Cumbo TJ, Kuritzky P, et al. Oral ciprofloxacin in the treatment of serious soft tissue and bone infections. Am J Med 1987; 82(suppl 4A):146–53.
304. Hoogkamp-Korstanji JAA, van Bottenburg HA, van Bruggen J, et al. Treatment of chronic osteomyelitis with ciprofloxacin. J Antimicrob Chemother 1989; 23:427–32.
305. Swedish Study Group. Therapy of acute and chronic gram-negative osteomyelitis with ciprofloxacin. J Antimicrob Chemother 1988; 22:221–8.
306. Wood MJ, Logan MN. Ciprofloxacin for soft tissue infections. J Antimicrob Chemother 1986; 18(suppl D):159–64.
307. Dan M, Siegman-Igra Y, Pitlik S, et al. Oral ciprofloxacin treatment of *Pseudomonas aeruginosa* osteomyelitis. Antimicrob Agents Chemother 1990; 34:849–52.
308. Dellamonica P, Etesse-Carsenti H, Bernard E, et al. Pefloxacin in the treatment of bone infections associated with foreign material. J Antimicrob Chemother 1990; 26(suppl B):199–205.
309. Lopitaux R, Hermet R, Sirot J, et al. Experience of ofloxacin in the treatment of osteoarticular infections. Pathol Biol 1988; 36:557–61.
310. Parish LC, Asper R. Systemic treatment of cutaneous infections. a comparative study of ciprofloxacin and cefotaxime. Am J Med 1987; 82(suppl 4A):227–32.
311. Valtonen V, Karppinen L, Kariniemi A-L. A comparative study of ciprofloxacin and conventional therapy in the treatment of patients with chronic lower leg ulcers infected with *Pseudomonas aeruginosa* or other gram-negative rods. Scand J Infect Dis 1989; Suppl 60:79–83.
312. Gentry LO, Koshdel A. Intravenous/oral ciprofloxacin versus intravenous ceftazidime in the treatment of serious gram-negative infections of the skin and skin structure. Am J Med 1989; 87(suppl 5A):132*S*–135*S*.
313. Ramirez-Ronda CH, Vazquez A, Zapata N, et al. Prospective, randomized, comparative study of oral enoxacin versus parenteral ceftriaxone in patients with skin and soft tissue infections. Proceedings of the Third International Symposium on New Quinolones, Vancouver, Canada, 1990, abstract 413.
314. Segev S, Rosen N, Pitlik SD, et al. Pefloxacin versus ceftazidime in therapy of soft tissue infections in compromised patients. J Antimicrob Chemother 1990; 26(suppl B):193–8.
315. Meunier F, Aoun M, Delhaye N, et al. Pefloxacin as therapy for non-neutropenic patients with gram-negative bacillary septicemia. Rev Infect Dis 1989; 11(suppl 5):*S*1175–*S*1176.
316. Gangji D, Jacobs F, de Jonckheer J, et al. Randomized study of intravenous versus sequential intravenous/oral regimen of ciprofloxacin in the treatment of gram-negative septicemia. Am J Med 1989; 87(suppl 5A):206*S*–208*S*.
317. Jourdan J, Barbuat C, and the Multicenter Study Group. Efficacy and tolerance of ofloxacin (OFX) compared with ceftriaxone (CFX) as first line therapy of septicemia caused by Enterobacteriaceae in immunocompetent patients. Proceedings of the Third International Symposium on New Quinolones, Vancouver, Canada, 1990, abstract 385.
318. Pien FD. Ciprofloxacin treatment of soft tissue and respiratory infections in a community outpatient practice. Am J Med 1987; 82(suppl 4A):236–8.
319. Maggiolo F, Bianchi W, Ohnmeiss H. Ciprofloxacin use in diabetic patients. Curr Ther Res 1988; 44:563–71.
320. Yangco BG, Kenyon VS, Halkias KD, et al. Oral ciprofloxacin treatment of infections in geriatric patients. Clin Ther 1989; 11:503–10.
321. Daly JS, Worthington MG, Razvi SA, et al. Intravenous and sequential intravenous and oral ciprofloxacin in the treatment of severe infections. Am J Med 1989; 87(suppl 5A):232*S*–234*S*.
322. Bianchi W, Maggiolo F, Ohnmeiss H. Ciprofloxacin in elderly patients with underlying chronic diseases. J Int Med Res 1988; 16:386–93.

323. Gibert CL, Seiler M, Joe L, et al. Intravenous and oral ciprofloxacin in the therapy of serious infections. Diagn Microbiol Infect Dis 1990; 13:173–6.
324. Naber K, Afschrift M, Bairos MA, et al. Fleroxacin (RO 23-6240) once daily in the intravenous therapy of serious bacterial infections. Proceedings of the Third International Symposium on New Quinolones, Vancouver, Canada, 1990, abstract 6.
325. Montalto Tentori T, Lombardi D, Mattu G, et al. A multicenter open study to evaluate the efficacy and safety of ofloxacin in the treatment of LRTI and UTI in the elderly. Proceedings of the Third International Symposium on New Quinolones, Vancouver, Canada, 1990, abstract 320.
326. Regamey C, Steinbach-Lebbin C. Severe infections treated with intravenous ofloxacin: a prospective clinical multicenter Swiss study. J Antimicrob Chemother 1990; 26(suppl D):107–14.
327. Levine DP, McNeil P, Lerner SA. Randomized, double-blind comparative study of intravenous ciprofloxacin versus ceftazidime in the treatment of serious infections. Am J Med 1989; 87(suppl 5A):160*S*–163*S*.
328. Gaut PL, Carron WC, Ching WTW, et al. Intravenous/oral ciprofloxacin therapy versus intravenous ceftazidime therapy for selected bacterial infections. Am J Med 1989; 87(suppl 5A):169*S*–175*S*.
329. Wauters E. Open randomized comparative multicenter trial of pefloxacin vs. cefotaxime for the treatment of patients with severe bacterial infections. Rev Infect Dis 1989; 11(suppl 5):*S*1171–*S*1172.
330. Sanders WE Jr. Adverse reactions to fluoroquinolones. In: Sanders WE Jr, Sanders CC, eds. Fluoroquinolones in the treatment of infectious diseases. Glenview, IL: Physicians & Scientists Publishing Co., Inc., 1990:233–48.
331. Grasela TH Jr, Dreis MW. An evaluation of the quinolone-theophylline interaction using the Food and Drug Administration Spontaneous Reporting System. Arch Intern Med 1992; 152:617–21.
332. Fraser AG, Harrower ADB. Convulsions and hyperglycemia associated with nalidixic acid. Br Med J 1977; 2:1518.
333. Anastasio GD, Menscer D, Little JM Jr. Norfloxacin and seizures. Ann Intern Med 1988; 109:169–70.
334. Christ W. Central nervous system toxicity of quinolones: human and animal findings. J Antimicrob Chemother 1990; 26(Suppl B):219–25.
335. Slavich IL, Gieffe RF, Haas EJ. Grand mal epileptic seizures during ciprofloxacin therapy. JAMA 1989; 261:558–9.
336. Schacht P, Arcieri G, Branolte J, et al. Worldwide clinical data on efficacy and safety of ciprofloxacin. Infection 1988; 16(suppl):*S*29–*S*43.
337. Shah PM, Frech K. Overview of clinical experience with the quinolones. In: Percival A, ed. Quinolones: their future in clinical practice. London: Royal Society of Medicine Services, 1986:29–43.
338. Halkin H. Adverse effects of the fluoroquinolones. Rev Infect Dis 1988; 10(suppl 1):*S*258–*S*261.
339. Monk JP, Campoli-Richards DM. Ofloxacin: a review of its antibacterial activity, pharmacokinetic properties and therapeutic use. Drugs 1987; 33:346–91.
340. Holmes B, Brogden RN, Richards DM. Norfloxacin: a review of its antibacterial activity, pharmacokinetic properties and therapeutic use. Drugs 1985; 30:482–513.
341. Tack KJ, Smith JA. The safety profile of ofloxacin. Am J Med 1989; 87(suppl 6C):78*S*–81*S*.
342. Paradiso LJ, McKay L. Tolerance of enoxacin in the elderly. Proceedings of the Thirtieth Interscience Conference on Antimicrobial Agents and Chemotherapy, Atlanta, GA, 1990, abstract 1320.
343. Pernet A. Temafloxacin: a safe antibiotic for the elderly, patients with comorbidities, and other special populations. Am J Med 1991; 91(suppl 6A):162*S*–165*S*.

344. Fostini R, Girelli M, Dalle Vedove P, et al. Safety profile of ofloxacin in elderly patients. Drugs Expt Clin Res 1988; 14:393–5.
345. Sanders WE Jr. Efficacy, safety, and potential economic benefits of oral ciprofloxacin in the treatment of infections. Rev Infect Dis 1988; 10:528–43.
346. Borner K, Lode H, Hoffken G, et al. Monitoring of ofloxacin after intravenous and oral administration. Rev Infect Dis 1989; 11(suppl 5):*S*1009.

15

Vancomycin

Burke A. Cunha and Natalie C. Klein
Winthrop-University Hospital, Mineola, and State University of New York School of Medicine, Stony Brook, New York

I. INTRODUCTION

Vancomycin is a bactericidal antibiotic that interferes with peptidogylcan biosynthesis and has a high degree of antimicrobial activity against gram-positive bacteria. Since its availability in 1956, vancomycin has been used primarily as an antistaphylococcal and antienterococcal antimicrobial agent, and during the past several years has become the mainstay of therapy for *Clostridium difficile*, i.e., antibiotic-associated diarrhea and colitis. Vancomycin was extensively used during the 1960s and was gradually supplanted by the introduction of the antistaphylococcal penicillins throughout the decade. Impurities associated with the initial lots of vancomycin resulted in a variety of side effects that limited its use on a wider scale (1,2). Since the 1970s, vancomycin's use has increased as an antistaphylococcal prophylactic antibiotic for foreign body implant surgery and as a therapeutic agent for patients with serious infections due to methicillin-resistant *Staphylococcus aureus* (MRSA). Vancomycin continues to be used extensively to treat *C. difficile* diarrhea and colitis, to prevent and treat gram-positive coccal infections in hemodialysis patients, and to treat patients with serious systemic enterococcal infections (31). Although a wide variety of side effects have been ascribed to vancomycin therapy, the incidence of serious side effects is relatively uncommon, and for this reason vancomycin continues to be used extensively in patients that have severe hypersensitivity reactions to penicillins or β-lactam antibiotics. The major use of vancomycin in elderly patients is in the prophylaxis or treatment of natural or prosthetic valve streptococcal endocarditis, the treatment of *C. difficile* diarrhea, the prevention and treatment of gram-positive coccal infections in hemodialysis patients, serious or systemic infections due to MRSA, and as an alternative to β-lactam therapy in patients with severe hypersensitivity reactions to this class of antibiotics (1–5).

II. CHEMISTRY

Vancomycin is a unique antibiotic that was isolated from *Nocardia orientalis* found in soil samples from Borneo. Vancomycin is a high molecular weight, complex glycopolypeptide (7).

III. MECHANISM OF ACTION

Vancomycin's antibacterial effects are related primarily to its ability to interfere with peptidoglycan biosynthesis in the cell walls of multiplying gram-positive organisms. Vancomycin also, to a lesser extent, interferes with cytoplasmic RNA synthesis. Vancomycin is bactericidal at clinically achievable concentrations against all gram-positive cocci except enterococci. The antimicrobial activity of vancomycin is optimal between pH 6.5 and 8.0. Vancomycin has a high molecular weight, and its structural formula is incompletely characterized (2,7).

IV. ANTIMICROBIAL SPECTRUM

At clinically achievable concentrations, vancomycin is active against only aerobic gram-positive organisms, e.g., staphylococci, streptococci, enterococci, pneumococci, as well as *Corynebacterium*, *Listeria*, and clostridia (1,8). Most of these organisms have been shown to be frequent and serious causes of infections in older adults (8a). Vancomycin is active against penicillin-sensitive and -resistant *S. aureus* and methicillin-sensitive and -resistant staphylococci. Vancomycin is uniformly active against methicillin-sensitive and -resistant *Staphylococcus epidermidis*, as well as JK diphtheroids and other less common gram-positive organisms. Gram-negative and anaerobic organisms, excluding clostridia, are resistant to vancomycin as are viruses, *Rickettsia*, *Chlamydia*, and fungi (5,9).

There is no cross-resistance between vancomycin and other classes of antibiotics. Resistance of susceptible organisms to vancomycin is fortunately very uncommon. Recently, a few strains of enterococci have been found to be resistant to vancomycin. Group D enterococci are also commonly "tolerant" to vancomycin, i.e., the organisms are inhibited but not killed by the drug, and consequently there is frequently a significant difference between the minimal inhibitory concentration (MIC) and minimal bactericidal concentration (MBC) for enterococci. Therefore, vancomycin is bacteriostatic for most enterococci. Antienterococcal bactericidal activity is achieved by adding an aminoglycoside to vancomycin. In vitro antistaphylococcal activity may be demonstrated with the addition of rifampin or aminoglycoside against some staphylococcal isolates. The clinical relevance of such in vitro observations remains controversial (10,11) (Table 1).

V. CLINICAL PHARMACOLOGY

A. Pharmacokinetics

Vancomycin is not well absorbed from the gastrointestinal tract after oral ingestion. Vancomycin should not be given by the intramuscular route but may be administered intravenously in 5% dextrose or 0.9% saline solution. The intravenous infusion should be given slowly over 30 or preferably 60 min. Vancomycin may be given together with β-lactams, monobactams, aminoglycosides, rifampin, or metronidazole. The elimination half-life (β-phase) of vancomycin is 6 h in adults. In a single study of vancomycin

Table 1 Antibacterial Spectrum of Vancomycin

Organisms	Minimal inhibitory concentration (μg/ml)	Median minimal inhibitory concentration (μg/ml)	Minimal bactericidal concentration (μg/ml)
Staphylococcus aureus	1.0–3.0	1.0	1.5–10.0
Methicillin-resistant *S. aureus* (MRSA)	0.3–12.0	1.5	
Staphylococcus epidermidis	1.0–6.3	3.1	
Streptococcus pyogenes (group A strep)	0.1–2.5	0.4	
Streptococcus pneumoniae	0.3–1.0	0.5	
Streptococcus viridans group	<1.0–1.25	0.8	<0.3–>10.0
Group D streptococci			
Enterococcal	1.5–100	3.1	>100
Nonenterococcal (*S. bovis*)	0.3–≥5.0	0.6	25–50
Clostridium spp.	0.5–5.0	1.25	≤1.0–≥10.0
Clostridium difficile	1.0–8.0		
Corynebacterium spp.	0.5–3.0	0.04	≤1.0–≥10.0
JK diphtheroids	0.2	6.25	
Bacillus spp.	0.5–5.0		≤1.0–≥10.0
Listeria monocytogenes	0.6	0.6–5.0	

Source: Adapted from Refs. 2–7.

pharmacokinetics in elderly subjects, Cutler et al. demonstrated that older subjects (mean age, 68.5 years; mean creatinine clearance, 97.7 ml/min) had a longer mean half-life (12.1 h) than younger subjects (7.2 h) (12). Approximately 55% of vancomycin is protein bound.

A two- or a three-compartment pharmacokinetic model best explains the behavior of vancomycin in vivo. The 500-mg dose of vancomycin hydrochloride results in a mean peak serum concentration of approximately 30 μg/ml immediately after the infusion. Concentrations after 1 h are approximately 6 μg/ml, and after 6 h are approximately 3 μg/ml. Concentrations are <1 μg/ml 24 h after the infusion. Following a 1 g slow intravenous infusion, vancomycin peak serum levels are approximately 48 μg/ml, with trough concentrations at 2 μg/ml 12 h after the infusion (4,7) (Table 2).

B. Distribution

Vancomycin given by the oral route concentrates intraluminally in the distal gastrointestinal tract, resulting in high intraluminal vancomycin concentrations—~10,000 μg/ml in the stool following a 2 g/day oral dose. Vancomycin is poorly absorbed from the gastrointestinal tract, and little, if any, enters the systemic circulation. Slightly higher but still low serum concentrations may occur in patients with a damaged intestinal mucosa, e.g., an inflammatory bowel disease. However, data on the impact of age on vancomycin gastrointestinal absorption are not available.

Table 2 Vancomycin Serum Concentrations Following IV Dosing

Patient	Dose	Time to sample	Mean serum concentration (μg/ml)
Normal patients	500 mg	30 min	33.4
Normal patients	500 mg	5 h	3.5
Anephric patients	1 g	30 min	48.0
	1 g	5 h	15.0
	1 g	7 days	7.0
	1 g	18 days	3.5

Source: Adapted from Ref. 4.

It is important to realize that intravenous vancomycin does not result in significant stool concentrations of vancomycin (13–15). After intravenous injection, vancomycin penetrates well into most tissues of the body. There are limited pharmacokinetic data on vancomycin penetration into various tissue sites; however, clinically useful concentrations are achieved in the lung, heart, synovial fluid, peritoneal fluid, bone, and kidney. Approximately 15% of simultaneous serum concentrations of vancomycin is the level achieved in most of the tissues of the body excluding the urine. Vancomycin does not penetrate the aqueous humor of the eye, nor does it penetrate into cerebrospinal fluid in the presence of noninflamed meninges (Table 3). Mean vancomycin concentration in the presence of inflamed meninges is approximately 2.5 μg/ml, or about 15% of simultaneous serum concentration. Since this concentration is inadequate for eradicating many gram-positive pathogens infecting the central nervous system, administration of intrathecal vancomycin may be necessary to achieve higher cerebrospinal fluid concentrations for the treatment of gram-positive meningitis (16,17). Intrathecal doses of vancomycin are 3–5 mg. Vancomycin may also be administered via an Omaya reservoir using a dose that achieves a concentration of 25 μg/ml.

Table 3 Vancomycin Concentrations in Body Fluids

Body/Fluid	Dose	Route of administration	Time to sample (h)	Mean concentrations (μg/ml)
Cerebrospinal fluid	40 mg/kg/day	IV	≈2	3.8
Urine	500 mg	IV	1	90–30
Pleural fluid	2 g	IV	4	50
	500 mg	IV	1	1.7–2.5
	500 mg	IV	3	2.9
Pericardial fluid	500 mg	IV	1.5–5.5	0.6–5.5
Synovial fluid	500 mg	IV	1	5.7
Ascitic fluid	500 mg	IV	1.5–5.2	3.6
Bile	500 mg	IV	1	3.1
Stools	500 mg	PO	6	100–350

Source: Adapted from Ref. 4.

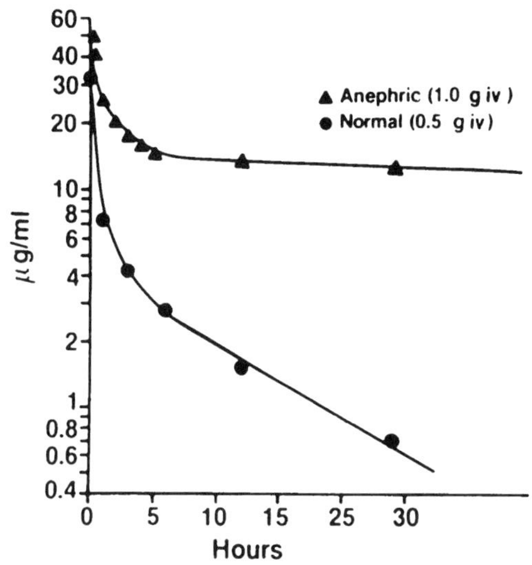

Figure 1 The elimination of vancomycin by anephric patients and by patients with normal renal function.

C. Elimination

Vancomycin is eliminated by glomerular filtration via the kidneys. Urine concentrations are ~300 μg/ml after a 500-mg intravenous dose. Tubular reabsorption is not important in the renal handling of vancomycin. Since vancomycin is eliminated via the renal route, vancomycin accumulates in the serum and tissues in the presence of renal insufficiency. Serum half-life of vancomycin in anuric patients is approximately 7 days in contrast to 6 h in adults with normal renal function (Figs. 1,2). The mechanism of elimination of vancomycin in anephric patients is not known at the present time. Vancomycin is not significantly removed by peritoneal or hemodialysis (18–22).

In the study noted earlier by Cutler et al., renal clearance of vancomycin was reduced in elderly subjects. However, the volume of distribution of the drug was increased in these older subjects. The authors concluded that the reduced clearance of vancomycin in older persons was due to enhanced tissue binding of the drug rather than differences in renal function (12).

D. Drug Interactions

Vancomycin should not be given to patients receiving cholestyramine since the resin binds the drug and results in decreased serum concentrations of vancomycin (7).

VI. CLINICAL INDICATIONS

A. Prophylaxis

Vancomycin has been used as an antimicrobial prophylactic agent for foreign body implants in orthopedic and cardiovascular surgery. Elderly patients commonly undergo surgery for

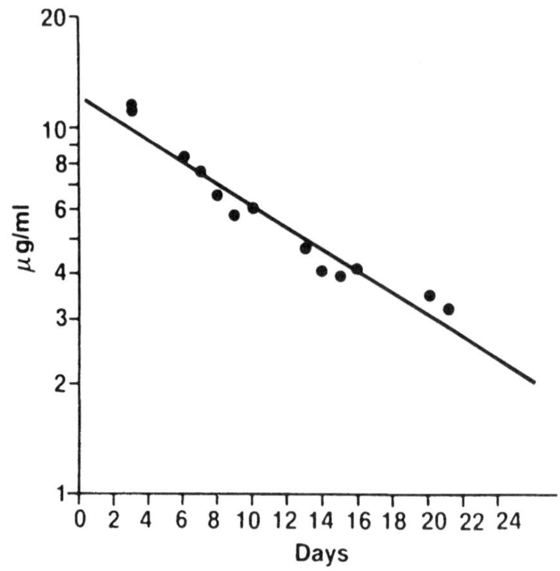

Figure 2 The elimination of vancomycin hydrochloride after a single 1-g IV dose in anephric patients undergoing hemodialysis at 3-day intervals.

such implants as artificial hip and knee joints, plates and nails for repair of fractural hips, prosthetic cardiac valves, and shunts for normal pressure hydrocephalus. Since the most common pathogens causing prosthetic implant surgery infection are gram-positive cocci, i.e., *S. epidermidis* and to a lesser extent *S. aureus*, vancomycin is an excellent chemoprophylactic agent against these potential gram-positive pathogens (23,24). An aminoglycoside is frequently added to vancomycin for surgical procedures involving prosthetic implants because an aminoglycoside provides coverage against potential aerobic gram-negative bacillary pathogens and, together with vancomycin, is synergistic and bactericidal against enterococci. Vancomycin has also been administered to prevent access site infections with central lines and in patients on chronic hemodialysis (4,26). Vancomycin is also used alone for prophylaxis against infective endocarditis in penicillin-allergic patients who undergo oral or upper respiratory tract procedures. Similarly, in patients allergic to ampicillin, vancomycin plus gentamicin is recommended for prophylaxis for older individuals at high risk for developing infective endocarditis while undergoing gastrointestinal/genitourinary procedures. Prophylactic oral vancomycin therapy to prevent antibiotic-associated diarrhea due to *C. difficile* is not recommended (2,4,7).

B. Therapy

Vancomycin has been used to treat serious gram-positive infections in patients with severe hypersensitivity reactions to β-lactam antibiotics (primarily penicillins and cephalosporins). A major use for vancomycin at the present time is in the treatment of serious MRSA infections. There is no convincing data that the addition of rifampin or an aminoglycoside enhances the in vivo activity of vancomycin against MRSA. MRSA colonization and infection is becoming an increasingly important problem in nursing homes and chronic care facilities (27). Thus, the use of vancomycin in frail elderly nursing home residents may increase in the future.

Vancomycin has been used extensively to treat infective endocarditis due to streptococci, enterococci, and staphylococci, as well as an alternative to β-lactam antimicrobials in the treatment of viridans group streptococcal endocarditis. An aminoglycoside or rifampin is commonly added to vancomycin therapy in serious infections caused by "tolerant" *S. aureus*, as well as by *S. epidermidis*. The latter organism may be resistant to antistaphylococcal penicillins (28). Vancomycin is commonly used for the empiric treatment of intravenous line sepsis, either alone or in combination with an aminoglycoside or aztreonam pending quantitative catheter tip cultures (4–7). Gram-positive meningitis may be treated with vancomycin alone, which is administered systematically, along with intrathecal doses by direct instillation or via an Omaya reservoir into the cerebrospinal fluid (16,17).

Oral vancomycin is perhaps the most effective therapy in the treatment of *C. difficile* diarrhea or colitis. However, oral vancomycin does not eliminate the organism from the gastrointestinal tract, and *C. difficile* may recur (13,14). It should be noted that *C. difficile* intestinal colonization and diarrhea are being reported in nursing home patients (29).

In summary, the majority of elderly patients receive vancomycin because of penicillin or cephalosporin allergies, methicillin-resistant staphylococcal infections, antibiotic-associated diarrhea, gram-positive intravenous line sepsis, or for prophylaxis or treatment of infective endocarditis (Table 4).

VII. ADMINISTRATION OF THE DRUG

For most older patients, oral vancomycin may be administered in a dose of 125 or 250 mg, given usually every 6 h for 5–7 days. Higher doses, e.g., 500 mg every 6 h, may occasionally be necessary in recurrent or severe cases of *C. difficile* colitis. Relapse may require retreatment with additional courses of oral vancomycin. Oral vancomycin may be administered via nasogastric or rectal tube in geriatric patients with antibiotic-associated colitis and ileus. In such patients, metronidazole is preferred since systemic administration will result in effective intraluminal metronidazole levels. The literature suggests that oral metronidazole and oral vancomycin are equally efficacious in the treatment of *C. difficile* diarrhea, but oral vancomycin is superior in the author's clinical experience (13,14).

The standard dosage of intravenous vancomycin is 500 mg every 6 h, but it may be given more cost effectively as a 1-g dose every 12 h. Because the serum half-life is longer in elderly patients, it may be prudent to decrease the dose of vancomycin in these individuals, e.g., 750 mg every 12 h. Serum levels should be monitored to determine if adequate or toxic concentrations are present. The volume of distribution of vancomycin is large. Thus, in patients with conditions resulting in abnormalities of their fluid compartments, dosage modifications may be needed. In such individuals, e.g., with ascites, burns, etc., dosing should be based upon the vancomycin serum levels desired (7,30).

Older patients with renal insufficiencies should receive a fraction of their daily vancomycin dose based upon the degree of renal insufficiency, which may be determined by the creatinine clearance of the patient. Dosing of vancomycin should not be based on the serum creatinine in elderly patients. Because of age-related decrease in muscle mass, serum creatinine in such individuals may not be a true indicator of renal function (19). For example, if the creatinine clearance is approximately 50 ml/min, then vancomycin may be administered either as a 500-mg intravenous dose every 12 h or as 1-g intravenous dose every 24 h (4,7). Usually it is more prudent to decrease the dose rather than to

Table 4 Clinical Prophylactic and Therapeutic Uses of Vancomycin

Prosthetic implant surgery	(vancomycin plus gentamicin)
Shunt infections in chronic hemodialysis caused by gram-positive cocci	(vancomycin alone)
Endocarditis	
Oral and upper respiratory tract procedures	(vancomycin alone)
Gastrointestinal/Genitourinary procedures	(vancomycin plus gentamicin)
Therapy gram-positive coccal IV line sepsis	
Serious methicillin-resistant *Staphylococcus aureus* infections	(vancomycin alone)
CNS or hemodialysis shunt infections caused by gram-positive cocci	(vancomycin plus rifampin)
Endocarditis caused by	
Viridans group streptococci	(vancomycin alone)
Staphylococcus epidermidis	(vancomycin plus rifampin)
Staphylococcus aureus	(vancomycin plus gentamicin)
Group D enterococci	(vancomycin plus gentamicin)
Group D nonenterococci (*S. bovis*)	
MBC $\leq$ 10 μg/ml	(vancomycin alone)
MBC $\geq$ 10 μg/ml	(vancomycin plus gentamicin)
JK diphtheroids	(vancomycin alone)
Clostridium difficile colitis	(oral vancomycin)
Meningitis caused by	
Gram-positive cocci	(intrathecal vancomycin)
Flavobacterium	(intrathecal vancomycin)
Other miscellaneous infections caused by gram-positive cocci	(vancomycin alone)

Source: Adapted from Ref. 4.

extend dosing intervals because it may leave the patient with subtherapeutic concentrations of antibiotic for variable periods of time. In anuric older patients, an initial 1-g loading dose of vancomycin is given, and a 500-mg dose is given weekly thereafter. Since vancomycin is not removed by peritoneal or hemodialysis, there is no need for a postdialysis supplementary dose (18).

If vancomycin is used to treat central nervous system infections, then 5 mg may be instilled directly into the cerebrospinal fluid. Alternatively, vancomycin may be administered via an Omaya reservoir, so that the concentration in the cerebrospinal fluid is 25 μg/ml (16,17).

VIII. ADVERSE EFFECTS

Except for the "red man" or "red neck" syndrome, adverse reactions to vancomycin are relatively uncommon (1,7). After impurities were removed from the early preparations in the early 1960s, the incidence of side effects remains low and is a function of the volume of use. Although a wide variety of side effects have been ascribed to vancomycin, it must be emphasized that vancomycin remains a relatively safe antibiotic when dosed and used appropriately (31–33).

Table 5 Vancomycin Side Effects

Side effects	Comments
Hematologic	
Neutropenia	Reversible and uncommon
Thrombocytopenia	Rare
Auditory nerve/ ototoxicity	
Tinnitus/High frequency loss	Usually reversible
Deafness	Permanent
Nephrotoxicity	Reversible if it occurs at all
Hypersensitivity reactions	
"Red neck" syndrome "Red man" syndrome	Usually related to too rapid injection/inadequate diluent volume
Drug fever	Uncommon
Hypotension	Rare
Cardiac arrest	Very rare
Rash	Rare
Urticarial anaphylaxis	Very rare

If vancomycin is administered too rapidly or is diluted in an inadequate volume of fluid, then a histaminelike reaction characterized by diffuse erythema and redness of the skin known as "red man" or "red neck" syndrome commonly occurs. Such reactions occur less frequently in patients given vancomycin using a 1-g (IV) 12 h dosing regimen rather than the 500 mg (IV) 6 h dosing regimen (7,32).

Reactions rarely associated with vancomycin use include hypotension, cardiac arrest, neutropenia, or thrombocytopenia (34–37). With pure vancomycin preparations and with proper administration, i.e., over 60 min with adequate volume of diluent, vancomycin is not irritating to the veins, even in elderly individuals (7).

The main concerns, in terms of toxicity, with respect to vancomycin, are renal dysfunction and ototoxic potential. Ototoxicity due to vancomycin is uncommon in patients with normal renal function receiving the usual doses of vancomycin. Vancomycin ototoxicity deafness is associated with prolonged serum concentrations exceeding 80 μg/ml. Transient tinnitus and/or high-tone hearing loss may occur with serum levels as low as 40 μg/ml (38,39). Ototoxicity may be reversible or permanent, is usually bilateral, and is more common in elderly persons.

Nephrotoxicity was ascribed to the impurities in the initial phases of drug production; there is no well-documented evidence of vancomycin nephrotoxicity when the drug is properly used alone. Conflicting data exist in terms of vancomycin's nephrotoxic potential when combined with other potentially nephrotoxic agents, e.g., aminoglycosides, loop diuretics, etc. Although clearly one should be aware of the nephrotoxic potential in administering nephrotoxic drugs with vancomycin, it is the author's opinion that clinically significant nephrotoxicity in patients dosed appropriately for their degree of renal function remains uncommon and is reversible (41–43). However, there is evidence that older patients are at increased risk for nephrotoxicity whether vancomycin is given alone (13% renal dysfunction) or in combination with an aminoglycoside (33% renal failure) (44) (Table 5).

REFERENCES

1. Alexander MR. A review of vancomycin after 15 years of use. Drug Intell Clin Pharm 1974; 8:520–5.
2. Cook FV, Farrar WE. Vancomycin. Ann Intern Med 1978; 88:813–8.
3. Fekety R. Vancomycin. Med Clin N Am 1982; 66:175–81.
4. Cunha BA, Ristuccia AM. Clinical usefulness of vancomycin. Clin Pharm 1983; 2:417–24.
5. Levine JF. Vancomycin: a review. Med Clin North Am 1987; 71:1135–45.
6. Hermans PE, Wilhelm MP. Vancomycin. Mayo Clin Proc 1987; 62:901–5.
7. Kucers A, Bennett N McK. The use of antibiotics. 4th ed. Philadelphia: Lippincott, 1988:1045–68.
8. Watanakunakorn C, Bakie C. The antibacterial action of vancomycin. Rev Infect Dis 1981; 3:210–5.

8a. Yoshikawa TT, Norman DC. Aging and clinical practice: infectious diseases. Diagnosis and treatment. New York: Igaku Shoin, 1987.

9. Kirby, WM. Vancomycin therapy of severe staphylococcal infections. J Antimicrob Chemother 1984; 14:73–8.
10. Mandell GL, Lindsey E, Hook EW. Synergism of vancomycin and streptomycin for enterococci. Am J Med Sci 1970; 259:346–9.
11. Besnier JM, Leport C, Bure A, et al. Vancomycin-aminoglycoside combinations in therapy of endocarditis caused by *Enterococcus* species and *Streptococcus bovis*. Eur J Clin Microbiol Infect Dis 1990; 9:130–3.
12. Cutler NR, Narang PK, Lesko LJ, et al. Vancomycin disposition: the importance of age. Clin Pharmacol Ther 1984; 36:803–10.
13. Bartlett JG. Antibiotic-associated pseudomembranous colitis. Rev Infect Dis 1979; 1:530–9.
14. Fekety R, Silva J, Armstrong J, et al. Treatment of antibiotic-associated enterocolitis with vancomycin. Rev Infect Dis 1981; 3:273–81.
15. Fekety R, Silva J, Kauffman C, et al. Treatment of antibiotic-associated *Clostridium difficile* colitis with oral vancomycin. Am J Med 1989; 86:15–9.
16. Congeni BL, Tan J, Salstrom SJ, et al. Kinetics of vancomycin after intraventricular and intravenous administration. Pediatr Res 1980; 13:459 (abstract).
17. Gump DW. Vancomycin for treatment of bacterial meningitis. Rev Infect Dis 1981; 3:289–92.
18. Cunha BA, Quintiliani R, Deglin JM, et al. Pharmacokinetics of vancomycin in anuria. Rev Infect Dis 1981; 3:269–72.
19. Moellering RC Jr, Krogstad DJ, Greenblatt DJ. Pharmacokinetics of vancomycin in normal subjects and in patients with reduced renal function. Rev Infect Dis 1981; 3:230–5.
20. Golper TA, Noonan HM, Elzinga L, et al. Vancomycin pharmacokinetics, renal handling, and nonrenal clearances in normal human subjects. Clin Pharmacol Ther 1988; 43:565–70.
21. Rodvoid KA, Blum RA, Fischer JH, et al. Vancomycin pharmacokinetics in patients with various degrees of renal function. Antimicrob Agents Chemother 1988; 32:848–52.
22. Eng RH, Wynn L, Smith SM, et al. Effect of intravenous vancomycin on renal function. Chemotherapy 1989; 35:320–5.
23. Ritter MA, Barzilauskas CD, Faris PM, et al. Vancomycin prophylaxis and elective total joint arthroplasty. Orthopedics 1989; 12:1333–6.
24. Wade JC, Schimpff SC, Newman KA, et al. *Staphylococcus epidermidis*: an increasing cause of infection in patients with granulocytopenia. Ann Intern Med 1982; 97:503–8.
25. Daschner FD, Frank U, Kümmel A, et al. Pharmacokinetics of vancomycin in serum and tissue of patients undergoing open-heart surgery. J Antimicrob Chemother 1987; 6:212–3.
26. Ranson MR, Oppenheim BA, Jackson A, et al. Double-blind placebo controlled study of vancomycin prophylaxis for central venous catheter insertion in cancer patients. J Hosp Infect 1990; 15:95–102.
27. Bradley SF. Methicillin-resistant *Staphylococcus aureus* infection. Clin Geriatr Med 1992; 4:853–68.

28. Karchmer AW, Archer GL, Desmukes WE. *Staphylococcus epidermidis* causing prosthetic-valve endocarditis: microbiologic and clinical observations as guides to therapy. Ann Intern Med 1983; 98:447–53.
29. Thomas DR, Bennett RG, Laughan BE, et al. Postantibiotic colonization with *Clostridium difficile* in nursing home patients. J Am Geriatr Soc 1990; 38:415–20.
30. Garrelts JC, Peterie JD. Altered vancomycin dose vs. serum concentration relationship in burn patients. Clin Pharmacol Ther 1988; 78:278–81.
31. Sorrell TC, Collignon PJ. A prospective study of adverse reactions associated with vancomycin therapy. J Antimicrob Chemother 1985; 16:235–41.
32. Holliman R. "Red man syndrome" associated with rapid vancomycin infusion [letter]. Lancet 1985; 1:1399.
33. Pau AK, Khakoo R. "Red-neck syndrome" with slow infusion of vancomycin [letter]. N Engl J Med 1985; 313:756–7.
34. Mayhew JR, Deutsch S. Cardiac arrest following administration of vancomycin. Can Anaesth Soc J 1985; 132:39–40.
35. Mackett RL, Guay DR. Vancomycin-induced neutropenia. Can Med Assoc J 1985; 132:39–40.
36. Dajee H, Laks H, Miller J, Oren R. Profound hypotension from rapid vancomycin administration during cardiac operation. J Thorac Cardiovasc Surg 1984; 87:145–6.
37. Stier GR, McGory RW, Spotnitz WD, et al. Hemodynamic effects of rapid vancomycin infusion in critically ill patients. Anesth Analg 1990; 71:394–9.
38. Bailie GR, Neal D. Vancomycin ototoxicity and nephrotoxicity. A review. Med Toxicol Adverse Drug Exp 1988; 3:376–86.
39. Mellor JA, Kingdom J, Cafferkey M, et al. Vancomycin ototoxicity in patients with normal renal function. Br J Audiol 1984; 18:179–80.
40. Rybak MJ, Bolke SC. Additive toxicity in patients receiving vancomycin and aminoglycosides [letter]. Clin Pharm 1983; 12:1609–10.
41. Rybak JH, Albrecht LM, Bolke SC, et al. Nephrotoxicity of vancomycin, alone and with an aminoglycoside. J Antimicrob Chemother 1991; 25:679–87.
42. Pauly DJ, Musa DM, Lestico MR, et al. Risk of nephrotoxicity with combination vancomycin-aminoglycoside antibiotic therapy. Pharmacotherapy 1990; 10:378–82.
43. EORTC and National Cancer Institute of Canada—Clinical Trials Group. Vancomycin added to empirical combination antibiotic therapy for fever in granulocytopenic cancer patients. J Infect Dis 1991; 163:951–8.
44. Downs NJ, Neihart RE, Dolezal JM, et al. Mild nephrotoxicity associated with vancomycin. Arch Intern Med 1989; 149:1777–81.

16

Tetracyclines

Natalie C. Klein and Burke A. Cunha
Winthrop-University Hospital, Mineola, and State University of New York School of Medicine, Stony Brook, New York

I. INTRODUCTION

The tetracyclines are broad-spectrum antibiotics with antimicrobial activity against many gram-positive and gram-negative facultative aerobic and anaerobic bacteria, as well as *Mycoplasma*, *Chlamydia*, rickettsiae, spirochetes, and some protozoa. The first tetracycline, chlortetracycline, was isolated in 1948 by Duggar, followed by the production of oxytetracycline 2 years later, and in 1952 tetracycline was released (1). The first of the second-generation tetracyclines, demeclocycline, was developed in 1959, and rolitetracycline, a soluble derivative of tetracycline, was produced soon afterwards, followed by methacycline in 1961, a derivative of oxytetracycline. The long-acting second-generation tetracycline doxycycline became available in 1966, while minocycline was released in 1972 (2).

The tetracyclines are relatively safe drugs for use in the elderly patient. The long half-life, efficient oral absorption, and hepatic excretion of the second-generation tetracyclines, especially doxycycline, make this drug an ideal therapeutic agent for a variety of infections in elderly patients. Unfortunately, there is a scarcity of information on the pharmacokinetics of antibiotics in elderly persons and the interaction of antibiotics with multiple drug regimens that the older patient may require.

II. CHEMISTRY

The structures of the tetracyclines, congeneric derivatives of the polycyclic naphthacene-carboxamide, are shown in Table 1. The tetracycline crystalline bases are only minimally soluble in water at pH 7 but form soluble salts and hydrochlorides (2).

III. MECHANISM OF ACTION

Tetracyclines, like aminoglycosides, inhibit protein synthesis by binding to the 30S ribosomal subunit. There are two processes necessary for tetracyclines to gain access to the

Table 1 Structures of Selected Tetracyclines

Tetracycline	Substituent(s)
Chlortetracycline	−Cl
Oxytetracycline	−OH, −H
Demeclocycline	−OH, −H; −Cl
Methacycline	−OH, −H; $-CH_2$
Doxycycline	−OH, −H; $-CH_3$, −H
Minocycline	−H, −H; $-N(CH_3)_2$

bacterial ribosomes of gram-negative bacteria (3). The first step is passive diffusion through hydrophilic pores in the outer cell membrane. The second step involves an energy-dependent active transport that pumps tetracycline through the inner cytoplasmic membrane. Once inside the cell, tetracyclines bind to the 30S ribosome and prevent access of aminoacyl transfer RNA to the acceptor site on the messenger RNA–ribosome complex (2). Resistance to tetracyclines in vitro occurs slowly, in incremental steps. Once microorganisms become resistant to one tetracycline, they frequently are also resistant to other tetracyclines. Plasmids mediate tetracycline resistance by coding for proteins that interrupt active transport of the antibiotic through the cytoplasmic membrane. Resistance may occur by chromosomal alteration as well (4).

IV. ANTIMICROBIAL SPECTRUM

The tetracyclines are active against many gram-positive and gram-negative bacteria as well as *Mycoplasma*, *Chlamydia*, rickettsiae, and amoebae (Table 2). The tetracyclines in vitro are bacteriostatic antibiotics; however, when present in high concentrations, they are frequently bactericidal (2). Gram-positive bacteria are more sensitive to tetracyclines than gram-negative bacteria in vitro. However, because of development of resistant strains, these drugs should not be used for *Streptococcus pyogenes* or *Streptococcus pneumoniae* infections. Tetracycline is bacteriostatic against *Staphylococcus aureus* and should not be used for serious staphylococcal infections. The usefulness of tetracyclines for the treatment of gram-negative bacteria such as *Salmonella* and *Shigella* is also limited by resistant strains. Tetracyclines have no activity against *Proteus mirabilis* or *Pseudomonas aeruginosa*. They remain active against some *Haemophilus* species, *Brucella*, *Vibrio*, *Pasteurella multocida*, *Chlamydia*, *Mycoplasma*, *Ureaplasma*, rickettsiae, and spirochetes.

The second-generation tetracyclines doxycycline and minocycline are more active than tetracycline against gram-positive bacteria, especially *S. aureus* and *S. pneumoniae*. They are both also quite active against *Bacteroides fragilis* and *Clostridium* in vitro (4).

V. CLINICAL PHARMACOLOGY

A. Pharmacokinetics

The tetracyclines are adequately but incompletely absorbed from the gastrointestinal tract, primarily from the stomach and the small intestine. The percentage of an oral dose absorbed on an empty stomach is lowest for chlortetracycline (25–30%), intermediate for oxytetracycline, demeclocycline, and tetracycline (58–80%), and highest for minocycline

Table 2 Antibiotic Sensitivities of Tetracycline, Doxycycline, and Minocycline

Organism	Mean minimal inhibitory concentration (μg/ml)		
	Tetracycline	Doxycycline	Minocycline
Gram-positive bacteria			
Staphylococcus aureus	3.1	1.6	0.78
Streptococcus pyogenes	0.78	0.39	0.39
Streptococcus pneumoniae	0.8	0.2	0.2
Viridans group streptococci	3.1	0.39	0.39
Enterococcus faecalis	>100	50	100
Gram-negative bacteria			
Escherichia coli	12.5	12.5	6.3
Enterobacter spp.	25	25	12.5
Klebsiella spp.	50	50	25
Serratia marcescens	200	50	25
Proteus mirabilis	>100	>100	>100
Neisseria gonorrhoeae	0.78	0.39	0.39
Neisseria meningitidis	0.8	1.6	1.6
Hemophilus influenzae	1.6	1.6	1.6
Legionella pneumophila	5.2	1.0	0.43
Mycoplasma/chlamydia			
Mycoplasma pneumoniae	1.6	1.6	1.6
Ureaplasma urealyticum	0.4	0.1	0.13
Chlamydia spp.	0.6	0.06	0.02

Source: Adapted from Ref. 4.

and doxycycline (93–100%) (2,5,6). Achlorhydria, a condition frequently found in older adults, does not impair absorption of tetracyclines. There was no difference in rate and extent of absorption in elderly achlorhydric patients from the control group given 250 mg tetracycline (7). However, the use of milk and milk products, aluminum hydroxide gels, sodium bicarbonate, calcium and magnesium salts, and iron preparations decreases the absorption of most tetracyclines by chelation and increasing gastric pH (2,8). Doxycycline and minocycline are the only tetracycline drugs that are well absorbed orally in the presence of food (9) (Table 3). Oral administration of 500 mg tetracycline or 200 mg doxycycline or minocycline produce peak serum concentrations of 3–5 μg/ml in about 2 h. Doxycycline and minocycline have a much longer half-life (18–20 h) compared to tetracycline (8.5 h) (2,11). Since intravenous tetracycline is associated with thrombophlebitis and hepatic toxicity, for practical purposes only intravenous doxycycline is used.

Plasma concentration of oral or intravenous administered doxycycline are equivalent, making doxycycline a convenient oral drug to use in geriatric patients when venous access is a problem (2). Tissue penetration of doxycycline appears unaffected by age. Serum levels in 12 geriatric patients given 200 mg doxycycline intravenously were not significantly different from those of young adults (12). However, Bocker et al. (13) found that the serum levels of doxycycline in 25 elderly patients were 50–100% higher than levels in young and middle-aged patients, probably due to an apparent lower volume of distribution from age-dependent changes in drug binding. Since doxycycline has a wide margin of safety and minimal toxicity, dose adjustment in elderly patients is not usually necessary.

Table 3 Oral Absorption of Tetracyclines

	% Absorbed Orally	
Drug	Fasting state	Effect with food
Chlortetracycline	25–30	NA
Oxytetracycline	58	Decreased
Methacycline	58	Decreased
Demethylchlortetracycline	66	Decreased
Tetracycline	77–80	Decreased
Doxycycline	93	Insignificant
Minocycline	100	Insignificant

NA = Not available.
Source: Adapted from Refs. 2 and 9.

B. Distribution

The volume of distribution of most tetracyclines is relatively larger than that of body water (2). Binding to plasma proteins occurs in varying degrees but is highest with doxycycline (82%), intermediate with minocycline (76%), and lowest with tetracycline (56%) (2,11). Lipid solubility also varies among the tetracyclines and is directly related to tissue penetration. Both doxycycline and minocycline are extremely lipid soluble, accounting for their superior tissue penetration. Doxycycline is five times more lipid soluble than tetracycline, while minocycline is five times more lipid soluble than doxycycline (10). The enhanced lipid solubility of doxycycline and minocycline allows these drugs to rapidly penetrate the secretions of the respiratory tract, lung tissue, and prostate (9,14–16) (Table 4). The lipid solubility of doxycycline allows for rapid and complete gastrointestinal absorption and excellent tissue penetration as well as persistence in secretions and tissue of respiratory tract and prostate, making doxycycline an ideal drug for atypical pneumonia and acute prostatitis. Tetracyclines cross the placenta and are found in relatively high concentrations in human milk. Because of the ability of tetracyclines to be stored in bone and the dentine and enamel of unerupted teeth, these drugs should not be used in pregnant women or children under age 8. Intravenously administered tetracyclines slowly penetrate cerebrospinal fluid in patients with both inflamed and noninflamed meninges, however, at approximately a fourth of the serum concentration.

Table 4 Penetration of Tetracyclines in Respiratory Tract and Prostate

	Extent of penetration			
Drug	Prostate	Lung	Sputum	Saliva
Tetracycline	+	++	+	+
Doxycycline	+++	+++	+++	++
Minocycline	+++	+++	+++	+++

+ = slight; ++ = moderate; +++ = excellent.
Source: Adapted from Refs. 6 and 9

Table 5 Drug Interactions with Tetracyclines

Drug	Effect
Oral antacid	Impaired absorption of tetracyclines
Ferrous sulfate	Impaired absorption of tetracyclines
Anticonvulsants (phenytoin, carbamazepine)	Shortens half-life of doxycycline
Barbiturates	Shortens half-life of doxycycline
Alcohol consumption	May reduce half-life of doxycycline
Anticoagulants	Intravenous tetracycline may cause enhanced anticoagulation
Methoxyflurane anesthesia	Renal failure after tetracycline use
Penicillin	Tetracyclines may interfere with bactericidal action of penicillin

C. Elimination

Except for doxycycline, the tetracyclines are excreted primarily in the urine by glomerular filtration. Up to 90% of doxycycline may be excreted in the feces as an inactive conjugate or as a chelate, while the renal clearance of doxycycline is from 19 to 23% of glomerular filtrate (5,17). Therefore, no alteration in dose is necessary for doxycycline when used in patients with renal insufficiency, making it an easy drug to use in elderly patients who frequently have some underlying renal impairment. All of the other tetracycline drugs must be given in reduced dosages to patients with renal insufficiency and should probably be avoided in patients with significant renal failure. Minocycline is excreted in the urine and feces in much lower amounts than the other tetracycline drugs, and the half-life is not prolonged in patients with hepatic failure. Minocycline appears to undergo considerable metabolism and is the safest of the tetracycline drugs for use in patients with liver failure (2).

D. Drug Interactions

A number of drugs may interact with tetracycline absorption or metabolism (Table 5). The concomitant use of oral antacids or other drugs containing calcium, magnesium, and aluminum impairs the oral absorption of tetracyclines (18,19). Gastrointestinal absorption of all tetracyclines is impaired by simultaneous administration of ferrous sulfate (18,20). Doxycycline may be less effective in patients receiving long-term therapy with phenytoin or carbamazepine because the half-life of doxycycline is shortened by 50% (21). Simultaneous use of barbiturates and doxycycline may also reduce the half-life of doxycycline from 15 to 11 h by the induction of doxycycline-metabolizing enzymes (22). Heavy alcohol consumption may also reduce the half-life of doxycycline by inducing more rapid metabolization of doxycycline (23).

Intravenous tetracycline, by reducing plasma prothrombin activity, may enhance the effects of anticoagulants (24). Severe renal failure has been reported in patients receiving tetracyclines after methoxyflurane anesthesia from the formation of calcium oxalate crystals (25,26). Finally, the tetracycline bacteriostatic drugs may interfere with bactericidal action of penicillins (27).

Table 6 Major Clinical Indications for Tetracyclines

Disease/Syndrome	Alternate Therapy
Rocky mountain spotted fever/Typhus	Chloramphenicol
Brucellosis	Streptomycin, TMP-SMX
Relapsing fever	Erythromycin, chloramphenicol
Lyme disease	Amoxicillin,[a] ceftriaxone[a]
Melioidosis	Chloramphenicol
Mycoplasma pneumonia	Erythromycin[a]
Syphilis	Benzathine penicillin[a]
Traveler's diarrhea	Ciprofloxacin[a] TMP-SMX[a]
Legionnaires' disease	Erythromycin[a]
Acute exacerbation of chronic bronchitis	Erythromycin, cephalosporin, TMP-SMX
Leptospirosis	Penicillin[a]
Tularemia	Streptomycin
Amebiasis	Metronidazole[a]
Actinomycosis	Penicillin[a]
Nocardiosis	TMP-SMX[a]
Whipple's disease	Penicillin, streptomycin
Acne	Topical erythromycin or clindamycin

TMP-SMX = trimethoprim sulfamethoxazole.
[a]Considered the drug of choice over tetracyclines.

VI. CLINICAL INDICATIONS

Tetracycline drugs are active against many commonly encountered pathogens as well as uncommon bacteria and are used to treat a variety of infections including pneumonia, diarrheal disease, prostatitis, sexually transmitted diseases, and acne. Tetracyclines are, however, prescribed less commonly in adult patients due in part to the availability of other more effective antimicrobial agents, as well as the lower occurrence of infections that require tetracyclines as primary therapy in elderly patients. Moreover, problems with tetracycline resistance have decreased the usefulness of tetracyclines for many infections. The tetracyclines, nevertheless, remain the treatment of choice for a number of less common but serious infections including rickettsial diseases, brucellosis, chlamydial infections, melioidosis, relapsing fever, cholera, Lyme disease, and atypical pneumonia (Table 6). Many, if not all, of these infections do occur in older adults, and, thus, clinicians who provide care to geriatric patients should be familiar with the indications for tetracycline drugs.

A. Respiratory Infections

Tetracyclines are useful in the management of acute exacerbations of chronic bronchitis, an infection that is common among elderly patients. Several studies have demonstrated doxycycline to be equally or slightly more efficacious than ampicillin for infective exacerbations of chronic bronchitis (28,29). Oral doxycycline and ampicillin were both found to be effective in the treatment of lower respiratory tract infections in patients with or without chronic lung disease (30,31). However, in many areas of the United States, the increasingly high rates of tetracycline resistance among pneumococci and *Haemophilus influenzae* make second-generation cephalosporins, trimethoprim-sulfamethoxazole, or erythromycin preferred drugs over tetracyclines for lower respiratory tract infections.

The tetracyclines have excellent activity against all the pathogens causing atypical pneumonia. Doxycycline is effective therapy for pneumonias caused by *Legionella pneumophila*, *Mycoplasma pneumoniae*, *Chlamydia pneumoniae*, *Chlamydia psittaci*, *Francisella tularensis*, and *Coxiella burnetti* (32,33). Of the pneumonias caused by these pathogens, *Legionella* pneumonia is especially important to older patients. However, currently, erythromycin remains the drug of choice for *Legionella* infection (33a) (see also Chap. 17). Several studies have demonstrated the efficacy of doxycycline in decreasing the number of febrile days and improving symptoms of patients with *Mycoplasma* pneumonia (34,35). Doxycycline has also been shown to be effective in the treatment of sinusitis because of its excellent penetration into sinus secretions (36,37). Sinusitis is also a relatively common infection of elderly persons (37a).

B. Gastrointestinal Infections

With the increasing number of retired persons, older adults are traveling abroad. The potential for acute gastroenteritis and diarrhea must be considered in this population. Some of these gastrointestinal infections may require tetracycline therapy.

Although the treatment of cholera is primarily rehydration, tetracyclines are effective therapy for eradicating cholera carrier state, for prophylaxis, and for decreasing duration and volume of diarrhea (38,39). However, tetracycline has no effect on epidemics of tetracycline-resistant strains of *Vibrio cholerae*. Tetracyclines are also effective in treating some *Shigella* infections. A single 2.5-g dose of tetracycline has been shown to be effective for adult shigellosis (40). Doxycycline, 100 mg daily, has been used to prevent traveler's diarrhea among Peace Corp volunteers.

C. Sexually Transmitted Diseases

In sexually active older persons, sexually transmitted disease should be considered in the differential diagnosis of genital lesions, penile or vaginal discharges, and inguinal adenopathy. The tetracyclines are excellent drugs for the treatment of nongonococcal urethritis caused by *C. trachomatis* or *Ureaplasma urealyticum*. Tetracyclines are also effective for the treatment of syphilis in a penicillin-allergic patient and are active against non–penicillinase-producing strains of pathogens causing gonorrhea, lymphogranuloma venereum, and granuloma inguinale, as well as a few strains of chancroid. However, because of widespread resistance of *Haemophilus ducreyi* to tetracyclines, ceftriaxone, erythromycin, or trimethoprim-sulfamethoxazole are now the preferred drugs.

VII. ADMINISTRATION OF DRUG

Tetracyclines are available for oral, topical, and parenteral administration (Table 7). Most tetracycline compounds are prescribed for oral use but they may be given intravenously. Intramuscular administration results in a high risk of sensitization. However, the risk of sensitization in older patients is unknown. Nevertheless, it would seem prudent to avoid both intramuscular administration and topical therapy in all patients, regardless of age. All tetracycline drugs except for doxycycline should be avoided in older patients with renal failure because their catabolic effect is associated with further deterioration of renal function. Minocycline, which is excreted primarily in the feces, can be used safely in elderly patients with minor renal failure but should be avoided in severe renal disease.

Table 7 Tetracycline Compounds, Routes of Administration, and Recommended Doses

Drug	Route of administration: Oral	Route of administration: Intravenous
Tetracycline	250–500 mg q6h	should not exceed 2 g/day
Oxtetracycline	250–500 mg q6h	should not exceed 2 g/day
Chlortetracycline	250–500 mg q6h	should not exceed 2 g/day
Doxycycline	100 mg q12h	100–200 mg q12 h
Minocycline	200 mg initially, then 100 mg q12h	same as oral
Demeclocycline	150–300 mg q6h	same as oral
Methacycline	150 mg q6h	same as oral

VIII. ADVERSE EFFECTS

Although tetracyclines are considered to be relatively safe drugs, a number of adverse effects can occur. Gastrointestinal irritation can occur with all orally administered tetracyclines, but it is more common with oxytetracycline and doxycycline when either are taken in large doses. Tetracycline and doxycycline may cause esophageal ulceration or stricture, especially in the elderly patient, but they can be prevented by taking capsules with food or copious water and not immediately before going to bed (42,43). Much of the gastric distress associated with tetracyclines can be alleviated by administration of the drug with food (not milk or milk products) or antacids that do not contain aluminum, magnesium, or calcium. Diarrhea due to the irritative effect of tetracyclines on the distal gastrointestinal tract must be distinguished from diarrhea due to candidal overgrowth or to pseudomembranous colitis secondary to *Clostridium difficile.*

Parenterally administered tetracycline has been associated with acute fatty necrosis of the liver. Most cases of severe hepatotoxicity have occurred in pregnant women receiving more than 2 g intravenous tetracycline per day. There does not appear to be increased risk of hepatotoxicity in the elderly patient.

All tetracyclines except doxycycline are antianabolic and are contraindicated in renal failure. This is especially relevant in elderly persons because they have a high prevalence of renal dysfunction, as well as protein-calorie malnutrition (43a). Tetracyclines worsen azotemia in patients with chronic renal failure by inhibiting protein synthesis so that the kidneys excrete an additional load from amino acid metabolism. Tetracyclines can cause renal tubular damage and a Fanconilike syndrome, while demethylchlortetracycline can induce nephrogenic diabetes insipidus.

Hypersensitivity reactions including morbilliform rashes, urticaria, asthma, and contact dermatitis are uncommon but may occur with all the tetracyclines. Demeclocycline and doxycycline may produce a mild to severe reaction in sun-exposed skin—called a phototoxic reaction (2). Some individuals will develop onycholysis and nail pigmentation. Although in children under the age of 8 tetracyclines cause brown discoloration of the teeth and may depress bone growth, these adverse effects do not occur in older adults. Minocycline is frequently accompanied by reversible vestibular toxicity characterized by dizziness, nausea, vomiting, and ataxia and is best avoided in the elderly patient (44).

Intravenous administration of first-generation tetracyclines is associated with frequent phlebitis, but this is less likely with doxycycline.

Despite the numerous reported side effects, the tetracyclines are relatively safe drugs for use in elderly patients. When a tetracycline is indicated, doxycycline is the preferred tetracycline compound for use in elderly patients. The long half-life of doxycycline makes it a more convenient drug to administer to the older patient and therefore assures better compliance with the therapeutic regimen. Oral absorption is rapid and not significantly decreased by food, tissue penetration is excellent, and doxycycline does not need to be dose adjusted in older patients with renal insufficiency.

REFERENCES

1. Duggar BM. Aureomycin: a product of the continuing search for new antibiotics. Ann NY Acad Sci 1948; 51:177–81.
2. Sande MA, Mandell GL. Antimicrobial agents. In: Goodman and Gilman's the pharmacological basis of therapeutics. 7th ed. New York: Macmillan, 1985:1170–98.
3. Chopra I, Howe TGB. Bacterial resistance to the tetracyclines. Microbiol Rev 1978; 42:707–24.
4. Cunha BA. Clinical uses of the tetracyclines. In: Hlavka JJ, Boothe JH, eds. The tetracyclines. Berlin: Springer-Verlag, 1985:393–404.
5. Fabre J, Milek E, Kalfopoulos P, et al. Kinetics of tetracycline in man. II. Excretion, penetration in normal and inflammatory tissues, behavior in renal insufficiency and hemodialysis. Schweiz Med Wochenschr 1971; 101:625–33.
6. Cunha BA. Pharmacokinetics of doxycycline. Postgrad Med Comm 1979; (suppl):63–72.
7. Kramer PA, Chapron DJ, Benson J, et al. Tetracycline absorption in elderly patients with achlorhydria. Clin Pharmacol Ther 1978; 23:467–72.
8. Neuvonen PJ, Gothoni G, Hackman R, et al. Interference of iron with the absorption of tetracyclines in man. Br Med J 1970; 4:532–4.
9. Fabre J, Milek E, Kalfopoulos P, et al. The kinetics of tetracycline in man. I. Digestive absorption and serum concentrations. Schweiz Med Wochenschr 1971; 101:593–8.
10. Cunha BA, Garabedian-Ruffalo SM. Tetracyclines in urology: current concepts. Urology 1990; 36:548–56.
11. Cunha BA, Comer JB, Jonas M. The tetracyclines. Med Clin North Am 1982; 66:293–302.
12. Simon C, Malerczyk V, Engelke H, et al. The pharmacokinetics of doxycycline in kidney insufficiency in geriatric patients compared to younger adults. Schweiz Med Wochenschr 1975; 105:1615–20.
13. Bocker R, Mühlberg W, Platt D, et al. Serum level, half-life and apparent volume of distribution of doxycycline in geriatric patients. Eur J Clin Pharmacol 1986; 30:105–8.
14. Thadepalli H, Huang JT. Treatment of anaerobic lung infections with intravenous doxycycline. Curr Ther Res 1977; 21:849–54.
15. Gartmann J. Doxycycline concentrations in lung tissue, bronchial wall and bronchial secretions. Schweiz Med Wochenschr 1972; 102:1484–6.
16. Garnes HA. Doxycycline levels in serum and prostatic tissue in man. Urology 1973; 1:205–7.
17. Merier G, Lawrencet FL, Rudhardt M, et al. Behaviour of doxycycline in renal insufficiency. Helv Med Acta 1969/1970; 35:124–34.
18. Neuvonen PJ. Interactions with absorption of tetracyclines. Drugs 1976; 11:45–54.
19. Barr WH, Adir JA, Barrettson L. Decrease of tetracycline absorption in man by sodium bicarbonate. Clin Pharmacol Ther 1971; 12:779–84.
20. Neuvonen PJ, Gothoni G, Hackman R, et al. Interference of iron with the absorption of tetracyclines in man. Br Med J 1970; 4:532–4.
21. Neuvonen PJ, Pentilla O, Lehtovaara R, et al. Effect of anti-epileptic drugs on the elimination of various tetracycline derivatives. Eur J Clin Pharmacol 1975; 9:147–54.

22. Neuvonen PJ, Pentilla O. Interaction between doxycycline and barbiturates. Br Med J 1974; 1:535–6.
23. Neuvonen PJ, Pentillo O, Roos M, et al. Effect of long-term alcohol consumption on the half life of tetracycline and doxycycline in man. Ont J Clin Pharmacol 1974; 14:303–7.
24. Searcy RL, Simms NM, Foreman JA, et al. Evaluation of the blood clotting mechanism in tetracycline-treated patients. Antimicrob Agents Chemother 1964;4:179–83.
25. Kuzacu EY. Methoxyflurane, tetracycline, and renal failure. JAMA 1970; 211:1162–4.
26. Cousins MJ, Mazze RI. Tetracycline, methoxyflurane anesthesia, and renal dysfunction. Lancet 1972; 1:751–2.
27. Jawetz E. The use of combinations of antimicrobial drugs. Annu Rev Pharmacol 1968; 8:151–70.
28. Chodosh S, Baigelman W. Doxycycline compared with amoxicillin in acute bacterial exacerbations of chronic bronchitis: preliminary report of a double-blind crossover study. In: Doxycycline (vibromycin): recent investigations and clinical experience, vol 3. New York: Excerpta Medica, 1977:1–11.
29. Aitchison WRC, Grant IWB, Gould JC. Treatment of acute exacerbations in chronic bronchitis. Br J Clin Pract 1968; 22:343–5.
30. Dalal A. Chronic bronchitis—a clinical trial of vibromycin and ampicillin. Med Digest 1969; 14:449–54.
31. Lyons HA, Thomas JS, Hewrich AE, et al. Efficacy of doxycycline in acute infections of the lower respiratory tract. Curr Ther Res Clin Exp 1976; 19:24–31.
32. Johnson DH, Cunha BA. The atypical pneumonias. Postgrad Med 1993;93:69–82.
33. Cunha BA, Jonas M. Legionnaires' disease treated with doxycycline. Lancet 1981; 2:1107.
33a. Yoshikawa TT. Antimicrobial therapy for the elderly patient. J Am Geriatr Soc 1990; 38:1353–72.
34. Gooch WM, Mogabgab WJ. Therapeutic effect of doxycycline upon *Mycoplasma pneumoniae* pneumonia. Antimicrob Agents Chemother 1971; 10:291–5.
35. Izumikawa K. Doxycycline treatment of mycoplasmal pneumonia. Postgrad Med Suppl 1979; 1:51–6.
36. Axelsson A, Brorson JE. Concentration of antibiotics in sinus secretions. Ann Otol 1973; 82:44–8.
37. Gnarpe H, Lundberg C. L-phase organisms in maxillary sinus secretions. Scand J Infect Dis 1971; 3:257–9.
37a. Slavin RG. Management of sinusitis. J Am Geriatr Soc 1991; 39:212–7.
38. De SA, Chauduri A, Duta D, et al. Doxycycline in the treatment of cholera. Bull WHO 1976; 54:177–9.
39. Rahman MM, Majid MA, Alam AK, et al. Effects of doxycycline in actively purging cholera patients: a double blind trial. Antimicrob Agents Chemother 1976; 10:610–2.
40. Pickering LK, DuPont HL, Olarte J. Single dose tetracycline therapy for shigellosis in adults. JAMA 1978; 239:853–4.
41. Sack DA, Kaminksy DC, Sack RB, et al. Prophylactic doxycycline for travelers diarrhea. Results of a prospective double-blind study of Peace Corps volunteers in Kenya. N Eng J Med 1978; 298:758–63.
42. Winckler K. Tetracycline ulcers of the oesophagus; endoscopy, histology, and roentgenology in two cases and review of the literature. Endoscopy 1981; 13:225–8.
43. Bonavina L, De Meester TR, McChesney L, et al. Drug-induced esophageal strictures. Ann Surg 1987; 206:173–83.
43a. Rudman D, Feller A. Protein-calorie undernutrition in the nursing home. J Am Geriatr Soc 1989; 37:173–83.
44. Fanning WL, Gump DW, Sofferman RA. Side effects of minocycline: a double blind study. Antimicrob Agents Chemother 1977; 11:712–7.

17

Erythromycin and Newer Macrolides

David M. Forrest and Anthony W. Chow
University of British Columbia, Vancouver, British Columbia, Canada

I. INTRODUCTION

The macrolide antibiotics represent a unique group of antimicrobial agents of increasing significance and expanding clinical utility. The parent compound, erythromycin, remains the most important. Erythromycin is the product of the Philippine soil actinomycete *Streptomyces erythreus* and was introduced into clinical practice by McGuire and associates in 1952 (1). Over the past 40 years, the drug has proven to be safe and effective for many common infections, and indications for its usage continue to increase (2,3). Unfortunately, however, erythromycin possesses certain characteristics that limit its use, thus stimulating the development of newer macrolide antibiotics (4). This heralds a new era in antibiotic therapy and will undoubtedly enhance further the stature of these agents in the antimicrobial armamentarium.

II. CHEMISTRY

The structure of macrolide antibiotics is based on a macrocyclic lactone ring (macrolide) to which various deoxy sugars are attached (5,6); erythromycin has two sugar moieties (Fig. 1). Erythromycin base is a crystalline compound with poor solubility in water. It has a pKa of 8.8 and is rapidly inactivated in an acid medium such as is found in the stomach. Consequently, it is absorbed erratically with inconsistent serum concentrations. Several modifications of the drug have been made in order to minimize the adverse effects of gastric acidity. This is achieved either by protecting the base with enteric or "film" coating, thus allowing passage through the stomach and absorption from the duodenum, or by development of more acid-resistant compounds (5–7). The latter include a salt (stearate), an ester (ethylsuccinate), and a salt of an ester (estolate). These compounds are converted before or after absorption to the base, which is the active form. Water-soluble salts (as lactobionate or gluceptate) are also available for intravenous use.

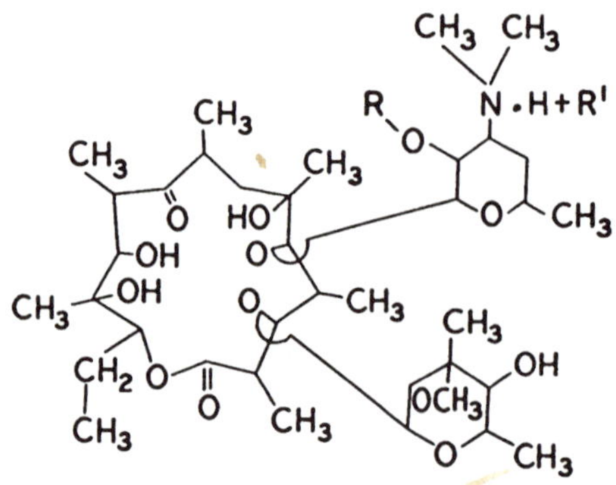

Figure 1 Chemical structure of erythromycin.

III. MECHANISM OF ACTION AND RESISTANCE

Erythromycin is variously described as a bacteriostatic or bactericidal agent. Indeed, its activity is variable depending on the organism to which it is directed, its susceptibility, density of inoculation and phase of growth, as well as the concentration of drug achievable at the site of infection (2,8). Moreover, it is apparent that even though erythromycin may only be bacteriostatic for a given organism in vitro, the agent may have bactericidal properties in vivo (9).

Macrolide antibiotics act by inhibiting RNA-dependent protein synthesis. The drugs bind reversibly to the 50S ribosomal subunit, preventing transpeptidation and/or translocation (10). In some instances, erythromycin shares a common ribosomal binding site with that of other macrolides, clindamycin and chloramphenicol, suggesting a common mechanism of action and antagonism if used in combination (3,5). Its effect is most pronounced in rapidly dividing bacteria and at increased pH (2,3). An interesting observation is that erythromycin may stimulate the immune system (11–13), a characteristic which may be of clinical import as suggested by Straughan and Anderson (9). It appears that erythromycin may enhance both cellular and humoral immune functions and facilitate neutrophil chemotaxis. This topic has been reviewed recently by Gemmell (14).

Resistance to erythromycin may be conferred in a variety of ways and may be constitutive or inducible, depending upon the organism. On a cellular level, resistance to erythromycin can occur by at least four mechanisms. First, there may be decreased cell envelope permeability to the drug. This is a chromosomally mediated, inherent characteristic of gram-negative bacilli (5,6); in *Staphylococcus epidermidis*, it has been found to be plasmid-mediated (15). Second, there can be a change in a single 50S ribosomal subunit protein at the macrolide-binding site (5). This is due to a chromosomal mutation and can occur in gram-positive and gram-negative organisms (5,6), including *Legionella* (16). Third, the 23S ribosomal RNA component of the 50S ribosomal subunit may also be modified so that binding of macrolides (and usually also of clindamycin and streptogramin type B antibiotics) is decreased (2,5,6,16). This is usually plasmid mediated, occurs in both gram-positive and gram-negative bacteria, and can either occur constitutively or be induced (5,6,17,18). This last characteristic may account for the "dissociated resistance" of staphylococci described by Garrod (19), in which organisms grown in the presence of low concentrations of erythromycin demonstrate resistance. Finally, erythromycin may be

Table 1 Antimicrobial Spectrum of Erythromycin

Organism	Minimum inhibitory concentration (μg/ml)		Frequency of resistance
	Median	Range	
Streptococcus pneumoniae	0.05	0.001–0.2[a]	Rare
Streptococcus pyogenes	0.04	0.005–0.2[a]	Rare
Viridans streptococci group	0.06	0.02–3.1[a]	10%
Enterococcus faecalis	1.5	0.1–>100	50%
Staphylococcus aureus	0.4	0.005–>100	10%
Staphylococcus epidermidis	0.6	0.2–>100	40%
Peptostreptococcus spp.	0.2	0.02–0.4	20%
Corynebacterium diphtheriae	0.02	0.003–3.1[a]	Rare
Listeria monocytogenes	0.2	0.1–0.3	Rare
Clostridum perfringens	0.8	0.1–6[a]	25%
Clostridum tetani	0.6	0.006–0.8	None
Actinomyces israelii	0.5	0.2–0.5	None
Nocardia asteroides	25	0.2–>200	Variable
Neisseria gonorrhoeae	0.1	0.005–0.5[a]	Variable
Neisseria meningitidis	0.4	0.1–2	Variable
Moraxella catarrhalis	0.07	0.03–0.125	None
Brucella spp.	5	0.3–10	Variable
Haemophilus influenzae	3.1	0.1–6	40%
Bordetella pertussis	0.4	0.02–1.6	Rare
Campylobacter jejuni	0.2	0.05–>50	Rare
Bacteroides fragilis	1.5	0.1–>100	35%
Bacteroides spp. (except *fragilis*)	0.4	0.02–3.1	Rare
Fusobacterium spp.	12.5	0.02–>25	10%
Legionella pneumophila	0.1	0.06–0.5	None
Mycoplasma pneumoniae	0.005	0.001–0.02	None
Chlamydia trachomatis	0.1	0.1–0.5	None
Mycobacterium kansasii	1	0.5–2	Variable

[a]Occasional clinical isolates are more resistant.
Source: Adapted from Refs. 2, 3, 5, 29.

inactivated by an esterase encoded by a plasmid-mediated determinant (20). Such enzymatic hydrolysis is characteristic of Enterobacteriaceae with high-level resistance (21).

Gram-negative bacilli generally have intrinsic resistance, probably due to inability of the drug to penetrate to the site of action (3), while gram-positive organisms accumulate the drug approximately 100 times more effectively (6). However, in an alkaline environment, the activity of erythromycin against gram-negative bacteria is increased, possibly because of enhanced cellular uptake of the unionized drug, which is more abundant at higher pH (3,5).

IV. ANTIMICROBIAL SPECTRUM

The spectrum of antimicrobial activity of erythromycin is broad. A summary of the susceptibility in vitro of a number of commonly encountered pathogens is presented in Table 1. In general, erythromycin is effective against streptococci, although there are a number of reports of resistance to group A beta-hemolytic streptococcus and pneumococcus, primarily related to increased use of the drug (22–26). Most clinical isolates of *Staphylococcus aureus* remain sensitive to erythromycin, but resistance may emerge during treatment due to induction as outlined above.

Of note, Enterobacteriaceae are usually resistant to erythromycin (2,3,5), although its activity is enhanced at an alkaline pH. Resistance to *Haemophilus influenzae* is reported in a large proportion of isolates (27). Erythromycin is effective against *Moraxella* and *Legionella* (2,3,5,28). In addition to those organisms listed in Table 1, erythromycin possesses clinically useful activity against *Rickettsia* species, *Treponema pallidum*, and a number of nontuberculous mycobacteria (2,3,5,7). It has no useful activity against fungi, parasites, or viruses (6).

V. CLINICAL PHARMACOLOGY

The pharmacological properties of the orally administered medication vary depending on the formulation. Only erythromycin base has antimicrobial activity, and therefore other salts of the drugs are generally inactive until hydrolyzed to the free base (29). Hence, analysis of pharmacokinetic data can be difficult, as reported serum levels tend to reflect the total drug concentration (including unhydrolyzed, protein-bound, and metabolized compound) and not solely the active, free base (2,3,5,6,29). Interpretation of pharmacological information is further complicated by the fact that serum levels may not correlate with those found in infected tissue.

A. Absorption

The peak serum level obtained with orally administered erythromycin is related to several factors: the specific formulation, its coating, temporal relation to food ingestion, and concomitant administration with other medications (5,7,29). In addition, there is considerable individual variability in absorption and achievable peak serum levels tend to increase with multiple doses (30). None of the oral preparations is completely absorbed (3). Peak serum levels rendered with a single dose of erythromycin are summarized in Table 2. It should be noted that these data are based on studies in young adults; in elderly subjects, peak concentrations are higher by approximately 1.5 times after a single dose in one study using the stearate preparation (31).

Erythromycin base is absorbed without alteration. The time course and total amount of absorption depends on the coating of the medication, with enteric-coated pellets providing somewhat more consistent serum concentrations than enteric coated tablets (32–34), although this has been disputed (35). The former have also compared favorably with other preparations (36,37). Food ingestion generally reduces absorption of both pelleted and enteric-coated tablet forms (33–35), though results are inconsistent and excellent bioavailability has been demonstrated in both the fasting and nonfasting states, which is largely dependent upon the particular preparation (38). In one report, absorption of the unprotected base was enhanced by co-administration with aluminum hydroxide (39).

Erythromycin stearate dissociates in the duodenum and is absorbed as the base. Like the base preparation, erythromycin stearate is acid-labile and thus absorption is reduced in the presence of food (which increases the acid content of the stomach), although it has also been suggested that absorption may in fact be enhanced in the nonfasting condition (40). Higher levels are also achieved if taken with a large volume of water (2).

Table 2 Achievable Serum Concentrations of Erythromycin in Adults

Preparation of erythromycin	Dose (mg)	Route	Hours after dose	Serum concentration (μg/ml)
Base	250	Oral	4	0.3–1.0
	500	Oral	4	0.3–1.9
	500	Rectal	1	0.9
Stearate	250 (fasting)	Oral	3	0.2–1.3
	500 (fasting)	Oral	3	0.4–1.8
	500 (nonfasting)	Oral	3	0.1–0.4
Estolate	250 (fasting)	Oral	2–4	1.4–1.7
	500 (fasting)	Oral	3.5–4	4.2[a] (1.1[b])
	250 (nonfasting)	Oral	2–4	1.1–2.9[a]
	500 (nonfasting)	Oral	2–4	1.8–5.2[a]
Ethylsuccinate	500	Oral	0.5–2.5	1.5[a] (0.6[b])
Lactobionate	500	Intravenous	1	9.9
Gluceptate	250	Intravenous	1	3.5–10.7
	1000	Intravenous	1	9.9

[a]Total drug (ester plus base).
[b]Free base.
Source: Adapted from Refs. 2,3,5,29.

Erythromycin estolate is not so acid-susceptible and absorption is largely unaffected when administered with food (2,5,6); again, it has been proposed that absorption may even be improved in the nonfasting state (7). The compound is absorbed mainly as the propionyl ester and achieves high serum levels, although the actual concentration of active free base represents only 20–30% of the total (6). There is some evidence that the ester form may have a modicum of clinical effect, but this remains unproven (6). New ester formulations are presently being studied (37,41); they proffer improved bioavailability and good clinical efficacy.

Like the estolate, erythromycin ethylsuccinate is stable in the presence of acid, although this is disputed. Despite this, it seems that the ethylsuccinate formulation is better absorbed in the absence of food (5,40). As with other preparations, however, various studies have produced differing results: one study has shown increased absorption with food (42). Erythromycin ethylsuccinate is partially hydrolyzed to the base prior to absorption so that the preparation is absorbed as both base and the ethylsuccinate with subsequent degradation of the latter to the active base (5). This may explain the variable results of bioavailability studies (36). Serum concentrations obtained are lower than those achieved with the estolate and higher than those with the base, but only 55% of the total circulating compound is in the form of the microbiologically active free base (5).

In sum, it appears that (1) virtually all oral preparations provide similar levels of active free base, no matter the composition of their formulation; (2) in general, all oral preparations are best absorbed in the fasting state (2,3,5,7); and (3) limited studies suggest that acid-labile forms of erythromycin are well absorbed orally in older adults. This may reflect the decreased gastric acid production associated with aging. The clinical equivalence of oral erythromycins has some support from studies in vivo (2,5,7).

The intravenous formulations are erythromycin lactobionate and gluceptate. Serum levels of the microbiologically active free base are much higher with parenteral administration (2,3,5,6).

B. Distribution

It is estimated that 40–90% of erythromycin is protein bound in serum (5,6), primarily to α-1-acid glycoprotein, but the significance of this is presently unclear (9). The serum half-life is typically approximately 1.5 h (3,6) with appreciable levels maintained for about 6 h. As noted above, peak serum concentrations with single and multiple doses are significantly higher in elderly persons than in younger adults, and the half-life is prolonged (twice that in younger subjects) with drug accumulation following repeated dosing (31).

Erythromycin is hydrophilic and therefore is well-distributed throughout body tissues and fluids (2,3,5,6,29); it persists in tissues longer than in serum (5). It does not cross the blood-brain barrier effectively, even in the presence of inflamed meninges, and achieves low central nervous system (CNS) and cerebrospinal fluid levels. It achieves high but variable urine concentrations, consistently good levels in prostatic tissue, and is concentrated in the liver and bile (2,3,5,29). It should be noted that while erythromycin penetrates sinus and bronchial secretions adequately for the treatment of streptococcal infections, levels are not sufficient to eradicate *H. influenzae* consistently (5,43). The drug is also concentrated in polymorphonuclear leukocytes (44) and alveolar macrophages (45). This last characteristic may have therapeutic implications (discussed below).

C. Excretion

A large proportion of orally administered erythromycin is not absorbed and is expelled unchanged in the feces, some of which represents that eliminated in bile (3,5,29), since the drug is concentrated in the liver and excreted by that route. Biliary clearance of the base form of erythromycin is substantially higher than that of the estolate form (5). There is some enterohepatic circulation, particularly if erythromycin is administered in a form other than the estolate (5), and biliary and fecal excretion is significantly reduced in the presence of biliary tract obstruction (3). A sizable amount of the drug is also converted to the inactive des-*N*-methyl moiety in the liver (2,3). Hepatic excretion, then, is thought to be the primary mode of clearance of the drug (2,3,5,46). The impact of biliary tract or hepatic disease on the elimination of erythromycin is not well known (3,46), but among cirrhotics, there is a reduction in hepatically generated α-1-acid glycoprotein resulting in a sharp rise in unbound, active erythromycin base and a prolonged half-life in vivo (46). Moreover, Miglioli et al. (31) recently showed significantly diminished clearance and accumulation of erythromycin in old age, primarily as a result of reduced hepatic biotransformation and possibly also of decreased hepatic blood flow, independent of demonstrable biochemical hepatic dysfunction; this is contradictory to results of an earlier study (46). Unlike cirrhotics, levels of α-1-acid glycoprotein are not depressed in older adults and may even be increased (47).

Only 2–6% of orally administered erythromycin is excreted unchanged in the urine (2,3,6). This level increases to approximately 15% following intravenous administration (2,5,29). Excretion is virtually solely dependent upon glomerular filtration, but some active transport and/or tubular reabsorption of the drug is also thought to occur (2). It has been recommended that in general no adjustment of the dose is necessary in the presence of impaired renal function (29,48,49). However, the drug half-life has been shown to increase in anuric patients from approximately 1.5 h to about 5 h, whether the drug is given orally or intravenously (2,3,50). This seems to result from enhanced bioavailability and may be more pronounced in elderly persons (51). Consequently, it has been suggested that the dose of erythromycin should be reduced in patients with severe renal impairment (52). Erythromycin is not removed by hemodialysis or peritoneal dialysis (2,3,5).

VI. CLINICAL INDICATIONS

Erythromycin is indicated as the antimicrobial agent of choice for a number of infections, as an alternative agent for select infections in penicillin-allergic patients, and as a prophylactic agent in certain situations (Table 3). Apart from its antimicrobial effects, there is evidence that erythromycin may have other therapeutic properties unrelated to its antimicrobial activity (see below).

A. Therapy

Perhaps one of the most important and common uses of erythromycin, in both young and older adults, is in the treatment of respiratory tract infections, particularly pneumonia (3). In the geriatric patient, erythromycin is especially indicated as therapy for pneumonia due to *Legionella* spp. Erythromycin is regarded as the most active agent and remains the treatment of choice for legionellosis (2,3,5,43). Some authorities recommend concurrent use of rifampin in severe cases, but the benefit of such an approach is unproven (6). The patient usually requires intravenous therapy initially, but treatment can be switched to oral agents in 5–7 days (53); a 3-week course is suggested (43,53). It should be noted that oral therapy alone has failed in the immunocompromised host (54).

Other agents of pneumonia that are well treated with erythromycin include *Chlamydia pneumoniae* (TWAR) (6,55), *Chlamydia psittaci* (psittacosis) (56), *Coxiella burnetii* (Q fever) (57,58), and *Mycoplasma pneumoniae* (2,3,5,6,59), although mycoplasma is an uncommon cause of pneumonia in elderly persons (43). Erythromycin treatment shortens the clinical course of mycoplasma pneumonia and hastens radiological clearing of pulmonary infiltrates (5), but does not accelerate eradication of the infecting pathogen (2). A 5- to 7-day course of therapy is generally recommended, but a more prolonged duration (such as 3 weeks) may be indicated in severe infections (2).

Erythromycin is commonly promulgated as excellent, broad-spectrum empirical treatment for young ambulatory patients with respiratory infections (3,60–62), but it is not an ideal choice for such infections in older patients (3,43). One reason for this is that most elderly patients with a significant respiratory infection, such as pneumonia, should probably be managed in a hospital setting (62). Furthermore, while erythromycin achieves excellent penetration of pulmonary tissues and secretions at bactericidal concentrations for susceptible organisms (9,29), resistance to erythromycin by *H. influenzae*, a common respiratory tract pathogen in elderly patients, is high (24–64%) (2,3,27). It is not recommended, therefore, to use erythromycin alone in the empirical therapy for respiratory infections in geriatric patients. The combination of erythromycin and ampicillin (63) or trimethoprim-sulfamethoxazole (2,3) has been suggested where empirical outpatient therapy is appropriate. Of course, in a desperately ill elderly patient who is hospitalized to receive intravenous antibiotic treatment for a pneumonia of unknown etiology, addition of erythromycin to the empiric antibiotic regimen is warranted (2,9,53). Some investigators have even

Table 3 Major Uses of Erythromycin

Indication	Doses of erythromycin for adults	Alternative choice
Infections in which erythromycin is the drug of first choice		
Mycoplasma pneumoniae infections	500 mg tid-qid po[a]	Tetracycline
Legionella pneumonia	0.5–1.0 g qid po[a]	Rifampin + erythromycin
Diphtheria[b]	Carrier state: 500 mg qid po for 10 days	Penicillin G
	Disease[a]: followed by 500 mg qid po for 10 days	Penicillin G
Pertussis	500 mg qid po	Ampicillin
Chlamydia pneumoniae or conjunctivitis	10 mg/kg qid po[a]	Trimethoprim-sulfamethoxazole
Chlamydia trachomatis pelvic infections in pregnancy	0.5–1.0 g qid po[a,c]	Sulfisoxazole
Campylobacter jejeuni gastroenteritis	250 mg qid po	Ciprofloxacin
Prevention of infection after colorectal surgery	1 g po each of neomycin and erythromycin base at 1, 2, and 11 p.m. on the day before surgery combined with purgation over the 2 days before surgery	Parenteral cephalosporin
Infections in which erythromycin is an alternative choice		Drug of first choice
Groups A, B, C, G streptococcal infection	250–500 mg qid po[a,d]	Penicillin G
Streptococcus pneumoniae infection	250–500 mg qid po[a]	Penicillin G
Rheumatic fever prophylaxis	250 mg bid po	Penicillin G
Prevention of bacterial endocarditis (in dental procedures)	1.0 g po 2 h before procedure, then 500 mg 6 h later	Penicillin G
Lymphogranuloma venereum	500 mg qid po for 21 days	Tetracycline
Chancroid	500 mg qid po for 7 days	Ceftriaxone
Nongonococcal urethritis	500 mg qid po for 7 days	Tetracycline
Bronchopulmonary anaerobic infections	500 mg qid po	Penicillin G; clindamycin
Acne vulgaris	250 mq qid po or topical preparation	Tetracycline po and a number of topical drugs
Urinary tract infection	500 mg qid po[e]	Many agents

[a]Intravenous therapy (2–4 g/day) should be used in serious illness or when oral therapy is not possible or reliable.
[b]Antitoxin is essential primary therapy for disease.
[c]Severe pelvic inflammatory disease is often polymicrobial in origin; treatment of such cases should include other agents more active against likely facultative and anaerobic enteric bacteria and/or *Neisseria gonorrhoeae*.
[d]Treatment should be continued for 10 days for Group A.
[e]Urine pH must be raised to greater than 8.0 with sodium bicarbonate.

suggested that intravenous erythromycin should be considered first-line therapy for respiratory infections in adults, including elderly patients (64,65).

For gastroenteritis due to *Campylobacter jejuni*, erythromycin treatment enhances elimination of the organism from feces, but the drug has not been shown to alter the course of illness if instituted more than 4 days after onset of symptoms (66). Approximately 8–10% of strains are resistant (2).

Erythromycin may also be indicated occasionally for the treatment of urinary tract infections. The generally poor activity of erythromycin against Enterobacteriaceae in this setting can be enhanced by the alkalinization of the urine. The drug may also have a role in the therapy of prostatitis (67). Erythromycin is an inferior alternative to penicillin in the treatment of syphilis. In penicillin-allergic patients with neurosyphilis, erythromycin is not indicated; use of penicillin after desensitization or treatment with other effective antibiotics is recommended. Erythromycin may also be used for the treatment of infective endocarditis due to organisms that are highly susceptible or for which it would otherwise be considered the treatment of choice (e.g., *Legionella*, *Coxiella*).

Other indications for erythromycin therapy are outlined in Table 3. It should be noted that, even if there is in vivo sensitivity, erythromycin should not be used as monotherapy for the treatment of serious staphylococcal infections because of the potential for emergence of resistance (2). Erythromycin, however, may be synergistic with penicillin against *S. aureus* (5). Erythromycin may also be considered as alternate therapy for anthrax, actinomycosis, and infections due to *Listeria monocytogenes* and *Eikenella corrodens* (5).

In combination with ampicillin, erythromycin has been found effective against *Nocardia asteroides* (2).

Erythromycin possesses unique properties unrelated to its antibacterial activity, which may be of therapeutic significance for older patients. It has been found that the drug mimics the effect of the gastrointestinal polypeptide motilin in stimulating gastrointestinal motility (68–71) and may thus have a role as a prokinetic agent (70,71). Specifically, erythromycin may have a role in the acute and chronic treatment of gastroparesis due to diabetes mellitus or other conditions (71) and for siting of nasogastric or oroduodenal tubes (70).

B. Prophylaxis

Erythromycin is the main alternative agent to penicillin as prophylaxis against endovascular infections following dental and upper airway procedures (72). Elderly persons are particularly at risk for the development of infective endocarditis because of degenerative or atherosclerotic cardiac valvular defects. Operative procedures, dental manipulations, and pressure ulcers are significant predisposing factors (73). It should be noted that even edentulous patients are still at increased risk for infective endocarditis. In the setting of penicillin allergy, the recommended prophylactic regimen for dental and upper airway procedures in older patients is 1 g of erythromycin 2 h prior to the procedure and 500 mg 6 h after the initial dose (72).

A second prophylactic use of erythromycin is in colorectal surgery. The drug is administered in combination with neomycin, 1 g of each, at 1300 h, 1400 h, and 2300 h on the day prior to surgery (74). Significant serum and wound levels of erythromycin are achieved with such a regimen, which contribute to its efficacy. It is not clear whether addition of parenteral antibiotics enhances the effectiveness of this regimen, as various studies have provided differing results (74).

VII. DRUG ADMINISTRATION AND DOSING

Erythromycin is administered most often orally, but intravenous preparations are available and are compatible with most intravenous solutions. Erythromycin can also be administered rectally, achieving concentrations that parallel those obtained after oral administration (2). Intramuscular injection is painful and is not recommended (2,5,6).

The typical adult dosage is 1–2 g per day in equally divided doses, usually every 6 h. With severe infections, a higher dosage, such as 1 g four times per day, can be used. Similar doses can be used intravenously (2,3). In elderly patients, in view of the known alteration in the pharmacokinetics of erythromycin, it is suggested that a maximum dosage of 1.5 g should be used even in the absence of hepatic or renal disease (31). Certainly this would seem prudent in the presence of severe hepatic disease or advanced renal failure. One author has advocated utilization of a more prolonged dosing interval instead of dose reduction (3). However, in the setting of a severe illness in which erythromycin is the drug of choice, it may be reasonable to administer a higher dose of the medication and monitor closely for toxicity; it must be recalled that erythromycin is still regarded as one of the safest antimicrobial agents (3,5,7,29).

VIII. ADVERSE EFFECTS AND DRUG INTERACTIONS

A. Adverse Effects

After 40 years of experience with erythromycin, it is clear that this agent is one of the safest antibiotics in current use (2,3,5,9), and this seems true for the newer macrolides as well (75). Many antibiotics in common use have some inhibitory action on the host immune system, but erythromycin does not seem to possess such properties (9). Adverse effects are generally not life threatening and are rare (2–3%), except for "irritative" adverse effects (2,3,5,6,29). Among these, the most common and troublesome is gastrointestinal intolerance with an incidence of approximately 40% following oral therapy (76,77), but sometimes the incidence is as high as 75% (78). Symptoms associated with gastrointestinal distress include abdominal pain, nausea, vomiting, and diarrhea. These side effects can occur with intravenously administered erythromycin as well, with an incidence reported as high as 84% (79). The occurrence of such reactions seems dose-related (2,7,29); the duration of infusion and concentration of the drug in the infusate appear to be the key predisposing factors with intravenously administered erythromycin (79). There is no clear advantage of one erythromycin preparation over another in this respect.

Several recent reports suggest that enteric-coated base formulations are better tolerated than uncoated forms (76), while others indicate that the ethylsuccinate formulation compares favorably with the stearate and both are better tolerated than the base (78). Interestingly, it has been suggested that the incidence of gastrointestinal side effects may be lower in elderly patients (76).

The mechanism of gastrointestinal disturbance is a matter of some debate. As discussed earlier, erythromycin has effects on the gastrointestinal tract similar to motilin and induces a migrating motor complex in the gastroduodenum in humans (68,69). While such properties may have implications for therapeutic uses of the drug, they may also explain at least in part the mechanism of gastrointestinal intolerance (70).

Various maneuvers have been suggested to minimize the gastrointestinal side effects of erythromycin. Tolerance seems to be increased if the drug is taken with food (7), but this may reduce bioavailability depending on the preparation. Other strategies include temporary, interruption of therapy and reduction of dose, more frequent administration of a diminished dose, and ingestion of medication with generous quantities of water (7). With regard to intravenous erythromycin, the dose should be diluted in a minimum of 250 ml of infusate and administered over at least 60 min (80).

Another common, irritative side effect of intravenously administered erythromycin is phlebitis (2,3,81). This can be minimized by adequate dilution of the drug and slow infusion. One author found slight alkalinization of the infusate was of value, but results were inconsistent (81).

The most serious toxic effect of erythromycin is cholestatic hepatitis, which was first reported in 1961 (82). The incidence is very low, perhaps 1 in 1000 or less (83). The syndrome usually starts 10–20 days after initiation of treatment and is characterized by nausea, vomiting, and abdominal cramps, followed by jaundice and fever, with hepatic enzyme abnormalities that are consistent with cholestasis, and leukocytosis and eosinophilia; a maculopapular rash may accompany these symptoms. Manifestations usually disappear within a few weeks after discontinuing the medication; they reappear if the patient is rechallenged (5–7), but chronic liver disease and death do not occur (3,83). The vast majority of cases are due to the estolate form and occur in adults (5). Minor transaminase elevation has been reported in 15% of patients administered the estolate preparation (84), however, hepatotoxic reactions can also occur with the ethylsuccinate and stearate compounds (85). The mechanism of hepatotoxicity is thought to be hypersensitivity to the propionyl ester linkage (3), but Keeffee et al. have suggested that there is cross-sensitivity between different preparations (86). Yet 93% of cases have occurred with the estolate form, which is, therefore, not recommended (3,29); other formulations should also be used with caution if there is a history of hepatotoxic reaction.

Another potentially serious complication of erythromycin therapy is ototoxicity. First reported in 1973, it is a relatively rare complication of treatment with erythromycin. However, a recent study suggests that the presence of subclinical ototoxicity may be considerably higher (87). Toxicity occurs when large doses are used (usually at least 4 g/day) and especially with the intravenous form, but adverse effects can occur with lower doses and with oral medication (88). Predisposing factors include older age; renal or hepatic (excretory) impairment; concurrent use of other ototoxic agents such as loop diuretics, aminoglycosides, and corticosteroids; and possibly female gender (87–89). Ototoxicity is manifested by bilateral sensorineural hearing loss, "blowing" tinnitus, and sometimes vertigo, usually several days after initiation of therapy (88). It is generally reversible within 2 weeks with discontinuation of the drug or even with a reduction in dose (88,89), but irreversible hearing loss has been reported (90). Disturbance of vestibular function has also been found (88). The mechanism is unclear, although one study has shown cochlear hair cell damage in an animal model and another demonstrated changes in brain stem function (89); it seems likely that the reaction is toxic and not immunological in nature. In order to minimize the risk of ototoxicity, authorities suggest limitation of the dose to 1.5 g/day in the presence of renal or hepatic dysfunction, audiometric testing (especially of high frequency) before, during, and after therapy in elderly patients, and avoidance of concomitant ototoxic medication where possible in the presence of renal or hepatic impairment. It is interesting to note that in a recent prospective study, only symptomatic patients had audiologically detectable ototoxicity (87). Indeed, this report challenges many of our suppositions regarding erythromycin ototoxicity, including the predisposition of older adults and persons with renal impairment; however, these results await confirmation.

A number of other adverse effects are reported with erythromycin. These include agranulocytosis (91), pancreatitis (in association with overdose) (92), allergy-induced fixed drug eruption (93), and other hypersensitivity reactions, such as fever, arthralgias, and eosinophilia. Confusion, paranoia, and psychosis have also been reported (94) and provide evidence for an effect by erythromycin on the central nervous system. Superinfection with other microorganisms is known to occur, and the gut flora is altered substantially with growth of erythromycin-resistant *Clostridium* species. Pseudomembranous colitis is a recognized complication (5). Life-threatening ventricular tachydysrhythmias can also occur in association with erythromycin-induced or -exacerbated prolonged QT syndrome similar to that due to Class IA antidysrhythmic agents (95,96).

B. Drug Interactions

Because many elderly patients are treated concomitantly with a number of medications, it behooves the clinician to anticipate possible interactions of any antibiotic added for short-term therapy to other medications, including those obtained over the counter. Furthermore, the potential for drug interactions is enhanced in the geriatric population as a result of physiological decline in renal and hepatic function, as well as serum albumin concentration (which may alter the ratio of free to bound drug in the bloodstream, although this may be of lesser importance with erythromycin, given that it is bound predominantly to α-1-glycoprotein and not to albumin). Erythromycin is oxidized in the liver by the cytochrome P-450 enzyme system with production of metabolites that form a stable complex with the enzymes, thus inhibiting metabolism of other drugs similarly oxidized by these enzymes (97).

Interaction of erythromycin and theophylline is well documented, but a multitude of case reports and studies has yielded conflicting results (98). Rieder and Spino (98) reviewed the literature and concluded that (1) there is considerable individual variability in the effects of erythromycin on theophylline clearance; (2) theophylline toxicity precipitated by concomitant erythromycin administration usually occurs after 7–10 days of therapy with the antibiotic; and (3) changes in theophylline clearance tend to occur particularly in patients in whom theophylline levels are maintained in the upper therapeutic range. Furthermore, interactions between theophylline and erythromycin appear also to depend upon the presence of underlying disease, cigarette smoking, and intravenous versus oral drug administration. Rieder and Spino recommend close monitoring of theophylline concentrations prior to and at 3-day intervals during erythromycin treatment (98). Where such intensive monitoring is impractical, they suggest routine reduction of theophylline dose by 25% on day 3 of erythromycin therapy (98). The validity of these recommendations in geriatric patients is unknown. Suffice it to say, close monitoring with decrease in theophylline dosing by 15–40% is prudent during erythromycin treatment of elderly patients. It should be noted further that the effects of erythromycin on theophylline metabolism may persist after antibiotic treatment is completed. Finally, there is some concern that co-administration of theophylline and erythromycin reduces erythromycin serum levels and thus may affect the efficacy of the antimicrobial agent (98,99).

Similarly, there is considerable clinical evidence that erythromycin potentiates the action of warfarin (100). This occurs most likely on the basis of erythromycin-induced inhibition of anticoagulant metabolism. Shepherd et al. (101) have demonstrated increased sensitivity to anticoagulant medication with reduced warfarin clearance among elderly persons, even in the absence of concomitant erythromycin administration, and consequently older persons may be especially predisposed to clinically significant alteration of the hypoprothrombinemic effect of warfarin by erythromycin.

Other interactions can also occur that are probably the result of inhibition of the cytochrome P-450 system by erythromycin. This antibiotic interferes with the metabolism of carbamazepine (102), cyclosporine (103), methylprednisolone (104), tricyclic antidepressants (105), and the calcium channel blocker felodipine (106). Much concern, too, has been raised regarding the possible precipitation of antihistamine-associated dysrhythmias when H2-antagonists are administered in conjunction with erythromycin as a consequence of the effect of the latter on hepatic metabolism. Such a mechanism has also been proposed for interference of erythromycin with glyburide metabolism, but this was not shown in one study (107).

Erythromycin also increases the bioavailability of a number of medications. Digoxin levels are elevated due to inhibition of breakdown of the drug by bacteria prior to its absorption (108). The effect of erythromycin on gastrointestinal motility is thought to enhance the delivery of some drugs to the proximal small bowel where they are rapidly absorbed. Such a mechanism has been postulated for clinical toxicity due to phenelzine and as a possible mechanism for an observed increase in glyburide levels in diabetic patients (107); the clinical significance of this latter finding is unknown, however. Coadministration of erythromycin with antacids (109) or sucralfate (110) does not appear to alter bioavailability of the antibiotic.

Sequential use of clindamycin and erythromycin is not recommended because of the possibility of the development of "dissociated resistance" (5). Dissociated resistance is the observation that prior exposure of some organisms to low concentrations of erythromycin results in resistance to erythromycin, lincosamide, and other macrolide antibiotics upon reexposure to these drugs.

Finally, because of incompatibility of intravenous preparations, administration of intravenous erythromycin should be avoided with cephalothin, tetracycline, chloramphenicol, colistin, heparin, diphenylhydantoin, vitamin B complex, vitamin C, and metaraminol (5).

IX. ROLE OF NEWER MACROLIDES: AZITHROMYCIN AND CLARITHROMYCIN

Despite the excellent clinical record of erythromycin, the drug is limited by its generally poor oral bioavailability, its high incidence of gastrointestinal side effects, and its suboptimal activity against *H. influenzae*, a common respiratory tract pathogen in elderly patients. A number of newer macrolides have been developed in an attempt to circumvent these deficiencies. These include trioleandomycin, josamycin, spiramycin, roxithromycin, and others. Another macrolide, FK506, was introduced in 1987 (111). It has been found to be a powerful immunosuppressive agent with potential applicability in transplantation. Two macrolide antibiotics—azithromycin and clarithromycin—have been approved recently for clinical use by the FDA. These drugs have been reviewed in detail by Piscitelli et al. (75). However, currently pharmacological data and clinical information on these two drugs in elderly persons are scant. One study showed maximal plasma concentrations and area under the curve of clarithromycin to be higher in elderly subjects (75a). Those findings were related to reduced renal clearance of the drug. Nevertheless, a brief review of azithromycin and clarithromycin will be provided.

Azithromycin is a 15-member derivative of the macrolide structure and is classified as an azalide antibiotic, while clarithromycin retains the 14-membered macrolide configuration. Their mechanism of action and resistance is similar to that of erythromycin, and they possess cross-resistance with other macrolide antibiotics (112). Both macrolides have the advantage of enhanced acid stability compared with erythromycin. They are thus better absorbed and consequently have increased bioavailability with good absorption characteristics when administered orally (113–116). The drugs are well distributed into tissues with high levels maintained in both serum and tissues with clarithromycin, while azithromycin administration is associated with low serum concentrations but achieves extensive distribution and persistence in tissues (75).

The half-life of both medications is long, allowing twice-daily dosing (114,115). They are eliminated primarily following hepatic metabolism; seven metabolites of clarithromycin have been identified with varying antimicrobial activity (115). Reduced clearance has been demonstrated in the presence of severe renal dysfunction, and a reduction in dose is suggested in this setting (75).

Against gram-positive bacteria, azithromycin possesses activity that is virtually as good as that of erythromycin. It is two to eight times more active than erythromycin against *H. influenzae*, has somewhat better activity against *Moraxella*, is approximately equipotent for *Legionella*, demonstrates enhanced activity compared with erythromycin against *Chlamydia*, and has comparable effects against anaerobic bacteria (75). Clarithromycin, on the other hand, has excellent activity against gram-positive microbes, is felt to have better in vitro activity than erythromycin against *Moraxella*, *Legionella*, and *Chlamydia*, and is similar to erythromycin in its effect on anaerobes (75). The parent compound is less active than erythromycin against *H. influenzae*, but it demonstrates excellent activity in combination with its metabolite (116). The clinical relevance of this observation is questionable, however. Clarithromycin has also shown the greatest activity of any macrolide against *Mycobacterium avium* complex (117); however, its role in the treatment of mycobacterial disease is still unclear.

Limited clinical data are available, but it seems both drugs are at least as efficacious as erythromycin in the treatment of most infections in which they are indicated (75). It should be noted, however, that there have been therapeutic failures reported for both macrolides against *H. influenzae* infections (118). Both antibiotics are well tolerated, generally better than erythromycin; the incidence of adverse effects has been reported as 12% for azithromycin in one report (119) and 4–30% for clarithromycin (75). As with erythromycin, the most common complaints are of gastrointestinal disturbance (75). Abnormalities of liver enzymes (120,121) and hepatic function (122) have also been found.

Since clarithromycin and azithromycin are metabolized largely via the cytochrome P-450 system, drug interactions are anticipated. Interestingly, initial animal studies indicate that clarithromycin does not form complexes with the enzymes in the same manner as erythromycin (123). Yet there are reports of increases in levels of carbamazepine and theophylline when clarithromycin is administered concurrently (118). Azithromycin has not been shown to affect the cytochrome P-450 system in rats (114).

X. CONCLUSION

The macrolide antibiotics represent an increasingly vital component of our antibiotic arsenal. Experience of over 40 years with erythromycin has proven it to be highly effective therapy for a wide variety of infectious conditions, and it remains the agent of choice for some; its unique nonantimicrobial properties are intriguing and indeed may have novel applicability in a variety of noninfectious situations. Erythromycin also retains its stature as one of the safest antibiotics with a very low incidence of life-threatening toxicity—a particularly significant consideration in elderly patients.

Yet the limitations of erythromycin are well recognized, especially its poor bioavailability orally, unreliable activity against *H. influenzae*, and inordinately common gastrointestinal side effects. These deficiencies have prompted the development of newer macrolide antibiotics. Among these, only clarithromycin and azithromycin are currently approved for clinical use. Limited experience to date has shown these drugs to have improved bioavailability and pharmacokinetic characteristics relative to erythromycin, with fewer adverse effects and at least comparable efficacy as erythromycin. However, experience in the treatment of *H. influenzae* infections has not shown the new macrolides to have a distinct advantage over erythromycin. Nonetheless, they represent major advances in antibiotic therapy of a number of conditions, including atypical mycobacterial disease, and hold promise for further refinement of this important class of antimicrobial agents. Until widespread pharmacological and clinical studies of these drugs are performed in older patients, the role of azithromycin and clarithromycin in this population will remain unclear.

REFERENCES

1. McGuire JM, Burch, RL, Anderson RC, et al. "Ilotycin," a new antibiotic. Antibiot Chemother 1952; 2:281–3.
2. Gribble MJ, Chow AW. Erythromycin. Med Clin North Am 1982; 66:79–89.
3. Brittain DC. Erythromycin. Med Clin North Am 1987; 71:1147–54.
4. Moellering RC, Jr. Introduction: revolutionary changes in the macrolide and azalide antibiotics. Am J Med 1991: 91(suppl 3A):1S–4S.
5. Steigbigel NH. Erythromycin, lincomycin, and clindamycin. In: Mandell GL, Douglas RG, Bennett JA, eds. Principles and practice of infectious diseases, 3rd ed. New York: Churchill Livingstone, 1990:308–17.
6. Sande MA, Mandell GL. Antimicrobial agents: tetracyclines, chloramphenicol, erythromycin, and various antibacterial agents. In: Gilman AG, et al., eds. Pharmacological basis of therapeutics, 8th ed. New York: Pergamon Press, 1990:1117–45.
7. Latare PA, Setness PA. Using erythromycin: some helpful observations. Postgrad Med 1990; 86:55–63.
8. Fraschini F, Braga, PC, Copponi V, et al. Bactericidal activity of erythromycin in the respiratory system. Curr Med Res Opin 1981; 7:429–39.
9. Straughan JL, Anderson R. Erythromycin—three decades later. South Afr Med J 1983; 64:197–201.
10. Brisson-Noel A, Trien-Cuot P, Courvalis P, et al. Mechanism of action of spiramycin and other macrolides. Antimicrob Agents Chemother 1988; 32(suppl B):13–23.
11. Van Rensburg CEJ, Anderson R, Joone, G, et al. Effects of erythromycin on cellular and humoral immune functions in vitro and in vivo. J Antimicrob Chemother 1982; 8:467–74.
12. Anderson R, Van Rensburg CEJ, Eftychis H, et al. Further studies on erythromycin effects on cellular immune functions in vitro and in vivo. Enhancement of neutrophil motility by erythromycin combined with ascorbate or thiamine. J Antimicrob Chemother 1982; 10:409–17.
13. Aho P, Mannisto PT. Effect of two erythromycins, doxycycline and phenoxymethylpenicillin on leucocyte chemotaxis in vitro. J Antimicrob Chemother 1988; 21(suppl D):29–32.
14. Gemmell CG. Macrolides and host defences to respiratory tract pathogens. J Hosp Infect 1991; 19(suppl A):11–19.
15. Lampson BC, von David W, Parisi JT, et al. Novel mechanism for plasmid-mediated erythromycin resistance by pNE24 from *Staphylococcus epidermidis*. Antimicrob Agents Chemother 1986; 30:653–8.

16. Dowling JN, McDevitt DA, Pasculle AW, et al. Isolation and preliminary characterization of erythromycin-resistant variants of *Legionella pneumophila*. Antimicrob Agents Chemother 1985; 27:272–4.
17. Matsuoka M, Endon K, Nakajima Y, et al. Localization of a determinant mediating partial macrolide resistance in *Staphylococcus aureus*. Microbiol Immunol 1990; 34:643–52.
18. Janosi L, Nakajima Y, Hashimoto H, et al. Characterization of plasmids that confer inducible resistance to 14-membered macrolides and streptogramin type B antibiotics in *Staphylococcus aureus*. Microbiol Immunol 1990; 34:723–35.
19. Garrod LP. The erythromycin group of antibiotics. Br Med J 1957; 2:57–63.
20. Ounissi H, Courvalin P. Nucleotide sequence of the gene ereA encoding the erythromycin esterase in *Escherichia coli*. Gene 1985; 35:271–8.
21. Barthelemy P, Autissier D, Gerband G, et al. Enzymatic hydrolysis of erythromycin by a strain of *Escherichia coli*. J Antibiot 1984; 37:1692–6.
22. Zackrisson G, Lind L, Roos K, et al. Erythromycin-resistant beta-haemolytic streptococci Group A in Goteberg, Sweden. Scand J Infect Dis 1988; 20:419–20.
23. Perez-Trallero E, Garcia-Arenzana JM, Urbieta-Ergana M, et al. Erythromycin resistance in streptococci. Lancet 1989; 2:444–5.
24. Scott RJD, Naidoo J, Lightfoot NF, et al. A community outbreak of Group A beta-haemolytic streptococci with transferable resistance to erythromycin. Epidemiol Infect 1989; 102:85–91.
25. Wittler RR, Yamada, SM, Bass, JW, et al. Penicillin tolerance and erythromycin resistance of Group A beta-haemolytic streptococci in Hawaii and the Philippines. Am J Dis Child 1990; 144:597–589.
26. Seppala H, Nissinen A, Jarvinen H et al. Resistance to erythromycin in Group A streptococci. N Engl J Med 1992; 326:292–297.
27. Tremblay LD, L'Ecuyer J, Provencher P, et al. Susceptibility of *Haemophilus influenzae* to antimicrobial agents used in Canada. Can Med Assoc J 1990; 143:895–901.
28. Hamedani P, Hafiz S, Menor R, et al. Respiratory symptoms due to *Branhamella catarrhalis* and other *Neisseria* species infections—response to erythromycin therapy. Clin Therapeut 1989; 11:633–9.
29. Nicholas P. Erythromycin: clinical review. I. Clinical pharmacology. NY State J Med 1977; 77:2088–94.
30. Birkett DJ, Robson RA, Grgurinovich N, et al. Single oral dose pharmacokinetics of erythromycin and roxithromycin and the effects of chronic dosing. Ther Drug Monit 1990; 12:65–71.
31. Miglioli PA, Pivetti P, Strazzabosco, M et al. Effect of age on single- and multiple-dose pharmacokinetics of erythromycin. Eur J Clin Pharmacol 1990; 39:161–4.
32. Graffner C, Josefsson K, Stockman O, et al. Intra- and inter-subject variation of erythromycin absorption from single-unit and multiple-unit enteric-coated products. Biopharm Drug Dispos 1986; 7:163–71.
33. Digranes A, Joseffson K, Schreiner A, et al. Influence of food on the absorption of erythromycin from enteric-coated pellets and stearate tablets. Curr Ther Res 1984; 35:313–20.
34. Hovi T, Heikinheimo M. Effect of concomitant food intake on absorption kinetics of erythromycin in healthy volunteers. Eur J Clin Pharmacol 1985; 28:231–3.
35. Randinitis EJ, Sedman AJ, Welling PG, et al. Effect of a high-fat meal on the bioavailability of a polymer-coated erythromycin particle tablet formulation. J Clin Pharmacol 1989; 29:79–84.
36. Tjandramago TB, Van Hecken A, Mullie A, et al. Relative bioavailability of enteric coated pellets, stearate and ethylsuccinate formulations of erythromycin. Pharmacology 1984; 29:305–11.
37. Mannisto PT, Taskinen J, Ottoila P, et al. Fate of single oral doses of erythromycin acistrate, erythromycin stearate and pelleted erythromycin base analyzed by mass-spectrophotometry in plasma of healthy human volunteers. J Antimicrob Chemother 1988; 21(suppl D):33–43.
38. Tuominen RK, Mannisto PT, Pohto P, et al. Absorption of erythromycin acistrate and erythromycin base in the fasting and non-fasting state. J Antimicrob Chemother 1988; 21(suppl D):45–55.

39. Josselyn LE, Sylvester JC. Absorption of erythromycin. Antimicrob Agents Chemother 1953; 3:63–7.
40. McCracken GH, Ginsburg CM, Clahsen JC, et al. Pharmacologic evaluation of orally administered antibiotics in infants and children: effect of feeding on bioavailability. Pediatrics 1978; 62:738–43.
41. DeBernardi M, Feletti F, Gazzani G, et al. Human pharmacokinetics of erythromycin propionate-N-acetylcystcinate: comparative evaluation with erythromycin stearate and N-acetylcystcine. Intern J Clin Pharmacol Ther Toxicol 1988; 26:444–7.
42. Coyne TC, Shum S, Chun A, et al. Bioavailability of erythromycin succinate in paediatric patients. J Clin Pharmacol 1978; 18:194–202.
43. Gleckman RA. Pneumonia: update on diagnosis and treatment. Geriatrics 1991; 46:49–56.
44. Miller MF, Martin JR, Johnson P, et al. Erythromycin uptake and accumulation by human polymorphonuclear leucocytes and efficacy of erythromycin in killing ingested *Legionella pneumophila*. J Infect Dis 1984; 149:714–18.
45. Hand WL, Corwin RW, Steinberg TH, et al. Uptake of antibiotics by human alveolar macrophages. Am Rev Respir Dis 1984; 129:933–7.
46. Barre J, Mallat A, Rosenbaum J, et al. Pharmacokinetics of erythromycin in patients with severe cirrhosis. Respective influence of decreased serum binding and impaired liver metabolic capacity. Br J Clin Pharmacol 1987; 23:753–7.
47. Verbeek RK, Cardinal JA, Wallace SM, et al. Effect of age and sex on the plasma binding of acidic basic drugs. Eur J Clin Pharmacol 1984; 27:91–7.
48. Bennet WM, Muther RS, Parber RA, et al. Drug therapy in renal failure: dosing guidelines for adults. Part I: antimicrobial agents, analgesics. Ann Intern Med 1980; 93:286–325.
49. Disse B, Gundert-Remy U, Weber E, et al. Pharmacokinetics of erythromycin in patients with different degrees of renal impairment. Int J Clin Pharmacol Ther Toxicol 1986; 24:460–4.
50. Kanfer A, Stamatakis G, Torlotin JC, et al. Changes in erythromycin pharmacokinetics induced by renal failure. Clin Nephrol 1987; 27:147–50.
51. Mery JP, Kanfer A. Letter to the editor. Am J Kidney Dis 1984; 4:95.
52. Bennett WM. Letter to the editor (reply). Am J Kidney Dis 1984; 4:95.
53. Nguyen MLT, Yu VL. Legionella infection. Clin Chest Med 1991; 12:257–68.
54. Saravolatz LD, Burch KH, Fisher E, et al. The compromised host and legionnaires' disease. Ann Intern Med 1979; 90:533–7.
55. Graystone JT. *Chlamydia pneumoniae* strain TWAR. Chest 1989; 95:664–9.
56. Covelli HD, Husky DL, Dolphin RE, et al. Psittacosis: clinical presentation and therapeutic observations. West J Med 1980; 132:242–5.
57. D'Angelo LJ, Hetherington R. Q fever treated with erythromycin. Br Med J 1979; 2:305–6.
58. Perez-del-Molino A, Aguado JM, Riancho JA, et al. Erythromycin and the treatment of *Coxiella burnetti* pneumonia. J Antimicrob Chemother 1991; 28:455–9.
59. McCracken GH, Jr. Current status of antibiotic treatment for *Mycoplasma pneumoniae* infections. Ped Infect Dis 1986; 5:167–71.
60. Dunlay J, Reinhardt R, Roi LD, et al. A placebo-controlled, double-blind trial of erythromycin in adults with acute bronchitis. J Fam Pract 1987; 25:137–41.
61. Brickfield FX, Carter WH, Johnson RE, et al. Erythromycin in the treatment of acute bronchitis in a community practice. J Fam Pract 1986; 23:119–22.
62. Siegel D. Management of community-acquired pneumonia in outpatients. West J Med 1985; 142:45–8.
63. Macfarlane JT, Finch RG, Ward MJ, et al. Erythromycin compared with a combination of ampicillin and amoxycillin as initial therapy for adults with pneumonia including Legionnaires' disease. J Infect 1983; 7:111–17.
64. Staniland DR, Glew C, Pechan J, et al. Legionnaires' disease in Staffordshire. Lancet 1985; 1:1329.

65. Di Sciacca A, Durante F, Cucchiara G, et al. Effects of intravenous erythromycin lactobionate in respiratory infections. J Internat Med Res 1987; 15:245–50.
66. Nolan CM, Johnson KE, Coyle MB, et al. *Campylobacter jejuni* enteritis: efficacy of antimicrobial and antimotility drugs. Am J Gastroenterol 1983; 78:621–6.
67. Mobley DF. Erythromycin plus sodium bicarbonate in chronic bacterial prostatitis. Urology 1974; 3:60–2.
68. Tomomasa T, Kuroume T, Arai H, et al. Erythromycin induces migrating motor complex in human gastrointestinal tract. Digest Dis Sci 1986; 31:157–61.
69. Sarna SK, Soergel KH, Koch TR, et al. Gastrointestinal motor effects of erythromycin in humans. Gastroenterology 1991; 101:1488–96.
70. Catnach SM, Fairclough PD. Erythromycin and the gut. Gut 1992; 33:397–401.
71. Janssens J, Peeters TL, Vantrappen G, et al. Improvement of gastric emptying in diabetic gastroparesis by erythromycin. Preliminary studies. N Engl J Med 1990; 322:1028–31.
72. Dajani AS, Dajani AS, Bisno AL, Chung KJ, et al. Prevention of bacterial endocarditis. Recommendations of the American Heart Association. JAMA 1990; 264:2919–22.
73. Friedlander AH, Yoshikawa TT. Pathogenesis, management, and prevention of infective endocarditis in the elderly dental patient. Oral Surg, Oral Med, Oral Pathol 1990; 69:177–81.
74. Berquist EJ, Murphy SA. Prophylactic antibiotics for surgery. Med Clin North Am 1987; 71:357–68.
75. Piscitelli SC, Danziger LH, Roduold KA, et al. Clarithromycin and azithromycin: new macrolide antibiotics. Clin Pharm 1992; 11:137–52.
75a. Chu SY, Wilson DS, Guay DR, et al. Clarithromycin pharmacokinetics in healthy young and elderly volunteers. J Clin Pharmacol 1992; 32:1045–9.
76. Ellsworth AJ, Christensen DB, Volpore-McMahon MR, et al. Prospective comparison of patient tolerance to enteric-coated vs. nonenteric-coated erythromycin. J Fam Prac 1990; 31:265–70.
77. Saloranta P, Roos L, Elonen R, et al. Erythromycin ethylsuccinate, base and acistrate in the treatment of upper respiratory tract infection: two comparative studies of tolerability. J Antimicrob Chemother 1989; 24:455–62.
78. Carter BL, Woodhead JC, Cole KJ, et al. Gastrointestinal side effects with erythromycin preparations. Drug Intell Clin Pharm 1987; 21:734–8.
79. Downey KM, de Saintonge C. Gastrointestinal side effects after intravenous erythromycin lactobionate. Br J Clin Pharmacol 1986; 21:295–9.
80. Seifert CF, Swaney RJ, Bellanger-McCleery RA, et al. Intravenous erythromycin lactobionate-induced severe nausea and vomiting. Drug Intell Clin Pharmacol 1989; 23:40–4.
81. David LM. Phlebitis with intravenous erythromycin. Am J Hosp Pharm 1987; 44:732–8.
82. Johnson DF, Hall WH. Allergic hepatitis caused by propionyl erythromycin ester of lauryl sulfate. N Engl J Med 1961; 265:1200–2.
83. Inman WHW, Rawson NSB. Erythromycin estolate and jaundice. Br Med J 1983; 286:1954–5.
84. Ginsburg CM, Eichenwald HF. Erythromycin: a review of its uses in paediatric practice. J Pediat 1976; 86:272.
85. Alcalay J, Halevy S, Theodor E, et al. Asymptomatic liver injury due to erythromycin stearate. Drug Intell Clin Pharm 1986; 20:601–2.
86. Keeffee EB, Reis TC, Berland JE, et al. Hepatotoxicity to both erythromycin estolate and erythromycin ethylsuccinate. Digest Dis Sci 1982; 27:701–4.
87. Swanson DJ, Surg RJ, Fine MJ, et al. Erythromycin ototoxicity: prospective assessment with serum concentrations and audiograms in a study of patients with pneumonia. Am J Med 1992; 92:61–8.
88. Schweitzer VG, Olson NR. Ototoxic effect of erythromycin therapy. Arch Otolaryngol 1984; 110:258–60.
89. Brummett RE, Fox KE. Vancomycin- and erythromycin-induced hearing loss in humans. Antimicrob Agents Chemother 1989; 33:791–6.

90. Fang GD, Fine MJ, Orloff J, et al. New and emerging etiologies for community-acquired pneumonia with implications for therapy—a prospective multicenter study of 359 cases. Medicine (Balt.) 1990; 69:309–16.
91. Pastor E, Linares M, Grau E, et al. Erythromycin-induced agranulocytosis. Drug Intell Clin Pharm 1991; 25:1136.
92. Gumaste VV. Erythromycin-induced pancreatitis. Am J Med 1989; 86:725.
93. Pigatto PD, Ribold A, Riva F, et al. Fixed drug eruption to erythromycin. Acta Derm Venereol 1984; 64:272–3.
94. Cohen IJ, Weitz R. Psychiatric complications with erythromycin. Drug Intell Clin Pharm 1981; 15:388.
95. Freedman RA, Anderson KP, Green LS, et al. Effect of erythromycin on ventricular arrhythmias and ventricular repolarization in idiopathic Long QT Syndrome. Am J Cardiol 1987; 59:168–9.
96. Nattel S, Ranger S, Talajic M, et al. Erythromycin-induced Long QT Syndrome: concordance with quinidine and underlying cellular electrophysiologic mechanism. Am J Med 1990; 89:235–8.
97. Danan G, Descatoire V, Pessayre D, et al. Self-induction by erythromycin of its own transformation into a metabolite forming an inactive complex with reduced cytochrome P-450. J Pharmacol Exp Ther 1981; 218:509–14.
98. Rieder MJ, Spino M. The theophylline-erythromycin interaction. J Asthma 1988; 25:195–204.
99. Paulsen O, Hoglund O, Nilsson L-G, et al. The interaction of erythromycin with theophylline. Eur J Clin Pharmacol 1987; 32:493–8.
100. Bachmann K, Schwartz JI, Forney R, et al. The effect of erythromycin on the disposition kinetics of warfarin. Pharmacology 1984; 28:171–6.
101. Shepherd AMM, Hewick DS, Moreland TA, et al. Age as a determinant of sensitivity to warfarin. Br J Clin Pharmacol 1977; 4:315–20.
102. Wroblewski BA, Singer WD, Whyte J, et al. Carbamazepine-erythromycin interaction. Case studies and clinical significance. JAMA 1986; 255:1165–7.
103. Sands M, Brown RB. Interactions of cyclosporine with a antimicrobial agents. Rev Infect Dis 1989; 11:691–7.
104. LaForce CF, Szefler JJ, Miller ME, et al. Inhibition of methylprednisolone elimination in the presence of erythromycin therapy. J Allergy Clin Immunol 1983; 72:34–9.
105. Amsterdam JD, Maislin G. Effect of erythromycin on tricyclic antidepressant metabolism. J Clin Psychopharmacol 1991; 11:203–6.
106. Liedholm H, Nordin G. Erythromycin-felodipine interaction. Drug Intell Clin Pharm 1991; 25:1007–8.
107. Fleishaker JC, Phillips JP. Evaluation of a potential interaction between erythromycin and glyburide in diabetic volunteers. J Clin Pharmacol 1991; 31:259–62.
108. Maxwell DL, Gilmar-White SK, Hall MR, et al. Digoxin toxicity due to interaction of digoxin with erythromycin. Br Med J 1989; 298:572.
109. Yamreudeewong W, Scavore JM, Paore RP, et al. Effect of antacid co-administration on the bioavailability of erythromycin stearate. Clin Pharm 1989; 8:352–3.
110. Miller LG, Prichard JG, White CA, et al. Effect of concurrent sucralfate administration on the absorption of erythromycin. J Clin Pharmacol 1990; 30:39–44.
111. Kino T, Hatanaka H, Hashimoto M, et al. FK506, a novel immunosuppressive isolated from *Streptomyces*. I. Fermentation, isolation and physicochemical and biological characteristics. J Antibiot (Tokyo) 1987; 40:1249–55.
112. Leclerq R, Courvalin P. Bacterial resistance to macrolide, lincosamide and streptogrammin antibiotics by target modification. Antimicrob Agents Chemother 1991; 35:1267–72.
113. Wise R. The development of macrolides and related compounds. J Antimicrob Chemother 1989; 23:299–300.

114. Foulds G, Shepard RM, Johnson RB, et al. The pharmacokinetics of azithromycin in human serum and tissues. J Antimicrob Chemother 1990; 25(suppl A):73–82.
115. Ferrero JL, Ferrero JL, Bopp BA, Marsh KC, et al. Metabolism and disposition of clarithromycin in man. Drug Metabol Dispos 1990; 18:441–6.
116. Jorgensen JH, Maher LA, Howell AW, et al. Activity of clarithromycin and its principal human metabolite against *Haemophilus influenzae*. Antimicrob Agents Chemother 1991; 35:1524–6.
117. Fernandes PB, Hardy DJ, McDaniel D, et al. In vitro and in vivo activities of clarithromycin against *Mycobacterium avium*. Antimicrob Agents Chemother 1989; 33:1531–4.
118. Bachand RT, Jr. Comparative study of clarithromycin and ampicillin in the treatment of patients with acute exacerbations of chronic bronchitis. J Antimicrob Chemother 1991; 27(suppl A):91–100.
119. Hopkins S. Clinical tolerance and safety of a azithromycin. Am J Med 1991; 91(suppl 3A):40–5.
120. Poirer R. Comparative study of clarithromycin and roxithromycin in the treatment of community-acquired pneumonia. J Antimicrob Chemother 1991; 27(suppl A):109–16.
121. Cassell GH, Drnec J, Waites KB, et al. Efficacy of clarithromycin against *Mycoplasma pneumoniae*. J Antimicrob Chemother 1991; 27(suppl A):47–59.
122. Levenstein JH. Clarithromycin versus penicillin in the treatment of streptococcal pharyngitis. J Antimicrob Chemother 1991; 27(suppl A):67–74.
123. Tinel M, Descatoire V, Larrey D, et al. Effects of clarithromycin on cytochrome P-450. Comparison with other macrolides. J Pharmacol Exp Ther 1989; 250:746–51.

18

Clindamycin

Haragopal Thadepalli
UCLA School of Medicine, Charles R. Drew University of Medicine and Science, and King/Drew Medical Center, Los Angeles, California

Daniel Hancz
Los Angeles County–USC Medical Center, Los Angeles, California

I. CHEMISTRY

Clindamycin is a 7 (S)-chloro-7-deoxy derivative of lincomycin (Fig. 1), which is produced by *Streptomyces linconensis*, a soil fungus obtained in Lincoln, Nebraska, in 1962. A review of our first 15 years of clinical experience with clindamycin was published in 1982 (1). Ten years later, this drug remains as a "gold-standard" for evaluation of any new antibiotic waiting to be tested in the treatment of anaerobic infections. The usage of clindamycin has declined since 1974 because of pseudomembranous colitis, a form of severe diarrhea proven to be caused by *Clostridium difficile* (2). This complication is reported to occur more frequently among elderly persons in the nursing homes than in younger adults (3).

II. MECHANISM OF ACTION

Clindamycin inhibits protein synthesis by acting on the 50S ribosomal subunits of bacteria. Its primary mode of inhibition is through interference with the initiation of peptide chain synthesis (1). Subinhibitory concentration of clindamycin suppresses streptolysin S production by bacteria.

III. ANTIMICROBIAL SPECTRUM

Clindamycin in vitro is about eight times more active than lincomycin against streptococci, including penicillin-resistant *Streptococcus pneumoniae*, but penicillin is 10 times more active than clindamycin against penicillin-susceptible (minimal inhibitory concentration [MIC] < 0.1 μg/ml) streptococci. Some streptococci are resistant to clindamycin; failure of eradicating streptococcal septicemia among elderly patients on clindamycin therapy has been reported (4). Against *Staphylococcus aureus*, clindamycin is more active than

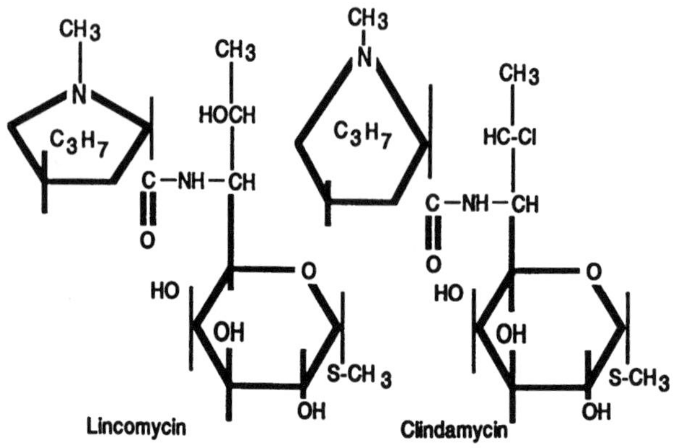

Figure 1 Chemical structures of lincomycin and clindamycin.

erythromycin and methicillin, but clindamycin should not be used to treat methicillin-resistant *S. aureus* (MRSA) because—even if it is susceptible in vitro—a high rate of therapeutic failure has been reported (5). Vancomycin is still the drug of choice for MRSA. *Staphylococcus aureus* can develop resistance to erythromycin and clindamycin during therapy, and, therefore, semisynthetic penicillins are preferred over these macrolide group of antibiotics. As a class, all species of enterococci, (group D streptococcus) and aerobic gram-negative bacilli except *Haemophilus influenzae* are resistant to clindamycin; Clindamycin is also ineffective against *Neisseria* species and other aerobic and facultative gram-negative cocci.

Clindamycin and metronidazole are active against anaerobic bacteria with the following exceptions.

Clindamycin is more active than metronidazole against *Peptococcus* and *Peptostreptococcus*, as well as other relatively more oxygen-tolerant strains of anaerobes such as *Bacteroides*. This is because metronidazole activity is directly proportional to the anaerobicity of the organism, i.e., bacteria that are strictly anaerobic are killed by metronidazole, but aerotolerant anaerobes are not as susceptible (6). Clindamycin is consistently bactericidal against all strains of *B. fragilis* tested in vitro at 2 μg/ml or less. Clindamycin-resistant *B. fragilis* (MIC = 25–100 μg/ml) has been reported, and these organisms are also resistant to chloramphenicol (MIC > 25 μg/ml) (7). Nationwide, clindamycin resistance among *B. fragilis* strains has not increased, although some hospitals are reporting increasing incidence of metronidazole- and clindamycin-resistant strains of *B. fragilis* (8,9). Clindamycin resistance in *B. fragilis* is plasmid mediated and transferable from one strain of *B. fragilis* to the other (10). In one study, clindamycin-resistant anaerobic gram-positive cocci increased in 55% of women 1–9 weeks after clindamycin therapy was discontinued (11). Certain species of *Clostridium*, such as *C. tertium*, *C. paraputrificum*, *C. sporogenes*, *C. subterminale*, and *C. difficile*, are resistant to clindamycin (12). Among *Bacteroides* species conjugal transfer of (non–plasmid-mediated) clindamycin and tetracycline resistance has been reported by a mechanism of genetic exchange (13).

Clindamycin is as active as erythromycin against *Chlamydia trachomatis* in vitro, the activity of clindamycin against *C. trachomatis* being potentiated by the addition of an aminoglycoside such as gentamicin. This finding supports the usage of a clindamycin plus gentamicin combination in the treatment of pelvic inflammatory disease due to chlamydia (14,15). Clindamycin is effective for the treatment of *Chlamydia pneumoniae* pneumonitis that occurs among elderly nursing home patients. The addition of an aminoglycoside enhances the efficacy of clindamycin against *S. aureus* as well, but it is not necessary. Moreover, this combination is not synergistic against facultative and aerobic gram-negative bacilli (16). Clindamycin in vitro enhances the bactericidal activity of cefoxitin and cefamandole against certain β-lactamase-producing aerobic gram-negative bacilli including *Pseudomonas*. This occurs via enzymatic derepression (17). Clindamycin with primaquin was found to be effective against *Pneumocystis carinii* infections (18). Clindamycin alone (without quinine) has cured *Plasmodium falciparum* but not *P. vivax* malaria (20). Clindamycin in combination with pyrimethamine is an alternative therapy for *Toxoplasma gondii* infections in patients with acquired immunodeficiency syndrome (AIDS) (19).

IV. CLINICAL PHARMACOLOGY

A. Pharmacodynamics

Like other macrolides, clindamycin uptake by polymorphonuclear neutrophils (PMNs) and pulmonary macrophages occurs rapidly and reach intracellular concentrations of 40 times serum levels (21,21a). It is a matter of controversy whether the increased intracellular uptake of antibiotic influences the clinical outcome in infections (22–24). In one study, PMNs pretreated with clindamycin failed to kill *S. aureus* in vitro. Similarly, clindamycin failed to kill certain gram-negative periodontal bacilli such as *Actinobacillus actinomycetemcomitans*, *Eikenella corrodens*, and *Capnocytophaga ochracea* despite high intracellular concentration of the antibiotic (25–27). In contrast, the peritoneal macrophages that were harvested during peritoneal dialysis from patients on clindamycin therapy showed increased phagocytosis and intracellular killing of *Staphylococcus epidermidis* (28).

The bacteria and host cell interaction may be dependent upon whether the bacteria or the host cell is preexposed to clindamycin before they interact with each other. For example, if *S. aureus* is exposed to clindamycin, it is killed by granulocytes. Untreated *S. aureus* is not killed by granulocytes previously exposed to clindamycin (29). *Streptococcus pyogenes* bearing M protein on its surface resists opsonization, but when pretreated with clindamycin, M protein is inhibited and the bacteria are readily opsonized by PMNs (30). Clindamycin inhibits the binding of fibronectin to bacteria, thus clearing bacteria from the vegetations in cases of infective endocarditis (31). Clindamycin also inhibits glycocalyx production, allowing for better antibiotic penetration into the infected cardiac vegetation (32). High intracellular clindamycin levels in T cells and macrophages and the antibiotic effect on *Bacteroides* cell wall might explain the efficacy of this drug in the treatment of *B. fragilis* infections.

B. Pharmacokinetics

Clindamycin can be given intravenously, intramuscularly, or by oral route. It is unnecessary to monitor clindamycin serum antibiotic levels because its toxicity is not well associated with its serum level. Serum levels can be measured if a patient is suspected of toxicity or in cases of severe hepato-renal failure. Clindamycin is available in three salt forms:

1. *Clindamycin phosphate*, by itself an inactive prodrug, is given parenterally by the intravenous (IV) or an intramuscular (IM) route and is rapidly hydrolyzed to its

free base. Its potency is equivalent to a minimum of 758 μg of clindamycin per mg, and it is commercially available as 150 mg/ml in various vial sizes.

2. *Clindamycin palmitate hydrochloride*, also an inactive prodrug, is hydrolyzed in the small bowel to active clindamycin. It is formulated into a suspension that may be considered in elderly patients when they have difficulty taking capsules. Potency is equivalent to no less than 540 μg of clindamycin per mg. It is commercially available as 75 mg/5 ml in a 100-ml suspension.
3. *Clindamycin hydrochloride* is a white bitter-tasting powder used in capsule form. This salt is active and is not hydrolyzed. Its potency is equivalent to a minimum of 800 μg of clindamycin per mg. It is available as 75-, 150-, and 300-mg capsules.

1. Onset and Duration

Peak levels of clindamycin occur 1–2 h following oral administration, and because clindamycin HCl is active, it is absorbed more quickly than clindamycin palmitate suspension (33). Peak levels occur 2 to 3 h following an IM injection and about 20 min after the start of an IV infusion (34). Following a single 500-mg oral dose, the duration of activity is less than 8 h (35).

2. Absorption

Oral clindamycin hydrochloride is rapidly and well absorbed, with about 90% of it entering the serum (35). Food delays but does not alter its total absorption (36). The peak serum levels following oral administration is slower than the peak following IV administration. One hour after a single dose of 150-, 300-, or 450-mg capsules, the mean peak serum concentrations in healthy adults were 2.5, 3.6, and 5.8 μg/ml, respectively, and after 6 h were 0.7, 1.1, and 1.9 μg/ml, respectively (34,35).

Clindamycin palmitate suspension is also absorbed rapidly and effectively following oral administration, however, serum levels are slightly lower than the HCl capsule. One hour after a single dose of 150, 300, or 600 mg, the mean peak serum concentrations were 1.8, 2.6, and 3.9 μg/ml, respectively (33).

Intravenous clindamycin in doses of 300, 600, 900, and 1200 mg given over 10–45 min reaches serum concentrations of 5.4, 8.4, 10.4, and 15.9 μg/ml, respectively. A continuous IV infusion of 900–1350 mg per day maintained serum concentrations consistently at 4–6 μg/ml with less fluctuation (33,34).

Clindamycin administered IM is well tolerated and produces good therapeutic levels; a single dose of 300, 450, or 600 mg achieves concentrations of 4.5, 5.3, and 6.2 μg/ml in the serum, respectively, after 2–4 h (33).

Clindamycin is generally well absorbed in elderly patients, but physiological changes associated with aging, such as elevated gastric pH, decreased blood flow, and decreased transmucosal transport, may delay or decrease the intestinal absorption of peroral clindamycin.

3. Distribution

Clindamycin distributes well throughout the body, except into the cerebrospinal fluid (CSF). CSF penetration is limited even in the presence of inflamed meninges. Clindamycin has good penetration into various sites of infection including tonsils, sputum, saliva, bronchus, bronchial secretions, lung, pleural fluid, muscle, sweat, sebum, pus, bone, synovial fluid, semen, prostate, peritoneal fluid, appendix, small intestine, liver, gallbladder, and bile (37–39).

Clindamycin concentrations peak in the synovial fluid and the bone 6 h after an infusion, reaching about 50% of serum levels regardless of the bone type (40). In patients with patent bile ducts the concentrations of total clindamycin in the liver, gallbladder, bile, and common duct bile at 60 min was approximately 2.5–3 times greater than in the serum. In contrast, in patients with obstructed common ducts the concentrations of clindamycin in the wall of the gallbladder were about half those in the serum (40a).

Significant sputum levels are achieved in patients with pneumonia. Sputum levels of clindamycin 3.2 and 4.7 μg/ml are reported 2 h after a 300-mg oral dose. (41). The drug does distribute into the saliva, and thus some patients complain of a metallic taste (38).

Clindamycin is approximately 94% protein bound, primarily to α-1-glycoprotein (42). It is the unbound clindamycin that exerts a pharmacological effect. Since the drug is so highly bound, small changes in binding will affect drug disposition. Some of the factors that may alter binding in elderly patients are the nutritional status and serum protein levels. Those elderly persons on low-protein diets and with low serum albumin may experience an increased pharmacological effect because of less available binding sites. The volume of distribution of clindamycin is 0.6 l/kg, but this volume may be altered in elderly persons because there is a decrease in total body water and lean body mass and an associated increase of body fat with aging(33).

4. Metabolism

Clindamycin is significantly metabolized by the liver into both active and inactive components, followed by excretion into the urine. The two primary metabolites found are *N*-demethyl-clindamycin, which is three times more potent than the parent, and clindamycin sulfoxide, which is less potent. These metabolites are primarily found in the bile, feces, and urine, but not in the serum. They increase the duration of antibacterial activity up to 5 days in the feces, which causes a major reduction of bacterial counts in the colon up to 14 days(43).

Clindamycin has no significant interactions with other drugs cleared by the liver, but liver diseases can affect clindamycin metabolism. Its half-life may be prolonged fivefold in cases of severe liver disease, and, therefore, higher serum levels are predicted in patients with hepatic failure (44). Patients with liver disease may need dose adjustment, but no specific guidelines exist for this. One study reports giving clindamycin 300 mg intravenously every 12 h in patients with chronic hepatitis and cirrhosis with no exacerbation of hepatotoxicity (45). We have used up to 600 mg IV every 6 h for about 2 weeks without any adverse effect in cases of severe liver failure.

5. Excretion

About 5–20% of clindamycin is excreted unchanged in the urine within 24 h. About 8% of an IM dose and 28% of an IV dose are excreted in the urine within an 8-h period (46). Other sources of excretion are milk, feces, and bile.

The half-lives of clindamycin in healthy adults are as follows: HCl capsule is 2–3.8 h; palmitate suspension, 3.2–3.4 h; phosphate IM, 4.5–5.3 h; and phosphate IV, 1.5–5.3 h. No specific dose adjustment is necessary for old age(36).

The half-life of clindamycin is not appreciably altered with impaired renal function, and thus minimal or no alteration in dosage is required (44–48). In anephric patients, clindamycin's half-life is increased from 2.4 to 6 h and peak levels are doubled, but the drug requires no dosage adjustment. Clindamycin is not dialyzable. Neither hemodialysis nor peritoneal dialysis removes it from the blood(49).

V. CLINICAL INDICATIONS

Clindamycin or metronidazole, when used along with an aminoglycoside, aztreonam, or a quinolone, are very effective in the treatment of mixed aerobic/anaerobic infection such as intraabdominal sepsis following intestinal surgery. However, it is no longer necessary to use two antibiotics to treat such infections. During the past two decades we tested several antibiotics for monotherapy of postoperative intraabdominal infections and found them to be as safe and as effective as clindamycin/aminoglycoside combination. Those single drug therapies are carbenicillin, mezlocilin, ticarcillin, piperacillin, cefoxitin, cefamandole, cefotetan, ceftizoxime, cefoperazone, moxalactam, imipenem, chloramphenicol, or doxycycline(50).

Clindamycin is effective in the treatment of anaerobic lung infections such as community-acquired aspiration pneumonia, lung abscess, and empyema. In anaerobic pulmonary infections, carbenicillin alone was found to be as effective as clindamycin/gentamicin combination (51). In an animal model of anaerobic lung abscess, clindamycin was found to be the most active drug compared to carbenicillin, doxycycline, or chloramphenicol because of high lung tissue concentrations of clindamycin (52,53). Penicillin, which is still considered the drug of choice in anaerobic lung infections, when tested in this animal model failed to treat *B. fragilis* lung abscess (53). This was substantiated by clinical observation as well. In cases of aspiration pneumonia in elderly patients in whom anaerobes, *S. aureus*, and hospital- or nursing home-acquired bacteria may be present, clindamycin/gentamicin therapy should be efficacious.

Clindamycin in combination with gentamicin is recommended by the Centers for Disease Control and Prevention for the treatment of pelvic inflammatory disease. This combination has been successful in the treatment of postoperative infections of the female genital tract in women above the age of 40 who underwent total hysterectomy for cancer of the cervix, *procedentia uteri*, and in the treatment of other female genital tract infections (54,55). Anaerobic bacteria are normal flora of cervix. They can become opportunistic pathogens when surgery is performed on the female genital tract. Elderly women with atrophic vaginitis have an elevated pH of the vagina when the normal resident flora such as lactobacili are being replaced by *Bacteroides* spp. and other anaerobes. This can be corrected by applying 1% clindamycin cream intravaginally. Only 10–15% of the antibiotic administrated as intravaginal cream is absorbed systemically (56).

Clindamycin therapy is very effective in the treatment of *Chlamydia trachomatis* in women (14,15). It is also useful for *Mycoplasma pneumoniae* infections, but for elderly patients, either doxycycline, erythromycin, or azithromycin are safer because of higher incidence of clindamycin-associated colitis among the older patients.

Among elderly patients, osteomyelitis can occur secondary to a fracture from a fall or due to postoperative prosthesis. Usually *S. aureus* and/or aerobic gram-negative bacilli are involved in such infections. Although cephalosporins are suitable, β-lactam drugs in general do not achieve as high a concentration as clindamycin in the bone. If the osteomyelitis is due to *S. aureus* and it is not methicillin resistant, clindamycin is the drug of choice because bone and synovial fluid levels of clindamycin are about 70% of the serum levels (57,58).

Clindamycin prophylaxis decreases the anaerobic microflora of the colon, and it was found to be effective for prophylaxis in colorectal surgery (59,60). The tissue samples of colon taken during surgery after a single 600-mg IV infusion showed 1.8–13.0 μg/g of tissue, and the corresponding serum levels were 6.8–37.9 μg/ml, respectively (60). In another study, clindamycin concentrations in the small intestinal wall tissue averaged 9.7 μg/g of tissue, with the corresponding serum levels around 11 μg/ml. The tissue concentrations observed in these studies are four to five times the MIC of 90% of *B. fragilis* tested, and therefore clindamycin is efficacious in *B. fragilis* intraabdominal infections (61). Intestinal tissue levels tend to increase in a "stepladder" fashion, with the highest peak level achieved after the third dose. Clindamycin penetrates well into the tissue of the normal as well as the inflamed appendix. About 1–5 h after a 600-mg dose, the concentration of clindamycin in the appendix tissue was about 154% of the serum level. Elderly patients with suspected appendicitis and other causes of intraabdominal sepsis caused in part by anaerobic bacteria may be best treated with clindamycin rather than any of the β-lactam antibiotics because the tissue/serum levels of β-lactam antibiotics are expected to be less than 50% of the serum level (61).

Clindamycin can be used by itself or in combination with other antibiotics in the treatment of skin and soft tissue infections. Oral clindamycin is as effective as penicillin for streptococcal pharyngitis. It can be used to eradicate penicillin-resistant *S. aureus* that are not methicillin resistant; clindamycin is effective against *S. aureus* infections of the lung and bone, however, it is not the drug of choice. Clindamycin efficacy is perhaps not affected by the "Eagle effect." Using an animal model, Eagle demonstrated that in streptococcal myositis, penicillin was effective when given early enough at the time the bacterial counts were low. But penicillin therapy, when started late while the bacterial counts were high, failed (mortality 100%). This phenomenon did occur with clindamycin; it prevented death even when therapy was delayed (63). Clindamycin was shown to be effective in the treatment of streptococcal and staphylococcal endocarditis, but we do not recommend any bacteriostatic antibiotic such as clindamycin to treat bacterial endocarditis. Clindamycin is relatively effective against cephalosporin-resistant but not against methicillin-resistant *S. aureus*. Clindamycin was effective for prophylaxis against experimental *S. aureus* endocarditis in rabbits (66).

About 90% of brain abscesses have anaerobic bacteria, mostly *Bacteroides* and anaerobic streptococci, in combination with aerobes (67). Chloramphenicol or metronidazole are the preferred drugs, although clindamycin was successful in an occasional case of *B. fragilis* brain abscess (68). However, it is not recommended because clindamycin penetration into the brain tissue is erratic (69).

VI. ADMINISTRATION

Normal dosage is 300–600 mg every 6 h. We have never used the maximum dose recommended for life-threatening anaerobic infections of 4800 mg per day and we do not recommend 12-h dosing in either normal or hepato-renal patients as recommended by others (44,70). Although no specific dose adjustments appear necessary, the elderly patients must be monitored for the onset of diarrhea for fear of pseudomembranous (antibiotic-associated) colitis. The incidence of diarrhea leading to pseudomembranous colitis is higher in elderly patients, particularly in females, and is not dose related (71–75).

VII. ADVERSE EFFECTS

A. Clindamycin-Associated Diarrhea

Any antibiotic may cause diarrhea as a side effect. Although ampicillin attracted initial attention, clindamycin was the first to be blamed for "antibiotic-associated diarrhea." Prior knowledge of lincomycin diarrhea led to special testing of peroral clindamycin of 1800 mg/day in 210 healthy men before it was introduced for clinical trials. The volunteers took the drug for 2 weeks, but none developed severe diarrhea (76). A cooperative study in Canada investigated the incidence of clindamycin-associated diarrhea and reported that it is increased with age; it occurred in 18 of 39 (46%) patients who were more than 60 years old, and it was not dose or duration related (77). In that study, diarrhea occurred in 5% of those on ampicillin and 18% of patients on clindamycin, but pseudomembranous colitis (PMC) developed in 2% of those on clindamycin and 0.3% of patients on ampicillin. An independent study from Stanford University reported an incidence of diarrhea of 6.6% in study subjects, but only 0.3% of cases had PMC. This study showed that in patients below the age of 20 the incidence of diarrhea was less than 5%, whereas it was 20–27% in patients above this age (78). They reported that PMC occurred more frequently among women over age 55, and it worsened when opiates such as diphenoxylate with atropine were prescribed for symptomatic therapy (79). Five out of seven cases of PMC that occurred in one study and four of six in another were in older patients (80,81). Clindamycin-associated diarrhea among older adults is even higher when the antibiotic is coadministered with cancer chemotherapeutic agents. This is because most anticancer drugs delay maturation of intestinal epithelium and increase bacterial colonization of the small intestinal epithelium (82). Peroral clindamycin given for soft tissue infections to 15,019 patients in one study conducted in Leeds, U.K., resulted in only 13 cases (0.1%) of severe diarrhea. Two of the patients developed PMC, an incidence of 1:30,000 (83). In contrast, in St. Louis, Missouri, the incidence of clindamycin-associated diarrhea was 20%, and 10% of the patients developed PMC as demonstrated on proctoscopy (84). Obviously, factors other than the "drug and the bug" are involved in developing this complication.

In 1978, antibiotic-induced pseudomembranous colitis was shown to be caused by toxin-producing clostridia identified as *C. difficile* (85,86). This organism appears to be the major cause of *colitis* (i.e., PMC) in humans, but it is not the major cause of antibiotic-induced diarrhea. Merely recovering *C. difficile* in cultures or detecting its toxins is not necessarily diagnostic of *C. difficile*-induced disease unless the clinical manifestations co-exist. Yet, volumes of data published are so overwhelming as to convince most clinicians that the devastating complication of PMC occurs only with clindamycin use (85). One of the co-authors of this chapter has been using clindamycin since it was still in clinical trials in 1971. The author's hospital to date has dispensed clindamycin to several thousand patients over the past two decades, but he has seen only one case of PMC so far, and it was not due to *C. difficile*. All cases of antibiotic-associated diarrhea in the author's hospital were self-limiting and corrected by discontinuing all antibiotics. Similarly, in a report from Sweden, of 2390 fecal samples cultured from patients with diarrhea, *C. difficile* was found in only 81 (3%). Most of the patients had pathogens such as *Salmonella*, *Campylobacter*, *Yersinia*, and *Shigella*, and their diarrhea resolved without specific therapy for *C. difficile* (87). Various published reports thus far suggest that the incidence of PMC associated with clindamycin occurs in such an absurdly wide range, as 3 in 1000 to 1 of 50,000 persons treated with this antibiotic (84–94).

B. Hospital-Acquired *C. difficile*

In one study, *C. difficile* was cultured in 36% of hospitalized patients without PMC and 0% of healthy controls (87). Long-term care facilities such as nursing homes have reported outbreaks of *C. difficile* infection and diarrhea (91,92). Asymptomatic patients need not be isolated just because they have positive stool cultures for *C. difficile* or have detectable enterotoxin. Cytotoxin assay alone by the latex aggluntination method without culture is not diagnostic because of the poor predictive value of this test when the disease incidence itself is very low (88). Conversely, isolation of *C. difficile* alone is not diagnostic because it has been cultured from the stool of 13% of adult hospitalized patients and from the stool of 5% of healthy adults who were not on antibiotics. In another study, 12% of patients with diarrhea but not on antibiotics and 13% with inflammatory bowel disease without diarrhea had their stools colonized with *C. difficile* (89,90). Hospitalization alone is the leading risk factor for *C. difficile* colonization.

C. Animal Models

Several animal models have been developed for *C. difficile*–associated colitis. Syrian hamsters given clindamycin developed colitis with *C. difficile*, and its toxin appeared in their stool (91,92). Animal models do not accurately represent human disease. For example, cefoxitin rarely causes PMC and *C. difficile* colitis in humans, but it can produce *C. difficile*–associated diarrhea in prairie dogs (92). Feeding infant hamsters with *C. difficile* causes abundance of cytotoxin in their stools. But the organism or toxin does not cause cecitis unless the animals also receive clindamycin, suggesting that *C. difficile* and its toxin alone are not enough to cause this disease and it is influenced by the antibiotic (91).

The toxin of *C. difficile* is inhibited by its antitoxin, and it is also neutralized by toxins produced by *C. glycolicum* and *C. sordelli*. Paradoxically, it is also inactivated by nontoxigenic strains of *C. difficile* (93). Such antagonism is known to exist in other diarrheagenic organisms such as *S. aureus* and *E. coli* as well. In hamster models, *C. difficile* can be a vivarium-acquired infection as it is a hospital-acquired infection in the human (94). Lactobacilli GG or a nonpathogenic strain of the yeast *Saccharomyces boulardii* did successfully terminate *C. difficile* colitis in some patients (95,96).

D. Susceptibility of *C. Difficile* to Antibiotics

Peroral vancomycin, given 2 g daily, resolves PMC in 7 days. The stool vancomycin levels are 3100 μg/g of stool, but little is found in the serum (97). Metronidazole 250 mg given four times daily is also effective, and it is 50 times cheaper than vancomycin (98). Most isolates of *C. difficile* that cause diarrhea are very susceptible to vancomycin, penicillin G, ampicillin, metronidazole, carbenicillin, ticarcillin, and piperacillin in vitro. Aztreonam, quinolones, and most cephalosporins including the third-generation cephalosporins are inactive against this organism (99,100). This organism is resistant to clindamycin (MIC 90 = 16 μg/ml) and cefoxitin. Paradoxically, the majority of patients with antibiotic-associated diarrhea due to this organism had *C. difficile* that was susceptible to the antibiotic the patient was receiving (100). This suggests that antibiotic-associated colitis due to *C. difficile* or its toxin and clindamycin may have other unknown host factors that trigger inflammation of the intestinal wall. For example, toxins produced by *C. difficile* are known to decrease the capacity of monocytes to stimulate T-cell proliferation (101).

Quinolones are inactive against *C. difficile* at serum concentrations achieved on therapeutic dose. However, certain quinolones such as ciprofloxacin, ofloxacin, pefloxacin, lomefloxacin, and norfloxacin are highly effective against the organism at stool concentrations achieved by these antibiotics, which are known to be 100- to 1000-fold higher than the serum levels (100,102). A single case of PMC associated with ciprofloxacin therapy has been reported (103) and is a cause for concern since quinolones are widely used for treatment of various types of bacterial diarrheas.

E. Diagnosis of *C. difficile* Colitis

The clinical diagnosis of PMC can be made by proctosigmoidoscopic examination, but some patients require colonoscopy for thorough examination of the colon for plaques. A computed tomographic scan of a barium-filled colon shows a characteristic thickening of the mucosa with contrast medium trapped in folds referred to as the "accordian sign" while the small bowel remains usually intact. Diagnosis of *C. difficile* diarrhea can be made by rectal swabs and stool cultures (for toxin and organisms). The most effective method (91%) for culturing *C. difficile* is ethanol-treated direct plating of the rectal swab on Carr-Scarborough cycloserine-cefoxitin fructose agar with horse blood (102,104,105). Detection of *C. difficile* toxin is required in most instances to confirm the diagnosis. The cytotoxin assay to detect toxin B of *C. difficile* has the best sensitivity and specificity and is the most accurate of all tests, but it requires almost 24 h to obtain the result. The latex particle agglutination method is not as sensitive but is more rapid. Enzyme immunoassay can detect toxin A and/or B within 2–4 h and is technically easier than the cytotoxin assay (106). The polymerase chain reaction method can be used to detect *C. difficile* and its toxin A gene (107,108).

REFERENCES

1. Dhawan VK, Thadepalli H. Clindamycin: review of fifteen years of experience. Rev Infect Dis 1982; 4:1133–53.
2. Bartlett JH, Chang TW, Gurwith M, et al. Antibiotic-associated pseudomembranous colitis due to toxin-producing clostridia. N Engl J Med 1978; 298:531–534.
3. Thomas DR, Bennett RG, Laughom B, et al. Post antibiotic colonization with *Clostridium difficile* in nursing home patients. J Am Geriatr Soc 1990; 38:415–20.
4. Drapkin MS, Karchmer AW, Moellering RC, Jr. Bacteremic infections due to clindamycin-resistant streptococci. JAMA 1976; 236:263–5.
5. Benner EJ, Adams PA, Jr. Unusual resistance of Staphylococcus aureus to lincomycin and 7-chlorolincomycin. Antimicrob Agents Chemother 1969; 9:100–3.
6. Ingham HR, Hall CG, Sisson PR, et al. The activity of metronidazole against facultative anaerobic bacteria. J Antimicrob Agents Chemother 1980; 6:343–7.
7. Salaki JS, Black R, Tally FP, et al. *Bacteroides fragilis* resistant to the administration of clindamycin. Am J Med 1976; 60:426–9.
8. Tally FP, Cuchural GJ, Jr., Jacobus NVC, et al. Nationwide study of the susceptibility of the *Bacteroides fragilis* group in the United States. Antimicrob Agents Chemother 1985; 28:675–8.
9. Kenneth SS. Emergence of antibiotic resistant strains of *Bacteroides fragilis*. Surg Gynecol Obstet 1988; 167:175–9.
10. Butler E, Joiner KA, Malamy M, et al. Transfer of tetracycline or clindamycin resistance among strains of *Bacteroides fragilis* in experimental abscesses. J Infect Dis 1984; 150:20–4.
11. Ohm-Smith MJ, Sweet RL, Hadley WK. Occurrence of clindamycin-resistant anaerobic bacreria isolated from cultures taken following clindamycin therapy. Antimicrob Agents Chemother 1986; 30:11–14.
12. Wilkins TD, Thiel T. Resistance of some species of Clostridium to clindamycin. Antimicrob Agents Chemother. 1973; 2:136–7.
13. Guiney DG, Jr., Hasegawa P, Stalker D, et al. Genetic analysis of clindamycin resistance in *Bacteroides fragilis* species. J Infect Dis 1983; 147:551–8.
14. Bowie WR. In vitro activity of clindamycin against *Chlamydia trachomatis*. Am Vener Dis Assoc 1981; 8:220–1.
15. Pearlman MD, Faro S, Riddle GD, et al. In vitro synergy of clindamycin and aminoglycoside against *Chlamydia trachomatis*. Antimicrob Agents Chemother 1990; 34:1399–401.
16. Zinner SH, Provonchee RB, Elias KS, et al. Effect of clindamycin on the in vitro activity of amikacin and gentamicin against gram-negative bacilli. Antimicrob Agents Chemother 1976; 9:661–4.

17. Sanders CC, Sanders WE, Jr., Goering RW. Influence of clindamycin on derepresion of B-lactamases in *Enterobacter spp.* and *Pseudomonas aeruginosa*. Antimicrob Agents Chemother 1983; 24:48–53.
18. Queener SF, Bartlett MS, Richardson JD, et al. Activity of clindamycin with primaquine against *Pneumocystis carinii* in vitro and in vivo. Antimicrob Agents Chemother 1988; 32:807–13.
19. Dannemann BR, Israelski DM, Remington JS. Treatment of toxoplasmic encephalitis with intravenous clindamycin. Arch Intern Med 1988; 148:2477–82.
20. Clyde DF, Gilman RH, McCarthy VC. Antimalarial effects of clindamycin in man. Am J Trop Med Hyg 1975; 24:369–70.
21. Klempner MS, Styrt B. Clindamycin uptake by human neutrophils. J Infect Dis 1981; 144:472–9.
21a. Hand WL, King-Thompson NL. Membrane transport of clindamycin in alveolar macrophages. Antimicrob Agents Chemother 1982; 21:241–7.
22. Steinberg TH, Hand WL. Effect of phagocyte membrane stimulation on antibiotic uptake and intracellular bactericidal activity. 1987; 31:660–2.
23. Milatovic D, Braveny I, Verhoef J. Clindamycin enhances opsonization of *Staphylococcus aureus*. Antimicrob Agents Chemother 1983; 24:413–17.
24. Faden H, Hong JJ, Ogra PL. In vivo effects of clindamycin on neutrophil function, a preliminary report. J Antimicrob Chemother 1983; 12:29–34.
25. Easmon CS, Crane JP. Cellular uptake of clindamycin and lincomycin. Br J Exp Path 1984; 65:725–30.
26. Baker PJ, Wilson ME. Effect of clindamycin on neutrophil killing of gram-negative periodontal bacteria. Antimicrob Agents Chemother 1988; 32:1521–7.
27. Wecke J, Johannsen L, Giesbrecht P. Reduction of wall degradability of clindamycin treated staphylococcus within macrophages. Infect Immun 1990; 58:197–204.
28. de Fijter CW, Verbrugh HA, Heezius HC, et al. Effect of clindamycin on the intracellular bactericidal capacity of human peritoneal macrophages. J Antimicrob Chemother 1990; 26:525–32.
29. Veringa EM, Verhoef J. Clindamycin at subinhibitory concentrations enhances antibody- and complement-dependent phagocytosis by human polymorphonuclear leukocytes on *Staphylococcus aureus*. Chemotherapy 1987; 33:243–9.
30. Gemmell CG, Peterson PK, Schmeling D, et al. Potentiation of opsonization and phagocytosis of *Streptococcus pyogenes* following growth in the presence of clindamycin. J Clin Invest 1981; 67:1249–56.
31. Doran JE, Rissing JP. Influence of clindamycin on fibronectin-staphylococcal interactions. J Antimicrob Chemother 1983; 12:75–83.
32. Dall L, Keihofner M, Herndon B, et al. Clindamycin effect on glycocalyx production in experimental viridans streptococcal endocarditis. J Infect Dis 1990; 161:1221–4.
33. Dehaan RM, Metzler CM, Schellenberg D, et al. Pharmacokinetic studies of clindamycin phosphate. J Clin Pharmacol 1973; 13:190–209.
34. Metzler C, Dehaan R, Schellenberg D, et al. Clindamycin dose-bioavailability relationships. J Pharm Sci 1973; 62:591–8.
35. McGehee RF Jr, Smith CB, Wilcox C, et al. Comparative studies of antibacterial activity in vitro and absorption and excretion of lincomycin and clindamycin. Am J Med Sci 1968; 256:279–92.
36. Dehaan RM, Vanden Bosch WD, Metzler CM. Clindamycin serum concentrations after administration of clindamycin palmitate with food. J Clin Pharmacol 1972; 12:205–11.
37. Thadepalli H, Mandal AK, Prabhala RH, et al. Antibiotic levels in the small intestine. Surg Gynecol Obstet 1986; 163:561–7.
38. Panzer JD, Brown DC, Epstein WL, et al. Clindamycin levels in various body tissues and fluids. J Clin Pharmacol 1972; 12:259–72.
39. Chin A, Gill MA, Ito MK, et al. Evaluation of two different dosage regimens of clindamycin and the penetration into human appendix. Therapeut Drug Monitoring 1989; 11:421–4.

40. Baird P, Hughes S, Sullivan M, et al. Penetration into bone and tissues of clindamycin phosphate. Postgrad Med J 1978; 54:65–7.
40a. Brown RB, Martyak SN, Barza M, et al. Penetration of clindamycin phosphate into the abnormal human biliary tract. Ann Intern Med 1976; 84:168–70.
41. Raeburn J, Devine JD. Clindamycin levels in sputum in a patient with purulent chest disease due to cystic fibrosis. Postgrad Med J 1971; 47:355–67.
42. Gordon RC, Regamey C, Kirby WM. Serum protein binding of erythromycin, lincomycin and clindamycin. J Pharm Sci 1973; 62:1074–7.
43. Manashil GB, Kern JA. Nonspecific colitis following oral lincomycin therapy. Am J Gastroenterol 1973; 60:394.
44. Flaherty JF, Rodondi LC, Guglielmo EJ, et al. Comparative pharmacokinetics and serum inhibitory activity of clindamycin in different dosing regimens. Antimicrob Agents Chemother 1988; 32:1825–9.
45. Hinthorn DR, Baker LH, Romig DA, et al. Use of clindamycin in patients with liver disease. Antimicrob Agents Chemother 1976; 9:498–501.
46. Joshi A, Stein RM. Altered serum clearance of intravenously administered clindamycin phosphate in patients with uremia. J Clin Pharmacol 1974; 14:140–4.
47. Bennett WM, Aronoff GR, Golper TA, et al., eds. Drug prescribing in renal failure. Philadelphia: American College of Physicians, 1987.
48. Anderson RJ, Gabertogolio JG, Schrier RW, eds. Clinical use of drugs in renal failure. Springfield, IL: Charles C Thomas, 1976.
49. Cimino JE, Tierno PM, Jr. Hemodialysis properties of clindamycin. Appl Microbiol 1969; 17:446.
50. Thadepalli H, Mandal AK. Antimicrobial therapy in abdominal surgery: precepts and practices. Boca Raton, FL: CRC Press, 1991.
51. Thadepalli H, Niden AH, Huang JT. Treatment of anaerobic pulmonary infections. Chest 1976; 49:743–6.
52. Kannangari DW, Thadepalli H, Bach VT, et al. Animal model for anaerobic lung abscess. Infect Immun 1981; 32:592–7.
53. Thadepalli H, Kannangara DW, Bach VT. Penicillin failure in the treatment of *Bacteroides fragilis* lung abscess. Chemotherapy 1983; 29:289–93.
54. Ledger WJ, Gee CL, Lewis WP, et al. Comparison of clindamycin and chloramphenicol in treatment of serious infections of the female genital tract. J Infect Dis 1977; 135:S30–S34.
55. Thadepalli H, Gorbach SL, Keith L. Anaerobic infections of the female genital tract: Bacteriologic and therapeutic aspects. Am J Obstet Gynecol 1973; 117:1034–40.
56. Borin MT. Systemic absorption of clindamycin following intravaginal application of clindamycin phosphate 1% cream. J Clin Pharmacol 1990; 30:33–8.
57. Dornbusch K, Carlstrom A, Hugo H, et al. Antibacterial activity of clindamycin and lincomycin in human bone. J Antimicrob Chemother 1977; 3:153–60.
58. Nicholas P, Myers BR, Levy RN, et al. Concentration of clindamycin in human bone. Antimicrob Agents Chemother 1975; 8:220–1.
59. Bartlett JG, Condon RE, Gorbach SL, et al. Veterans Administration cooperative study on bowel preparation for elective colorectal operations: Impact of oral antibiotic regimen on colonic flora wound irrigation, cultures and bacteriology of septic complications. Ann Surg 1978; 188:249–54.
60. Kager L, Liljeqvist L, Malmborg AS, et al. Effect of clindamycin prophylaxis on the colonic microflora in patients undergoing colorectal surgery. Antimicrob Agents Chemother 1981; 20:736–40.
61. Thadepalli H, Lou MA, Prabhala RH, et al. Human intestinal tissue antibiotic concentrations Am Surg 1990; 56:655–8.
62. Berger SA, Barza M, Leslie SW, Raciti A, Kazarian KK, Kane A. Penetration of clindamycin into the human appendix. Arch Surg 1978; 113:1094–5.

63. Stevens DL, Gibbons AE, Bergstrom, et al. The Eagle effect revisted: Efficacy of clindamycin, erythromycin, and penicillin in the treatment of streptococcal myositis. J Infect Dis 1988; 158:23–8.
64. Menda, KB, Gorbach SL. Favorable experience with bacterial endocarditis in heroin addicts. Ann Intern Med 1973; 78:25–32.
65. Burch KH, Quinn EL, Cox F, et al. Intramuscular clindamycin for therapy of infective endocarditis. Am J Cardiol 1976; 38:899–903.
66. Dhawan VK, Thadepalli H, Rao B, et al. Chemoprophylaxis of experimental endocarditis caused by *Staphylococcus aureus*. J Antimicrob Chemother 1982; 9:319–24.
67. Heineman HS, Braude AI. Anaerobic infections of the brain. Ann J Med 1963; 35:682–97.
68. Khuri-Bulos N, McIntosh K, Ehret J. Bacteroides brain abscess treated with clindamycin. Am J Dis Child 1973; 126:96–8.
69. Picardi JL, Lewis HP, Tan JS, et al. Clindamycin concentrations in the central nervous system of primates before and after head trauma. J Neurosurg 1975; 43:717–20.
70. Product information: cleocin phosphate (R), clindamycin. Kalamazoo, MI: The Upjohn Company, 1989.
71. Hoberman LJ, Eigenbrodt EH, Kilman WJ, et al. Colitis associated with oral clindamycin therapy. A clinical study of 16 patients. Am J Dig Dis 1976; 21:1–17.
72. Neu HC, Prince A, Neu CO, et al. Incidence of diarrhea and colitis associated with clindamycin therapy. J Infect Dis 1977; 135 (suppl):S120–S125.
73. Swartzberg JE, Maresca RM, Remington JS. Clinical study of gastrointestinal complications associated with clindamycin therapy. J Infect Dis 1977; 135 (suppl):S99–S103.
74. Townsend RJ, Baker RP. Pharmacokinetic comparison of three clindamycin phosphate dosing schedules. Drug Intell Clin Pharmacol 1987; 21:279–81.
75. Wells RF, Cohen LE. Clindamycin and pseudomembranous colitis. Lancet 1974; 1:66.
76. De Haan RM, Schellenberg D, Vanden Bosch WD, et al. Clindamycin palmitate in healthy men: General tolerance and effect on stools. Curr Ther Res 1972; 14:80–90.
77. Gurwith MJ, Rabin HR, Love K, and Cooperative Diarrhea Study Group. Diarrhea associated with clindamycin and ampicillin therapy: preliminary results of a cooperative study. J Infect Dis 1977; 135:S104–S10.
78. Swartzberg JE, Maresca RM, Remington JS. Gastrointestinal side effects associated with clindamycin. Arch Intern Med 1976; 136:876–9.
79. Ramirez-Ronda CH. Incidence of clindamycin-associated colitis. Ann Intern Med 1974; 81:860.
80. Viteri AL Howard PH, Dyck WP. The spectrum of lincomycin-clindamycin colitis. Gastroenterology 1974; 66:1137–44.
81. Weinrib M, Sheehy TW. Colitis associated with clindamycin therapy. South Med J 1975; 68:1471–4.
82. Cudmore MA, Silva J, Jr, Fekety R, et al. *Clostridium difficile* colitis associated with cancer chemotherapy. Arch Intern Med 1982; 142:333–5.
83. Wilson DH. Clindamycin in the treatment of soft tissue infections: a review of 15019 patients. Br J Surg 1980; 67:93–96.
84. Tedesco FJ, Anderson CB, Ballinger WF. Drug-induced colitis mimicking an acute surgical condition of the abdomen. Arch Surg 1975; 110:481–4.
85. Bartlett JG. *Clostridium difficile*: clinical considerations. Rev Infect Dis 1990; 12:S243–50.
86. Pierce PF, Jr, Wilson R, Silva J, Jr, et al. Antibiotic-associated pseudomembranous colitis: an epidemiologic investigation of a cluster of cases. J Infect Dis 1982; 145:269–74.
87. Falsen E, Kaijser B, Nehls L, Nygren B. Svedhem A. *Clostridium difficile* in relation to enteric bacterial pathogens. J Clin Microbiol 1980; 12:297–300.
88. Bennett RG, Laughon BE, Mundy LM, et al. Evaluation of latex agglutination test for *Clostridium difficile* in two nursing home outbreaks. J Clin Microbiol 1989; 27:889–93.
89. Varki NM, Aquino TI. Isolation of *Clostridium difficile* from hospitalized patients without antibiotic-associated diarrhea or colitis. J Clin Microbiol 1982; 16:659–62.

90. Greenfield C, Aguilar Ramirez, Jr, Pounder RE, et al. *Clostridium difficile* and inflammatory bowel disease. Gut 1983; 24:713–17.
91. Rolfe RD, Iaconis JP, Kim PH. Symptomatic and asymptomatic colonization of infant hamsters by *Clostridium difficile*. Microecol Ther 1986; 16:217–30.
92. Muller EL, Pitt HA, George WL. Prairie dog model for antimicrobial agent-induced *Clostridium difficile* diarrhea. Infect Immun 1987; 55:198–200.
93. Wilson KH, Sheagren JN. Antagonism of toxigenic *Clostridium difficile* by nontoxigenic *C. difficile*. J Infect Dis 1983; 147:733–6.
94. Larson HE, Price AB, Borriello SP. Epidemiology of experimental enterocecitis due to *Clostridium difficile*. J Infect Dis 1980; 142:408–13.
95. Gorbach SL, Chang TW, Goldin B. Successful treatment of relapsing *Clostridium difficile* colitis with lactobacillus GG. Lancet 1987; 2:1519.
96. Surawicz CM, Elmer GW, Speelman P, et al. Prevention of antibiotic-associated diarrhea by *Saccharomyces boulardii*: a prospective study. Gastroenterology 1989; 96:981–8.
97. Tedesco F, Gurwith M, Markham R, et al. Oral vancomycin for antibiotic-associated pseudomembranous colitis. Lancet 1978; 1:226–8.
98. Teasley DG, Olson MM, Gebhard RL, et al. Prospective randomized trial of metronidazole versus vancomycin for *Clostridium difficile*-associated diarrhea and colitis. Lancet 1983; 2:1043–6.
99. Chow AW, Cheng N, Bartlett KH. In vitro susceptibility of *Clostridium difficile* to new B-lactam and quinolone antibiotics. Antimicrob Agents Chemother 1985; 28:842–4.
100. Dzink J, Bartlett JG. In vitro susceptibility of *Clostridium difficile* isolates from patients with antibiotic-associated diarrhea or colitis. Antimicrob Agents Chemother 1980; 17:695–8.
101. Daubener W, Leiser E, von Eichel-Streiber C, et al. *Clostridium difficile* toxins A and B inhibit human immune response in vitro. Infect Immun 1988; 56:1107–12.
102. Delmee M, Avesani V. Comparative in vitro activity of seven quinolones against 100 clinical isolates of *Clostridium difficile*. Antimicrob Agents Chemother 1986; 29:374–5.
103. Bates CJ, Wilcox MH, Spencer RC, et al. Ciprofloxacin and *Clostridium difficile* infection. Lancet 1990; 336:1193.
104. George WL, Sutter VL, Citron D, et al. Selective and differential medium for isolation of *Clostridium difficile* J Clin Microbiol 1979; 9:214–19.
105. McFarland LV, Coyle MB, Kremer WH, Stamm WE. Rectal swab cultures for *Clostridium difficile* surveillance studies. J Clin Microbiol 1987; 25:2241–2.
106. Bartlett JG. Antibiotic-associated diarrhea. Clin Infect Dis 1992; 15:573–81.
107. Kato Naoki, Ou CY, Kato H, Bartley SL, et al. Identification of toxigenic *Clostridium difficile* by the polymerase chain reaction. J Clin Microbiol 1991; 29:33–7.
108. Wren B, Clayton C, Tabaqchali S. Rapid identification of toxigenic *Clostridium difficile* by polymerase chain reaction. Lancet 1990; 1:423.

19

Metronidazole

Kimberly A. Shriner
Huntington Memorial Hospital, Pasadena, California

Glenn E. Mathisen
Olive View–UCLA Medical Center, Sylmar, California

I. INTRODUCTION

Metronidazole is a nitroimidazole that was developed in the late 1950s as therapy for *Trichomonas vaginalis.* Since the 1960s, metronidazole has been prescribed for a wide range of clinical conditions. Its utility against parasites has been well described, and it remains the mainstay of therapy for giardiasis and amebic infections. Ironically, the activity of metronidazole against anaerobic bacteria, currently one of its most important properties, was a somewhat serendipitous discovery, when Shinn noted improvement in ulcerative gingivitis in a patient being treated for trichomonal vaginitis (1). The increased frequency of age-related conditions such as diabetes mellitus, ischemic vascular disease, malignancy, and pulmonary disease, as well as surgical interventions predispose the elderly patient to infections with anaerobic pathogens. In this patient population, metronidazole plays a pivotal role in the primary therapy of local abscesses and anaerobic bacteremia. It may also be important for prophylaxis in colorectal surgery and as an adjunctive chemotherapeutic agent in the treatment of certain malignancies.

II. CHEMISTRY

The nitroimidazole compounds were originally isolated from *Streptomyces* species and were noted to exhibit activity against *T. vaginalis.* Cosar and Julou were the first to describe in vivo and in vitro activity of 1-(β-hydroxy-ethyl)-2-methyl-5-nitroimidazole or metronidazole (Fig. 1) (2). Other nitroimidazoles with bacterial and parasitic properties similar to those of metronidazole include tinidazole and nimorazole.

III. MECHANISM OF ACTION

Although metronidazole is concentrated in both aerobic and anaerobic bacteria, its bactericidal activity is reserved for those organisms that possess anaerobic metabolic pathways.

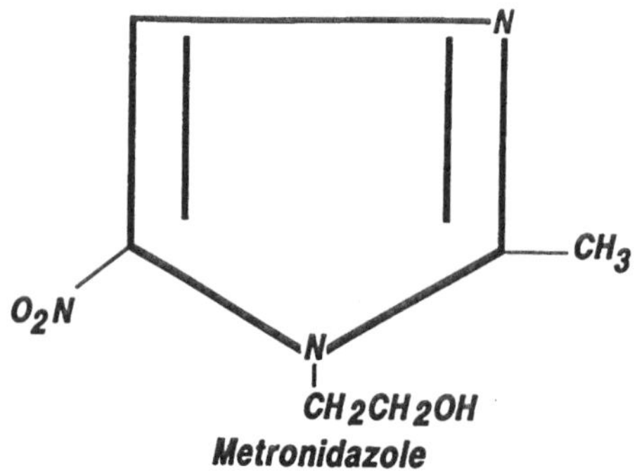

Figure 1 Chemical structure of metronidazole.

Indeed, metronidazole is unusual in its activity against both prokaryotic and eukaryotic organisms, provided they rely on anaerobic metabolism.

Metronidazole exists as a small, uncharged molecule that passively diffuses into the target cell. This process occurs with equal efficacy in both aerobic and anaerobic environments. A linear relationship between intracellular and extracellular drug concentrations has been shown in trichomonads and appears not to be inhibited by high concentrations of nitroimidazoles or their derivatives (3). Maintenance of high intracellular concentrations of metronidazole is dependent upon the fate of the parent compound. In aerobic organisms, the intracellular drug remains unchanged. With passive diffusion, an equilibrium will eventually be reached between intracellular and extracellular drug concentrations. In organisms utilizing anaerobic metabolism, the parent compound undergoes reduction of the nitro group, forming cytotoxic intermediates. This modification decreases intracellular concentrations of unchanged drug and perpetuates extracellular to intracellular diffusion (4,5).

After entry into the anaerobic organism, the nitro side chain of metronidazole is quickly reduced by donation of electrons from ferrodoxinlike electron transport proteins (see Fig. 2) (5). This active reduction leads to the formation of short-lived but cytotoxic intermediates that include nitroso-free radicals and nitroso and hydroxylamine derivatives. Metronidazole's mechanisms of cytotoxicity are poorly understood in part due to the difficulty in isolating these cytotoxic intermediates. The most frequently cited explanation for metronidazole's microbicidal activity is that the cytotoxic intermediates interfere with the deoxyribonucleic acids of target cells (4,6,7). This is supported by experiments, which show that while reduced metronidazole metabolites interfere with DNA synthesis unchanged drug does not (8). The reduced intermediates may attach directly to nucleic acids or cause single-stranded or double-stranded breaks in cellular DNA (9,10). Further metabolism of the cytotoxic intermediates of metronidazole leads to the production of acetamide and 2-hydroxyethyl oxamic acid as well as other equally inactive end products (4).

IV. ANTIMICROBIAL SPECTRUM

Metronidazole exhibits antimicrobial activity against a wide variety of protozoal and bacterial pathogens. Originally utilized as therapy for infections with *T. vaginalis*, it has become one of the most important antimicrobial agents for most anaerobic and some facultatively anaerobic pathogens.

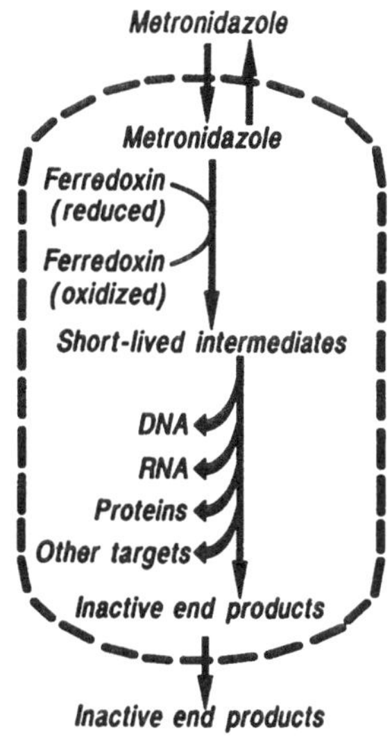

Figure 2 Pharmacological activity of metronidazole in an anaerobic organism. (From Ref. 65.)

A. Protozoa

Most anaerobic protozoa are susceptible to metronidazole. These would include *T. vaginalis*, *Entamoeba histolytica*, *Giardia lamblia*, and *Balantidium coli*. Metronidazole resistance has been reported in *T. vaginalis*, but it is rare (11). Although in vitro studies have shown that other nitroimidazoles such as tinidazole are more active against *G. lamblia* than metronidazole, the latter still exhibits adequate protozoal killing at concentrations well below that which is achievable in human serum (12). Variation in metronidazole sensitivity among isolates of *Giardia* has been recognized and may account for periodic treatment failures (13,14). Definite metronidazole resistance has not been shown in *E. histolytica* infections.

B. Bacteria

The most commonly encountered obligate anaerobic pathogens and many facultatively anaerobic organisms are susceptible to metronidazole (Table 1). These would include pathogens associated with intraabdominal sepsis and abscesses, genital tract infections, and suppurative anaerobic pulmonary abscesses; all of these infections occur commonly in older patients. Gram-negative anaerobic bacteria such as *Bacteroides* and *Fusobacterium* species are nearly always sensitive to metronidazole. A nationwide 3-year study of *Bacteroides fragilis* at New England Medical Center showed that while resistance to clindamycin (6%) and piperacillin (12%) was present and to cephalosporins such as cefoxitin, cefotaxime, and cefuroxime was increased no metronidazole-resistant isolates could be identified (15). *Bacteroides* species are capable of producing β-lactamases; this may account for the cephalosporin resistance but does not explain the rare clinical reports of *B. fragilis* resistance to metronidazole (16). Metronidazole-resistant isolates of *B. fragilis* produced in the laboratory show diminished pyruvate dehydrogenase activity. This, in turn, may decrease intracellular drug uptake and attenuate bacterial killing (17).

Table 1 Spectrum of Activity of Metronidazole Against Anaerobic and Microaerophilic Organisms.

Bacteria	No. strains	Cumulative % susceptible to indicated concentration (μg/ml)			
		<4	8	16	32
Bacteroides fragilis	161	90	9	100	—
Bacteroides melaninogenicus	60	98	100	—	—
Other Bacteroides and Selenomonas species	154	95	98	100	—
Fusobacterium species	65	100	—	—	—
Anaerobic gram negative cocci	24	92	96	100	—
Anaerobic gram positive cocci	124	98	—	—	—
Clostridium perfringens	18	94	100	—	—
Other Clostridium species	73	97	99	—	100
Gram positive nonsporulating bacilli	87	57	60	62	66
Capnocytophaga species	27	52	70	93	—

Source: Ref. 66. (With permission. From Sutter VL: In vitro susceptibility of anaerobic and microaerophilic bacteria to metronidazole and its hydroxy metabolite. In Finegold SM, Mathisen GE. "Metronidazole," Principles and Practice of Infectious Disease, edited by G Mandel, RG Douglas, J Bennett. New York: Churchill Livingston, 1990.

Many gram-positive anaerobic bacteria are also susceptible to metronidazole. These include obligate anaerobes such as *Peptococcus*, *Peptostreptococcus*, and *Eubacterium spp*. Nearly all clostridial pathogens, including *C. perfringens* and *C. difficile*, are sensitive to metronidazole (18,19). Organisms that are not strict obligate anaerobes, such as *Proprionibacterium*, *Actinomyces*, *Lactobacillus*, and many microaerophilic streptococci, are usually resistant to metronidazole (20).

Metronidazole has also been shown to have some activity against commonly encountered Enterobacteriaceae, including *Escherichia coli*, *Klebsiella*, and *Proteus*. This activity appears to be especially evident in the presence of mixed anaerobic/gram-negative aerobic infections where a reciprocal synergism in bactericidal activity has been noted between *E. coli* and *B. fragilis* (21,22). The mechanism may be due in part to bactericidal metabolites excreted by coexistent anaerobes (23).

V. CLINICAL PHARMACOLOGY

Metronidazole may be administered orally, intravenously, or by rectal suppository. Interestingly, each of these routes appears to be equally efficacious in delivering high systemic concentrations of the drug. After oral administration, metronidazole is rapidly absorbed by the gastrointestinal mucosa, achieving rates as high as 80% within 1 h. Indeed, some studies have shown bioavailabilities of 93–99% after oral administration of metronidazole (24). Although gut motility per se may not affect metronidazole metabolism, some studies have shown higher plasma concentrations of the drug in patients with ileostomies and intestinal disorders such as Crohn's disease (25,26). Thiercelin et al. have shown changes in metronidazole kinetics in patients who receive oral therapy after gastrointestinal surgery (27). Although definitive evidence is lacking, these studies suggest that in an elderly patient population where gastrointestinal motility disorders and diseases are common, a decrease in oral dosage of metronidazole may be needed to compensate for altered drug kinetics. Absorption of metronidazole does not appear to be altered by food.

Peak serum concentrations of 20–25 μg/ml are reached after intravenous or oral administration of 7.5 mg/kg of metronidazole. The drug has a large volume of distribution (approximately 80% of body weight) and an estimated serum half-life of 8 h. Less than 20% of the drug is protein bound (28). Bactericidal levels of metronidazole are reached in cerebrospinal fluid, bile, vitreous humor, abscesses, and all tissues.

Metronidazole has two principal routes of metabolism. It is metabolized in the liver via oxidation to its primary metabolites, the biologically active 1-(2-hydroxyethyl)-2-hydroxymethyl-5-nitroimidazole and biologically inactive 1-acetic acid-2-methyl-5-nitroimidazole. Both are subsequently excreted in the urine. Unaltered drug may circumvent hepatic metabolism and be excreted unchanged via the kidneys (29,30). Pharmacokinetic studies in patients with liver disease have shown a reduction in drug elimination and total body clearance as well as an increase in serum half-life of metronidazole and its metabolites (30,31). Roux et al. examined metronidazole kinetics in patients undergoing hemodialysis for acute renal failure and found no accumulation of metronidazole or its metabolites, although approximately 25% of the drug was eliminated at the beginning of dialysis (32). In their examination of metronidazole pharmacokinetics in critically ill patients, Plaisance et al. found a prolonged serum half-life of the drug and accumulation of the hydroxy metabolite in three patients with creatinine clearances of <15 ml/min. Patients with obstructive liver disease in this study, however, exhibited the longest half-lives and lowest clearances of metronidazole (33). Hepatic and renal dysfunction are commonly encountered in the elderly patient population. Liver disease may be the more significant abnormality in altered metronidazole metabolism, although the importance of renal elimination cannot be ignored. Pending further studies, it is safe to say that both clinical entities warrant appropriate dosage adjustment to prevent accumulation of potentially toxic metabolites.

Phase I oxidative drug metabolism may be impaired in elderly persons. Impaired clearance of drugs such as antipyrine, quinidine, diazepam, and theophylline has been shown in the aged patient population (34). In spite of the fact that metronidazole undergoes hepatic oxidation, Loft et al. have shown that the elimination of metronidazole is maintained in elderly patients. With the exception of minor alterations in accumulation of the hydroxy metabolite, no age-related differences could be found between elderly patients and young controls (35). Thus, in the absence of hepatic or renal pathology, age itself appears to have very little effect on metronidazole metabolism.

Metronidazole's dependence upon hepatic oxidation may interfere with the metabolism of other drugs such as warfarin, theophylline, and quinidine (5,34,35). Since these are drugs commonly prescribed in the elderly population, rigorous monitoring of serum levels is warranted. The structural similarity of metronidazole with disulfuram accounts for its well-documented antabuse effect when used with alcohol.

VI. CLINICAL INDICATIONS

A. Parasitic Infections

Metronidazole is recognized as an effective agent against many anaerobic protozoa including *T. vaginalis*, *E. histolytica*, *G. lamblia*, and *B. coli*. Trichomonal infections are most frequently encountered in the younger, more sexually active patient population. Intestinal parasite infections are a function of exposure and endemicity and therefore may occur in any age group including the elderly population. Metronidazole is effective in the treatment of symptomatic and asymptomatic intestinal amebiasis and amebic liver abscess, but should be used in conjunction with a luminally active agent such as iodoquinol (5,36). Oral metronidazole is active against intestinal giardiasis and may be better tolerated than quinacrine (5).

B. Anaerobic Infections

Metronidazole is active against most anaerobic bacteria, the notable exceptions being *Actinomyces* and *Proprionibacterium acnes*. Because of reports of clindamycin resistance, it may be the drug of choice for infections caused by *B. fragilis*. Nevertheless, clinical trials of intraabdominal sepsis comparing metronidazole with cefoxitin, clindamycin, and chloramphenicol in combination with an aminoglycoside have failed to show superiority of any regimen (37,38).

Lower respiratory infections are a common clinical problem in older adults. Although anaerobic bacteria often play a significant role in these infections, metronidazole alone may not be adequate therapy (39). The presence of other pathogens such as facultative streptococci and aerobic bacteria warrant the addition of other antimicrobial agents with activity against these organisms. Metronidazole in conjunction with penicillin G, amoxicillin, or erythromycin often provides excellent coverage in these clinical situations.

C. Abscesses

Intraabdominal, pulmonary, and pleuropulmonary abscesses are primary sources of anaerobic bacteremia in elderly patients (40). In these clinical situations, metronidazole may be used as a single agent or in conjunction with other antimicrobials and/or surgical interventions.

Bacteroides spp., *Fusobacterium* spp. and other gram-negative anaerobes are important pathogens in intraabdominal and pelvic abscesses. Most spontaneous and postsurgical abdominal infections, however, are composed of mixed aerobic and anaerobic organisms. In their experimental model of intraabdominal sepsis, Bartlett et al. showed that metronidazole alone cured 80% of polymicrobial infections (41). This may be due in part to metronidazole metabolites, which have antibacterial activity against Enterobacteriaceae (23,28). Nevertheless, because polymicrobial infections are more common in the elderly population and may carry a higher mortality, it is necessary to use metronidazole in conjunction with an aminoglycoside or antimicrobial agent with similar gram-negative activity (41).

Pulmonary and pleuropulmonary abscesses in elderly patients frequently involve odontogenic sources. *Peptococcus*, *Peptostreptococcus* spp., and microaerophilic streptococci are the predominant pathogens, organisms against which metronidazole lacks antimicrobial activity. In spite of this observation, *Fusobacterium nucleatum* and *Bacteroides* species, including *B. fragilis*, have been isolated in up to 15% of anaerobic lung infections and may account for occasional penicillin failures (42,43). This, in addition to the occasional presence of β-lactamase–producing *B. fragilis*, would support the use of metronidazole in conjunction with penicillin G or a cephalosporin in necrotizing pulmonary infections. As a single agent, clindamycin is more effective than metronidazole in pleuropulmonary disease (44).

Although anaerobic bacteria are an uncommon cause of meningitis in elderly patients they frequently account for brain abscesses and cerebritis in this patient population. Odontogenic, otitic, and sinusitic sources are important in geriatric patients and necessitate the use of antibiotics that are active against microaerophilic streptococci as well as anaerobes. Metronidazole penetrates well into cerebrospinal fluid and, when used in conjunction with penicillin G, cephalosporins, or chloramphenicol, provides adequate coverage for most pathogens involved in anaerobic cerebral abscesses. Surgical drainage in addition to adequate antimicrobial coverage is frequently necessary in these patients (45,46).

D. Osteomyelitis

Diabetes mellitus, peripheral vascular disease, osteoarthritis, and the presence of various prosthetic devices may predispose the elderly patient to anaerobic bone infections (40). Metronidazole has been used successfully in the treatment of osteomyelitis due to *B. fragilis*, *C. difficile*, and other anaerobic pathogens (47,48). For odontogenic sites, such as mandibular osteomyelitis, it may be used in conjunction with antibiotics active against facultative streptococci.

E. Other Infections

Metronidazole can be used in a wide variety of other infections afflicting the geriatric patient population, including anaerobic infections of soft tissues, sinuses, and other head and neck regions. Metronidazole has proven to be effective in the occasional case of *B. fragilis* endocarditis and other endovascular infections (49). It has excellent activity against *Clostridium perfringens* and may have an advantage over cefoxitin and clindamycin in treating infections due to other clostridial species. It is as effective as oral vancomycin in the treatment of *C. difficile*–associated pseudomembranous colitis, and it is considerably less expensive than vancomycin (50). Metronidazole is a well-recognized treatment for pelvic and genitourinary infections including vaginosis, urethritis, cystitis, and pelvic abscess. Controversy exists over the role of metronidazole in inflammatory bowel disease. While some studies have shown a decrease in bacterial, inflammatory, and fistular complications in patients treated with the drug, others have found no significant advantage in adjuvant metronidazole therapy (51–53). Topical metronidazole has been used effectively in the treatment of rosacea (54).

F. Surgical Prophylaxis

Antibiotic prophylaxis prior to surgical procedures has significantly decreased postsurgical wound infections. Colorectal, gynecological, and other intraabdominal procedures are common in geriatric patients. Postoperative abdominal wound infections are commonly due to mixed aerobic and anaerobic flora. Metronidazole in conjunction with an agent active against aerobic gram-negative bacteria may decrease the incidence of postoperative infections in elective intraabdominal surgeries (55–57). The use of perioperative metronidazole in elective gynecological surgeries is less conclusive. Vincelette et al. showed no difference in the incidence of postoperative pelvic infections between patients receiving metronidazole and those who received placebo (58).

VII. ROUTES OF ADMINISTRATION

Metronidazole may be administered orally, intravenously, and by rectal suppository. Topical administration can be used for the treatment of rosacea. Standard doses for various

Table 2 Dosages and Administration of Metronidazole for Various Infections

Indication	Route of administration	Dosage
Susceptible anaerobic infections	IV	Loading dose of 15 mg/kg, then 7.5 mg/kg q6h
	PO	1–2 g/day in 2–4 doses q6–12h
Nonspecific vaginitis	PO	500 mg bid for 7 days
Trichomonas vaginitis	PO	250 mg tid for 7 days or 500 mg bid for 5 days or 2 g in single dose
Amebiasis (intestinal or extraintestinal)	IV or PO	750 mg tid for 10 days
Giardiasis	PO	250 mg bid or tid for 5–7 days or 2 g/day for 3 days

Source: In Finegold SM, Mathisen GE. "Metronidazole," Principles and Practice of Infectious Disease, edited by G Mandel, RG Douglas, J Bennett. New York: Churchill Livingston, 1990.

infections are listed in Table 2. The high systemic concentration after oral administration of metronidazole is a particular advantage, allowing for a noninvasive and inexpensive treatment modality. The standard oral regimen for anaerobic infections in adults is 500–750 mg three times daily. Parasitic infections such as *Trichomonas* can often be treated with a single 2-g oral dose. Intestinal giardiasis usually requires at least 3 days of oral therapy.

Rectal suppositories can be used when oral administration is not feasible. This may be a particularly useful modality in nursing home residents or other chronic care patients in whom intravenous or oral therapy is problematic. A 1-g suppository can be inserted every 8 h for 3 days, followed by every 12 h for the duration of therapy.

Serious anaerobic infections usually warrant intravenous therapy initially. The standard regimen is 15 mg/kg loading dose, followed by 7.5 mg/kg every 6 h. Dosage adjustment is probably not warranted in the otherwise healthy elderly patient but should be considered in patients with underlying renal and/or hepatic disease (see Sec. V). The maximum daily dose of metronidazole should not exceed 4 g. A premixed intravenous metronidazole preparation (Flagyl IV RTU) is available, or metronidazole hydrochloride can be reconstituted and diluted with intravenous solution to a concentration not exceeding 8 mg/ml. Metronidazole is not compatible with 10% dextrose or sodium lactate solutions.

VIII. ADVERSE REACTIONS

Metronidazole is a relatively safe and well-tolerated antibiotic. Gastrointestinal effects include an unpleasant metallic taste, furred tongue, stomatitis, and dry mouth. Abdominal pain, nausea, and occasionally vomiting may be encountered, especially in cancer patients receiving high-dose metronidazole as adjunctive chemotherapy. Although a proven therapy for *Clostridium difficile* infections, rare cases of pseudomembranous colitis have been reported with metronidazole use (59).

Neurological side effects of metronidazole are of concern, especially in the aged population where preexisting neuropathies and central nervous system disorders are common. Stocking/glove sensory neuropathies are well described with prolonged or high-dose metronidazole use (60). Dysesthesias usually abate with dose reduction or discontinuation of the drug, though resolution may be slow. Metronidazole should be used cautiously in older patients with serious seizure disorders and other central nervous system diseases.

The mutagenic potential of metronidazole is controversial. Bacterial reduction products of the drug may have mutagenic activity in animals (61,62). Data concerning carcinogenicity in humans are less convincing. Anecdotal reports exist of various solid tumors that developed after prolonged metronidazole use. An increased incidence of colorectal carcinoma has been noted in patients taking metronidazole for Crohn's disease, although it is difficult to separate mutagenicity of drug from that of intrinsic disease (63). The possible teratogenic effects of the drug during pregnancy add further concern for metronidazole's mutagenic potential. Nevertheless, a large study of women receiving metronidazole for vaginal trichomoniasis failed to show an association between malignancy and the drug (64). In elderly persons who already have a high incidence of carcinoma, it may be impossible to assess the direct mutagenicity of metronidazole. Pending further investigations, mutagenic concerns should not be the exclusive reason for withholding the drug when treating serious anaerobic infections in elderly patients.

Reversible neutropenia, maculopapular rash, urticaria, ototoxicity, and gynecomastia are other minor and uncommon adverse reactions associated with metronidazole use. The disulfuram reaction with alcohol has been previously noted.

When one compares the serious and occasionally life-threatening side effects associated with other common antibiotics, metronidazole is remarkably safe. Unlike aminoglycosides and other drugs frequently used in geriatric patients, it does not usually require monitoring of serum levels. Its excellent bioavailability and multiple routes of administration add to metronidazole's clinical versatility. Finally, and perhaps most importantly, its efficacy in treating serious anaerobic infections makes metronidazole a useful antimicrobial agent in the elderly patient population.

REFERENCES

1. Shinn DLS. Metronidazole in acute ulcerative gingivitis. Lancet 1962; 1(7240):1191.
2. Cosar C, Joulou L. Activite de L' (hydroxy-2-ethyl)-1-methyl-2-nitro-5-imidazole (8823 R.P.) vis-à-vis des infections experimentales à Trichomonas vaginalis. Ann Inst Pasteur Microbiol 1959; 96(2):238–41.
3. Muller M, Lindmark DG. Uptake of metronidazole and its effect on viability in trichomonads and *Entamoeba invadens* under anaerobic and aerobic conditions. Antimicrob Agents Chemother 1976; 9:696–700.
4. Muller M. Mode of action of metronidazole on anaerobic bacteria and protozoa. Surgery 1983; 93:165–71.
5. Scully B. Metronidazole. Med Clin North Am 1988; 72:613–21.
6. Ings RMJ, McFadzean JA, Ormerod WE. The mode of action of metronidazole in *Trichomonas vaginalis* and other microorganisms. Biochem Pharmacol 1974; 23:1421–9.
7. Goldman P. Metronidazole. N Engl J Med 1980; 303:1212–18.
8. Edwards DI. The action of metronidazole on DNA. J Antimicrob Chemother 1977; 3:43–8.
9. Plant CW, Edwards DI. The effect of tinidazole, metronidazole and nitrofurazone on nucleic acid synthesis in Clostridium bifermentans. J Antimicrob Chemother 1976; 2:203–9.
10. LaRusso NF, Tomasz F, Muller M, et al. In vitro interaction of metronidazole with nucleic acids. Mol Pharmacol 1977; 13:872–82.
11. Muller M, Meingassner JG, Miller WA, et al. Three metronidazole resistant strains of *Trichomonas vaginalis* from the United States. Am J Obstet Gynecol 1980; 138:808–12.

12. Jokipii L, Jokipii AMM. In vitro susceptibility of Giardia lamblia trophozoites to metronidazole and tinidazole. J Infect Dis 1980; 141:317–25.
13. Borecham PFL, Phillips RE, Sheperd RW. Heterogeneity in the response of clones of *Giardia intestinalis* to anti-giardial drugs. Trans R Soc Trop Med Hyg 1987; 81:406–7.
14. McIntyre P, Boreham PFL, Phillips RE, et al. Chemotherapy in giardiasis: clinical responses and in vitro drug sensitivity of human isolates in axenic culture. J Pediatr 1986; 108:1005–10.
15. Tally FP, Cuchural GJ, Jacobus NV, et al. Nationwide study of the susceptibility of the *Bacteroides fragilis* group in the United States. Antimicrob Agents Chemother 1985; 28:675–7.
16. Gabay EL, Sutter VL, Finegold SM. Rapid β-lactamase testing in bacteroides. J Antimicrob Chemother 1981; 8:413–66.
17. Britz ML, Wilkinson RG. Isolation and properties of metronidazole resistant mutants of *Bacteroides fragilis*. Antimicrob Agents Chemother 1979; 16:19–27.
18. Appelbaum PC, Chatterton SA. Susceptibility of anaerobic bacteria to ten antimicrobial agents. Antimicrob Agents Chemother 1978; 14(3):371–6.
19. Brazier JS, Levett PN, Stannard AJ. Antibiotic susceptibility of clinical isolates of *Clostridia*. J Antimicrob Chemother 1985; 15(2):181–5.
20. Goldstein EJC, Sutter VL, Finegold SM: Comparative susceptibilities of anaerobic bacteria to metronidazole, ornidazole and SC-28538. Antimicrob Agents Chemother 1978; 14:609–13.
21. Chrystal EJT, Koch RL, McLafferty MA, et al. Relationship between metronidazole metabolism and bactericidal activity. Antimicrob Agents Chemother 1980; 18:566–73.
22. Ingham HR, Hall CJ, Sisson PR, et al. The activity of metronidazole against facultatively anaerobic bacteria. J Antimicrob Chemother 1980; 6:343–7.
23. Onderdonk AB, Louie TJ, Tally FP, et al. Activity of metronidazole against *Escherichia coli* in experimental intra-abdominal sepsis. J Antimicrob Chemother 1979; 5:201–10.
24. Bergan T, Leinbo O, Blom-Hagen T, et al. Pharmacokinetics and bioavailability of metronidazole after tablets, suppositories and intravenous administration. Scand J Gastroenterol 1984; 91(suppl):45–60.
25. Bergan T, Bjerke PEM, Fansa O. Pharmacokinetics of metronidazole in patients with enteric disease compared to normal volunteers. Chemotherapy 1981; 27:233–8.
26. Melander A, Kahlmeter G, Kamme C, et al. Bioavailability of metronidazole in fasting and nonfasting healthy subjects and in patients with Crohn's disease. Eur J Clin Pharmacol 1977; 12:69–72.
27. Thiercelin JF, Diquet B, Levesque C, et al. Metronidazole kinetics and bioavailability in patients undergoing gastrointestinal surgery. Clin Pharmacol Ther 1984; 35:510–19.
28. Rosenblatt JE, Edson R. Metronidazole. Mayo Clin Proc 1983; 58:154–7.
29. Ljungberg B, Nilsson-Ehle I, Ursing B. Metronidazole: pharmacokinetic observations in severely ill patients. J Antimicrob Chemother 1984; 14:275–83.
30. Lau AH, Evans R, Chang CW, et al. Pharmacokinetics of metronidazole in patients with alcoholic liver disease. Antimicrob Agents Chemother 1987; 31:1662–4.
31. Farrell G, Lambert JB, Cvejic M, et al. Disposition and metabolism of metronidazole in patients with liver failure. Hepatology 1984; 4:722–6.
32. Roux AF, Moirot E, Delhotol B, et al: Metronidazole kinetics in patients with acute renal failure on dialysis: a cumulative study. Clin Pharmacol Ther 1984; 36:363–8.
33. Plaisance KI, Quintiliani R, Nightingale CH. The pharmacokinetics of metronidazole and its metabolites in critically ill patients. J Antimicrob Chemother 1988; 21:195–200.
34. Greenblatt DJ, Sellers EM, Shader RI. Drug disposition in old age. N Engl J Med 1982; 306:1081–7.
35. Loft S, Egsmose C, Sonne J, et al. Metronidazole elimination is preserved in the elderly. Human Exp Toxicol 1990; 9(3):155–9.
36. Peterson PO, Bengtsson E. A long term following up study of amoebiasis treated with metronidazole. Scand J Infect Dis 1984; 16:195–8.

37. Bartlett JG. Recent developments in the management of anaerobic infections. Rev Infect Dis 1983; 5:235–45.
38. Tally FP, Sullivan CE. Metronidazole: in vitro activity, pharmacology and efficacy in anaerobic bacterial infections. Pharmacotherapy 1981; 1:28.
39. Sanders CV, Hanna BJ, Lewis AC, et al. The use of metronidazole in the treatment of anaerobic pleuropulmonary infections. In: Phillips I, Collier J, eds. Metronidazole Conference, Proc Symp, Tarpon Springs, Florida, February 1982. New York: Biomedical Information Corp, 1982:371.
40. Terpenning MS. Anaerobic bacteremia in the elderly. Gerontology 1989; 35:130–6.
41. Bartlett JG, Louie TS, Gorbach SL, et al. Therapeutic efficacy of 29 antimicrobial regimens in experimental intra-abdominal sepsis. Rev Infect Dis 1981; 3:535–42.
42. Bartlett JG, Gorbach SL, Tally FP, et al. Bacteriology and treatment of primary lung abscess. Am Rev Resp Dis 1974; 109:510–18.
43. Panwalker AP. Failure of penicillin in anaerobic necrotizing pneumonia. Chest 1982; 82:500–1.
44. Collier J, Colhoun EM, Hill PL. A multicenter comparison of clindamycin and metronidazole in the treatment of anaerobic infections. Scand J Infect Dis 1981; 26(suppl):96–100.
45. DeLouvois J, Gortrai P, Henley R. Antibiotic treatment of abscess of the central nervous system. Br Med J 1977; 2:985–7.
46. Mathisen GE, Meyer RD, George WL, et al. Brain abscess and cerebritis. Rev Infect Dis 1984; 6(suppl):101–6.
47. Templeton WC III, Wawrukiewicz A, Melo JC, et al. Anaerobic osteomyelitis of long bones. Rev Infect Dis 1983; 5:692–712.
48. Riley TV, Karthigasu KT. Chronic osteomyelitis due to *Clostridium difficile*. Br Med J 1982; 284:1217.
49. Galgiani JN, Busch DF, Brass C, et al. *Bacteroides fragilis* endocarditis, bacteremia and other infections treated with oral or intravenous metronidazole. Am J Med 1978; 65:284–9.
50. Teasley DG, Olson MM, Gebbard RL, et al. Prospective randomized trial of metronidazole versus vancomycin for *Clostridium difficile*-associated diarrhoea and colitis. Lancet 1983; 2(8358):1043–6.
51. Keighley MRB. Infection and the use of antibiotics in Crohn's disease. Can J Surg 1984; 27:438–41.
52. Jakobovitis J, Schuster M. Metronidazole therapy for Crohn's disease and associated fistulae. Am J Gastroenterol 1984; 79:533–40.
53. Chapman RW, Selby WS, Jewell DP. Controlled trial of intravenous metronidazole as an adjunct to corticosteroids in severe ulcerative colitis. Gut 1986; 27:1210–12.
54. Aronsen IK, Rumsfield JA, West DP, et al. Evaluation of topical metronidazole gel in acne rosacea. Drug Intell Clin Pharm 1987; 21:346–51.
55. Beggs FD, Jobanputra RS, Holmes JT. A comparison of intravenous and oral metronidazole as prophylaxis in colorectal surgery. Br J Surg 1982; 69:226–7.
56. Hinckey EJ, Richards GK, Prentiss J. Metronidazole as a prophylactic agent in wound infections after colon surgery. Surgery 1983; 93:204–8.
57. Bell CA, Smith JA, Murphy J. Prophylactic antibiotics in elective colorectal surgery. Surgery 1983; 93:204–8.
58. Vincelette I, Finkelstein F, Aoki FY, et al. Double-blind trial of perioperative intravenous metronidazole prophylaxis for abdominal and vaginal hysterectomy. Surgery 1983; 93:185–9.
59. Saginur R, Hawley CR, Bartlett JG. Colitis associated with metronidazole therapy. J Infect Dis 1980; 141:772–4.
60. Stahlberg D, Barany F, Einarsson K, et al. Neurophysiologic studies of patients with Crohn's disease on long term treatment with metronidazole. Scand J Gastroenterol 1991; 26:219–24.
61. Rust JR. An assessment of metronidazole tumorigenicity studies in mouse and rats. In: Finegold SM, McGadzean JA, Roe FJC, eds. Metronidazole—Proceedings of the International Metronidazole Conference, Montreal, Quebec, Canada, 1977:138–44.

62. Cohen SM, Enturk E, Von Esch AM, et al. Carcinogenicity of 5-nitrofurins, 5-nitroimidazoles, 4-nitrobenzenes and related compounds. J Natl Cancer Inst 1973; 51:403–17.
63. Krause JR, Ayunyang HQ, Ellis LD. Occurrence of three cases of carcinoma in individuals with Crohn's disease treated with metronidazole. Am J Gastroenterol 1985; 80:978–82.
64. Beard CM, Noller KL, O'Fallan WM, et al. Cancer after exposure to metronidazole. Mayo Clin Proc 1988; 63:147–53.
65. Muller M. Mode of action of metronidazole on anaerobic organisms. In: Finegold SM, George WL, Rolfe RD, eds. Proceedings First United States Metronidazole Conference, Tarpon Springs, FL. New York: Biomedical Information Corp., 1982:67.
66. Sutter VL. In vitro susceptibility of anaerobic and microaerophilic bacteria to metronidazole and its hydroxy metabolite. In: Finegold SM George WL, Rolfe RD, eds. Proceedings First United States Metronidazole Conference, Tarpon Springs, FL. New York: Biomedical Information Corp., 1982:61–6.

20

Chloramphenicol

Haragopal Thadepalli
UCLA School of Medicine, Charles R. Drew University of Medicine and Science, and King/Drew Medical Center, Los Angeles, California

Daniel Hancz
Los Angeles County–USC Medical Center, Los Angeles, California

I. CHEMISTRY

Chloramphenicol contains organically bound chlorine and a nitro group, not usually found in compounds occurring in nature. It was originally observed in 1947 by Burkholder in a soil organism found in Caracas, Venezuela, and later named *Streptomyces venezuelae* (1). Chloramphenicol was the first naturally occurring antibiotic that was later chemically synthesized. Of several structurally similar compounds, the D(−)Threo isomer (not D + Threo isomer) was found to be microbiologically active. The reduction of the nitro group to an amino group rendered the chloramphenicol molecule microbiologically inactive, the basic mechanism of chloramphenicol resistance.

II. MECHANISM OF ACTION

Chloramphenicol inhibits microbial growth by binding to the 50S subunit of the 70S ribosome of the organism, which interferes with the attachment of aminoacetyl transfer RNA to the ribosome. Thus, peptide bond formation is prevented (1a,3).

III. ANTIMICROBIAL SPECTRUM

Chloramphenicol is the first of the broad-spectrum antibiotics with therapeutic efficacy against both aerobic and anaerobic gram-positive and gram-negative bacteria and *Rickettsia* (1). Although chloramphenicol has "broad-spectrum" activity, it has a limited number of in vivo indications because of known in vitro and in vivo discrepancies. Chloramphenicol is still the drug of choice for *Salmonella*, *Shigella*, *Campylobacter*, *Escherichia coli*, *Yersinia*, and *Vibrio cholerae* infections in some parts of the world. It is now being replaced largely by quinolones for these indications in adults and elderly persons but not in children. Chloramphenicol is ineffective against *Pseudomonas*, *Citrobacter*, *Providencia*,

Acinetobacter, and certain types of *Klebsiella* and fungi. For rickettsial and chlamydial infections, either tetracyclines or chloramphenicol and more recently the azalide group of antibiotics are being used.

Anaerobic bacteria that are susceptible to chloramphenicol in vitro may in fact be resistant in vivo. Chloramphenicol failed to combat experimentally created *Clostridium welchii* infection in guinea pigs when therapy was delayed for 4 h after the initiation of infection (2,3). The growth of clostridia such as *C. difficile* and *C. acetobutylicum*, although susceptible to chloramphenicol by plate-assay at 0.6 μg/ml, was uninhibited when the antibiotic was added to the actively growing culture, even at a concentration of 100 μg/ml. Furthermore, even killed extracts of these bacteria reduced the nitro group in chloramphenicol ring via a ferredoxin-dependent enzyme reaction with pyruvates serving as electron donors (4). Indeed, clostridia can inactivate other nitro compounds such as metronidazole by a similar mechanism (5). Chloramphenicol can be inactivated by other anaerobes such as *Eubacterium*, *Peptococcus*, *Fusobacterium*, and *Bacteroides* in broth cultures (6). However, another study of more than 300 clinical isolates of *Bacteroides* belonging to different species showed not even a single isolate that was resistant to chloramphenicol by disc diffusion method (7). In fact, none of the 3076 strains of *B. fragilis* group tested in the United States between 1981 and 1985 were resistant to either chloramphenicol or metronidazole (8). Yet, patients with severe anaerobic infections have failed on large doses of intravenous chloramphenicol therapy (9).

In vitro, chloramphenicol is also effective against mycoplasmas and *Ureaplasma* (minimal inhibitory concentration [MIC] = <1.0 μg/ml) as well as *Chlamydia trachomatis* (MIC = <10 μg/ml) and *Rickettsia prowazeki* (MIC = <1.0 μg/ml); however, macrolides, azalides, and doxycycline are the preferred drugs today for these infections in the United States (10). In vitro, chloramphenicol is very active against pneumococci and even mycobacteria but is not the drug of choice for these infections.

IV. CLINICAL PHARMACOLOGY

A. Pharmacokinetics

The bioavailability of chloramphenicol is quite variable depending on its preparation; it is available in three forms:

1. Chloramphenicol base, a bitter-tasting powder in a capsule. This salt is active and has better bioavailability than the intravenous form.
2. Chloramphenicol palmitate suspension, an inactive prodrug hydrolyzed in the intestine to active chloramphenicol (11).
3. Chloramphenicol sodium succinate, a parenteral prodrug which is hydrolyzed by the liver to active chloramphenicol (12).

The peak serum concentrations of chloramphenicol given by mouth and by the intravenous route are similar, although it takes longer to reach peak levels by peroral route. An average peak level of 11.2 μg/ml is achieved in 1 h after a 1-g dose of peroral chloramphenicol. However, when the same dose is given intravenously, a peak serum level of 11 μg/ml is achieved within 30 min (13).

Data from the intramuscular route are mixed; some studies indicate incomplete absorption, while others show peak therapeutic levels. Despite this, the studies are convincing that the IM route is as efficacious as IV therapy (14,15).

The efficacy and toxicity (Type I, reversible) of chloramphenicol correlates with its serum levels, and the drug has a narrow therapeutic index. Therapeutic peak and trough levels range from 10 to 20 μg/ml and 5 to 10 μg/ml, respectively.

1. *Absorption*

When the palmitate ester form of chloramphenicol is given perorally, it is hydrolyzed in the duodenum by pancreatic lipase and only about 75–90% of it is absorbed (16). However, chloramphenicol base, when given by mouth, shows complete absorption that is similar to the intravenous route (17). Peroral absorption of chloramphenicol among elderly and malnourished patients can be quite erratic, and this can be due to increased pH, delayed gastric emptying, slow intestinal transit, or a decreased level of serum albumin. Regardless, peroral chloramphenicol should be avoided in elderly as well as in malnourished patients. If chloramphenicol is required, it should be given intravenously.

2. *Distribution*

Chloramphenicol is well distributed in all body sites, with the highest concentrations being in the liver and kidney; the lowest concentrations are in the brain and the cerebrospinal fluid (CSF) (18). Chloramphenicol levels in the CSF are not significantly modified by the presence or absence of meningeal swelling. In fact, concentrations of chloramphenicol in the CSF may reach 70–80% of plasma levels, thus making it an extremely useful drug in the treatment of bacterial meningitis (18).

About 60–80% of chloramphenicol is protein bound, which can affect the drug's distribution. It is the unbound chloramphenicol that exerts a pharmacological effect. Changes in protein binding may have an adverse effect in elderly or malnourished patients when the serum albumin is low. This may be intensified when they are receiving other concomitant medications. The elderly patient with low serum albumin levels will have less protein-bound drug, and therefore an increased pharmacological effect of chloramphenicol can be expected. The volume of distribution of chloramphenicol is about 40 L, and it is distributed well in fatty tissue. This volume of distribution may be increased in elderly persons since there is less muscle mass and an increase in connective tissue and fat with aging (16).

3. *Metabolism*

About 90% of chloramphenicol is metabolized by glucuronidation to an inactive monoglucuronide, which is excreted in the urine (18a). Chloramphenicol interacts with many drugs that are cleared by the liver (18b). Chloramphenicol is an enzyme inhibitor of tolbutamide, chlorpropamide, phenytoin, and warfarin, and, therefore, increased levels of these drugs are expected with concomitant administration (19–21). Coadministration of chlorpropamide with chloramphenicol increases the half-life of chlorpropamide from 30–36 h to as long as 40–146 h; thus, simultaneous administration of these two drugs could produce unwanted hypoglycemia (20). Similarly, chloramphenicol was shown to retard biotransformation of tolbutamide (19). This observation is of relevance when treating elderly patients with diabetes mellitus and foot infections, which are usually caused by anaerobic and aerobic bacteria (see Chap. 27). In these patients chloramphenicol may be coadministered with oral antidiabetic drugs. Phenobarbital, phenytoin, and rifampin have been shown to be enzyme inducers, thus decreasing the levels of chloramphenicol (21).

Liver disease can affect the metabolism of chloramphenicol, and consequently higher serum levels can be expected under these circumstances. Certain physiological changes that occur in the liver with aging, such as decreased blood flow and decrease in the total liver mass, may result in higher serum levels of chloramphenicol. Patients with liver function test abnormalities (e.g., increased bilirubin levels) need dose modification of chloramphenicol, but no specific guidelines exist for this purpose. It seems prudent to monitor liver function tests and serum antibiotic levels among elderly patients receiving chloramphenicol therapy (18b).

4. Excretion

Approximately 5–15% of chloramphenicol is excreted unchanged in the urine, and about 85% of the drug is excreted as an inactive glucuronide metabolite (16,18a).

The renal clearance of chloramphenicol decreases in patients with compromised renal function as measured by creatinine clearance. High serum levels of chloramphenicol (primarily its metabolites) are found in patients with impaired renal function. Although renal function declines with aging, dose adjustment is not routinely recommended because the metabolites of chloramphenicol (which increase in serum with renal failure) are considered to be nontoxic (22).

B. Renal Failure

The average serum half-life of chloramphenicol is 2.7 h, and thus a dosage interval of 6 h in healthy adults is recommended. In patients with anuria the half-life increases to 3.2–4.3 h and the half-life of chloramphenicol metabolites increases to a much greater extent. Fortunately, its metabolites do not appear to be as toxic. (22).

V. CLINICAL INDICATIONS

A. Experimental Animal Models

Although chloramphenicol therapy has shown good results in salmonella infections in mice and leptospira infections produced in hamsters, typhus fever in mice, and plague model created in monkeys (1), usage of this antibiotic to treat these infections is limited.

In an experimental model of intraabdominal abscess, which was produced by inoculating a combination of *B. fragilis* and *E. coli*, chloramphenicol cured 41% of the animals compared to 94% achieved by clindamycin, despite the excellent in vitro efficacy of chloramphenicol against these organisms (MIC = 1.0 μg/ml) (23). In an anaerobic lung abscess model in rabbits created by transtracheal inoculation of a mixture of anaerobes, i.e., *B. fragilis, Peptococcus morbillorum, Eubacterium lentum*, and *Fusobacterium nucleatum*, chloramphenicol therapy failed to eliminate the lung abscess. Presumably this failure was due to *B. fragilis* producing acetyl transferase, which destroyed chloramphenicol (24,25). Paradoxically, in the lung abscess model, the concentration of chloramphenicol was 12 μg/g of lung tissue at 1 hour and 6 μg/g at 4 h, after three injections of chloramphenicol given 75 mg twice daily. Although the pus in the lung abscess was sterile, in most animals purulent inflammation persisted presumably due to suppression of host factors, i.e., T-cell formation suppressed by either *B. fragilis* or chloramphenicol or both (26).

B. Current Clinical Indications

Woodward and Wisseman, in their treatise on Chloromycetin® (chloramphenicol) published in 1958, 10 years after the release of this antibiotic, made the following observation, which continues to be true 34 years later (1):

> chloramphenicol is effective in the treatment of typhoid fever but (1) relapses occur (2) *S. typhi* may persist in feces and biliary tract (3) carrier state in typhoid is not cured and (4) intestinal hemorrhage and perforation continues to occur—although this antibiotic fails to eradicate *S. typhosa* from the host promptly, chloramphenicol therapy quickly brings down fever, abdominal symptoms and other signs of toxicity within 3 to 5 days. Bacteremia may persist in some cases. Chloramphenicol therapy does not free the urinary tract of *S. typhosa*.

During earlier days, the relapse rate of typhoid fever was between 20 and 30% and chloramphenicol therapy had not decreased the intestinal perforation rate of 3–5% that occurred before the chloramphenicol era (27). Without question, chloramphenicol decreased the then high typhoid fever mortality of 13% to 1% to date. Chloramphenicol is also very effective against paratyphoid fever caused by *S. paratyphi* type A and B as well as salmonellosis caused by other species of *Salmonella*. It is also very effective against shigellosis, including *Shigella dysenteriae* infection.

Chloramphenicol is as effective as penicillin and tetracycline in the treatment of pneumococcal pneumonia, and the mortality was 5% with either drug (28). Pneumococcal pneumonia in penicillin-allergic patients may be treated with the first- or second-generation cephalosporins provided they do not have an allergic reaction that includes urticaria, angioedema, anaphylaxis, or hypotension. With such severe allergic reactions, chloramphenicol could be considered an alternative choice for pneumococcal pneumonia. However, most clinicians prefer erythromycin, clindamycin, trimethoprim-sulfamethoxazole, or vancomycin under these circumstances.

Chloramphenicol and congeners of tetracycline such as doxycycline remain the drugs of choice for the treatment of rickettsial infections, i.e., Q fever, Rocky Mountain spotted fever, and other typhus infections. Prompt clinical response is expected with chloramphenicol therapy of these infections, and a 10-day course almost always ensures cure (29).

Until recently, chloramphenicol has been a time-honored therapeutic choice for intraabdominal sepsis due to the mixed anaerobic-aerobic flora (see Chap. 26). Chloramphenicol made a profound impact in the treatment of intraabdominal sepsis and stayed in usage for about four decades. Chloramphenicol prophylaxis was effective in preventing sepsis following intestinal surgery in cases of abdominal trauma (30). However, therapeutic failure with chloramphenicol seems to be common when it is given in combination with other antibiotics. Nethertheless, no other antibiotic has been proven to be superior to chloramphenicol when it is the sole antibiotic used for treating intraabdominal sepsis. Chloramphenicol alone was shown to be as effective as clindamycin and gentamicin in the treatment of anaerobic infections (31). In another study of 175 patients with anaerobic intraabdominal infections treated with either chloramphenicol alone or clindamycin plus gentamicin combination, chloramphenicol alone was as effective as the combination (32). Even today, chloramphenicol is used as an alternative antibiotic in patients that fail on clindamycin or metronidazole therapy.

Intravenous chloramphenicol has long been the drug of choice for meningitis in adults when identification of the etiological agent is pending. Chloramphenicol quickly achieves cerebrospinal fluid concentrations high enough to kill *Streptococcus pneumoniae*, *Haemophilus influenzae*, *Neisseria meningitidis*, and facultative and aerobic gram-negative bacilli. These organisms together constitute nearly 80% of the causes of bacterial meningitis. Among those patients 65 years and older, *S. pneumoniae*, *Listeria monocytogenes*, and enteric gram-negative bacilli are important meningo-pathogens. Third-generation cephalosporins have replaced the usage of chloramphenicol in the empiric treatment of meningitis of elderly patients. This is not because chloramphenicol is ineffective against these bacteria

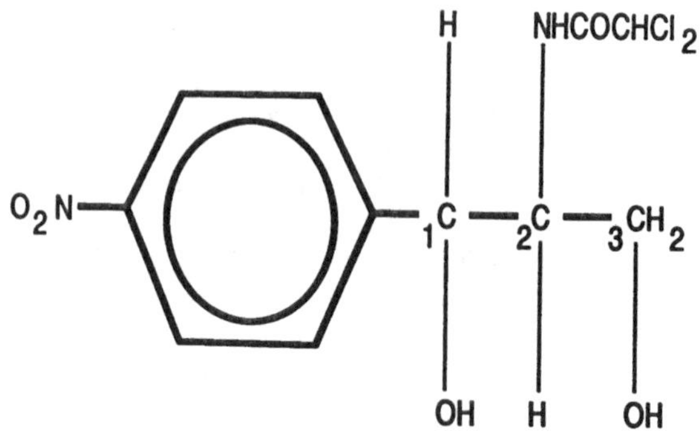

Figure 1 Structure of chloramphenicol.

but because of the highly dreaded but rare toxicity of aplastic anemia. The third-generation cephalosporins have not been shown to be superior to chloramphenicol for empiric therapy of meningitis. Furthermore, chloramphenicol is more active than any of the third-generation cephalosporins against pneumococcus, which is the leading cause of bacterial meningitis among elderly patients. In countries that cannot afford the cost of third-generation cephalosporins, intravenous chloramphenicol remains the drug of choice for the treatment of meningitis.

Chloramphenicol and/or metronidazole are the recommended regimens for treatment of brain abscess where aerobic/anaerobic bacterial synergism is involved (33). Chloramphenicol levels in brain abscess vary from 0 to 90% (34,35). Surgical drainage and antibiotic therapy have improved the outcome of this disease; without surgery deaths can occur despite high concentrations of chloramphenicol in the brain abscess.

The usage of chloramphenicol is declining. In 1978, 0.4% of patients admitted to general medical wards and 5.5% admitted to general surgery received this antibiotic (36). In 1980, only 1.2% of hospitalized patients were prescribed chloramphenicol, 98% of which was given intravenously. Chloramphenicol was considered inappropriate in 92% of these patients because equally efficacious alternate therapies were available (37).

C. Causes of Therapeutic Failures

The nitro group of chloramphenicol (see Fig. 1) is the active part of the drug that can be reduced to an amino group by cell-free extracts of *Streptococcus hemolyticus* and *Pseudomonas aeruginosa* by enzymatic action (38,39). Chromosomally mediated acetylation of chloramphenicol, a transferable R factor, was found in *E. coli* and *Staphylococcus aureus*. They were susceptible to chloramphenicol, but grew in the presence of this antibiotic. The organisms showed an initial lag phase of growth while the antibiotic in the medium was being inactivated followed by an uninhibited logarithmic growth phase (40). This acetyl transferase enzyme is also produced by *Streptococcus (Enterococcus) faecalis*, but the products inactivated by this organism revert to active chloramphenicol (see Fig. 2) (41). It is also important to note that chloramphenicol and tetracycline-resistant pneumococci have been reported (28,42).

Chloramphenicol-resistant *Salmonella* species are a constant threat in countries where typhoid is prevalent and chloramphenicol is used indiscriminately. These two factors favor

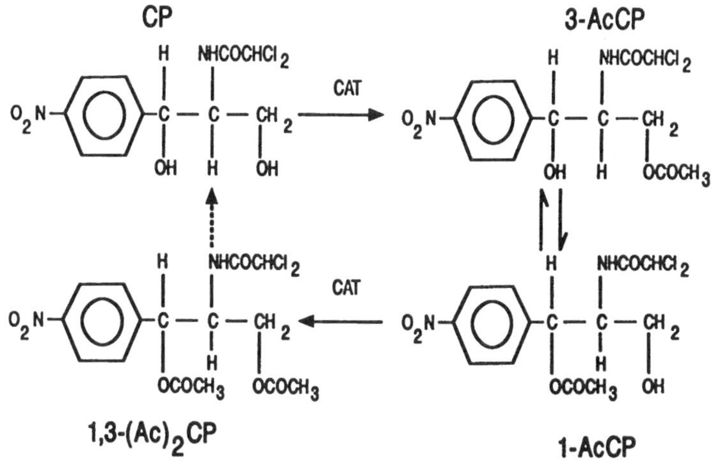

Figure 2 Proposed formula of inactivation of chloramphenicol.

transfer of the R factors to other Enterobacteriaceae bacteria. Chloramphenicol-resistant *S. typhi*, *S. newport*, and other species of *Salmonella* imported from Mexico have caused havoc in the state of California (43,44). One such strain, *S. typhi* in Los Angeles, had the R factor mediated through degraded Vi antigen, which is similar to the chloramphenicol-resistant *Shigella dysenteriae*-1 that caused an epidemic in Central America (45). Indiscriminate use of antibiotics, including chloramphenicol, used in animal feeds is one of the causes of antimicrobial-resistant salmonellae in humans.

Haemophilus influenzae, a common cause of acute exacerbations of pulmonary symptoms among elderly patients with chronic obstructive pulmonary disease, can develop multidrug resistance to, for example, ampicillin, chloramphenicol, tetracycline, and even rifampin. This resistance is transferable from one strain to the other (46). Therefore, it should not be assumed that ampicillin-resistant strains of *H. influenzae* can be automatically treated with tetracycline, chloramphenicol, or rifampin. This resistance is usually mediated by a conjugative plasmid, but some strains of *H. influenzae* acquire resistance by developing permeability barriers due to the loss of the bacterial cell wall protein (47). Chloramphenicol resistance among *Bacteroides* is transferable from one species to the other, e.g., from *B. uniformis* to *B. fragilis* (48).

D. Therapeutic Drug Interactions

The current trend to treat meningitis with ampicillin and chloramphenicol combination can be questioned. Chloramphenicol alone is as effective as this combination (49,50). Addition of ampicillin to chloramphenicol is either antagonistic or indifferent but not synergistic (51). Furthermore, chloramphenicol alone was shown to be preferable over ampicillin or any other antibiotic for empiric therapy of bacterial meningitis in children and young adults (52).

Elderly patients with suspected bacterial meningitis are best treated with a third-generation cephalosporin plus penicillin. Chloramphenicol may be used as an alternative agent, but chloramphenicol should not be added to the third-generation cephalosporin or a penicillin. Chloramphenicol is antagonistic to third-generation cephalosporins such as cefotaxime, moxalactam, ceftriaxone, and cefoperazone when used against *Klebsiella pneumoniae* and other gram-negative bacilli(53). The antagonism of ceftazidime to chloramphenicol in the treatment of gram-negative meningitis is known (54). Addition of clindamycin or erythromycin to chloramphenicol is not recommended because these antibiotics act by competitive inhibition of the 50S ribosomal subunit in the bacteria and therefore exert antagonism (3).

Co-administration of rifampin lowers chloramphenicol serum levels by increasing the metabolic clearance of chloramphenicol in the liver (55). Among antiepileptic drugs, phenobarbital will lower chloramphenicol levels by a similar mechanism, whereas phenytoin increases chloramphenicol serum levels. Therefore, older patients receiving chloramphenicol and anticonvulsant therapy may require monitoring of chloramphenicol serum levels (56).

VI. ADVERSE EFFECTS

A. Toxicity

Chloramphenicol is the leading cause of drug-induced aplastic anaemia in humans. The first case was reported in 1949, a year after chloramphenicol was released (57). Of 607 cases of aplastic anemia reviewed in 1954, 279 had a history of drug exposure and 92 received chloramphenicol (58). Based on chloramphenicol sales during 1958 and 1959, the incidence of aplastic anemia in the United States was estimated to be from 1:156,000 to 1:227,000 prescriptions. This was an underestimate, because the death rate due to aplastic anemia in California between 1963 to 1964 was 1:20,000 to 1:30,000 prescriptions written for chloramphenicol (59).

Aging plays a detrimental role in chloramphenicol toxicity. One per million below the age of 50, 1:500,000 above the age of 50, and 1:52,000 above the age of 80 died with aplastic anemia related to chloramphenicol. Chloramphenicol toxicity, therefore, is 10–20 times higher among elderly persons. Indeed, 7 of every 10 cases of aplastic anemia associated with chloramphenicol in the state of California occurred among those 58 years of age and above. The precise percentage of users of chloramphenicol among African American elderly patients in California was not studied, but there was a higher clustering of chloramphenicol-associated deaths among African Americans than among white Americans (56:4), and it was higher among females (36:24). About 75% of all chloramphenicol manufactured today is consumed in third world countries, where it is sold without prescription and, in some places, without the warning about aplastic anemia. The precise incidence of this complication in these countries is not known (60). In Hong Kong, where the per capita sale of chloramphenicol is estimated to be several hundred–fold higher than the United Kingdom, aplastic anemia deaths due to any cause were only 40 per 100,000 compared to 100 per 100,000 in the United Kingdom (61). The cause for this discrepancy is not known.

Chloramphenicol can produce two types of bone marrow toxicity: Type I normocellular and Type II hypoplastic/or aplastic. Type I manifests as anemia without leukopenia or thrombocytopenia, whereas Type II exhibits pancytopenia. There is no dose relationship to Type II, whereas Type I is dose related, usually large doses given within a short period. Type I toxicity occurs while on therapy, whereas Type II can occur long after completion of therapy—2 weeks to 5 months after therapy is discontinued. Anemia and pallor typify Type I; Type II can herald with purpura or hemorrhage. Recovery is the rule with Type

I, but Type II is often associated with death. Paradoxically, Type II toxicity almost always occurs with peroral chloramphenicol, but it is extremely rare with intravenous chloramphenicol (62,63).

Human volunteers on chloramphenicol developed reversible anemia associated with depressed erythropoiesis (Type I defects), elevated plasma iron levels, and abnormally high saturation of plasma iron binding globulin associated with failure of iron uptake by erythrocytes for 8 days or more. Such erythropoietic defects induced by chloramphenicol are not to be construed as a warning of impending aplastic anemia. Marrow aplasia has been reported with such paltry doses such as topical application of chloramphenicol eye ointment (64). Chloramphenicol toxicity may be related to its effect on human DNA, as it is known to damage bacterial DNA. Nitro bond-containing drugs such as chloramphenicol and metronidazole are associated with mutagenicity and carcinogenicity in animals. It was shown that chloramphenicol at therapeutically achievable levels damages DNA as a result of reduction of the nitro group that occurs in mammalian cells (65,66). Chloramphenicol inhibits cytochrome P-450, protein synthesis, and mitochrondria in eukaryotes, and it has profound teratogenic effect on several sea urchins, zebrafish, and such. Weighing all the available data, however, chloramphenicol per se does not present an unacceptably high genetic or genotoxic risk (66).

B. Drug Monitoring

Type I effects of chloramphenicol are dose related and common when the serum level exceeds 25 μg/ml, which is considered to be the maximum desirable and safe level. Therapeutic levels of chloramphenicol are between 10 and 20 μg/ml in the serum. We strongly feel that all patients with severe hepatic or renal impairment and all elderly patients require monitoring of serum chloramphenicol levels. Modifying the dose or time interval to achieve serum levels no less than 5–10 μg/ml (trough levels) and no more than 25 μg/ml has been shown to be efficacious. However, not all clinicians recommend routine serum chloramphenicol levels in these patients.

REFERENCES

1. Woodward TE, Wisseman CL, eds. Chloromycetin: antibiotic monographs No. 8. New York: Med Encyclopedia Inc., 1958.

1a. Shalit I, Marks MI. Chloramphenicol in the 1980s. Drugs 1984; 28:281–91.

2. Altemeir WA, McMurrin JA, Alt LP. Chloromycetin and areomycin in experimental gas gangrene. Surgery 1950; 28:621–31.

3. Vasquez D. Binding of chloramphenicol to ribosomes: the effect of a number of antibiotics. Biochem Biophys Acta 1965; 114:277–9.

4. O'Brien RW, Morris JG. The ferredoxin-dependent reduction of chloramphenicol by *Clostridium acetobutylicum*. J Gen Microbiol 1971; 67:265–71.

5. O'Brien RW, Morris JG. Reduction of aryl and heterocyclic nitro compounds by clostridia. Proc Aust Biochem Soc 1972; 5:24–7.

6. Kanazawa Y, Kuramata T, Miyanura S. Inactivation of chemotherapeutic agents by anaerobes. Progress in antimicrobial and anticancer chemotherapy. Proceedings of VI Int'l Congress Chemotherapy. Tokyo: University of Tokyo Press, 1975:388–93.

7. Bach VT, Thadepalli H. Susceptibility of anaerobic bacteria, in vitro to 23 antimicrobial agents. Chemotherapy 1980; 26:344–53.

8. Cuchural GJ Jr, Tally FP, Jacobus NV, et al. Susceptibility of the *Bacteroides fragilis* group in the United States: analysis by site of isolation. Antimicrob Agents Chemother 1988; 32:717–22.

9. Thadepalli H, Gorbach SL, Bartlett JG. Apparent failure of chloramphenicol in the treatment of anaerobic infections. Curr Ther Res 1977; 22:421–6.
10. Jones RB. Antimicrobial susceptibility testing for some atypical microorganisms: mycoplasma, chlamydiae and rickettsia. In: Lorian V, ed. Antibiotics in laboratory medicine, 2nd ed. Baltimore: Williams and Wilkins; 1986:246–50.
11. Glazko AS, Dill WA, Kazenko A, et al. Physical factors affecting the rate of absorption in chloramphenicol esters. Antibiot Chemother 1958; 8:516–27.
12. Kauffman RE, Thirumoorthi MC, Buckley JA. Relative bioavailability of chloramphenicol succinate and chloramphenicol palmitate. J Pediatr 1981; 99:963–7.
13. McCrumb FR Jr, Snyder MJ, Hicken WJ. The use of chloramphenicol acid succinate in the treatment of acute infections. Antibiot Annu 1957–1958; 837–41.
14. Glazko AJ, Dill WA, Kirkel AW, et al. Absorption and excretion of parenteral doses of chloramphenicol sodium succinate in comparison with peroral doses of chloramphenicol. Clin Pharmacol Ther 1977; 21:104–6.
15. Shann F, Barker J, Poore P. Absorption of chloramphenicol sodium succinate after intramuscular administration in children. N Engl J Med 1985; 313:410–14.
16. Glazko AJ, Kinkel AW, Alegnani WC, et al. An evaluation of the absorption characteristics of different chloramphenicol preparations in normal human subjects. Clin Pharmacol Ther 1968; 9:472–83.
17. Product information: Chloramphenicol (R), Parke-Davis, 1992.
18. Schoenbach EB, Spencer HC, Monnier J. Treatment of *Haemophilus influenzae* meningitis with aureomycin and chloramphenicol. Am J Med 1952; 12:263–5.
18a. Kunin C, Finland M. Persistence of antibiotics in blood of patients with acute renal failure III. Penicillin, streptomycin, erythromycin and kanamycin. J Clin Invest 1959; 38:1498–519.
18b. Narang APS, Datta DV, Nath N, et al. Pharmacokinetic study of chloramphenicol in patients with liver disease. Eur J Clin Pharmacol 1981; 20(6):479–83.
19. Christensen KK, Skovsted L. Inhibition of drug metabolism by chloramphenicol. Lancet 1969; 2:1397–9.
20. Petipierre B, Fabre J. Chlorpropamide and chloramphenicol. Lancet 1970; 1:789.
21. Powell DA, Nahata MC, Durrell DC, et al. Interactions among chloramphenicol, phenytoin and phenobarbital in a pediatric patient. J Pediatr 1981; 98:1001–3.
22. Pankey GA, Horton JM. Choramphenicol. In: Ristuccia DM, Cunha BA, eds. Antimicrobial therapy. New York; Raven Press, 1984:249–53.
23. Bartlett JG, Louie TJ, Gorbach SL, et al. Therapeutic efficacy of 29 antimicrobial regimens in experimental intra-abdominal sepsis. Rev Infect Dis 1981; 3:535–42.
24. Thadepalli H, Kannangara DW, Bach VT. Penicillin failure in the treatment of *Bacteroides fragilis* lung abscess. Chemotherapy 1983; 29:289–93.
25. Britz ML, Wilkinson RG. Chloramphenicol acetyltransferase of *Bacteroides fragilis*. Antimicrob Agents Chemother 1978; 15:105–11.
26. Zaleznik DF, Finberg RW, Shapiro ME, et al. Soluble suppressor T Cell factor protects against experimental intra-abdominal abscesses. J Clin Invest 1985; 75:1023–7.
27. Woodward TE, Smadel JE, Ley HL, Jr. Chloramphenicol and other antibiotics in the treatment of typhoid fever and typhoid carriers. J Clin Invest 1950; 29:87–99.
28. Dowling HF, Lepper MH. The effect of antibiotics (penicillin, aureomycin, and terramycin) on the fatality rate and incidence of complications in pneumococcic pneumonia. A comparison with methods of therapy. Am J Med Sci 1951; 222:396–403.
29. Knight V, McDermott W, Ruiz-Sanchez F. Aureomycin and chloramphenicol use in typhus, typhoid and brucellosis. J Clin Invest 1949; 28:1052–8.
30. Fullen WD, Hunt J, Altemeier WA. Prophylactic antibiotics in penetrating wounds of the abdomen. J Trauma 1972; 12:282–9.

31. Van Scoy RE, Wilkowske CJ, O'Fallon WM, et al. Clindamycin versus chloramphenicol in treatment of anaerobic infections: a prospective, randomized, double-blind study. Mayo Clin Proc 1984; 59:842–6.
32. Harding GKM, Buckwold FJ, Ronald AR, et al. Prospective, randomized comparative study of clindamycin, chloramphenicol, and ticarcillin, each in combination with gentamicin, in therapy for intraabdominal and female genital tract sepsis. J Infect Dis 1980; 142:384–93.
33. Laferriere CI, Marks MI. Chloramphenicol: properties and clinical use. Pediatr Infect Dis 1982; 1:257–64.
34. De Louvois J, Gortvai P, Hurley R. Bacteriology of abscesses of the central nervous system; a multicentre prospective study. Br Med J 1977; 2:981–4.
35. De Louvois J, Gortvai P, Hurley R. Antibiotic treatment of abscesses of central nervous system. Br Med J 1977 2:985–8.
36. Fink TJ, Gump DW. Chloramphenicol: an inpatient study of use and abuse. J Infect Dis 1978; 138:690–4.
37. Feder HM Jr, Osier, C, Maderazo EG. An audit of chloramphenicol use in a large community hospital. Arch Intern Med 1981; 141:597–8.
38. Smith GN, Worrel CS. Enzymatic reduction of chloramphenicol (chloromycetin). Arch Biochem 1949; 24:216–23.
39. Egami F, Ebata M, Sato R. Reduction of chloromycetin by a cell-free bacterial extract and its relation to nitrite reduction. Nature 1951; 167:118–19.
40. Shaw WV, Brodsky RF. Chloramphenicol resistance by enzymatic acetylation: comparative aspects. Antimicrob Agents Chemother. 1968; 7:257–63.
41. Nakagawa Y, Nitahara Y, Miyamura S. Kinetic studies on enzymatic acetylation of chloramphenicol in *Streptococcus faecalis*. Antimicrob Agents Chemother 1979; 16:719–23.
42. Dang-Van A, Tiraby G, De La Maza L, et al. Use of commercially available rapid chloramphenicol acetyltransferase test to detect resistance in salmonella species. J Clin Microbiol 1990; 28:1867–9.
43. Overturf G, Marton KI, Mathies AW, Jr. Antibiotic resistance in typhoid fever: chloramphenicol resistance among clinical isolates of *Salmonella typhosa* in Los Angeles, 1972-epidemiologic and bacteriologic characteristics. N Engl J Med 1973; 289:463–6.
44. Spika JS, Waterman SH, Soo Hoo GW, et al. Chloramphenicol resistant *Salmonella newport* traced through hamburger to dairy farms. N Engl J Med 1987; 316:563–70.
45. Gangarosa EJ, Bennett JV, Wyatt, C, et al. An epidemic associated episome? J Infect Dis 1972; 126:215–18.
46. Bryan LE. Transferable chloramphenicol and ampicillin resistance in a strain of *Haemophilus influenzae*. Antimicrob Agents Chemother 1978; 14:154–6.
47. Roberts MC, Swenson CD, Owens LM, et al. Characterization of chloramphenicol-resistant *Haemophilus influenzae*. Antimicrob. Agents Chemother. 1980; 18:610–15.
48. Martinez-Suarez JV, Baquero F, Reig M, et al. Transferable plasmid-linked chloramphenicol acetyltransferase conferring high-level resistance in *Bacteroides uniformis*. Antimicrob Agents Chemother 1985: 28:113–17.
49. Shann F, Barker V, Poore P. Chloramphenicol alone versus chloramphenicol plus penicillin for severe pneumonia in children. Lancet 1985; 2:684–5.
50. Shann F, Barker J, Poore P. Chloramphenicol alone versus chloramphenicol plus penicillin for bacterial meningitis in children. Lancet 1985; 2:681–4.
51. Coles FS, Daum RS, Teller L, et al. Effect of ampicillin and chloramphenicol alone and in combination on ampicillin-susceptible and-resistant *Haemophilus influenzae*. Antimicrob Agents Chemother 1979; 15:415–19.
52. Pecoul B, Varaine F, Keita M, et al. Long-acting chloramphenicol versus intravenous ampicillin for treatment of bacterial meningitis. Lancet 1991; 338:862–6.
53. Brown TH, Alford RH. Antagonism of chloramphenicol of broad-spectrum β-lactam antibiotics against *Klebsiella pneumoniae*. Antimicrob Agents Chemother 1984; 25:405–7.

54. Mathies AW Jr, Leedom JW, Ivler D, et al. Antibiotic antagonism in bacterial meningitis. Antimicrob Agents Chemother 1968; 7:218–24.
55. Kelly HW, Couch RC, Davis RL, et al. Interaction of chloramphenicol and rifampin. Clin Lab Observ 1987; 112:817–20.
56. Krasinski K, Kusmiesz H, Nelson JD. Pharmacologic interactions among chloramphenicol, phenytoin and phenobarbital. Pediatr Infect Dis 1982; 1:232–5.
57. Rich ML, Ritterhof RJ, Hoffman RJ. A fatal case of aplastic anaemia following chloramphenicol therapy. Ann Intern Med 1950; 33:1459.
58. Welch H, Lewis CN, Kerlin I. Blood dyscrasias, a nationwide survey. Antibiot Chemother 1954; 4:607–11.
59. Wallerstein RO, Condit PK, Kasper CK, et al. Statewide study of chloramphenicol therapy and fatal aplastic anemia. JAMA 1969; 208:2045–50.
60. Dunne M, Herxheimer A, Newman M, et al. Indications and warnings about chloramphenicol. Lancet 1973; 1:781–3.
61. Kumana CR, Li KY, Chau PY. Worldwide variation in chloramphenicol utilization: should it cause concern? J Clin Pharmacol 1988; 28:1071–5.
62. West BC, DeVault GA Jr, Clement JC, et al. Aplastic anemia associated with parenteral chloramphenicol: review of 10 cases, including the second case of possible increased risk with cimetidine. Rev Infect Dis 1988; 10:1048–51.
63. Yunis AA, Bloomberg GR. Chloramphenicol toxicity: Clinical features and pathogenesis. Prog Haematol 1964; 4:138–50.
64. Abrams SM, Degnan TJ, Vinciguerra V. Marrow aplasia following topical application of chloramphenicol eye ointment. Arch Intern Med 1980; 140:576–7.
65. Skolimowski IM, Rowley DA, Knight RC, et al. Reduced chloramphenicol-induced damage to DNA. J Antimicrob Chemother 1981; 7:593–7.
66. Rosenkranz HS. Chloramphenicol: magic bullet or double-edge sword? Mutation Res 1988; 196:1–16.

21

Nitrofurans

Keith Beck
Harbor-UCLA Medical Center, Torrance, and UCLA School of Medicine, Los Angeles, California

Hearee Chung Julius
Harbor-UCLA Medical Center, Torrance, and University of Southern California School of Pharmacy, Los Angeles, California

I. NITROFURANTOIN

Nitrofurantoin is an antimicrobial agent that is prescribed primarily for the treatment of urinary tract infection. However, there are little data on the pharmacology and clinical experience of this drug in elderly patients. Nevertheless, because of the importance of urinary tract infections in the geriatric population, a discussion of nitrofurantoin is appropriate.

A. Chemistry

Nitrofurantoin is a synthetic nitrofuran antibacterial agent [*O*-(*t*-nitrofur-furylideneamino)-hydantoin] with a pKa of 7.2. Nitrofurantoin is commercially available as an oral suspension, tablets, capsules containing microcrystals, capsules containing macrocrystals, and hard gelatin capsules containing a mixture of macrocrystals and nitrofurantoin monohydrate (Table 1) (1–3).

B. Mechanism of Action

The exact mechanism of nitrofurantoin is not well understood. It has been postulated that the drug may inhibit acetylcoenzyme A, thus interfering with bacterial carbohydrate metabolism; it may also disrupt bacterial cell wall formation (4,5). Nitrofurantoin is bacteriostatic in low concentrations and bactericidal in higher concentrations. The antibacterial activity of nitrofurantoin is highest at pH 5.8 and reduced at alkaline pH (6).

C. Antimicrobial Spectrum

Nitrofurantoin has activity against a broad spectrum of gram-positive and gram-negative bacteria, with susceptibility defined as a minimal inhibitory concentration (MIC) ≤ 32

Table 1 Preparations of Nitrofurantoin

Macrocrystals		
Oral Capsules:	25 mg	Macrodantin (Norwich Eaton)
	50 mg	Macrodantin (Norwich Eaton)
		Macrodantin MACPAC (Norwich Eaton)
	100 mg	Macrodantin (Norwich Eaton)
		Macrodantin MACPAC (Norwich Eaton)
Microcrystals		
Oral capsules:	50 mg	Nitrofan (Major)
		Nitrofurantoin (Various)
	100 mg	Nitrofan (Major)
		Nitrofurantoin (Various)
Oral Tablets:	50 mg	Furadantin (Norwich Eaton)
		Furaian (Lannett), Furan (American Urologicals), Furanite (Major), Nitrofurantoin (Various)
	100 mg	Furadantin (Norwich Eaton), Furaian (Lannett), Furan (American Urologicals), Furanite (Major)
		Nitrofurantoin (Various)
Oral Suspension:	25 mg/5 ml	Furadantin (Norwich Eaton)
Nitrofurantoin Monohydrate/Macrocrystals		
Oral Capsule:	75 mg/25 mg	Macrobid (Norwich Eaton)

μg/ml. A nitrofurantoin concentration of 32 μg/ml (or more) is only achievable in the urine, making nitrofurantoin clinically useful only against organisms in the lower urinary tract. More than 90% of *Escherichia coli* are susceptible, while *Pseudomonas aeruginosa* and *Proteus* spp. are usually resistant. *Klebsiella* and *Enterobacter* spp. are more variable, with 35–50% of strains being susceptible. Urinary levels of nitrofurantoin are above the MIC for 96% of *Enterococcus faecalis*. Development of bacterial resistance to nitrofurantoin during therapy is rare (7). While many other gram-negative and some gram-positive organisms are susceptible to nitrofurantoin by the above definition, this is of little clinical significance, since its levels achieved in other body fluids, tissues, and blood are negligible (8,9). Such low drug levels are beneficial in that nitrofurantoin alters perineal and bowel flora less than most antimicrobial agents, which may lower the risk of superinfections, e.g., vaginal candidiasis (10).

D. Clinical Pharmacology

1. Pharmacokinetics

The oral suspension and tablets of nitrofurantoin are well absorbed in the small intestine. Particle size influences the bioavailability of nitrofurantoin. The macrocrystalline form is absorbed more slowly and causes less gastrointestinal (GI) irritation. Conversely, the microcrystals are absorbed faster, reach higher peak serum concentrations and produce high urine levels in a shorter period of time (11). Nitrofurantoin monohydrate, upon exposure to intestinal fluids, forms a gel matrix that releases nitrofurantoin slowly (1). The impact of age on GI absorption of nitrofurantoin is unknown.

Food increases the overall bioavailability of nitrofurantoin; both the amount of drug absorbed and the duration of effective urinary drug concentrations are increased significantly when it is taken with a meal (12,13). Anticholinergic drugs may also increase the bioavailability by slowing GI motility, which allows increased dissolution of nitrofurantoin before its arrival in the small intestine for absorption (14).

After an oral dose of nitrofurantoin, the serum concentration is negligible (≤1.5 μg/ml) (15). Serum concentrations are only modestly increased in the presence of severe renal failure, usually not exceeding 6 μg/ml (16). Urinary nitrofurantoin levels of 50–150 μg/ml are achieved within 30 min after an oral dose of 100 mg, while multiple doses of nitrofurantoin produce peak urine levels of 50–250 μg/ml in patients with normal renal function (11).

Nitrofurantoin is 90% bound to plasma protein. Approximately two thirds of absorbed nitrofurantoin is rapidly metabolized, mainly in the liver. The half-life in normal individuals is 20 min and is prolonged in patients with impaired renal function. Drug levels are lower than those achieved in blood in body fluids and tissues outside the urinary tract (2,17,18). Nitrofurantoin does not penetrate significantly into prostatic secretions, aqueous humor, or cerebrospinal fluid.

Nitrofurantoin and its metabolites are excreted in urine and bile. Approximately one-third of absorbed drug rapidly appears unchanged in the urine; it is excreted by glomerular filtration and is both secreted and reabsorbed in the tubules (18,19). The amount of drug excreted is directly related to creatinine clearance (ClCr) (16). With reduced glomerular filtration, therapeutic concentrations of nitrofurantoin are decreased. While the clearance of nitrofurantoin in acid urine is lower than in alkaline urine, optimal antimicrobial activity occurs at a pH of 5.8; thus alkalinization of the urine is not recommended during nitrofurantoin therapy (19,20).

Because the amount of excretion of nitrofurantoin is directly related to creatinine clearance, in patients with ClCr < 60 ml/min, serum concentrations of nitrofurantoin are increased, which enhance the potential for increased adverse effects. Furthermore, subtherapeutic urinary levels of the drug may occur when the ClCr falls below 60 ml/min. Nitrofurantoin is therefore contraindicated in the presence of significant renal impairment (2,11,18). It would be anticipated that in many older adults, the renal excretion of nitrofurantoin would be reduced.

2. *Drug Interactions*

Any agent that decreases GI motility may increase absorption, thereby enhancing nitrofurantoin bioavailability. This has the potential to increase both therapeutic efficacy and dose-related adverse effects of nitrofurantoin. Anticholinergic agents, narcotics, metoclopramide, and food may have this effect (11–14). Probenecid and sulfinpyrazone inhibit renal excretion of nitrofurantoin, resulting in reduced efficacy and increased toxicity (2).

Concomitant administration of nitrofurantoin and magnesium trisilicate reduces absorption of nitrofurantoin as a result of adsorption of nitrofurantoin onto magnesium trisilicate (21). In vitro antagonism of quinolones by nitrofurantoin has been observed. Although the clinical significance of this has not been determined, it is recommended that nitrofurantoin should not be used concomitantly with a quinolone (2,22). Plasma phenytoin levels and clinical response should be monitored in patients who are receiving phenytoin and nitrofurantoin (14,21).

Nitrofurantoin causes false-positive results for urine glucose determinations utilizing cupric sulfate solution (Benedict's reagent, Clinitest®), making this form of monitoring unsuitable during therapy. However, glucose oxidase methods (Clinistix®, Tes-Tape®) are not affected by the drug. Serum levels of glucose, bilirubin, alkaline phosphatase, and blood urea nitrogen may be spuriously elevated with use of nitrofurantoin (2,23).

E. Clinical Indications

Nitrofurantoin has been in clinical use since 1953. Its use has declined somewhat, due to the advent of newer agents and clinician concerns over the toxicity of nitrofurantoin. Nitrofurantoin's current role is in the treatment and prevention of lower urinary tract infections (UTI) (24–27). Because nitrofurantoin reaches therapeutic levels only in the urine, it has no role in the therapy of pyelonephritis, prostatitis, perinephric abscess, or other infections. It is contraindicated in those older patients with a decrease in ClCr to 60ml/min or less, and should be used with caution in the setting of any degree of renal impairment. Patients receiving prolonged therapy should be monitored for the appearance of early signs of toxicity, as discussed below. Indications and dosages are summarized in Table 2.

1. Acute Lower Urinary Tract Infection

Nitrofurantoin is very effective in the treatment of acute cystitis, but should be limited to use in the patient with uncomplicated infection and ClCr > 60 ml/min. In some patients, bladder organisms will be eliminated with a single dose of 200 mg; others will require 50 mg four times daily (100 mg twice daily of the monohydrate gelatin capsule, Macrobid®) for 3–7 days. Patients with a high risk of resistant organisms causing the (UTI) (e.g., recent hospitalization, genitourinary (GU) instrumentation, receiving other antibiotics) should empirically receive an agent more likely to cover such resistant organisms (e.g., a fluoroquinolone or ampicillin/clavulanate) until the results of susceptibility testing are known.

2. Asymptomatic Bacteriuria

Persistent asymptomatic urinary carriage of potential pathogens is relatively common in the elderly patient and usually should not be treated. While a thorough discussion of this issue is beyond the scope of this chapter, treatment should be considered in the setting of obstruction, nephrolithiasis, papillary necrosis, frequent symptomatic UTIs, or immune-compromised state (28–30). If treatment is elected, nitrofurantoin may be chosen if the organisms have been shown to be susceptible by culture. Dosage of the drug is the same as for cystitis. The more complex clinical issue of prolonged antibiotic suppression is discussed below.

Table 2 Nitrofurantoin Dosages

Indication	Dosage
Asymptomatic bacteriuria	200 mg (one dose) or 50 mg qid × 5–7 days
Acute cystitis	200 mg (one dose) or 50 mg qid × 5–7 days
Relapse of cystitis	50 mg qid (100 mg bid) × 7–10 days, followed by 50 mg bid
Prophylaxis	Treat as for acute cystitis, followed by 50 mg qd or bid

3. *Relapsing Urinary Tract Infection*

Relapse of UTI with the same organism in an older patient within a week or two after an appropriate course of therapy should prompt the clinician to evaluate for renal involvement with bacteria, structural abnormalities of the GU tract, and prostatitis. Upper tract infection and prostatitis should be treated with antibacterial agents other than nitrofurantoin. If surgical correction of structural abnormalities is not feasible, or if such abnormalities are not found, prolonged antimicrobial suppressive therapy—weeks to months—may be indicated. This decision involves a complex evaluation of relative risks and benefits, especially in elderly patients, who are at risk not only for urosepsis but for severe adverse drug reactions as well. Nitrofurantoin should be considered as an alternative choice under these circumstances. The dose of nitrofurantoin would be 50 mg four times daily for 7–10 days followed by 50 mg twice daily for the duration of suppressive therapy. The increased incidence of nitrofurantoin toxicity in the elderly patient, however, makes other agents, such as trimethoprim/sulfamethoxazole (TMP/SMX) or TMP alone, more appropriate treatment for prolonged suppressive therapy.

4. *Recurrent Urinary Tract Infection*

Frequent discrete episodes of symptomatic lower tract infection is common in older women and may indicate a need for prolonged prophylactic therapy. As discussed earlier, the decision for prolonged chemotherapy involves a thorough consideration of the risks and benefits. Nitrofurantoin is an effective prophylactic agent for lower tract bacteriuria, as are methenamine, TMP, and TMP/SMX (31–33). After treatment of the acute urinary infection with the doses mentioned earlier, prophylaxis with nitrofurantoin may be continued with a dosage of 50 mg once daily. Urine cultures should be done at least once each month during long-term prophylaxis, and patients should be monitored for any adverse drug reactions.

Nitrofurantoin is an effective agent for the short-term prophylaxis of UTI related to bladder instrumentation. Prophylaxis against bacteremia following GU instrumentation in patients with abnormal or prosthetic valves should be with systemically active antimicrobials rather than nitrofurantoin (34). Transurethral resection of the prostate is a common procedure in elderly men. The urine should be sterile at the time of instrumentation; bacteriuria prior to the procedure may be treated with nitrofurantoin. Also, some clinicians have recommended antimicrobial prophylaxis from the time of instrumentation until the bladder catheter is removed (35).

Long-term antibiotic prophylaxis against UTI in patients with long-term indwelling bladder catheters is generally doomed to failure. Invariably, bacteriuria returns, which is generally associated with organisms resistant to the prophylactic antibiotic. If intermittent catheterization of the neurogenic bladder causes symptomatic UTI and the clinical situation warrants prophylaxis for a few days, nitrofurantoin (50 mg twice daily) may decrease the incidence of symptomatic infection (36).

5. *Helicobacter Pylori Infections*

Helicobacter pylori (HP) has emerged as an etiological agent in a variety of syndromes of gastroduodenal inflammation (37–40). While there is evidence that antimicrobial therapy can eradicate the organism, definition of the precise indications for treatment must await the results of current trials (41,42). At present, a possible indication for antimicrobial therapy is the treatment of HP-infected patients with relapse of duodenal ulceration or type B antral gastritis in spite of conventional therapy. A currently acceptable regimen is at least 2 weeks of therapy with the combination of amoxicillin 500 mg three times daily, metronidazole 250 mg two or three times daily, and bismuth 525 mg four times daily. While nitrofurantoin has activity against HP and has been effective in eradicating the organism from patients with gastritis, it cannot be recommended until results of ongoing investigations are analyzed (40,43,44).

F. Administration

The available preparations of nitrofurantoin are shown in Table 1. Table 2 summarizes dosages for nitrofurantoin for specific clinical indications. When the ClCr is less than 60 ml/min, the urinary concentration of nitrofurantoin is reduced to a level below the MIC of many uropathogens. Thus, nitrofurantoin should not be used in patients with a decrease in renal function to this level (16,23).

Nitrofurantoin is administered orally and should be administered with food to improve absorption and tolerance. The commercially available oral suspension is readily miscible with water, milk, or fruit juice (2).

G. Drug Monitoring and Adverse Effects

Adverse reactions to nitrofurantoin are relatively common, with 5% of therapeutic courses in elderly patients being associated with severe enough reactions to lead to cessation of therapy. Almost all these adverse reactions subside rapidly upon discontinuation of the drug. However, there are occasional serious reactions (45). The most common adverse reactions are benign, involving the gastrointestinal tract, i.e., nausea, vomiting, and diarrhea. Skin reactions are seen in approximately 1% of treatment courses and range from urticarial to macular eruptions. Neurological reactions, including lethargy, diplopia, dizziness, headache, and peripheral sensorimotor neuropathy, are rare ($<0.01\%$). However, neuropathy has an increased incidence in patients with uremia and may be severe (46,47). Hematological reactions are also rare, but hemolytic anemia may occur in those with patients glucose-6-phosphate dehydrogenase deficiency. Leukopenia and megaloblastic anemia and aplastic anemia have also been reported. Cholestatic and autoimmune hepatitis are well described but quite uncommon, and pancreatitis is a very rare complication. Other reactions include drug fever, various hypersensitivity manifestations, and a lupuslike syndrome (48–51).

Considerable attention has been paid to pulmonary reactions, although the overall incidence is less than 0.001% of therapeutic courses. This toxicity is slightly increased, however, in elderly patients and in women. The reactions are immunological in nature, and cause interstitial inflammation and alveolar septal thickening. The typical reaction includes fever, chills, cough, and dyspnea. Radiographic findings include diffuse interstitial markings and pleural effusions. These reactions usually occur hours to days after starting the medication, although there is a rare chronic form that may appear much later. While most symptoms resolve after discontinuation of the agent, there have been a few fatal cases (17,22,51).

Although uncommon, acute hepatitis, which is a cholestatic form of liver injury, does occur with short courses of treatment with nitrofurantoin. The injury does reverse with cessation of therapy (52,53). However, long-term administration of nitrofurantoin (>6 months) may result in chronic active hepatitis. Clinical symptoms of hepatitis may last as long as 4 months after withdrawal of the drug; death has been reported in two patients (54). It appears that the pathogenesis is immune mediated (54,55). It is important to note that these earlier reports of chronic active hepatitis occurred only in women, with nearly one half of all cases in one report of 20 patients being found in patients age 60 years and older. Therefore, prolonged therapy with nitrofurantoin, especially in elderly women, must be carefully assessed in terms of risks and benefits. If the drug is prescribed for prolonged periods, careful monitoring for all potential adverse effects—particularly hepatic and pulmonary—is essential.

II. FURAZOLIDONE (FUROXONE®)

A. Chemistry

Furazolidone is a synthetic, nitrofuran-derivative antibacterial and antiprotozoal agent. Furazolidone occurs as a yellow, crystalline powder with a bitter aftertaste. The drug is practically insoluble in water and in alcohol (2).

B. Mechanism of Action

Furazolidone is bactericidal due to its interference with several bacterial and protozoal enzyme systems, the precise nature of which is not well understood (2).

C. Antimicrobial Spectrum

Furazolidone is active against *Giardia lamblia* and somewhat active against *Isospora belli.* It is active in vitro against numerous bacteria that can cause diarrhea, including *Escherichia coli* (enterotoxigenic), *Vibrio parahaemolyticus* and *V. cholerae*, *Campylobacter jejuni*, *Yersinia enterocolitica*, *Salmonella* spp., and *Shigella* spp. (56,57).

D. Clinical Pharmacology

1. Pharmacokinetics

Furazolidone is approximately 75% absorbed and is rapidly and extensively metabolized. The particle size appears to affect the kinetics of absorption; microcrystal tablets are absorbed more rapidly than capsules containing macrocrystals as reflected in the urinary drug recovery (58,59). The primary metabolic pathway of furazolidone is nitro-reduction to aminofuran, which is pharmacologically inactive, followed by further degradation to several other metabolites.

Clinically insignificant amounts of furazolidone appear transiently in various biological fluids. Inactive metabolites are excreted in the urine, whereas significant amounts of intact drug are appear in the feces (58,60). Pharmacokinetic data for furazolidone in elderly persons are not available.

2. Drug Interactions

Furazolidone acts as a monoamine oxidase (MAO) inhibitor, with numerous potential adverse interactions when taken with other drugs. Amphetamines together with furazolidone may induce a hypertensive response, and the alpha-adrenergic effects of indirect- and mixed-acting sympathomimetics may be increased (61). Concurrent use of levodopa and furazolidone may cause an increase in the therapeutic and/or toxic effects of levodopa, specifically hypertensive crisis (60). An uncommon but potentially fatal reaction—characterized by agitation, seizures, diaphoresis, fever, apnea, and coma—has been observed in some patients receiving a MAO inhibitor and meperidine. While this has not been reported with furazolidone, the potential may exist. Caution should be used in combining tricyclic antidepressants and furazolidone, since the combination of an antidepressant and a MAO inhibitor can produce serious adverse reactions including hypertension, hyperpyrexia, seizures, tachycardia, and acute psychosis. For similar reasons, amine-containing foods should be avoided (61). A disulfiramlike reaction may occur when patients taking furazolidone ingest alcohol (14). Because older patients are often taking many different drugs, special caution must be exercised if furazolidone is to be prescribed in this population.

Furazolidone metabolites that are excreted in the urine following oral administration of the drug may interfere with tests performed with cupric sulfate reagent (Benedict's Qualitative Reagent®, Clinitest®, Fehling's Solution®), yielding false-positive results for urine glucose (2).

E. Clinical Indications

At present, furazolidone is not the agent of choice for any illness in adults, but it may be considered as an alternative chemotherapeutic drug for infections described below (62).

1. Giardiasis

Furazolidone is clinically active against the parasite causing giardiasis, but it is less effective than quinacrine or metronidazole (drugs of choice for this infection). It is an alternative for patients with contraindications to the latter two agents. The suspension of furazolidone is more palatable than crushed tablets for patients unable to ingest tablets. The recommended dosage is 100 mg four times daily for 7–10 days; the relapse rate is lower with the longer (10-day) course of therapy (62–64).

2. Traveler's Diarrhea

Furazolidone may be considered at best a tertiary alternative for the empiric treatment of traveler's diarrhea. The availability of much more effective agents such as TMP/SMX and ciprofloxacin make this indication doubtful. It should only be considered if there are clear contraindications to other therapies. The dosage is 100 mg four times daily. For diarrhea with documented bacterial etiology—such as *Shigella*, *Salmonella*, *Campylobacter*—furazolidone would be inferior to the agent(s) that would be considered the treatment of choice.

3. Helicobacter Pylori Infections

Furazolidone has activity against *Helicobacter pylori* and has shown favorable effect on the healing of peptic ulcers and gastritis (65–67). Definitive conclusions await further study, and furazolidone cannot be recommended at this time for this clinical condition.

F. Administration of Drug

Furazolidone is available in scored tablets of 100 mg and as a suspension of 16.7 mg/5 ml. Both are marketed as Furoxone®. Administration with food enhances absorption and decreases gastrointestinal side effects. Dosage is discussed above.

G. Drug Monitoring and Adverse Effects

Approximately 8% of patients treated with furazolidone have gastrointestinal side effects, which include nausea, vomiting, abdominal pain, and diarrhea; there is no specific information about toxicity in elderly persons. Ingestion with food and/or lowering the dose can minimize these reactions. Hepatitis or jaundice occurs in less than 1% of patients taking the drug. Approximately 1–2% of patients complain of neurological side effects; headache and vertigo are most common, with insomnia and agitation less so. Hematological reactions—anemia, leukopenia—are overall reported in less than 1% of patients, but it should be noted that furazolidone may cause hemolysis in patients with glucose-6-phosphate dehydrogenase deficiency. Pulmonary, dermatological, renal, and hypersensitivity reactions occur in less than 1% of patients (68).

REFERENCES

1. Manufacturer's information. Norwich, NY: Norwich Eaton Pharmaceuticals, 1991.
2. McEvoy GK, Litvak K, Welsh OH, eds. American Hospital Formulary Service (AHFS) drug information. Bethesda, MD: American Society of Hospital Pharmacists, 1992.
3. Budavari S, O'Neil MJ, Smith A, eds. The Merck index. 11th ed. Rahway, NJ: Merck & Co., 1989.
4. Lorian V, Popoola B. The effect of nitrofurantoin on the morphology of gram negative bacilli. J Infect Dis 1972; 125:187–8.
5. Green MN. The effect of furacin (5-nitro 2-furaldehyde semicarbazone) on the metabolism of bacteria. Arch Biochem 1948; 19:397–406.
6. Richards WA, Riss E, Kass EH, et al. Nitrofurantoin: clinical laboratory studies in urinary tract infections. Arch Intern Med 1955; 96:437–50.
7. Cunha BA. Nitrofurantoin—current concepts. Urology 1988; 32:67–71.
8. Turck M, Ronald AR, Petersdorf RG. Susceptibility of Enterobacteriaceae to nitrofurantoin correlated to eradication of bacteriuria. Antimicrob Agents Chemother 1966; 446–52.
9. Kucers A, Bennett NM. Nitrofurans. In: Kucers A, Bennett NM, eds. The use of antibiotics: a comprehensive review with clinical emphasis. 4th ed. 1987:1276–89.
10. Brumfitt W, Hamilton-Miller JMT. Development of bacterial resistance during the treatment of urinary tract infections: a constant clinical challenge. In: L'Etang, ed. Recent advances in the treatment of urinary tract infections. London: Royal Society of Medicine Services, 1985:13–24.
11. Mannisto P. The effect of crystal size, gastric content and emptying rate on the absorption of nitrofurantoin in healthy human volunteers. Int J Clin Pharmacol Biopharm 1978; 16:223–8.
12. Rosenberg HA, Bates TR. The influence of food on nitrofurantoin bioavailability. Clin Pharmacol Ther 1976; 20:227–32.
13. Bates TR, Sequeira JA, Tembo AV. The effect of food on nitrofurantoin absorption. Clin Pharmacol Ther 1974; 16:63–8.
14. Hansten PD, Horn JR. Drug interactions and updates. Malvern: Lea-Febiger, 1990.
15. Albert KS, Sedman AJ, Wilkinson P, et al. Bioavailability studies of acetaminophen and nitrofurantoin. J Clin Pharmacol 1974; 14:264–70.
16. Sachs J, Geer J, Noell P, et al. Effect of renal function on urinary recovery of orally administered nitrofurantoin. N Engl J Med 1968; 278:1032–5.
17. Pekka M, Lamminsivu U. Nitrofurantoin is highly bound to plasma protein. J Antimicrob Chemother 1982; 9:327–8.
18. Reckendorf HK, Castringius RG, Spingler HK. Comparative pharmacodynamics, urinary excretion and half-life determination of nitrofurantoin sodium. Antimicrob Agents Chemother 1962; 2:531–7.
19. Conklin JD. Biopharmaceutics of nitrofurantoin. Pharmacology 1972; 8:178–81.
20. Schirmeister J, Stefani F, Willmann H, Hallauer W. Renal handling of nitrofurantoin in man. Antimicrob Agents Chemother 1965; 223–6.
21. Naggar VF, Khalil SA. Effect of magnesium trisilicate on nitrofurantoin absorption. Clin Pharmacol Ther 1979; 25:857–63.
22. D'Arcy PF. Nitrofurantoin. Drug Intell Clin Pharm 1985; 19:540–7.
23. Gleckman R, Alvarez S, Joubert DW. Drug therapy reviews: nitrofurantoin. Am J Hosp Pharm 1979; 36:342–51.
24. Gleckman RA. Urinary tract infection. Clin Geriatr Med 1992; 8:793–803.

25. Warren JW. Catheter-associated bacteriuria. Clin Geriatr Med 1992; 8:805–19.
26. Sobel JD, Kaye D. Urinary tract infections. In: Mandell GL, Douglas RG Jr., Bennett JE, eds. Principles and practice of infectious diseases. New York: Churchill Livingstone, 1990:582–611.
27. Stamey TA. Pathogenesis and treatment of urinary tract infections. Baltimore: Williams & Wilkins. 1980.
28. Boscia JA, Abrutyn E, Kay D. Asymptomatic bacteriuria in elderly persons: treat or do not treat? Ann Intern Med 1987; 106:764–6.
29. Boscia JA, Kobase WD, Knight RA, et al. Therapy versus no therapy for bacteriuria in elderly ambulatory nonhospitalized women. JAMA 1987; 257:1067–71.
30. Zhanel GC, Harding GKM, Guay DRP. Asymptomatic bacteriuria: which patients should be treated? Arch Intern Med 1990; 150:1389–96.
31. Stamm WE, Counts GW, Wagner KF, et al. Antimicrobial prophylaxis of recurrent urinary tract infections. Ann Intern Med 1980; 92:770–5.
32. Cronberg S, Welin CO, Henricksson L, et al. Prevention of recurrent acute cystitis by methenamine hippurate: double-blind crossover long-term study. Br Med J 1987; 294:1507–8.
33. Bailey RR, Roberts AP, Gower PL, et al. Prevention of urinary-tract infection with low-dose nitrofurantoin. Lancet 1971; 2:1112–14.
34. Dajani AS, Bisno AL, Chung KJ, et al. Prevention of bacterial endocarditis. Recommendations by the American Heart Association. JAMA 1990; 264:2919–22.
35. Weiss J, Wein A, Jacobs J, et al. Use of nitrofurantoin macrocrystals after transurethral prostatectomy. J Urol 1983; 130(3):479–80.
36. Anderson RU. Prophylaxis of bacteriuria during intermittent catheterization of the acute neurogenic bladder. J Urol 1980; 123:364–6.
37. Blaser MJ. *Helicobacter pylori* and the pathogenesis of gastroduodenal inflammation. J Infect Dis 1990; 161:626–33.
38. Jones DM, Lessels AM, Eldridge J. *Campylobacter*-like organism on the gastric mucosa: culture, histological, and serological studies. J Clin Pathol 1984; 37:1002–6.
39. Marshal BJ. *Campylobacter pyloridis* and gastritis. J Infect Dis 1986; 153:650–7.
40. Blaser MJ. *Helicobacter pylori.* In: Mandell GL, Douglas RG Jr, Bennett JE, eds. Principles and practice of infectious diseases. Update 9. New York: Churchill Livingstone, 1991:1–10.
41. Marshal BJ, Goodwin CS, Warren JR, et al. Prospective double-blind trial of duodenal ulcer relapse after eradication of *Campylobacter pylori.* Lancet 1988; 2:1437–45.
42. Rauws EAJ, Tytgat GNJ. Eradication of *Helicobacter pylori* cures duodenal ulcer. Lancet 1990; 1:1233–5.
43. Morgan D, Kraft W, Bender M, et al. Nitroflurans in the treatment of gastritis associated with *Campylobacter pylori.* Gastroenterology 1988; 95:1178–84.
44. Goodwin CS, Blake P, Blincow E. The minimum inhibitory and bactericidal concentrations of antibiotics and anti-ulcer agents against *Campylobacter pyloridis.* J Antimicrob Chemother 1986; 17:309–14.
45. Shah RR, Wade G. Reappraisal of the risk/benefit of nitrofurantoin: review of toxicity and efficacy. Adverse Drug React Acute Poisoning Rev 1989; 8(4):183–201.
46. Ellis FG. Acute polyneuritis after nitrofurantoin therapy. Lancet 1962; 2:1136–8.
47. Felts JH, Hayes DM, Gergen JA, et al. Neural, hematologic and bacteriologic effects of nitrofurantoin in renal insufficiency. Am J Med 1971; 51:331–9.
48. Swanson M, Cook R. Drugs, chemicals, and blood dyscrasias. Hamilton, IL: Drug Intelligence Publications, 1990:685–95.
49. Young TL, Achkar E, Tuthill R, et al. Chronic active hepatitis induced by nitrofurantoin. Cleve Clin Q 1985; 52:253–6.
50. Nelis GF. Nitrofurantoin-induced pancreatitis: report of a case. Gastroenterology 1983; 84:1032–4.
51. Holmberg L, Boman G, Bottiger LE, et al. Adverse reactions to nitrofurantoin: Analysis of 921 reports. Am J Med 1980; 69:733–8.

52. Ernaesteen D, Williams R. Jaundice due to nitrofurantoin. Gastroenterology 1961; 4:590–2.
53. Jokela A. Liver disease due to nitrofurantoin. Gastroenterology 1967; 53:306–11.
54. Sharp JR, Ishak KG, Zimmerman HJ. Chronic active hepatitis and severe hepatic necrosis associated with nitrofurantoin. Ann Intern Med 1980; 92:14–19.
55. Black M, Rabin L, Schatz N. Nitrofurantoin-induced chronic active hepatitis. Ann Intern Med 1980; 92:62–4.
56. Carlson JR, Thornton SA, DuPont HL, et al. Comparative *in vitro* activities of ten antimicrobial agents against bacterial enteropathogens. Antimicrob Agents Chemother 1983; 24:509–13.
57. Phillips KR, Hailey FJ. The use of furoxone: a perspective. J Int Med Res 1986; 14:19–29.
58. White AH. Absorption, distribution, metabolism, and excretion of furazolidone: a review of the literature. Scan J Gastroenterol 1989; 25(suppl 169):4–10.
59. Hollifield RD, Conklin JD. Method specific for determination of furazolidone in urine: evidence for drug-related metabolites. J Pharm Sci 1968; 57:2:325–8.
60. Tatsumi K, Nakabeppu H, Takahashi Y, et al. Metabolism *in-vivo* of furazolidone: evidence for formation of an open-chain carboxylic acid and alpha-ketoglutaric acid from the nitrofuran in rats. Arch Biochem Biophys 1984; 234:112–16.
61. Olin BR, Hebel SK, Dombek CE, eds. Drug facts and comparisons. St. Louis: Facts and Comparisons, 1992.
62. Drugs for parasitic infections. Med Lett Drugs Ther 1988; 30:15–24.
63. Bassily S, Farid Z, Makhail JW, et al. The treatment of *Giardia lamblia* infection with mepacrine, metronidazole, and furazolidone. J Trop Med Hyg 1970; 73:15–18.
64. Wolfe MS. Giardiasis. JAMA 1975; 233:1362–3.
65. Xiao SD, Liu WZ, Xia DH, et al. The efficacy of furazolidone and metronidazole in the treatment of chronic gastritis associated with *Helicobacter* (*Campylobacter*) *pylori*—a randomized double-blind placebo-controlled clinical trial. Hepato-gastroenterology 1990; 37:503–6.
66. Huai-yu, Guozhen L, Jundong G, et al. Furazolidone in peptic ulcer (letter). Lancet 1985; 2:276–7.
67. Zhi-tian Z, Zheng-ying W, Ya-xian C, et al. Double-blind short-term trial of furazolidone in peptic ulcer (letter). Lancet 1985; 1:1048–9.
68. Altamirano A, Bondani A. Adverse reactions to furazolidone and other drugs: a comparative review. Scand J Gastroenterol 1989; 24(suppl 169):70–80.

22

Methenamine

William L. Quinn
Department of Veterans Affairs Medical Center, Waco, and Texas A&M School of Medicine, College Station, Texas

I. CHEMISTRY

Methenamine (hexamethylenetetramine, hexamethyleneamine, hexamine) is a unique synthetic tertiary amine used as an antimicrobial agent. Its chemical structure is unrelated to other currently available anti-infectives (Fig. 1). According to the American Hospital Formulary Service's Drug Information, methenamine is a colorless, practically odorless compound, having the properties of a monoacidic base in its salt formation (1). It has the

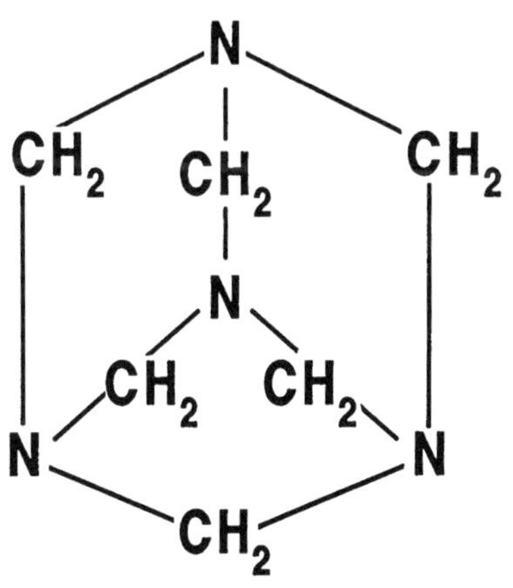

Figure 1 Chemical structure of methenamine.

capacity to combine with an unlimited number of organic and inorganic compounds. The two organic salts that have been commonly combined with methenamine as urinary anti-infectives are hippuric and mandelic acids. Methenamine hippurate contains approximately 44% methenamine and 56% hippuric acid, and methenamine mandelate contains approximately 48% methenamine and 52% mandelic acid; both compounds are readily soluble in water.

II. MECHANISM OF ACTION

In and of itself methenamine has no known antibacterial action. In an acid medium with a pH of less than 6.7, e.g., gastric juice or urine, methenamine hydrolyzes to ammonia and formaldehyde by the following reaction:

$$N_4\,(CH_2)_6 + 6H_2O + 4H^+ \rightleftharpoons 4NH_4 + 6HCHO$$

Formaldehyde is bactericidal; therefore, the effectiveness of methenamine as an antibacterial agent is dependent on its acid hydrolysis liberating free formaldehyde. The generation of formaldehyde from methenamine is dependent on three factors: (1) urinary pH, (2) the concentration of methenamine, and (3) the length of time urine remains in the bladder (2–4). Under most circumstances urine is sufficiently acidic, i.e., less than pH 6.0, to initiate the acid hydrolysis of methenamine. According to Gleckman et al., peak concentrations of formaldehyde are best achieved in urine at pH 5.6 (3). Further, the authors provide data on urinary concentrations of liberated formaldehyde from increasing methenamine urinary concentrations. An effective concentration of formaldehyde, ≥25 μg/ml, could be achieved from 0.7 μg/ml of methenamine. Lower concentrations of methenamine would not generate sufficient concentrations of formaldehyde to be an effective antibacterial agent in urine. It takes approximately an hour to generate 25 μg/ml of free formaldehyde in an acid urine. Within 3 h, 90% of the formaldehyde would be hydrolyzed from methenamine (4). The bactericidal mechanism of action for formaldehyde is slow. With an effective concentration of formaldehyde in the urine, a minimum of 2 h of exposure of the bacteria to the formaldehyde is necessary for it to be effectively bactericidal (2–4). Insufficient concentrations of formaldehyde (i.e., <25 μg/ml) with exposure of bacteria to the agent for 4–8 h or adequate concentrations of formaldehyde (35–50 μg/ml) for less than 2 h of exposure by the bacteria failed to cause discernible bacteriostasis (2). In a 0.5% (5 mg/ml or 5000 μg/ml) concentration of formaldehyde, it may take 2–4 days to kill spores; even at 8% concentration, it may take formaldehyde as much as 18 h to destroy bacterial spores.

III. ANTIMICROBIAL SPECTRUM

The antimicrobial action of methenamine is dependent upon its acid hydrolysis generating free formaldehyde. Almost all bacterial (gram-positive and gram-negative) and fungal organisms usually found in the urinary tract of elderly patients are susceptible to formaldehyde (4). Table 1 lists the common organisms isolated from urinary tract infections of elderly patients, which may be acquired in both community and institutional settings. Boscia and Kaye studied asymptomatic bacteriuria in a geriatric population and found that Enterobacteriaceae were the most common organisms isolated from women with gram-positive organisms predominating in men (5).

Due to the cidal mechanism of formaldehyde, i.e., protein denaturing and precipitation, there are no reported cases of resistance to formaldehyde by fungi or bacteria (6). Therefore,

Table 1 Common Organisms Causing Institutional and Community-Acquired Urinary Tract Infection in Elderly Persons

Gram-positive	Gram-negative	Miscellaneous
Staphylococcus epidermidis	*Providencia stuartii*	*Candida albicans*
Staphylococcus aureus	*Proteus mirabilis*	*Mycobacterium tuberculosis*
Enterococcus	*Escherichia coli*	
	Pseudomonas aeruginosa	
	Morganella morganii	
	Klebsiella pneumoniae	
	Serratia marcescens	

it would not be cost effective or meaningful to perform bacteriological sensitivity tests in urine with methenamine.

However, there is disagreement in the literature regarding the efficacy of methenamine being bactericidal against *Proteus* species. *Proteus* is a urea-splitting organism producing ammonia from urea. Infections with *Proteus* are characterized by very alkaline urine, with pH values up to 9.5. Theoretically, methenamine would not generate formaldehyde in an alkaline medium. Andriole concludes that urinary tract infections with urea-splitting organisms such as *Proteus* species may not respond to methenamine in the absence of an acidic urine (7). One study recommends acetohydroxamine acid, an inhibitor of urease, to establish urinary acidity to promote therapeutic efficacy of methenamine when *Proteus* species is isolated from the urine (3). In a recent study in which spinal cord injury patients with positive urine cultures were treated with an appropriate antibiotic, according to the sensitivity of the microorganism(s), it was found that methenamine might have more potent suppressive antimicrobial activity against *Proteus* species than against some other bacteria (i.e., *Pseudomonas* and *Acinetobacter*) (8). These findings support previous observations by Hamilton-Miller and Brumf (9) and Pearman (10) that methenamine might have more potent antimicrobial activity against *Proteus* species than against other bacteria.

Banovac et al. utilized methenamine hippurate, 1 g twice daily, as a suppressive treatment. They had recurrent positive cultures in 23.4% of patients when methenamine was used as preventive therapy, compared to 57.5% recurrence rate in the control group, which received no suppressive therapy. Banovac et al.'s study was carried out in a rehabilitation hospital with a cohort of spinal cord injury patients. Table 2 lists the frequency of microorganisms isolated from these patients with recurrent bacteriuria after appropriate antibiotic therapy for an episode of acute urinary tract infection followed by suppressive therapy with methenamine. In addition to bacteria, there were four positive urine cultures (4%) in which the causative microorganism was *Candida* despite suppressive therapy with methenamine hippurate. The data from Table 2 emphasize the greater success in suppressing *Proteus* species and *Klebsiella* compared with *Acinetobacter* and *Pseudomonas*. There were no positive cultures for *Proteus* species following suppressive therapy with methenamine hippurate, while 8% of the control group that were not administered suppressive therapy were positive for *Proteus*. Differences in design of previous studies and patient population may explain the inconsistencies in reporting the effectiveness of methenamine in suppressing *Proteus* species.

Table 2 Frequency and Profile of Different Microorganisms in the Urine of Patients with Spinal Cord Injury

Microorganism	Methenamine group	Control group	*p*
Acinetobacter	11 (11.3%)	5 (3.3%)	<0.001
Candida	4 (4.0%)	2 (1.3%)	n.s.
Citrobacter	2 (2.0%)	1 (0.6%)	n.s.
Enterobacter	12 (12.4%)	8 (5.3%)	n.s.
Enterococcus	10 (10.3%)	17 (11.6%)	n.s.
Escherichia	16 (16.5%)	25 (16.6%)	n.s.
Klebsiella	8 (8.2%)	28 (18.6%)	<0.025
Proteus	0 —	12 (8.0%)	<0.005
Pseudomonas	23 (23.7%)	19 (12.6%)	<0.025
Serratia	1 (1.0%)	6 (4.0%)	n.s.
Staphylococcus	10 (10.3%)	20 (13.3%)	n.s.
Streptococcus	0 —	7 (4.7%)	<0.005
Total	97	150	

Statistical analysis by χ^2 test. n.s. = not significant
Source: Ref. 8.

It has been postulated that *Candida* and other fungi would be susceptible to the cidal action of formaldehyde (4,7). However, the results of studies of Banovac et al. (8) and Gandelman (11) raise questions as to the effectiveness of methenamine against fungi colonizing the lower urinary tract. The effectiveness of methenamine against mycobacteria is unknown.

IV. CLINICAL PHARMACOLOGY

Methenamine and the methenamine salts are well absorbed from the gastrointestinal tract. Ten to thirty percent of an oral dose of methenamine is hydrolyzed by gastric juices to formaldehyde and ammonia. If an enteric-coated tablet is ingested, the percentage of the amount of drugs hydrolyzed in the gastrointestinal tract and the rate and amount of absorption of the agent are reduced; drug absorption is reduced by 30% (3) (methenamine mandelate has an enteric-coated tablet available). The distribution of methenamine throughout the body parallels the distribution of total body water. Because most normal body fluids are physiologically neutral, blood, cerebrospinal fluid, aqueous and vitreous humors of the eye, saliva, bile, synovial and pericardial fluids will not sustain antibacterial effect from methenamine; formaldehyde should not be generated from methenamine in a neutral medium (4). In the first 24 h 70–90% or more of a single oral dose of methanamine, or one of its salts, is excreted intact in the urine by glomerular filtration and tubular secretion. Only about 20% of the methenamine that reaches the bladder is converted to free formaldehyde. Concentrations of formaldehyde are found in the bladder urine within 1–2 h of a single oral dose in a fasting healthy adult. If the enteric-coated methenamine mandelate is used, it may require 3–8 h after oral ingestion to reach peak urine levels of formaldehyde.

V. CLINICAL INDICATIONS

Methenamine was first used almost 100 years ago, in 1895, by Nicolaier for the treatment of urinary tract infections. In 1935 Rosenheim observed that mandelic acid is excreted in the urine unchanged and, when given in large doses, renders the urine bactericidal (7). This observation led to the development of the combination of methenamine with mandelic acid and hippurate. In elderly persons the only indication for methenamine and the methenamine salts is as chemoprophylaxis against or suppressive therapy of bacteria in the urine.

Chemoprophylaxis is for the prevention of bacteriuria using antimicrobial therapy and would be indicated for older persons who have frequent recurrent urinary infections due to reinfection. Chemoprophylaxis should be used when there is a relatively normal genitourinary tract and the absence of an indwelling catheter.

Suppressive therapy has been shown to be effective in preventing symptomatic disease by decreasing the concentration of organism(s) in the urine. Suppressive therapy does not imply rendering the urine sterile. However, if bacteriuria progresses to a symptomatic urinary tract infection and is successfully treated with organism-specific antibiotic therapy and the urine is rendered sterile, suppressive therapy would be appropriate in an attempt to provide a hostile environment for bacterial growth and possibly decreasing the incidence of acute recurrent urinary tract infections.

There is no indication for the use of methenamine or the methenamine salts in acute pyelonephritis or in an acute lower urinary tract infection. It takes a minimum of 1 h to generate free formaldehyde from methenamine. Peak concentrations may take up to 3 h in an acid medium. There would not be sufficient time for an infected foci of the kidneys or the calyces for the bacteria to be exposed to the free formaldehyde in a sufficient concentration to be bactericidal. For lower urinary tract infections the same principle is true with urine in the bladder. With irritative symptoms, e.g., urgency, frequency, and frequent nocturia, bladder emptying would occur, resulting in insufficient antibacterial concentrations and duration of formaldehyde in the bladder to reduce the number of invading microorganisms.

Older men with obstructive uropathy (e.g., prostatic enlargement) that may be the etiology of their asymptomatic bacteriuria, who are unable or refuse to undergo appropriate therapeutic procedures should be considered for treatment for up to 14 days with an appropriate antibiotic (12). If there is sterilization of the urine, chronic suppressive therapy with methenamine may be appropriate in an attempt to prevent bacteriuria or reduce the concentration of organisms.

Most of the literature discourages the use of methenamine and its compounds in patients with chronic indwelling catheters, as well as in intermittent catheterized patients (12,13). Patients who have urine continuously draining through an indwelling catheter would not generate formaldehyde in the bladder in sufficient concentrations to be bactericidal. Nor would there be adequate exposure time of the bacteria to formaldehyde (2 h) to be effective. This concept might be applicable to catheterized patients if one were to clamp the catheter and allow the urine to remain in the bladder until sufficient concentrations of formaldehyde have been generated and ample exposure of the bacteria to the formaldehyde has been adequately provided. However, such an approach would be labor intensive as well as creating a potential for excessively prolonged duration of formaldehyde in the bladder (if unclamping and drainage is delayed), which could result in chemical damage to bladder mucosa.

VI. ADMINISTRATION OF DRUG

Methenamine and the methenamine salts are administered orally. Methenamine mandelate (Mandelamine®) is available in tablet form, as an enteric-coated tablet, in an oral suspension or as 1-g granule packets, which are dissolved in water just prior to administration of the drug. For chronic suppressive therapy of bacteriuria in elderly patients, the recommended dose is 1 g four times a day. Methenamine hippurate (Hiprex® and Urex®) is available in 1-g tablets. The recommended dose of methenamine hippurate for the same purpose is 1 g twice a day.

VII. DRUG MONITORING AND ADVERSE EFFECTS

Other than for research purposes, there is no indication to monitor therapeutic urinary concentrations of free formaldehyde.

The most common side effects of methenamine and its salts have been minor gastrointestinal disturbances including nausea, vomiting, diarrhea, abdominal cramps, and anorexia. Headache, dyspnea, a generalized edema, tinnitus, muscle cramps, microscopic or gross hematuria all have on rare occasions been reported to be side effects from methenamine or its two salts. With protracted use or with higher dosages than normally recommended, formaldehyde can alter tissue proteins, causing local toxicity, which may lead to bladder irritation with dysuria, frequency, hematuria, and generalized bladder discomfort. Freeman et al. (14) reported that after 25 months of suppressive therapy with methenamine mandelate, 10 of 19 men had sterile urines in which antibiotic therapy was instituted for seemingly symptomatic infections. It was postulated that a number of the reported symptoms from the lower urinary tract were due to bladder irritation from protracted use of methenamine mandelate and the prolonged exposure of the bladder mucosa to free formaldehyde since cultures were negative. Overall side effects of methenamine and its salts have an incidence of 3.5% or less.

Methenamine may be contraindicated in elderly individuals with hepatic insufficiency or chronic alcohol abuse. Gastric acidity hydrolyzes 10–30% of methenamine in the stomach, releasing formaldehyde and ammonia. Elderly individuals with confusion and chronic bacteriuria may have their deteriorating mental status exacerbated by increasing plasma ammonia levels.

Older adults with gout should avoid methenamine and its salts because of the possibility of precipitating urate crystals in the urine. Also, patients with azotemia should avoid the methenamine salts; the acid salts may precipitate crystalluria. However, methenamine alone is not contraindicated in renal insufficiency. If the acidifying ability of the renal tubules still functions, these patients can hydrolyze methenamine to formaldehyde and ammonia.

Sulfamethizole, and possibly other sulfonamides, reacts with formaldehyde to form an insoluble precipitate in acid urine. Neither methenamine nor methenamine salts should be prescribed with the sulfonamides.

There is one report of two elderly nursing patients with dysphagia developing lipoid pneumonia after receiving methenamine mandelate suspension. Mandelamine suspension forte has an oil base (13).

REFERENCES

1. American Hospital Formulary Service: Drug Information. 1991, p. 458.
2. Musher DM, Griffith DP, Richie Y. The generation of formaldehyde from methenamine: effect of urinary flow and residual volume. Invest Urol 1976; 13:380–2.
3. Gleckman R, Alvarez S, Joubert DW, et al. Drug therapy reviews: methenamine mandelate and methenamine hippurate. Am J Hosp Pharm 1979; 34:1509–12.
4. Mayrer AR, Andriole VT. Urinary tract antiseptics. Med Clin North Am 1982; 66:199–208.
5. Boscia JA, Kaye D. Asymptomatic bacteriuria in the elderly. Infect Dis Clin North Am 1987; 1:893–905.
6. Tyreman NO, Andersson PO, Kroon L, et al. Urinary tract infection after vaginal surgery: effect of prophylactic treatment with methenamine hippurate. Acta Obstet Gynecol Scand 1986; 65:731–3.
7. Andriole VT. Urinary tract agents: quinolones, nitrofurantoin, and methenamine. In: Mandell GL, Douglas, Jr., RG, Bennett JE, eds. Principles and practice of infectious diseases. 2nd ed. New York: John Wiley and Sons, 1985:249–52.
8. Banovac K, Wade N, Gonzales F, et al. Decreased incidence of urinary tract infections in patients with spinal cord injury: effect of methenamine. J Am Paraplegia Soc 1991; 14:52–4.
9. Hamilton-Miller JMT, Brumfitt W. Methenamine and its salts as urinary tract antiseptics. Invest Urol 1977; 14:287–91.
10. Pearman JW. Prevention of urinary tract infection following spinal cord injury. Paraplegia 1971; 9:95–104.
11. Gandelman AL. Methenamine mandelate: antimicrobial activity in urine and correlation with formaldehyde levels. J Urol 1967; 97:533–6.
12. Yoshikawa TT, Norman DC. Aging and clinical practice: infectious diseases. Diagnosis and treatment. New York: Igaku-Shoin, 1987:178.
13. Timmerman RJ, Schroer JA. Lipoid pneumonia caused by methenamine mandelate suspension. JAMA 1973; 225:1524–5.
14. Freeman RB, Richardson JA, Thurm RH, et al. Long-term therapy for chronic bacteriuria in men. Ann Intern Med 1975; 83:133–47.

23

Antituberculosis Agents

Asim K. Dutt
Alvin C. York Veterans Affairs Medical Center, Murfreesboro, and Meharry Medical College, Nashville, Tennessee

Hope Marlow
Alvin C. York Veterans Affairs Medical Center, Murfreesboro, Tennessee

I. INTRODUCTION

Chemotherapy with antituberculosis drugs originated in 1944 with the discovery of streptomycin (SM) by Waksman and Associates (1) and the observations of Feldman and Hinshaw (2) that the drug was remarkably effective against tubercle bacilli. The introduction of isoniazid (INH) in 1952 made a major impact and set the stage for modern chemotherapy. The major problems of SM were its parenteral administration and high toxicity, which were unacceptable to many patients. Para-aminosalicylic acid (PAS) was used as an accompanying drug to INH, but its troublesome gastrointestinal side effects frequently caused patients to stop the drug and take INH alone, resulting in emergence of INH resistance. In 1968, ethambutol (EMB) was introduced to replace PAS, which reduced the problems of patient unacceptability and drug resistance. Although the cure rate was 90%, the therapy had to be given for 18–24 months, which made patient compliance difficult.

The introduction of rifampin (RIF) in the United States in 1971 revolutionized tuberculosis therapy. Several clinical trials confirmed the potency and efficacy of the combination of INH and RIF in curing tuberculosis in a relatively short period of time—the duration of therapy was shortened by half. During that time, pyrazinamide (PZA) was reintroduced in lower therapeutic doses to minimize its toxic effects. The drug potentiated the efficacy of INH and RIF combination to further reduce the duration of therapy to 6 months. At present, INH, RIF, and PZA are first-line drugs in the therapy of tuberculosis. Several other antituberculosis drugs are available, which are often bacteriostatic, less potent, and less toxic. They are second-line drugs employed mostly in the treatment of drug-resistant tuberculosis.

With the increasing incidence of *Mycobacterium avium* complex infections, particularly in acquired immunodeficiency syndrome (AIDS) patients, the list of antituberculosis drugs has expanded to include many newer drugs not commonly used for *Mycobacterium tuberculosis* infections. The quinolones, macrolides, azalides, and amikacin have proven useful in the treatment of *M. avium* complex infections. The major properties of antituberculosis drugs are summarized in Table 1.

II. ISONIAZID

Isonicotinic acid hydrazide (INH) remains the most effective and important antimycobacterial drug in use today. The drug has high bactericidal activity, very low toxicity, and high patient acceptability. INH is the cornerstone of modern chemotherapy for tuberculosis.

A. Chemistry and Mechanism of Action

INH is a hydrazide of isonicotinic acid. It inhibits the synthesis of mycolic acid and its incorporation into cell walls (3). The action is both bacteriostatic and bactericidal. Resistance occurs with the loss of the active uptake mechanism for isoniazid by tubercle bacilli. A recent study indicates that INH resistance is due to deletion of the catalase-peroxidase gene from the chromosome of *M. tuberculosis*, which is a discovery with exciting potential for newer therapeutic approaches (4).

B. Antimicrobial Spectrum

Isoniazid is highly active against *M. tuberculosis* (5). The drug kills both actively multiplying extracellular bacilli and slowly or intermittently replicating intracellular organisms as well as those in closed caseous lesions. *M. kansasii* (5) and *M. xenopi* (6) are generally susceptible. Many strains of *M. avium* complex are resistant, but some are moderately susceptible (7).

C. Clinical Pharmacology

INH is well absorbed orally. It is primarily metabolized by undergoing acetylation in the liver, the metabolite being excreted in the urine. There is a genetic variation in the rate of acetylation, both slow and fast. Clinically significant changes in serum levels occur with fast acetylators undergoing intermittent therapy (8,9). Age is not a factor in the acetylator phenotype of an individual (9). However, in one study, total body clearance in slow acetylators decreased significantly with age, as did the volume of distribution of the drug (9a). INH is distributed in all body fluids and tissues, including the central nervous system (CNS). It readily penetrates caseous tissues and macrophages. INH crosses the placenta and is excreted into milk. Protein binding is low. Hepatic metabolism is the primary means of elimination of INH with excretion of metabolites in the urine (8,9).

INH inhibits the metabolism of carbamazepine and phenytoin causing clinically significant increases in serum levels. These anticonvulsants are not infrequently prescribed for older patients. Serum levels should therefore be carefully monitored when either of these drugs and INH are given together. Coordination difficulties and psychotic episodes occur when INH and disulfiram are used together, probably due to altered dopamine metabolism. Antacids interfere with the absorption of INH and should be given at least 1 h after the dose of INH (10).

D. Administration of Drug

Most elderly patients without severe renal or hepatic disease should receive the standard dose regimen of INH that is reasonable for adults. The usual adult dose is 5 mg/kg/day,

Table 1 Antituberculosis Drugs: Dosage, Side Effects, and Mode of Action

Drug	Dosage: Daily	Dosage: Twice weekly	Side effects	Mode of action
Bactericidal drugs				
Streptomycin and other aminoglycosides	10–15 mg/kg (usually 0.5–1.0 g) 5 days/week IM	20–25 mg/kg (usually 1.0–1.5 g) IM	Cranial nerve VIII damage (vestibular and auditory) nephrotoxicity, allergic fever, rash	Active against rapidly multiplying bacilli in neutral or slightly alkaline extracellular medium
Capreomycin	Same as above	Same as above	Same as above	Same as above
Isoniazid (INH)	5 mg/kg (usually 300 mg) PO or IM	15 mg/kg (usually 900 mg) PO	Peripheral neuritis, hepatotoxicity, allergic fever and rash, lupus erythematosus phenomenon	Acts strongly on rapidly dividing extracellular bacilli; acts weakly on slowly multiplying intracellular bacilli
Rifampin (RIF)	10 mg/kg (usually 450–600 mg) PO	10 mg/kg (usually 450–600 mg) PO	Hepatotoxicity, nausea and vomiting, allergic fever and rash, flulike syndrome, petechiae with thrombocytopenia or acute renal failure during intermittent therapy	Acts on both rapidly and slowly multiplying bacilli either extracellular or intracellular, particularly on slowly multiplying "persisters"
Rifabutin (Ansamycin)	150–300 mg PO		Same as above	Same as above
Pyrazinamide (PZA)	25–30 mg/kg (usually 2.5 g) PO	45–50 mg/kg (usually 3.0–3.5 mg) PO	Hyperuricemia, hepatotoxicity, allergic fever and rash	Active in acid pH medium on intracellular bacilli
Ethambutol (EMB)	15–25 mg/kg (usually 800–1600 mg) PO	50 mg/kg PO	Optic neuritis, skin rash, hyperuricemia	Weakly active against both extracellular and intracellular bacilli to inhibit the development of resistant bacilli
Bacteriostatic drugs				
Ethionamide	10–15 mg/kg (usually 500–750 mg) in divided doses PO	Not used	Nausea, vomiting, anorexia, allergic fever and rash, hepatotoxic, neurotoxic	Same as above
Cycloserine	15–20 mg/kg (usually 0.75–1.0 g) in divided doses with 200 mg of pyridoxine PO	Not used	Personality changes, psychosis, convulsions, rash	Same as above
Para-aminosalicyclic acid (PAS)	150 mg/kg (usually 12 g) in divided doses PO	Not used	Nausea, vomiting, diarrhea, hepatotoxicity, allergic rash and fever	Weak action on extracellular bacilli; inhibits development of drug-resistant organisms
Thiacetazone (not available in the United States)	150 mg daily PO	Not used	Allergic rash and fever, Stevens-Johnson syndrome, blood disorders, nausea and vomiting	Same as above
Clofazimine (antileprosy)	100 mg tid, PO	Not used	Pigmentation of skin, abdominal pain	Against *Mycobacterium intracellulare*

Table 1 Continued

Drug	Dosage		Side effects	Mode of action
	Daily	Twice weekly		
Newer agents				
Ofloxacin	400 mg q 12	Not used	Gastrointestinal: diarrhea, nausea, abdominal pain, anorexia CNS effects: dizziness, restlessness, nightmares, ataxia, seizures	Rapidly multiplying bacilli at neutral or alkaline pH
Ciprofloxacin	750 mg q 12	Not used	Same as above	Same as above
Azithromycin	500 mg/day for up to 30 days	Not used	Gastrointestinal: diarrhea, nausea, abdominal pain, elevation of liver enzymes	Rapidly multiplying bacilli in macrophages, against *M. intracellulare*
Clarithromycin	1 g q 12	Not used	Same as above	Same as above

IM = intramuscular; PO = oral.

up to 300 mg taken as a single dose. For intermittent twice-weekly administration, the dose of INH is increased to 900 mg. The prophylactic dose for tuberculosis is 300 mg/day, which can also be given twice weekly in 900-mg doses. The drug is available parenterally in 100 mg/ml vials and in tablets of 50, 100, and 300 mg. A liquid form of 50 mg/5 ml is also available. The drug is usually given orally but can be given by intramuscular (IM) injection. Combination tablets containing 150 mg RIF and 300 mg INH (Rifamate) are strongly recommended when both drugs are prescribed for treatment.

E. Drug Monitoring and Adverse Effects

Approximately 10% of patients on INH therapy develop abnormalities of liver function tests. Only 1–3%, however, develop clinical hepatitis, which in some instances may lead to jaundice and hepatic failure and on rare occasions to death. INH and RIF given together may increase the incidence of hepatotoxicity, the effect being additive, not synergistic (11). Elderly patients are at increased risk for hepatotoxicity (6).

Neurotoxicity is a result of pyridoxine deficiency due to inhibition of pyridoxine metabolism by INH. It is uncommon in patients treated with recommended doses. Elderly, alcoholic, malnourished, or pregnant patients and patients with cancer, uremia, or chronic liver disease are at increased risk of neurotoxicity and should receive pyridoxine supplementation (10). Peripheral neuritis is the most common form of neurotoxicity. More serious effects of optic neuritis, seizures, toxic encephalopathy, and mental impairment are rare (10).

Other uncommon adverse effects are hypersensitivity reactions of rash, fever, lymphadenopathy, vasculitis, and lupus erythematosus phenomenon. The hematological effects of anemia, agranulocytosis, thrombocytopenia, and eosinophilia are rare.

III. RIFAMPIN (RIFADIN)

RIF was introduced in the late 1960s and made a major impact on the chemotherapy of tuberculosis and other mycobacterial diseases. The drug has high bactericidal activity. In combination with INH, therapy of tuberculosis with RIF is very effective, and the duration of the disease is shortened.

A. Chemistry and Mechanism of Action

The rifamycins were isolated from the microorganism *Nocardia mediterranci*. Rifamycin B was modified to produce RIF. The chemical name is 3-4(4-methylpiperazinyl-iminomethylidine)-rifamycin SV (9).

RIF inhibits bacterial DNA-dependent RNA polymerase, the enzyme responsible for DNA transcription. The action is bactericidal. RIF penetrates cell membranes and kills intracellular organisms. Resistance occurs with decreased binding to the polymerase due to structural changes in RNA polymerase or decreased cellular permeability (12).

B. Antimicrobial Spectrum

M. tuberculosis is very susceptible to RIF (5). Other mycobacteria that are often susceptible are *M. avium* complex, *M. kansasii*, *M. scrofulaceum*, and *M. xenopi* (5,13).

C. Clinical Pharmacology

RIF is well absorbed (75–80%) from the gastrointestinal (GI) tract with a peak level of 4–32 μg/ml occurring in 2–4 h. RIF is lipid soluble and penetrates well into most tissues. Levels greater than serum concentrations are found in the liver, lung, ascitic fluid, pleural effusion, wall of the stomach, and in bone. With inflamed meninges, therapeutic levels are obtained in the central nervous system. Significant levels are found in tears, saliva, and vitreous humor. RIF is metabolized in the liver by undergoing deacetylation to form the less active desacetylrifampin metabolite. Both RIF and its metabolite are excreted in the bile. The half-life is 2–3 h. RIF induces liver enzymes, which increases its own metabolism and decreases serum level. It is approximately 80% protein bound (9).

The pharmacokinetics of RIF has been studied in six elderly subjects aged 78–95 years (13a). The maximal plasma concentration and elimination half-lives of both RIF and desacetylrifampin were comparable to those reported in younger adults. However, renal excretion of RIF and its metabolite were reduced in elderly subjects, most likely because of decreased renal function in these individuals. It is probable that excretion of RIF and desacetylrifampin is enhanced through the liver in these elderly subjects since the plasma concentration, half-lives, and total drug clearances did not change with age (13a).

RIF, a potent inducer of hepatic P-450 oxidative enzymes, causes clinically significant drug interactions—many of these drugs are frequently prescribed in older adults. Those of clinical significance include oral anticoagulants, digitoxin, cyclosporine, glucocorticoids, ketoconazole, methadone, phenytoin, quinidine, theophylline, and verapamil. Other clinically significant drug interactions are with beta-blockers, chloramphenicol, sulfonylureas, haloperidol, antiarrhythmics (tocainide and disopyramide), and calcium channel blockers (nifedipine and diltiazem) (14).

D. Administration of Drug

The recommended dose of RIF for patients weighing 50 kg or more is 600 mg (in single dose before breakfast) or 450 mg for patients weighing less than 50 kg (9). The same dose is recommended for twice-weekly administration. There is no evidence that a reduction in dose is necessary in elderly patients (13a). Food decreases the oral absorption and serum level of RIF (10). The oral form is available in 150-mg and 300-mg capsules. Parenteral RIF is also available in 600-mg vials.

E. Drug Monitoring and Adverse Effects

RIF is generally well tolerated with low incidence of adverse effects in both young and older adults. Common side effects are nausea and vomiting and hypersensitivity reactions of rash and fever. Another hypersensitivity reaction, the "cutaneous syndrome," causes flushing and/or itching with or without a rash. Redness and watering of eyes may also occur. Other GI effects include anorexia, abdominal pain, and diarrhea. Severe GI side effects may require withdrawal of the drug (10,15).

Hepatitis is an uncommon but serious adverse effect of RIF. Use of RIF with INH may increase the hepatotoxicity of either drug. Despite mild and transient abnormalities in liver function tests, which commonly occur early in the course of RIF treatment, the risk of hepatitis is low (10,15). The relationship of age and risk of RIF-induced hepatic has not been described.

Intermittent administration of RIF may cause hepatorenal syndrome and a "flulike" syndrome. The hepatorenal syndrome consists of a sudden onset of fever and lumbar pain followed by oliguria and later anuria. The anuria may last for several days, but recovery is usual. The "flulike" syndrome consists of fever, headache, malaise, and bone pain shortly after a dose of RIF with symptoms disappearing several hours later. Intermittent RIF may give rise to thrombocytopenia and petechiae due to immunological reaction, which occurs more often with dose of the drug higher than 600 mg. A less common respiratory syndrome of dyspnea with and without wheezing also occurs with intermittent therapy. Shock may be associated with this syndrome (10,15).

RIF causes a reddish color in the urine, sputum, sweat, and other body fluids. With overdoses, the skin and other tissue may turn pink. This is referred to as "red man syndrome" (10,15).

IV. RIFABUTIN (ANSAMYCIN)

A. Chemistry and Mechanism of Action

Rifabutin is a spiropiperidyl derivative of rifamycin S similar in structure and activity to rifampin (16). The drug inhibits DNA-dependent RNA polymerase. It may also inhibit DNA synthesis. The action is bactericidal (16).

B. Antimicrobial Spectrum

Rifabutin is more active than rifampin against *M. tuberculosis* (16). It also has activity against *M. kansasii* (17) and *M. fortuitum* (18). It is effective against 70–80% of *M. avium* complex bacilli (19). The activity is attributed to its lipophilic properties and its ability to penetrate *M. avium* complex cell walls (16). A particularly useful property of rifabutin when treating mycobacterial infections in AIDS patients is the drug's ability to inhibit replication of human immunodeficiency virus (HIV) at achievable serum concentrations (16). There is cross-resistance with rifampin (16,17).

C. Clinical Pharmacology

Oral absorption is 12–20%. Peak levels are reached in 3–4 h. The drug is well distributed to all tissues, with levels greater than serum levels found in the lungs, bile, and urine.

The half-life is 16 h, and protein binding is 71%. The volume of distribution is very large at 8–9 L/kg. The drug is metabolized to an active 25-deacetyl derivative, which is excreted in high concentration in the urine. Approximately 44% of the drug and its metabolite are excreted in urine, the rest being excreted in feces (16,18). Little is known about the impact of age on the pharmacokinetics of rifabutin.

D. Administration of Drug

The usual dose of rifabutin is 150–300 mg/day (16). At this time, it would be reasonable to give older adults the same dose.

E. Drug Monitoring and Adverse Effects

The most frequently reported side effects are hepatotoxicity and hematological changes (neutropenia and thrombocytopenia). Hypersensitivity reactions and GI disturbance also occur (16).

V. PYRAZINAMIDE

Pyrazinamide (PZA) was enthusiastically used in the early 1960s for treatment of tuberculosis. However, it was soon abandoned because of excessive side effects as a result of the high dosage (50–75 mg/kg) prescribed at that time. PZA was reintroduced in the 1970s in lower doses to become the third most important drug used in tuberculosis chemotherapy today. It has the capacity to further reduce the duration of chemotherapy when used in combination with other potent bactericidal drugs (INH and RIF).

A. Chemistry and Mechanism of Action

PZA (pyrazinoic acid amide) is a derivative of nicotinamide. It is converted by the amidase activity present in the mycobacteria to the active drug pyrazinoic acid (20). The drug easily penetrates the cell wall of macrophages, where it is highly active against phagocytosed tubercle bacilli in the acid intracellular milieu. It is a bactericidal drug.

B. Antimicrobial Spectrum

The action of PZA is specific for *M. tuberculosis. M. avium* complex is generally resistant, and the drug is not effective in the treatment of infections caused by this organism.

C. Clinical Pharmacology

PZA is rapidly and completely absorbed from the GI tract after oral administration. It distributes well into lungs, liver, and kidneys, with peak level occurring in about 2 h. Therapeutic levels are obtained in the CNS. The drug is hydrolyzed in the liver to its active metabolite pyrazinoic acid. Less than 5% is excreted unchanged in the urine. Renal tubular reabsorption of the unchanged drug is high. The half-life is 9–10 h, and protein binding is 50% (9). Although pharmacokinetic data on PZA and aging are not available, it would appear that because the drug is metabolized primarily by the liver, age should not have a major impact on drug levels and clearance.

D. Administration of Drug

The usual dose is 25–30 mg/kg given once a day. For intermittent twice-weekly therapy, the dose is increased to 45–50 mg/kg/day (3). It is available in 500-mg tablets.

E. Drug Monitoring and Adverse Effects

PZA is a hepatotoxic drug. With the use of lower doses and shorter duration of therapy, hepatotoxicity is rare (10). It has become a first-line drug in tuberculosis chemotherapy. Transient abnormalities in liver function tests are common early in the course of therapy, which do not require discontinuance of therapy unless symptomatic. Although elderly patients are at greater risk, routine biochemical monitoring is not necessary without other risk factors (10). However, other authors have recommended routine monitoring of liver function tests in older patients receiving INH, RIF, and/or PZA (20a,20b).

Up to 40% of patients experience hyperuricemia as a result of the inhibition of urate excretion by PZA. Arthralgia occurs in 7–10% of patients. Acute gout is rare (20).

Photosensitivity, hematological side effects, and hypersensitivity reactions are rare. Flushing is sometimes troublesome. GI side effects of anorexia, nausea, and vomiting may occur.

VI. AMINOGLYCOSIDES: STREPTOMYCIN, KANAMYCIN, AND AMIKACIN

The discovery of streptomycin SM in 1944 was a landmark in the history of chemotherapy for tuberculosis. For many years, SM and INH were the primary therapeutic agents in the therapy of tuberculosis. With the introduction of RIF and PZA the importance of SM has decreased, mostly due to its side effects and need for parenteral administration. Although it is a "powerful" antimycobacterial agent, it is currently available only through the Centers for Disease Control and Prevention (CDC) in the United States.

A. Chemistry and Mechanism of Action

The aminoglycosides are amino sugars in glycoside linkages. They inhibit protein synthesis. They are rapidly bactericidal. Their action depends on their transport into the cell across cell membrane. The transport of aminoglycosides is inhibited by low pH, with the active process requiring oxygen (21). The drugs are active in neutral or slightly alkaline medium. (See also Chap. 13.)

There are three mechanisms by which bacteria are resistant or acquire resistance to the aminoglycoside. The most common and important cause of acquired resistance is the plasmid-mediated enzymatic inactivation of the antibiotic by acetylation, adenylation, and phosphorylation (21). Amikacin is the least likely to acquire resistance by this mechanism, as it only undergoes acetylation (21). A second mechanism for resistance is low affinity for the ribosomes in the cell of the bacteria. This may occur as a result of a change in structure of the ribosome, as is the case with SM. Binding of SM only occurs at the 30S ribosome. Kanamycin, amikacin, and other aminoglycosides bind to multiple sites on the ribosomes including the 50S ribosome and hence do not exhibit this type of resistance (21). The third method involves changes in permeability of the drug and decreased transport into the cell. Anaerobic bacteria are resistant to the aminoglycosides because their environment lacks oxygen necessary for the transport of the aminoglycoside across cell membranes (21).

B. Antimicrobial Spectrum

M. tuberculosis is very susceptible to SM (22), as are some strains of *M. kansaii* (17). Other strains showing susceptibility to SM are *M. malmoense* (23), *M. scrofulaceum* (5), and *M. xenopi* (6). Approximately one-third of *M. avium* complex strains tested are susceptible to SM (7,22).

M. tuberculosis (22), *M. marinum* (24), and most strains of *M. kanasasii* (17), *M. fortuitum* (5), and some strains of *M. chelonae* (5) are susceptible to amikacin. *M. avium* complex is sometimes susceptible. Amikacin has been used for treating these infections (22,25).

M. tuberculosis (22), *M. marinum* (24), and *M. chelonei* (26) are usually susceptible to kanamycin, whereas *M. fortuitum* is moderately susceptible (26). Kanamycin is moderately active against *M. avium* complex in approximately one-third of the strains tested (7,21).

C. Clinical Pharmacology

Poor oral absorption of aminoglycosides requires their parenteral administration. The volume of distribution of aminoglycosides is approximately equal to 25% of body weight in kilograms; distribution in intravascular spaces is rapid. Good penetration of the drugs into the walls of tuberculous abscesses provides adequate levels, even in caseous tissue. Urine levels can be 100 or more times the serum level (9). Aminoglycoside levels reached in respiratory secretions are low, but therapeutic levels in pleural fluid are attained after repeated administration (27). Inadequate levels are achieved in purulent fluid of low pH. Aminoglycosides penetrate the cerebrospinal fluid (CSF) very poorly, even with inflamed meninges. Protein binding is low. Aminoglycosides are excreted unchanged in the urine with the exception of SM, which undergoes some metabolism. Clearance of the drugs is reduced in elderly patients, even those with normal creatinine levels (9). However, in healthy elderly subjects with normal creatinine clearances, studies of gentamicin, tobramycin, and amikacin showed no influence of age on the pharmacokinetics of aminoglycosides (27a).

D. Administration of Drug

All aminoglycosides must be given by the parenteral route.

Streptomycin: The usual dose is 1 g daily (15 mg/kg/day) as a single dose. Individual dosing with monitoring of serum levels provides for optimum dosing regimens. In elderly patients the dosage should not exceed 0.5–0.75 g 5 days a week. The drug may also be given twice weekly. Dosing adjustment must be made with renal impairment. Doses may be decreased or dosing interval prolonged. Streptomycin is usually given by deep IM injections.

Amikacin: The usual dosage is 15 mg/kg/day given as divided doses every 8 or 12 h. Peak and trough levels of amikacin should be drawn to adjust the dosage, as there is considerable interpatient variations. A peak level of 20–30 μg/ml and a trough level up to 10 μg/ml are considered therapeutic. Dosing adjustments must be made for renal impairment, preferably by prolongation of the dosing interval. The drug is available for intravenous (IV) infusion or IM injections in 100 mg/2 ml, 500 mg/2 ml, and 1 g/4 ml vials.

Kanamycin: The usual adult dose is 15 mg/kg/day in divided doses. Dosing adjustments must be made for renal impairment. Kanamycin is available in 250 mg/ml, 500 mg/ml and 1000 mg/3 ml vials for deep IM injections or IV infusion.

E. Drug Monitoring and Adverse Effects

All aminoglycosides share three toxicities: nephrotoxicity, ototoxicity, and neuromuscular blockade. The latter, which can cause acute muscular paralysis and apnea, is now quite rare since the effect is well known and the precipitating factors are avoided, which include judicious use of anesthetics, eliminating other neuromuscular blocking agents and avoiding administration of large doses into body cavities. The neuromuscular effects are reversed by the administration of calcium (28).

Ototoxicity occurs with all aminoglycosides, and is enhanced by prolonged high levels of the drug and co-administration of other ototoxic drugs such as ethacrynic acid. Ototoxicity is primarily vestibular with SM, while that of amikacin and kanamycin is hearing loss. Elderly patients are at increased risk of the ototoxic effects of these drugs (10).

Nephrotoxicity of the aminoglycosides involves acute tubular necrosis. The toxicity is generally reversible with regeneration of renal cells after withdrawal of the drug. However, permanent damage and loss of function can occur (10). Nephrotoxicity is increased by the co-administration of other nephrotoxic drugs, such as vancomycin and amphotericin B. Other factors increasing the toxicity are prolonged therapy, high trough concentrations, high daily doses, age, shock with oliguria, and preexisting renal disease (29).

Streptomycin: Rash, eosinophilia, and drug fever are common hypersensitivity reactions. However, exfoliative dermatitis, angioedema, and blood dyscrasias do occur. Anaphylactic shock is rare.

Amikacin: Hypersensitive reactions are rare. Other uncommon reactions are tremor, headache, nausea and vomiting, paresthesia, anemia, and mild abnormalities in liver function tests.

Kanamycin: Uncommon neurological side effects are blurred vision, paresthesias, acute brain syndrome, restlessness, headaches, and tachycardia. Hypersensitivity reactions are rare, eosinophilia being the most frequently reported reaction (30).

VII. CAPREOMYCIN

Capreomycin is a bactericidal antimycobacterial drug. It is mainly used to replace SM in treatment when organisms are resistant to the drug.

A. Chemistry and Mechanism of Action

Capreomycin is a cyclic polypeptide. The mechanism of action is unknown. It is bactericidal to extracellular bacilli in neutral or slightly alkaline pH medium of tuberculous cavities.

B. Antimicrobial Spectrum

Capreomycin is used for *M. tuberculosis* infections (10). *M. kansasii* is also sensitive to the drug (31). Viomycin, kanamycin, and SM show cross-resistance to capreomycin. The drug is used mostly in drug-resistant tuberculosis.

C. Clinical Pharmacology

Capreomycin is poorly absorbed orally. A peak level is attained 1–2 h after IM injection. Protein binding and drug distribution of the drug are unknown. It does not reach therapeutic levels in the CNS. Approximately 50–60% of capreomycin is excreted unchanged in the urine. Some is excreted in the bile. The half-life ranges from 10–20 h (9). Adequate pharmacokinetic data of capreomycin in elderly persons is not available. Because the drug is excreted primarily by renal mechanisms, the clearance of capreomycin may be reduced in older patients with altered renal function.

D. Administration of Drug

Capreomycin is given by deep IM injection. The usual dose is 15–20 mg/kg up to 1 g per day. The dose is adjusted for age, with 1 g daily for patients under 50 years, 0.75 g for 50–59 years, and 0.5 g for patients older than 60 years (32). Dosing adjustment must be made in renal failure. Patients undergoing hemodialysis should receive reduced doses at 5- to 7-day intervals. The drug is available in 1-g vials.

E. Drug Monitoring and Adverse Effects

Nephrotoxicity is a serious adverse effect of capreomycin, particularly in older adults, who frequently already have reduced renal function. If blood urea nitrogen (BUN) and serum creatinine concentrations rise or creatinine clearance decreases, the drug should be discontinued. The renal toxicity is usually reversible. Tubular dysfunction may give rise to alkalosis, hypokalemia, hypocalcemia, or hypomagnesemia. These deficiencies may cause lethargy, muscle weakness, and tetany. Electrolytes should be monitored (32).

Ototoxicity, both auditory and vestibular, occurs with capreomycin. Tinnitus, hearing loss, and vertigo occur, but deafness is rare. Elderly patients are at increased risk of ototoxicity (32,33).

Hematological effects are rare except for eosinophilia, which may occur in approximately 5% of patients (33). Hypersensitivity reactions are rare. Rash, fever, and photosensitivity have occurred (33).

VIII. ETHAMBUTOL

Ethambutol (EMB) in the early 1960s replaced the use of the para-aminosalicylic acid (PAS), a drug with considerable side effects. The use of EMB improved patient acceptability of antituberculosis therapy. In low doses (15 mg/kg) the drug prevents emergence of drug-resistant organisms, but in high doses (25 mg/kg) EMB is bactericidal, which contributes to shortening the duration of therapy.

A. Chemistry and Mechanism of Action

EMB is a synthetic compound. Its chemical name is dextro-2,2′-(ethylenediimino)-di-1-butanol dihydrochloride.

EMB inhibits the incorporation of mycolic acid into cell walls. Its action is weakly bactericidal (34).

B. Antimicrobial Spectrum

M. tuberculosis (8) is highly susceptible to EMB, as well as most strains of *M. kansasii* (5), *M. scrofulaceum* (5), *M. malmoense* (23), and *M. marinum* (35). Some strains of *M. avium* complex are also susceptible to EMB (25).

C. Clinical Pharmacology

Approximately 75–80% of EMB is rapidly absorbed from the GI tract after an oral dose. It distributes well into all tissues and fluids. EMB crosses the placenta and is excreted into milk, but its CNS penetration is poor. However, high doses (25 mg/kg/day) can achieve therapeutic levels in patients with meningitis. About 20% of EMB is metabolized in the liver, with approximately 60% excreted unchanged in the urine. Renal failure greatly increases the 4-h half-life (9). The pharmacokinetics of EMB is not well understood in elderly persons because of the paucity of data.

D. Administration of Drug

The recommended dose of EMB is 15–25 mg/kg daily. It is bactericidal in high doses (25 mg/kg) and bacteriostatic at low doses (15 mg/kg). The drug is available in 100- and 400-mg tablets. Dosing adjustments must be made for renal failure. In patients requiring hemodialysis the dose should be reduced to 5 mg/kg/day (36). Because of the high prevalence of renal dysfunction and visual impairment in older adults (see next section), the benefits of EMB in elderly patients must be weighed against its risks (36a).

E. Drug Monitoring and Adverse Effects

Optic neuritis is the most important side effect of EMB, and it appears to be dose related. The side effect is experienced in 15% of patients on 50 mg/kg/day, 5% of patients on 25 mg/kg/day, and less than 1% on 15 mg/kg/day. The symptoms are decreased visual acuity, central and peripheral scotomas, and color blindness (loss of red-green discrimination). Regular eye examinations are essential for elderly patients during therapy. The eye effects are reversible if the drug is stopped early. Full recovery may take months, or permanent impairment of vision may occur (10).

Hypersensitivity reactions of rash, fever, pruritus, and joint pain are rare. GI effects are few and uncommon. Neurological effects of mental confusion, disorientation, dizziness, and peripheral neuropathy have occurred, but rarely. An increase in uric acid level in the serum is common (10).

IX. ETHIONAMIDE

Ethionamide is mainly a second-line drug for retreatment of drug-resistant tuberculosis. The drug may be included in the multidrug regimens for treatment of *M. avium* complex disease.

A. Chemistry and Mechanism of Action

Ethionamide is a derivative of isonicotinic acid. It inhibits mycolic acid synthesis and, hence, its incorporation into cell walls (34). Depending on the dose and the sensitivity of the organism, ethionamide may be bacteriostatic or bactericidal. Except for thiacetazone, cross-resistance of ethionamide to other tuberculosis agents is rare (34).

B. Antimicrobial Spectrum

Ethionamide is active against *M. tuberculosis* and *M. leprae* (34). Many strains of *M. avium* complex (37) have shown substantial susceptibility to the drug. Other mycobacteria such as *M. kansasii* (5), *M. simiae* (38), *M. asiaticum* (39), *M. malmoense* (23), and *M. xenopi* (6) are also susceptible to ethionamide.

C. Clinical Pharmacology

Ethionamide is well absorbed orally, reaching a peak in 2–3 h. It is widely distributed into all tissues and fluids of the body, including the CNS. The drug is nearly 100% metabolized in the liver. Ethionamide sulfoxide is an active metabolite, which is further metabolized to an inactive form (9). The effect of age on the pharmacokinetics of ethionamide is unknown.

D. Administration of Drug

The recommended dose is 500–1000 mg daily, given in divided doses two to four times a day. Patients seldom tolerate a 1000-mg dose due to excessive GI side effects. Because of potential serious side effects, ethionamide should be prescribed in elderly patients only if there are no alternative drugs available.

E. Drug Monitoring and Adverse Effects

Many of adverse effects of ethionamide (GI and neurological side effects) may be particularly devastating to older patients, especially those who are frail and/or have multiple chronic conditions. Careful monitoring is essential. GI effects are common, resulting in frequent discontinuation of the drug. Such effects include anorexia, nausea, abdominal pain, vomiting, diarrhea, and excessive salivation (10). The drug has a garliclike taste. These effects are dose related, the frequency and severity decrease with lower doses. Administration of the drug with the main meal or just prior to retiring may decrease the GI effects.

Neurotoxicity such as depression, psychosis, anxiety, headache, and drowsiness may occur. Less frequently, optic neuritis, seizures, and a pellagralike encephalopathy are seen. Vitamin B complexes may decrease these adverse effects. Olfactory disturbances, tremors, blurred vision, and diplopia can occur (10).

Hepatotoxicity occurs in less than 5% of patients. The liver damage may occur more often in patients with diabetes mellitus, and thus the diabetes may be more difficult to manage. Hypersensitive reactions include rash, photosensitivity, and thrombocytopenia. Goiter and hypothyroidism have occurred (10). Incidences of impotence, gynecomastia, and menorrhagia have been reported.

X. CYCLOSERINE

Cycloserine is mostly used as a bacteriostatic companion to other drugs in retreatment regimens for drug-resistant tuberculosis. It has also gained a place in treatment of nontuberculous mycobacterial diseases.

A. Chemistry and Mechanism of Action

Cycloserine is a synthetic analog of d-alanine. It inhibits the incorporation of d-alanine into cell walls. The action is bacteriostatic (40). Resistance is a result of decreased uptake of cycloserine into cells.

B. Antimicrobial Spectrum

Cycloserine is effective against *M. tuberculosis*. It is used when organisms have become resistant to other drugs. The drug also has activity against *M. kansasii* (41), *M. xenopi* (6), *M. simiae* (38), and *M. asiaticum* (39). Some strains of *M. marinum* (42), and *M. avium* complex are also susceptible to cycloserine (37,41).

C. Clinical Pharmacology

Cycloserine is well absorbed orally. Distribution into body tissues and fluids is extensive, including therapeutic levels in the CNS. It crosses the placenta and is excreted into milk. The half-life of cycloserine ranges between 10 and 25 h. Cycloserine undergoes almost no protein binding. The drug is primarily excreted (50–70%) unchanged in the urine (9). Little is known of the pharmacology of cycloserine in geriatric patients.

D. Administration of Drug

The usual dose is 500–1000 mg per day usually divided into an every 6- to 12-h schedule. The total daily dose should not exceed 1 g. Pyridoxine 200–300 mg per day is recommended to decrease the incidence of neurotoxicity. Cycloserine is available in 250-mg capsules. Dosing adjustments are necessary for renal impairment. Like ethionamide, careful evaluation should be made before prescribing cycloserine to older patients.

E. Monitoring and Adverse Effects

Neurotoxicity is the most common and important adverse effect of cycloserine. Depression, nervousness, irritability, anxiety, confusion with disorientation, memory loss, and psychotic states are some of the symptoms. Seizures occur in up to 8% of patients taking the drug. Other manifestation of the CNS effects include headache, dizziness, lethargy, vertigo, and visual disturbances. The drug should be avoided in patients with mental instability or epilepsy. Monitoring serum level to keep level below 30 μg/ml is recommended. High-risk patients include those with renal dysfunction and CNS disease (10). Elderly patients are at high risk for experiencing the neuropsychiatric adverse effects of cycloserine. Therefore, not only should careful assessment of the risks and benefits of cycloserine be made in older patients, appropriate patient selection for treatment and careful monitoring are essential.

Rarely, hypersensitivity reactions including rash and photosensitivity may occur. Electrolyte abnormalities (hypocalcemia and hypomagnesia) and cardiac arrhythmias have occurred occasionally.

XI. PARA-AMINOSALICYLIC ACID

In the past para-aminosalicylic acid (PAS) was frequently used for the treatment of tuberculosis. The drug was poorly tolerated due to its side effects. Its use has been abandoned due to availability of more potent drugs. PAS is now limited to treatment of drug-resistant tuberculosis. The drug is available only through the CDC.

A. Chemistry and Mechanism of Action

PAS is a structural analog of para-aminobenzoic acid. A competitive antagonist of *p*-aminobenzoic acid, PAS inhibits *p*-aminobenzoic acid's reaction with dihydropteroic acid to form folic acid. DNA synthesis is thereby blocked, folic acid being essential for its synthesis. Its action is bacteriostatic (8).

B. Antimicrobial Spectrum

M. tuberculosis is susceptible to PAS. As a bacteriostatic drug PAS prevents development of drug resistance when used with other drugs. Nontuberculous mycobacteria are generally resistant (5).

C. Clinical Pharmacology

PAS is available only in an oral preparation. It is readily absorbed in the GI tract and undergoes acetylation in the liver. It is well distributed into body fluids including the pleural fluid and caseous tissue but has very poor CNS penetration. Protein binding is approximately 15% (9). The half-life is only 1 h (8). Greater than 40% is excreted in the urine as the acetyl metabolite, with up to 33% excreted unchanged in the urine (8). Data on PAS pharmacokinetics with aging are not available. Precautions are necessary to prevent crystalluria. Dose adjustment is necessary in renal failure (9), hence, care must be exercised in prescribing and monitoring PAS in older patients.

D. Administration of Drug

At present, PAS is available only through the CDC. The dose ranges from 10 to 15 g daily in divided doses. Generally, the drug is taken with food or antacid to minimize GI intolerance (9). Use in renal failure is not recommended. The drug is known to increase uremic acidosis and GI adverse effects (36).

E. Drug Monitoring and Adverse Effects

Nausea, vomiting, abdominal cramps, epigastric pain, diarrhea, and anorexia are extremely common side effects. The severity of the symptoms may cause the discontinuation of the drug (10).

Hypersensitivity reactions to PAS occur in up to 10% of patients; fever, rash, pruritus, and conjunctivitis are common. Exfoliative dermatitis may occur, but hepatitis with jaundice occurs rarely. Other forms of hypersensitivity include joint pain, sore throat, lymphadenopathy, hepatosplenomegaly, and very rarely myocarditis, encephalopathy, and anaphylaxis (10).

Hematological side effects are rare. Neutropenia, agranulocytosis, acute hemolytic anemia, hypothrombinemia, and thrombocytopenia can occur. Hypokalemia may occur due to severe diarrhea and other GI effects (10).

XII. THIACETAZONE

Thiacetazone is a toxic but very inexpensive drug, which is mostly used in economically developing countries. It is not available in this country.

A. Chemistry and Mechanism of Action

Thiacetazone is a thiosemicarbazone. The mechanism of action is unknown. Its action is bacteriostatic.

B. Antimicrobial Spectrum

M. tuberculosis is susceptible to thiacetazone.

C. Clinical Pharmacology

Thiacetazone is well absorbed orally, undergoing hepatic metabolism. Approximately one-fifth of the absorbed drug is excreted unchanged in the urine. Little is known about the effect of age on the pharmacology of thiacetazone.

D. Administration of Drug

The usual adult dosage is 150 mg/day (2.5 mg/kg/day).

E. Drug Monitoring and Adverse Effects

There are considerable racial and geographical differences in the side effects of thiacetazone (43). Severe, even fatal cutaneous reactions to thiacetazone have occurred. Stevens–Johnson syndrome is not an uncommon serious reaction to the drug (44). Nausea, vomiting, diarrhea, and abdominal pain are very frequent GI adverse effects (43).

Adverse hematological effects of leukopenia, agranulocytosis, anemia, and thrombocytopenia occur as well as ototoxic effects of vertigo, ataxia, tinnitus, and hearing loss. Severe liver damage with jaundice has been reported (43).

XIII. CLOFAZIMINE

Clofazimine is an antileprosy drug that was introduced in the late 1950s. In recent years the drug has been used for the treatment of disseminated *M. avium* complex infection in AIDS and drug-resistant tuberculosis.

A. Chemistry and Mechanism of Action

Clofazimine is a bright red phenazone dye. It inhibits the template function of DNA by binding to DNA at the guanine base, thus inhibiting bacteria cell growth (45).

B. Antimicrobial Spectrum

One of clofazimine's primary uses, other than treating *M. leprae*, is for the treatment of *M. avium* complex (7,25,46). The activity of clofazimine against this organism has been shown to be pH dependent with activity decreasing as pH decreases (48). Other mycobacteria are also reported to be susceptible to this drug.

C. Clinical Pharmacology

Clofazimine is slowly absorbed in the GI tract, with an absorption rate of 70%. It is widely distributed in tissues but does not penetrate the CNS. The drug crosses the placenta and is excreted into milk. The metabolism of clofazimine is not fully known. More than 50% is excreted unchanged in the feces. The drug exhibits two compartment pharmacokinetics. In low-dose, short-term therapy, the drug has a half-life of about 10 days. With high-dose, long-term therapy, it has a half-life of about 70 days. Approximately 30 days are needed to reach steady-state concentrations unless loading doses are given (10). Data are not available on the pharmacokinetics of clofazimine in older adults.

Clofazimine decreases estrogen levels in women. Estrogen replacement may be necessary. Plasma levels of vitamin A are decreased with long-term use and may cause ichthyosis. The dermal adverse effects may be decreased by the use of vitamin A (10).

D. Administration of the Drug

Clofazimine is available in 50- and 100-mg capsules. The usual dose for *M. avium* infections is 100–300 mg per day. To increase absorption, clofazimine should be taken with food.

E. Drug Monitoring and Adverse Effects

Clofazimine is usually well tolerated with doses of 100 mg per day. Side effects are more frequent at the higher dose of 300 mg per day (48). The most common side effect of clofazimine is a reddish-brown discoloration of the skin, conjunctiva, sweat, hair, sputum, urine, and feces found in well over 50% of patients. Discolorations take months to completely clear after stopping the drug (10,48).

Abdominal pain is the most common adverse effect. Nausea, diarrhea, anorexia, and weight loss occur frequently. These effects may be sufficiently severe for discontinuation of the drug (10,48).

Rashes, ichthyosis, pruritus, xeroderma, acneiform eruptions, and exfoliative dermatitis have been reported (10,48).

XIV. QUINOLONES: CIPROFLOXACIN AND OFLOXACIN

Quinolones are newer chemotherapeutic agents that show antimycobacterial activity. Their use is mostly confined to the treatment of drug-resistant tuberculosis and nontuberculous mycobacterial diseases. More experience is needed to firmly establish their role in the treatment of mycobacterial diseases. (See also Chap. 14.)

A. Chemistry and Mechanism of Action

The quinolones, analogs of nalidixic acid, are 4-fluoroquinolones. Quinolones inhibit DNA synthesis by inhibiting DNA gyrase, the enzyme responsible for the cleavage and rejoining of DNA chains during supercoiling. Low pH slows the bactericidal activity and increases the minimal inhibitory concentration (MIC) as well as decreasing the postantibiotic effect of the quinolones (49,50).

B. Antimicrobial Spectrum

Most strains of *M. tuberculosis* (51), *M. fortuitum* (52), *M. kansasii* (52,53), *M. marinum* (54), and *M. xenopi* (52,53) are sensitive. *M. avium* has been reported to be both resistant and susceptible at achievable serum levels (7,46,54). The resistance or susceptibility is method dependent. Ciprofloxacin has much greater activity than ofloxacin. In clinical studies, response has been observed using ciprofloxacin with other antituberculous drugs (25,46,55). RIF and the quinolones, when both are ineffective alone, are effective when used in combination (52).

C. Clinical Pharmacology

The quinolones are rapidly and extensively absorbed. Peak levels are reached in 1–3 h. Ciprofloxacin undergoes hepatic metabolism and renal elimination (40–50% excreted unchanged in the urine). Ofloxacin undergoes less hepatic metabolism, with 70–80% excreted unchanged in the urine. Their half-lives are between 3 and 6 h. The volume of distribution is approximately equal to the total body water. Both are widely distributed in tissues and body fluids. For either, protein binding is less than 40%. Neither drug is removed well by peritoneal dialysis. Both cross the placenta and are excreted in milk. Oral absorption, hepatic metabolism, and renal elimination of quinolones are decreased in elderly persons but have no clinical significance (49,50). (See Chap. 14 for more detailed data on pharmacokinetics of quinolones with aging.)

Aluminum, calcium, and iron decrease the oral absorption of quinolones (49,50). Ofloxacin has minimal effect on theophylline levels, while ciprofloxacin may increase levels by 23%. Theophylline levels should be monitored when used with ciprofloxacin (49,50). Caffeine may increase the incidence and severity of CNS adverse effects of the quinolones (49,50). Some nonsteroidal anti-inflammatory drugs (indomethacin, ketoprofen, naproxen, ibuprofen, pranoprofen) used with quinolones may cause seizures by inhibiting select neurotransmission (56). Ciprofloxacin has been reported to cause a clinically significant rise in coumadin levels (57). Cyclosporine levels may also increase with the concomitant use of the quinolones.

D. Administration of Drug

Both quinolones are administered by the oral and parenteral routes.

Ofloxacin: The usual adult oral and parenteral dose is 200–400 mg every 12 h. In severe renal failure, this should be changed to every 24 h. To prevent hypotensive episodes, intravenous infusions over 60 min are recommended. Orally, ofloxacin is available in 200-, 300-, and 400-mg tablets and parenterally in 200- and 400-mg vials.

Ciprofloxacin: The recommended oral adult dose is 250–750 mg every 12 h. Parenterally, 200 mg is equivalent to an oral dose of 250 mg, and 400 mg parenterally is equivalent to 500 mg given orally. Only IV infusions over 60 min are recommended. Tablets containing 250, 500, and 750 mg are available. The recommended dose for *M. avium* complex infections is 750 mg every 12 h.

E. Drug Monitoring and Adverse Effects

The predominant adverse effects of the quinolones involve the GI tract, the CNS, and hypersensitivity reactions. The most frequent adverse effects are nausea, upper GI tract discomfort, headache, and dizziness. Anorexia, vomiting, insomnia, mood alteration, restlessness, tremors, lightheadedness, mental confusion, pruritus, and rash are also part of this triad. The incidence of reported side effects have been around 10%, with 3–4% of patients requiring discontinuation of the drug. Photosensitivity occurs rarely. Serious side effects have included seizures, crystalluria, allergic nephritis, and hematological effects (49,50). Elderly patients, especially with CNS disorders or cerebral arteriosclerosis, are more likely to experience the neurological effects of the quinolones. Quinolones are not recommended in children because of arthralgic side effects.

XV. MACROLIDES: AZITHROMYCIN AND CLARITHROMYCIN

The role of the newer macrolide antibiotics in the treatment of mycobacterial diseases is not yet established. Antimycobacterial activity is seen in in vitro studies. At the present time, these drugs are experimental in the therapy of tuberculosis. (See Chap. 17.)

A. Chemistry and Mechanism of Action

Clarithromycin is a 6-methyl analog (of the 14-membered lactone ring) of erythromycin. Azithromycin with the addition of a nitrogen atom to the lactone ring of erythromycin is a 15-membered derivative known as an azalide.

The macrolides inhibit bacteria protein synthesis by reversibly binding to ribosomes, thus inhibiting RNA. Azithromycin and clarithromycin are bactericidal or bacteriostatic depending on the concentration of the drug at the site of action (58). Both drugs are highly concentrated in macrophages and are effective against bacteria in these cells.

B. Antimicrobial Spectrum

Azithromycin and clarithromycin are not active against *M. tuberculosis*. However, both drugs have activity against *M. fortuitum* and *M. chelonae* (59). Clarithromycin is also active against *M. kansasii* and *M. xenopi* (60). Clarithromycin and azithromydin are bactericidal against *M. avium* complex and have been used to treat infection caused by these organisms. Generally, clarithromycin has shown greater activity than azithromycin against *M. avium* complex (61–63).

C. Clinical Pharmacology

Azithromycin and clarithromycin have distinct pharmacokinetic properties.

Clarithromycin: Clarithromycin is 55% absorbed orally. Peak concentration occurs in 2–4 h. The half-life increases from 4.39 to 11.27 h with high doses. Urinary excretion of clarithromycin and its metabolites is 35–43%, with 18–29% excretion of unchanged drug. Fecal excretion of clarithromycin and its metabolites is 27–38%. Clarithromycin is distributed widely into tissue and fluids, with high concentration occurring in lungs. CNS penetration is not known (58). Limited pharmacokinetic data of clarithromycin in elderly persons indicate high plasma concentrations and area under the curve, which are due to decreased renal clearance of the drug. However, dosage adjustment is not necessary unless severe renal impairment is present (63a).

Clarithromycin significantly decreases the metabolism of carbamazepine. Clarithromycin should be used with caution with drugs undergoing significant liver metabolism (58).

Azithromycin: Azithromycin is 37% absorbed orally. The drug is rapidly distributed and highly concentrated in tissues. Tissue concentrations of azithromycin are much greater than serum concentrations; intracellular levels far exceed extracellular levels. Very low levels of the drug are found in the CNS. The terminal half-life of azithromycin is 68 h. Most is excreted unchanged. Approximately 20% is excreted unchanged in the urine, but the majority is excreted in the bile and eliminated unchanged in the feces. Azithromycin is highly concentrated in macrophages resulting in high concentrations at the site of infection (64).

Aluminum- and magnesium-containing antacids decrease peak levels of azithromycin. The drug should be taken 1 h before or 2 h after such antacids.

D. Administration of Drug

Both clarithromycin and azithromycin are only available for oral use. It is unknown if either drug has greater risks in elderly persons than in young adults.

Clarithromycin: The drug is available in 250- and 500-mg tablets. The usual reported dosage for *Mycobacterium avium* complex infections is 1 g twice a day. Dose adjustment is required for severe renal impairment. It does not appear that a dose reduction is necessary for elderly patients without serious renal dysfunction (63a).

Azithromycin: Azithromycin's absorption is affected by food. It should be given 1 h before or 2 h after eating. The drug is available in 250-mg capsules. For *M. avium* complex infections, the recommended dose of azithromycin is 500 mg per day for up to 30 days. If duration of therapy is greater than 30 days, caution should be exercised due to reported complexing of the drug with phospholipid in the liver of animals (62). The proper dose for older patients has not been determined, but the standard adult dose is currently acceptable.

E. Drug Monitoring and Adverse Effects

Both azithromycin and clarithromycin are well tolerated. The most common side effects are diarrhea, nausea, and abdominal pain (58). Other adverse effects noted with clarithromycin have been dyspepsia, abnormal taste, and headache. Hyperbilirubinemia and elevations in liver enzymes have been reported (58).

Angioedema and cholestatic jaundice may occur with azithromycin. Elevations of liver enzyme, serum creatinine, and BUN have also been reported. Leukopenia, neutropenia, and thrombocytopenia have occurred (58).

Other uncommon adverse effects of azithromycin are palpitations, chest pain, vaginitis, nephritis, headache dizziness, vertigo, somnolence, and photosensitivity (58).

XVI. PRESENT DRUG TREATMENT OF TUBERCULOSIS

With the advent of the bactericidal drugs INH and RIF and the reintroduction of PZA in the therapeutic armamentarium, treatment of tuberculosis has been revolutionized during the past two decades. Therapy for tuberculosis has become very effective, with decreased duration and reduced cost (65). However, appropriate choice of drugs and duration of therapy is necessary for successful outcome.

A. Bacteriological Basis of Therapy

Mycobacterium tuberculosis is an aerobic organism that survives best at physiological pH of 7.40 and in a PO_2 of 100–140 mmHg (66). Even under normal conditions tubercle bacilli divide only every 16–20 h. Because of slow replication time, the disease is chronic and indolent. For this reason, medications are effective in single daily doses initially, as well as intermittent doses after the infection is controlled.

Another characteristic of the organisms is the natural occurrence of resistant mutants, irrespective of exposure to drugs. In a virgin population of bacilli, mutants resistant to one drug occur in a frequency of 1×10^{-5} to 1×10^{-6} (67). Fortunately, resistance to one drug is independent of resistance to others. The incidence of resistance to two drugs is only about 1×10^{-12}. Thus, at least two effective drugs should be given simultaneously to avoid selective emergence of drug-resistant mutants.

B. Bacterial Population in Tuberculosis

Bacilli in tuberculous lesions are located extracellularly in cavitary lesions, in closed caseous lesions, and intracellularly within macrophages (Fig. 1). An understanding of this fact is necessary for the appropriate choice of chemotherapy:

1. The large actively dividing extracellular population in cavitary lesions often numbers 1×10^7 to 1×10^9 bacilli, which may contain a significant number of mutants resistant to a single drug (68). Therefore, it is necessary to kill rapidly multiplying extracellular bacilli in the cavitary lesions and eliminate drug-resistant mutants.
2. A smaller population (1×10^2 to 1×10^5) of bacilli is located in closed caseous lesions, where they multiply slowly and intermittently.

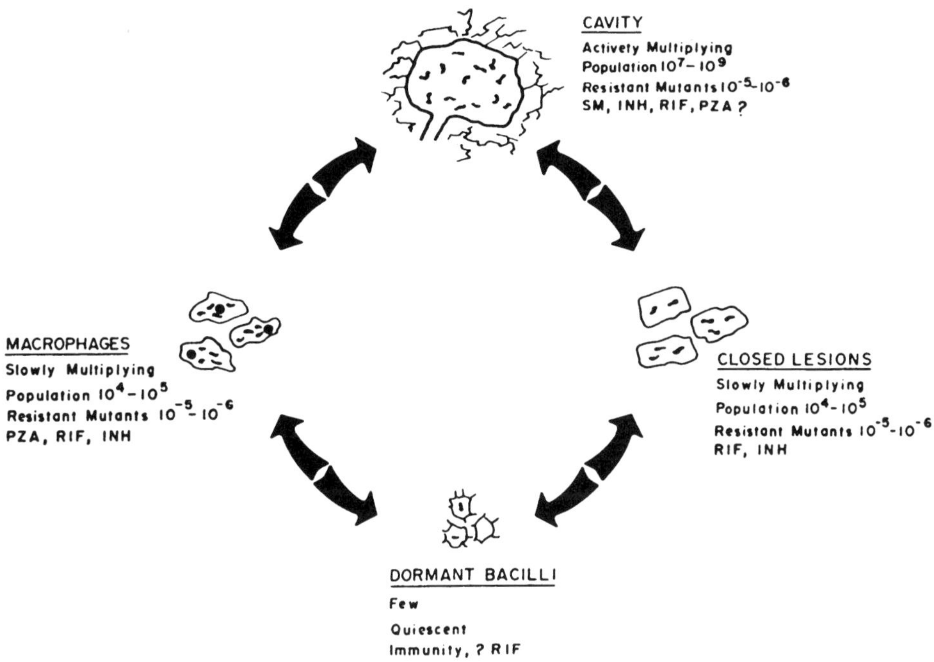

Figure 1 Bacterial populations in human tuberculous lesions.

3. A similar small number of bacilli lies within macrophages and multiplies infrequently.

The significance of the latter two populations is their persistence in lesions that require prolonged therapy for elimination of these "persisters." For effective chemotherapy, drugs must be capable of eliminating the above three populations of bacilli (69). Failure to eliminate the rapidly multiplying organisms in cavitary lesions results in continued positive cultures, often with development of drug-resistant organisms. If the slowly multiplying "persisters" are not eradicated, late relapse may occur after stopping therapy, usually with susceptible organisms.

C. Antituberculosis Drugs

The available antituberculosis drugs are classified as bactericidal or bacteriostatic. The bactericidal drugs are INH, RIF, PZA, and EMB in higher doses (25 mg/kg). INH and RIF are potent bactericidal drugs, which act on both rapidly multiplying extracellular bacilli and slowly dividing bacilli in closed lesions and intracellular organisms within macrophages (70). PZA is generally effective in an acid medium in the milieu within macrophages (71). SM acts best in a neutral or slightly alkaline medium on rapidly multiplying extracellular bacilli in cavitary lesions. EMB is generally a bacteriostatic drug but in higher concentration is weakly bactericidal, both for extracellular and intracellular organisms.

Bacteriostatic drugs contribute very little to the bactericidal regimen because they inhibit only multiplication of resistant mutants. Chemotherapy regimens containing bacteriostatic

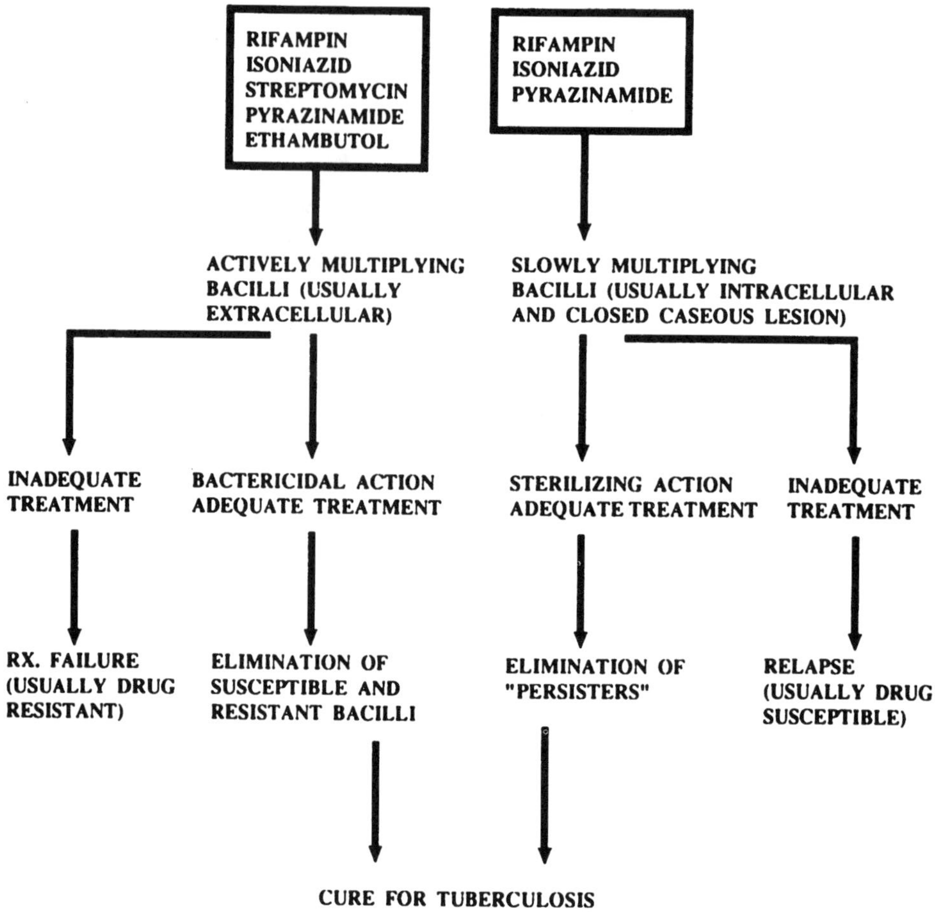

Figure 2 Principles of modern chemotherapy based on the action of drugs on the characteristics of bacilli in tuberculous lesions and causes of treatment failure vs. relapse.

drugs must be administered for a longer period (18–24 months) to ensure eradication of both groups of bacilli and prevent late relapses.

D. Principles of Chemotherapy

Present chemotherapy regimens are bactericidal, which renders the patient rapidly "smear negative" by eliminating extracellular organisms in the lesions. The patient soon becomes noninfectious. Moreover, due to their effective action on "persisters," relapses are uncommon after discontinuation of therapy. As shown in Figure 2, the combination of INH and RIF is a potent bactericidal regimen, which kills actively multiplying organisms rapidly, rendering the patient bacteriologically negative. Due to early elimination of the bacillary population, failure is uncommon. However, when therapy fails, it is usually due to selection of resistant organism. The combination of INH and RIF has a potent sterilizing action on slowly or intermittently replicating "persisters," for which relapses are infrequent after

Table 2 Chemotherapy Regimens for Treatment of Tuberculosis

Nine-Month Regimen
- ☐ INH 300 mg + RIF 600 mg daily for 9 months or
- ☐ INH 300 mg + RIF mg daily for 1 month followed by INH 900 mg + RIF 600 mg twice weekly for 8 months

Six-Month Regimen
- ☐ INH 300 mg + RIF 600 mg + PZA 25–30 mg/kg/body weight daily for 2 months followed by INH 300 mg + RIF 600 mg daily or INH 900 mg + RIF 600 mg twice weekly for 4 months
- ☐ For three smears negative but culture positive: INH + RIF for 6 months (one month daily and five months twice weekly)
- ☐ For three smears negative and culture negative suspected active tuberculosis: INH + RIF for 4 months (one daily and 3 months twice weekly)

For Suspected Drug Resistance
- ☐ Add ethambutol (EMB) 25 mg/kg/daily or streptomycin 0.5–0.75 g (five times/week) initially for 2 months to above INH + RIF + PZA regimen or until drug susceptibility results are known
- ☐ Follow with two or three drugs (preferably bactericidal) to which the organisms are susceptible for 9–12 months

INH = isoniazid; RIF = rifampin; PZA = pyrazinamide; EMB = ethambutol.

stopping chemotherapy. Occasional relapses are generally responsive to both drugs (70).

Addition of other bactericidal drugs such as PZA and/or SM or EMB (25 mg/kg) to INH and RIF therapy further potentiates the bactericidal activity of the regimen. The patients are rendered noninfectious sooner, and the duration of therapy is further reduced.

E. Regimens of Therapy

Drugs are selected to which bacilli are expected to be susceptible. Present chemotherapy regimens are summarized in Table 2. In developed countries most of the newly diagnosed patients have susceptible bacilli for which two-drug regimens with INH and RIF do not pose any problem. The duration of INH and RIF therapy is 9 months. The drugs (INH 300 mg and RIF 600 mg) may be given daily for 9 months or daily for 1 month in the same doses followed by INH 900 mg and RIF 600 mg twice weekly for another 8 months (72).

In elderly populations, the disease is primarily due to recrudescence of an old infection acquired many years ago, and the bacilli are usually susceptible to most antituberculous drugs. Use of combination capsules of INH and RIF (Rifamate: INH 150 mg, RIF 300 mg) is strongly recommended. The regimen should consist of two combination capsules daily for 1 month followed by two Rifamate capsules and two 300-mg tablets of INH twice weekly for another 8 months. Pyridoxine (25–50 mg daily) is also prescribed during therapy in elderly persons. The regimen has a success rate of 95%. Two capsules of Rifamate may be given daily for the full period (9 months) with equal, but not superior results.

Rifamate therapy permits monotherapy and minimizes error for patients. Also, it is easier to remember to take two capsules and two white tablets during twice-weekly therapy. Twice-weekly therapy is easier for health care providers to supervise in elderly patients.

The duration of therapy can be reduced if the bacterial population is small. If the initial three specimens of bronchial secretion have negative smears but the cultures are positive, indicating fewer bacilli, 6 months of therapy with INH and RIF is adequate (73). When three smears, as well as cultures, are negative, active disease may still be present but with very small numbers of organisms. Total therapy for only 4 months is then sufficient (74).

In geographic areas where the incidence of drug resistance is high, a two-drug regimen has a high risk of failure and relapse and is therefore inappropriate. Drug resistance should be suspected in a patient who has received chemotherapy in the past or who acquired the infection in an area with a high prevalence of drug resistance, e.g., Southeast Asia, the Philippines, Mexico, Africa, or large cities in the United States. Therapy in such patients should include additional bactericidal drugs (PZA, EMB, or SM) until the drug susceptibilities of the bacilli are known.

Generally, a third drug is not necessary in the regimen of newly diagnosed disease of elderly patients. The chance of drug resistance is extremely low. However, the addition of PZA (25–30 mg/kg) to INH and RIF regimen for the first 2 months of daily therapy, followed by INH and RIF daily or twice weekly (INH dose is 900 mg) for another 4 months reduces the total duration of therapy to 6 months (20b). Addition of another potentially hepatotoxic drug to the regimen may increase toxicity in elderly persons. More experience with this regimen in elderly patients is needed and is only cautiously recommended.

F. Retreatment Regimens

Two-drug therapy is potentially dangerous in patients whose organisms may be resistant to one of the drugs. Such therapy may lead to the development of resistance to the other drugs, which is a tragedy for patients as well as the community. The clinician should be aware of situations where the presence of drug resistance may be suspected. There is a possibility that a patient may harbor INH-resistant bacilli if (1) prior chemotherapy was given, (2) the patient received previous INH preventive therapy, (3) the patient acquired the infection in areas with high prevalence of INH resistance (Asia, Latin America, Africa, and large cities of certain geographical areas of the United States), or (4) the patient acquired the disease through contact with an INH-resistant patient.

A good history is essential before initiation of chemotherapy. In the above situations, further development of resistance to another drug can be avoided by initiating therapy with a combination of INH, RIF, PZA, and EMB, or SM for a minimum of 8 weeks or until the drug susceptibility results are known. With this combination, two bactericidal drugs are always active against the bacilli in all three populations, even if INH resistance is present. EMB (25 mg/kg) or SM, RIF, and PZA are bactericidal for large extracellular bacterial populations, whereas RIF and PZA are active against organisms that are intracellular or present in closed caseous lesions. After the results of susceptibility tests are known, therapy should be modified accordingly. If INH susceptibility is found, the therapy can be completed with INH and RIF for another 4 months. When INH resistance is demonstrated, therapy may be completed with RIF and EMB (25 mg/kg) or PZA for a total period of 12 months or at least 6 months beyond the time of conversion. These drugs can be given twice weekly with equal effectiveness (75).

In a patient whose resistance to two or more drugs has been demonstrated, the drug regimen must consist of two or three drugs to which the bacilli are susceptible. The drugs should be administered in full tolerable doses. Generally, these drugs are more toxic, hence close monitoring for side effects and compliance is necessary. Duration of therapy is extended to 18–24 months.

Patients with AIDS should be given INH, RIF, and PZA for 2 months followed by INH and RIF for 7 months or for 6 months after they have remained negative, whichever is longer (75a,75b).

Older patients with tuberculous meningitis may suffer severe neurological sequelae. Some experts recommend that INH, RIF, *and* PZA be administered for the full 9 months of therapy (75a).

In older patients with mild to moderate renal impairment, INH, RIF, and PZA do not require dose reduction. However, with severe kidney dysfunction, the dosage of INH and PZA should be decreased; RIF dosage may remain the same (75a).

G. Monitoring of Adverse Effects

Diligent and frequent monitoring of drug toxicity is required. Elderly patients may fail to identify and communicate adverse symptoms. Therapy in geriatric patients should be supervised by dependable persons who are knowledgeable about adverse signs and symptoms of the drugs. Patients should also be acquainted with the side effects to facilitate early detection. Although periodic liver function testing during therapy of elderly patients is advised by some (20a,20b), routine testing, except baseline studies, is not recommended by the authors because levels are often elevated in an asymptomatic patient, which can be misleading. When a patient is symptomatic with anorexia, nausea, and vomiting, the drug should be immediately discontinued and the liver function tests performed. If the transaminase levels are found to be normal, the drugs are prescribed in full doses. When the transaminases are elevated, the drugs are reintroduced one at a time after the enzyme levels return to normal. The drug is started with one half of the doses and gradually increased every third day under close clinical and biochemical monitoring until the full dose is tolerated. In this manner, the drugs may be reintroduced in more than half of the patients and tolerated. When INH or RIF is not tolerated, a third bactericidal drug is substituted and the treatment is completed.

H. Preventive Therapy

Due to risk of developing age-related hepatitis, INH preventive therapy is usually not recommended in elderly persons unless risk factors are identified. In persons with long-standing positive tuberculin reactivity, the risk of developing active tuberculosis is only 2–3%, while the chances of developing hepatitis with INH is greater (76,77). However, presence of risk factors such as diabetes mellitus, upper lobe scarring, and long-term corticosteroid therapy are considered indications for preventive therapy.

Regardless of age, recent conversion of a tuberculin test (an increase of 15 mm or more over previously tested as negative) is associated with greater incidence of tuberculosis and constitutes a strong indication of preventive therapy with INH 300 mg daily for 6–12 months (76). Studies have shown that 12 months of therapy confer a protection of 98% against tuberculosis when compared to converters who were not treated. When properly supervised, the therapy is quite safe. In a large number of patients so treated, incidence of nonfatal toxic hepatitis was 4.5% (77). Clinical monitoring for toxic side effects must be intensive. The most common symptoms are anorexia, nausea, and vomiting. When symptomatic, blood should be drawn for liver function test. If the transaminases are elevated 500 units/ml or more, the drugs should not be continued. However, if the enzymes are modestly elevated, a 3-day challenge with 150 mg of INH is appropriate after the enzyme levels return to normal. If tolerated, then full doses are started. In this manner, 50% of patients may restart the therapy. Generally pyridoxine 25–50 mg daily is recommended in elderly persons to prevent the neurological and hematological side effects of INH.

I. Compliance with Therapy

For successful treatment outcome, drug compliance is essential and should be monitored carefully. Elderly patients may show specific problems during drug therapy. Some are unreliable in taking medicines due to mental confusion, failing memory, and poor vision. Treatment must be supervised by some reliable family members, friends, domestic help, or by nurses in the nursing homes. Supervisors and patients must be educated in the signs and symptoms of drug toxicities. An elderly person may not recognize and communicate adverse symptoms. Monitoring of drug toxicity should be frequent and careful to facilitate early recognition (78).

REFERENCES

1. Waksman SA, Bugie E, Schatz A. Isolation of antibiotic substance from soil microorganisms with special reference to streptothricin and streptomycin. Mayo Clin Proc 1944; 19:537–48.
2. Feldman WH, Hinshaw HC. Effects of streptomycin on experimental tuberculosis in guinea pigs. Mayo Clin Proc 1944; 19:593–603.
3. Van Scoy RE, Wilkowske CJ. Antituberculous agents. Mayo Clin Proc 1992; 67:179–87.
4. Zhang Y, Heym B, Allen B, et al. The catalase-perioxidase gene and isoniazid resistance of mycobacterium tuberculosis. Nature 1992; 358:591–3.
5. Kuze F, Kurasawa T, Bando K, et al. In vitro and in vivo susceptibility of atypical mycobacteria to various drugs. Rev Infect Dis 1981; 3:885–97.
6. Simor AE, Salit IE, Vellend H. The role of *Mycobacterium xenopi* in human disease. Am Rev Resp Dis 1984; 129:435–8.
7. Heifets L. MIC as a quantitative measurement of the susceptibility of Mycobacterium avium strains to seven antituberculosis drugs. Antimicrob Agents Chemother 1988; 32:1131–6.
8. Robson JM, Sullivan FM. Antituberculosis drugs. Pharmacol Rev 1963; 15:169–223.
9. Holdiness MR. Clinical pharmacokinetics of antituberculosis drugs. Clin Pharmacokin 1984; 9:511–44.

9a. Kergueris MF, Bourin M, Larousse C. Pharmacokinetics of isoniazid: influence of age. Eur J Clin Pharmacol 1986; 30:335–40.

10. Girling DJ. Adverse effect of antituberculosis drugs. Drugs 1982; 23:56–74.
11. Steele MA, Burk RF, Des Prez RM. Toxic hepatitis with isoniazid and rifampin: a meta-analysis. Chest 1991; 99:465–71.
12. Wehrli W. Rifampin: mechanism of action and resistance. Rev Infect Dis 1983; 5(suppl):407–11.
13. David HL. Basis for lack of drug susceptibility of atypical mycobacteria. Rev Infect Dis 1981; 3:878–84.

13a. Advenier C, Gobert C, Houin G, et al. Pharmacokinetic studies of rifampicin in the elderly. Ther Drug Monitor 1983; 5:61–5.

14. Borcherding SN, Baciewicz AM, Self TH. Update on rifampin drug interactions. Arch Intern Med 1992; 152:711–16.
15. Girling DJ. Adverse reactions to rifampicin in antituberculosis regimens. J Antimicrob Chemother 1977; 3:115–32.
16. O'Brien RJ, Lyle MA, Snider DE Jr. Rifabutin (Ansamycin LM427): a new rifamycin-S derivative for the treatment of mycobacterial disease. Rev Infect Dis 1987; 9:519–30.

17. Ahn CH, Wallace RJ, Steele LC, et al. Sulfonamide-containing regimens for disease caused by rifampin-resistant Mycobacterium kansasii. Am Rev Resp Dis 1987; 135:10–16.
18. Skinner MH, Hsieh M, Torseth J, et al. Pharmacokinetics of rifabutin. Antimicrob Agents Chemother 1989; 33:1237–41.
19. Woodley CL, Kilburn JO. In vitro susceptibility of Mycobacterium avium complex and M. tuberculosis strains to a spiro-piperidyl rifamycin. Am Rev Resp Dis 1982; 126:586–7.
20. Sarma GR, Acharyulu GS, Kannapiran M, et al. Role of rifampin in arthralgia induced by pyrazinamide. Tubercle 1983; 64:93–100.
20a. Yoshikawa TT. Tuberculosis in aging adults. J Am Geriatr Soc 1992; 40:178–87.
20b. American Thoracic Society. Treatment of tuberculosis and tuberculous infections in adults and children. Am Rev Resp Dis 1986; 134:355–63.
21. Moellering RC. In vitro antibacterial activity of the aminoglycoside antibiotics. Rev Infect Dis 1983; 2(suppl):212–31.
22. Heifets L, Lindholm-Levy P. Comparison of bactericidal activities of streptomycin, amikacin, kanamycin and capreomycin against *Mycobacterium avium* and *Mycobacterium tuberculosis*. Antimicrob Agents Chemother 1989; 33:1298–301.
23. Banks J, Smith AP, Jenkins PA. Mycobacterium malmoense-problems with treatment and diagnosis—a case report. Tubercle 1983; 64:217–19.
24. Sanders WJ, Wolinsky E. In vitro susceptibility of mycobacterium marinum to eight antimicrobial agents. Antimicrob Agents Chemother 1980; 18:525–31.
25. Benson CA, Kessler HA, Pottage JC, et al. Successful treatment of acquired immunodeficiency syndrome-related *Mycobacterium avium* complex disease with a multiple drug regimen including amikacin. Arch Intern Med 1991; 151:582–5.
26. Wallace RJ Jr, Dalovisio JR, Pankey GA. Disk diffusion testing of susceptibility of *Mycobacterium fortuitum* and *Mycobacterium chelonei* to antibacterial agents. Antimicrob Agents Chemother 1979; 16:611–14.
27. Hawley HB, Lewis RM, Swartz DB, et al. Tobramycin therapy of pulmonary infections in patients with cystic fibrosis. Curr Ther Res 1974; 6:414–23.
27a. Yoshikawa TT. Antimicrobial therapy in the elderly patient. J Am Geriatr Soc 1990; 38:1353–72.
28. Argov Z, Mastaglia FL. Disorders of neuromuscular transmission caused by drugs. N Engl J Med 1979; 301:409–13.
29. Lietman PS, Smith CR. Aminoglycoside nephrotoxicity in humans. Rev Infect Dis 1983; 5(suppl):284–92.
30. Finegold SM. Toxicity of kanamycin in adults. Ann NY Acad Sci 1966; 132:942–56.
31. Sutton WB, Gordee RS, Wick WE, et al. In vitro and in vivo laboratory studies on the antituberculous activity of capreomycin. Ann NY Acad Sci 1966; 135:947–59.
32. Aquinas M, Citron KM. Rifampicin, ethambutol, and capreomycin in pulmonary tuberculosis, previously treated with both first and second line drugs: the results of 2 years' chemotherapy. Tubercle 1972; 53:153–65.
33. Miller JD, Popplewell AG, Landwehr A, et al. Toxicology studies in patients on prolonged therapy with capreomycin. Ann NY Acad Sci 1966; 135:1047–56.
34. Takayama K, Armstrong EL, Kunugi KA, et al. Inhibition by ethambutol of mycolic acid transfer into the cell wall of *Mycobacterium smegmatis*. Antimicrob Agent Chemother 1979; 16:240–2.
35. Yates MD, Collins CH. Sensitivity of opportunist mycobacteria to rifampicin and ethambutol. Tubercle. 1981; 62:117–21.
36. Cheigh JS. Drug administration in renal failure. Am J Med 1977; 62:555–63.
36a. Yoshikawa TT, Nagami PH. Adverse drug reactions in TB therapy: Risks and recommendations. Geriatrics 1982; 7:61–8.
37. Dutt AK, Stead WW. Long term results of medical treatment in *Mycobacterium intracellulare* infection. Am J Med 1979; 67:449–53.

38. Weiszfeiler JG, Karasseva J, Karczag E. *Mycobacterium simiae* and related mycobacteria. Rev Infect Dis 1981; 3:1040–5.
39. Blacklock ZM, Dawson DJ, Kane DW, et al. *Mycobacterium asiaticum* as a potential pulmonary pathogen for humans. Am Rev Resp Dis 1983; 127:241–4.
40. Strominger JL, Tipper DJ. Bacteria cell wall synthesis and structure in relation to the mechanism of action of penicillins and other antibacterial agents. Am J Med 1965; 39:708–12.
41. Hejny J. A drug sensitivity strategy for atypical mycobacteria. Tubercle 1982; 62:63–9.
42. Engbaek HC, Thormann J, Vergmann B. Aquarium borne *Mycobacterium marinum* granulomas. Scand J Infect Dis 1980; 12:74–8.
43. Miller AB, Fox W, Tall R. An international co-operative investigation into thiacetazone (thiocetazone) side-effects. Tubercle 1966; 47:33–6.
44. Nunn P, Kibuga D, Gathua S, et al. Cutaneous hypersensitivity reactions due to thiacetazone in HIV-1 seropositive patients treated for tuberculosis. Lancet 1991; 337:627–38.
45. Morrison NE, Marley GM. The mode of action of clofazimine. DNA binding studies. Int J Lepr 1976; 44:133–4.
46. Kemper Carol A, Meng Tze-Chiang, Nussbaum J, et al. Treatment of *Mycobacterium avium* complex bacteremia in AIDS with a four-drug oral regimen. Ann Intern Med 1992; 116:466–72.
47. Garrelts JC. Clofazimine: a review of its use in leprosy and *Mycobacterium avium* complex infection. DICP Ann Pharmacother 1991; 25:525–31.
48. Lindholm-Levy PJ, Heifets LB. Clofazimine and other rimino-compounds: minimal inhibitory and minimal bactericidal concentrations at different pHs for *Mycobacterium avium* complex. Tubercle 1988; 69:179–86.
49. Newman M. Clinical pharmacokinetic of the newer antibacterial 4-quinolones. Clin Pharmacokinet 1988; 44:96–121.
50. Neu HC. The quinolones. Infect Dis Clin North Am 1989; 3:625–39.
51. Rastogi N, Goh KS. In vitro activity of the new difluorinated quinolone sparfloxacin (AT=4140) against *Mycobacterium tuberculosis* compared with activities of ofloxacin and ciprofloxacin. Antimicrob Agent Chemother 1991; 35:2933–6.
52. Young LS, Berlin OG, Inderlied CB. Activity of ciprofloxacin and other fluorinated quinolones against mycobacteria. Am J Med 1987; 82:23–6.
53. Leysen DC, Haemers A, Pattyn SR. Mini-review. Mycobacteria and the new quinolones. Antimicrob Agents Chemother 1989; 33:1–5.
54. Yajko DM, Nassos PS, Hadley WK. Therapeutic implications of inhibition versus killing of *M. avium* complex by antimicrobial agents. Antimicrob Agents Chemother 1987; 31:117–20.
55. Chiu J, Nussbaum J, Bozzette S, et al. Treatment of disseminated *Mycobacterium avium* complex infection in AIDS with amikacin, ethambutol, rifampin and ciprofloxacin. Ann Intern Med 1990; 113:358–61.
56. Akaike N, Shirasaki T, Yakushiji TJ. Quinolones and fenbufen interact with GABA(A) receptor in dissociated hippocampal cells of rat. Neurophysiology 1991; 66:497–504.
57. Renzi R, Finkbeiner S. Ciprofloxacin interaction with sodium warfarin: a potentially dangerous side effect. Am J Emerg Med 1991; 9:551–2.
58. Piscitelli SC, Danziger LH, Rodvold KA. Clarithromycin and azithromycin: new macrolide antibiotics. Clin Pharm 1992; 11:137–52.
59. Brown BA, Wallace RJ, Onyl GO, et al. Activities of four macrolides, including clarithromycin against *Mycobacterium fortuitum*, *Mycobacterium chelonae* and *Mycobacterium chelonae*-like organisms. Antimicrob Agents Chemother 1992; 36:180–4.
60. Berlin OGW, Young SA, Floyd-Reising SA, et al. Comparative in vivo activity of the new macrolide A56268 against mycobacteria. Eur J Clin Microbiol 1987; 4:486–7.
61. Bernudez LEM, Young LS. Activities of amikacin, roxithromycin and azithromycin alone or in combination with tumor necrosis factor against *Mycobacterium avium* complex. Antimicrob Agents Chemother 1988; 32:1149–53.

62. Young LS, Wiviott L, Wu M, Kolonoski P, et al. Azithromycin for treatment of mycobacterium avium intracellulare complex infection in patients with AIDS. Lancet 1991; 338:1107–9.
63. Fernandez PBD, Hardy D, McDaniel D, et al. In vitro and in vivo activities of clarithromycin against *Mycobacterium avium*. Antimicrob Agents Chemother 1989; 33:1531–4.
63a. Peters DH, Clessold Sp. Clarithromycin. A review of its antimicrobial activity, pharmacokinetic properties and therapeutic potential. Drugs 1992; 44:117–64.
64. Schentag JJ, Ballow CH. Tissue-directed pharmacokinetics. Am J Med 1991; 91(suppl 3A):5–11.
65. Dutt AK, Stead WW. Medical perspective: present chemotherapy for tuberculosis. J Infect Dis 1982; 146:698–704.
66. Fox W, Mitchison DA. Short-course chemotherapy for pulmonary tuberculosis. Am Rev Resp Dis 1973; 111:325–53.
67. Cannetti G. The J Burns Amberson Lecture: present aspects of bacterial resistance in tuberculosis. Am Rev Resp Dis 1965; 92:667–703.
68. Grosset J. Bacteriologic basis of short course chemotherapy for tuberculosis. Clin Chest Med 1980; 1:231–42.
69. Mitchison DA, Dickinson JM. Bactericidal mechanism in short course chemotherapy. Bull Int Union Tuberc 1978; 53:254–9.
70. Fox W. The current status of short course chemotherapy. Tubercle 1979; 60:177–90.
71. Grosset J. The sterilizing value of rifampicin and pyrazinamide in experimental short-course chemotherapy. Bull Int Union Tuberc 1978; 53:5–12.
72. Dutt AK, Moers D, Stead WW. Short-course chemotherapy for tuberculosis with mainly twice-weekly isoniazid and rifampin. Community physicians' seven-year experience with mainly outpatients. Am J Med 1984; 77:233–42.
73. Dutt AK, Moers D, Stead WW. Smear-negative, culture-positive tuberculosis: six-month therapy with isoniazid and rifampin. Am Rev Resp Dis 1990; 141:1232–5.
74. Dutt AK, Moers D, Stead WW. Smear and culture negative pulmonary tuberculosis: four-month short course chemotherapy. Am Rev Resp Dis 1989; 139:867–70.
75. Castello A, Gothmans C, Dalbori MA, et al. Comparison of daily and twice-weekly regimens to treat pulmonary tuberculosis. Lancet 1989; 2:1173–6.
75a. Davidson PT, Le HQ. Drug treatment of tuberculosis—1992. Drugs 1992; 43:651–73.
75b. Barnes PF, Bloch AB, Davidson PT, et al. Tuberculosis in patients with human immunodeficiency virus infection. N Engl J Med 1991; 364:1641–50.
76. Stead WW, To T. The significance of the tuberculin test in elderly persons. Ann Intern Med 1987; 107:837–42.
77. Stead WW, To T, Harrison RW, et al. Benefit-risk consideration in preventive treatment for tuberculosis in elderly persons. Ann Intern Med 1987; 107:843–5.
78. Centers of Disease Control. Prevention and control of tuberculosis in facilities providing long-term care to the elderly: recommendations of the advisory committee for elimination of tuberculosis. MMWR 1990; 39:7–20.

24

Antifungal Agents

Carol A. Kauffman
Department of Veterans Affairs Medical Center and University of Michigan Medical School, Ann Arbor, Michigan

I. INTRODUCTION

In past decades, treatment of fungal infections could be characterized by lack of choice of different drugs, significant toxicity of existing drugs, and little available data on the most efficacious way to treat different fungal infections. Major changes have occurred in the past decade since new oral antifungal drugs have been developed and are now available for use. Also, new information about decreasing the toxicity of amphotericin B has been reported. Individual reports on the use of newer antifungal drugs have been published, and most importantly, the Mycoses Study Group has systematically studied and reported on their efforts to determine the most appropriate drugs and most efficacious dosages for a variety of different fungal infections.

In certain areas of the country, the endemic mycoses are common infections, and certain disease manifestations are particularly likely to occur in elderly persons (1). For several of these infections, such as chronic cavitary pulmonary histoplasmosis, treatment is mandatory and knowledge of the use of the new azole antifungal drugs is essential.

In recent years, an increase in infections with the opportunistic fungi, especially *Candida* and *Aspergillus,* has been noted in elderly patients, especially those in the intensive care unit setting (2,3). In this situation, treatment is not only required, but must be given promptly and expertly to prevent a fatal outcome. Most often, amphotericin B is the drug of choice, and knowledge of how to administer this drug, with its frequent toxicities in older patients, is essential.

More commonly, elderly persons have local fungal infections, such as denture stomatitis or tinea infections, which are not serious, but tend to recur and are annoying. Several options now exist for therapy of these types of fungal infections. In these circumstances, efficacy, absence of toxicity, and cost are important factors to be considered in choosing the most appropriate antifungal drug.

II. AMPHOTERICIN B (FUNGIZONE)

A. Chemistry and Mechanism of Action

Amphotericin B is a member of the polyene macrolide family of drugs resulting from fermentation of *Streptomyces nodosus.* The drug binds to ergosterol, a major component of fungal cell membranes, leading to changes in membrane permeability, subsequent leakage of cell constituents, and cell death (4).

B. Antifungal Spectrum

Amphotericin B is active against most classes of fungi, including dermatophytes, all of the dimorphic organisms causing the major endemic mycoses (histoplasmosis, blastomycosis, sporotrichosis, coccidioidomycosis), the yeastlike opportunists (*Candida, Torulopsis,* and *Cryptococcus*), and the filamentous opportunists (*Aspergillus, Rhizopus, Mucor,* and many others) (5). One opportunist against which it is not active is *Pseudallescheria boydii* (6).

C. Clinical Pharmacology

Amphotericin B is not water soluble and is not absorbed when given orally. It has been developed for use by the addition of sodium desoxycholate, giving a colloidal dispersion for intravenous infusion (7). The drug is rapidly taken up by cell membranes, and serum levels are low (7,8). The drug is highly protein bound and achieves only very low concentrations in body fluids, such as urine, cerebrospinal fluid, and synovial fluid (8). Tissues with the highest concentration of drug are kidney, liver, spleen, and lung (7). Amphotericin B is very slowly eliminated, and the mechanisms of elimination have not been elucidated. Active drug can be detected in urine for as long as one month after discontinuation (9).

D. Clinical Indications

Amphotericin B remains the drug of choice for many different fungal infections seen in elderly patients. One definite indication is the treatment of the opportunistic infections aspergillosis and mucormycosis (10). The total dose and length of therapy will vary depending on the manifestations of infection, but as a general rule, aggressive use of high doses of amphotericin B is required for these difficult-to-treat infections.

Amphotericin B continues to remain the drug of choice for therapy of disseminated candidiasis and candidemia, the most common nosocomial fungal infection encountered in elderly patients (4,5,10). The question is frequently asked whether an elderly patient who has preexisting renal insufficiency should be treated for candidemia with fluconazole instead of amphotericin B. Although less toxic, only anecdotal reports on the use of fluconazole are available. Both failures (11) and successes (12) have been described with fluconazole. It seems prudent to use amphotericin B, at least initially, in these cases to ensure the best possible antifungal effect.

The initial therapy of cryptococcal meningitis remains amphotericin B combined with flucytosine (13). However, after the patient is stabilized and cultures are negative, it is probably reasonable to switch to fluconazole (14).

Even though the oral azoles have supplanted amphotericin B as primary treatment of many of the endemic mycoses (histoplasmosis, blastomycosis, sporotrichosis, and coccidioidomycosis), amphotericin B remains useful for acute, life-threatening manifestations, such as overwhelmingly pulmonary infection and meningitis. It is now unlikely, however, that the entire course of therapy for any of the endemic mycoses will require amphotericin B as the only drug. Azoles are often used after initial therapy with amphotericin B is completed.

In a patient with candiduria, bladder irrigation with amphotericin B for 3–5 days usually eliminates colonization of the bladder but is probably not effective for invasion of the bladder and certainly does not treat upper tract infection (15,16). Whether it is necessary to eliminate colonization and whether amphotericin B irrigation is preferable to fluconazole in the elderly diabetic patient or elderly patient in the intensive care unit is not known.

E. Administration of Drug

Amphotericin B is available as a powder containing 50 mg amphotericin B and 41 mg sodium desoxycholate. Ten milliliters of sterile water is added to the vial giving a concentration of 5 mg/ml, which is further diluted in 5% dextrose in water to a concentration of 0.1 mg/ml. A test dose of 1 mg in 50 ml 5% dextrose in water is infused over 20–30 minutes to ensure that the patient will tolerate the drug. Rarely, an anaphylactic reaction or arrhythmia will occur, precluding therapy with amphotericin B (5).

Amphotericin B is generally infused slowly over approximately 4 h. Some patients can tolerate a faster infusion, but generally 2 h should be the minimum time of infusion in elderly patients, who often have cardiac and/or renal problems (17). The solution does not have to be covered to protect it from light (5).

The daily dose, length of therapy, and rapidity with which the daily dose is attained depend on the infection being treated, the use of concomitant antifungals, such as flucytosine, and toxicity manifested by the patient (5). The specifics of administration often require consultation with an infectious diseases specialist. However, the following general points can be made. If the infection is a life-threatening opportunistic infection for which there is no other antifungal therapy, high-dose amphotericin B (0.7–1.0 mg/kg/day) is attained quickly (within 2–3 days) and continued while trying to prevent nephrotoxicity, as suggested below. If the patient has a chronic endemic mycotic infection, for which amphotericin B is the treatment of choice, then the daily dose can be lower (~0.5 mg/kg/day), can be achieved after a slow increase in the daily dose over 1 week, and therapy can be changed to alternate days if nephrotoxicity intervenes. It has been shown that the addition of a drug, such as flucytosine, causing synergistic killing of organisms such as *Cryptococcus neoformans,* will allow a lower daily dose of amphotericin B (e.g., 0.3 mg/kg/day) to be used (13).

The major side effect of amphotericin B is nephrotoxicity, making it sometimes difficult to give to elderly patients (18–21). Careful attention to hydration of the patient can obviate some of this toxicity. It has been shown that nephrotoxicity is enhanced when a patient is dehydrated or salt-depleted (20). With an elderly patient, who may have cardiac failure, a balance needs to be achieved between the consequences of salt and water loading and the nephrotoxity of amphotericin B.

Some patients tolerate the infusion of amphotericin B very poorly, developing rigors, fever, nausea, and vomiting (5,21). Premedication with acetominophen, diphenhydramine hydrochloride, and prochlorperazine can abort many of the above symptoms. Some patients will require intravenous meperidine to stop rigors (22), and rarely, corticosteroids, such as methylprednisolone, may be required.

For use as a bladder irrigant, 50 mg amphotericin B is suspended in 1000 ml of sterile water for irrigation and infused over 24 h through a triple-lumen catheter (5,15,16).

F. Drug Monitoring and Adverse Effects

Nephrotoxicity is the major side effect of amphotericin B (18–21). It is presumably related to vasoconstriction of the afferent renal arterioles (18). Although usually reversible (21), renal insufficiency may persist if the patient has had a large cumulative dose of amphotericin B or has been given several nephrotoxic drugs concomitantly (5). Other toxicities include hypokalemia, hypomagnesemia, renal tubular acidosis, and nephrogenic diabetes insipidus related to effects on the renal tubules (23); anemia, which occurs in most patients but rarely requires transfusion (24); and immediate effects related to the infusion, including chills or rigors, fever, nausea and vomiting, and phlebitis (5,7). Less commonly, thrombocytopenia, hepatotoxicity, and arrhythmias have been reported (5).

Neither minimal inhibitory concentrations (MICs) nor serum levels of amphotericin B are readily obtained. However, those parameters altered by amphotericin B need to be monitored carefully. Thus, serum creatinine, blood urea nitrogen, serum potassium, and serum magnesium should be monitored 2–3 times weekly, and a complete blood count should be obtained weekly.

III. FLUCYTOSINE (5-FLUOROCYTOSINE, 5-FC, ANCOBON)

A. Chemistry and Mechanism of Action

Flucytosine is a synthetic fluorinated pyrimidine compound. Yeast cells selectively take up the drug and convert it to 5-fluorouracil (5-FU), which interferes with RNA synthesis. In addition, a second action inhibits DNA synthesis in yeast (4,7). There is minimal uptake by mammalian cells; however, it has been postulated that some conversion from 5-FC to 5-FU in humans might occur by normal gut flora. Nanogram amounts of 5-FU can sometimes be measured in serum (25).

B. Antifungal Spectrum

The antifungal activity of flucytosine is more limited than that of most other commonly used antifungal agents. It has excellent activity against yeasts, including *Candida albicans* and other *Candida* species, *Torulopsis glabrata, C. neoformans,* and other yeasts (4,10). When combined with amphotericin B, synergistic killing of many strains of yeast occurs (4,13). Although flucytosine may have synergistic activity with amphotericin B against some *Aspergillus* strains, it generally is inactive against filamentous fungi, dimorphic fungi, and the dermatophytes. When used alone, fungi quickly develop high-level resistance to flucytosine, rendering the drug useless (4).

C. Clinical Pharmacology

Flucytosine, only available as an oral preparation, is well absorbed from the gastrointestinal tract and distributes into all body fluids, including cerebrospinal fluid, vitreous humor, and synovial fluid (7,26). The drug is excreted almost totally unchanged in the urine, and the half-life is 3–6 h (26).

The most important pharmacological consideration when using this drug in elderly patients is the effect of the reduced glomerular filtration rate of these individuals on flucytosine excretion. With reduced creatinine clearance, the excretion of flucytosine is diminished, serum levels rise, and toxicity is increased (27). When amphotericin B is

Table 1 Flucytosine Dosing in Patients with Renal Insufficiency

Creatinine clearance (ml/min)	Flucytosine dosage (mg/kg)	Dosing interval (h)
>40	35	6
20–40	35	12
10–20	35	24
<10	35	>24
hemodialysis	20	after each dialysis

used in conjunction with flucytosine, as is almost always the case, creatinine clearance usually falls even further, and the risk of flucytosine toxicity is high (27).

D. Clinical Indications

Except in rare circumstances, flucytosine is an adjunctive drug, which should be used in combination with another antifungal drug, almost always amphotericin B (4,27). The two main indications for using flucytosine are treatment of cryptococcal meningitis and candidiasis, including *Torulopsis* infections.

In the elderly patient with cryptococcal meningitis, the treatment of choice is amphotericin B combined with flucytosine (13). Although fluconazole has proved very useful in treating this infection in acquired immunodeficiency syndrome (AIDS) patients (28), it cannot be recommended as primary therapy in non-AIDS patients with cryptococcal meningitis until further studies are done.

Although no studies have been carried out to show whether combined therapy with amphotericin B and flucytosine is superior to amphotericin B alone for treating serious *Candida* infections, many authorities recommend combination therapy for disseminated candidiasis, endophthalmitis, and meningitis (27). In an elderly patient with multiple medical problems who develops disseminated candidiasis, it seems reasonable to try to obtain synergistic killing of the organism with a two-drug regimen.

On rare occasions, flucytosine can be used as a single agent to treat *Candida* urinary tract infections. This can only be recommended in a patient in whom short-course therapy for 2 weeks or less is likely to eradicate the infection (27).

E. Administration of Drug

Flucytosine is available in 250-mg and 500-mg capsules, which can be given with food or on an empty stomach. The total daily dose is 150 mg/kg, which is given in divided doses every 6 h when the creatinine clearance is normal. With reduced creatinine clearance, the drug should be given as suggested in Table 1. In older patients it is uncommon to be able to give full-dose flucytosine; a general rule of thumb is to begin therapy every 8 h and then regulate the dose according to serum flucytosine levels.

F. Drug Monitoring and Adverse Effects

The most serious toxicity of flucytosine is bone marrow suppression, which is reversible if the drug is stopped, but which may progress to aplasia (29). Toxicity is directly related to serum levels of >100 μg/ml (29) and is especially common in elderly patients if the dose given is not appropriate for a reduced creatinine clearance. Other side effects include nausea and vomiting and hepatotoxicity, which usually are dose-related also. Rash can occur and usually requires that the drug be stopped.

When flucytosine is used, it is essential that serum levels be measured weekly to prevent toxicity. Side effects generally can be avoided if peak serum levels remain between 50 and 75 μg/ml.

IV. AZOLE DRUGS: KETOCONAZOLE (NIZORAL), ITRACONAZOLE (SPORANOX), FLUCONAZOLE (DIFLUCAN), AND MICONAZOLE (MONISTAT)

The systemic azole drugs will be discussed together since many of their properties are similar. Two of these drugs are available only as oral formulations (ketoconazole and itraconazole); one is available as both an oral and an intravenous preparation and has many differences from the other two oral drugs (fluconazole); and miconazole is only available for systemic use as an intravenous drug.

A. Chemistry and Mechanisms of Action

Azole antifungal drugs are multiringed compounds, which have in the 5-membered azole ring either two nitrogen atoms (imidazoles, such as ketoconazole and miconazole) or three nitrogen atoms (triazoles, such as itraconazole and fluconazole) (30).

The mechanism of action of all of the azoles is similar. They inhibit ergosterol synthesis in the fungal cell membrane and appear to do this by inhibition of the fungal cytochrome P-450 enzyme system (30–32). Different azoles bind with different avidity to fungal or mammalian cytochrome P-450 enzymes, influencing both the antifungal activity and the toxicity of the drugs (33). In addition to inhibition of sterol synthesis, azoles may have other direct effects on cell membrane fatty acids and oxidative enzyme systems and appear to inhibit the formation of pseudohyphae in *Candida* species (32,34).

B. Antifungal Spectrum

As a class of antifungals, the azoles have a broad range of activity, which includes dermatophytes, the dimorphic fungi causing the endemic mycoses, opportunistic yeasts, and opportunistic filamentous fungi (30). Several important differences exist among the four azole drugs in regard to antifungal activity. For example, itraconazole is the only azole with good activity against *Aspergillus* species (35), and it also appears to have better activity against *Sporothrix schenckii* (36). Miconazole has established activity against *P. boydii* (6).

It is important to note that in vitro susceptibility testing using azoles is not standardized and not always predictive of activity in vivo (30). Thus, much of the data showing the usefulness of these drugs derives from results in experimental infections using animal models and subsequent trials in humans.

C. Clinical Pharmacology

1. *Ketoconazole*

Ketoconazole is available only as an oral preparation. It is insoluble in water and requires gastric acid for absorption (7,37). In elderly patients one must be concerned that absorption

Table 2 Effects of Azole Antifungal Drugs on Serum Levels of Concomitantly Administered Drugs

Drug affected by azole	Azole antifungal drug		
	Ketoconazole	Itraconazole	Fluconazole
Cyclosporine	↑[a]	↑[a]	↑[a]
Warfarin	↑[a]	None known	↑[a]
Phenytoin	↑[a]	None known	↑[a]
Carbamazepine	None known	None known	↑[a]
Terfenadine	↑[b]	↑[b]	None known
Astemizole	↑[b]	↑[b]	None known
Digoxin	None known	↑[a]	None known
Oral hypoglycemics	↑	None known	↑
Isoniazid	↓[a]	None known	None known
Rifampin	↓[a]	None known	None known

[a] Significant interaction, monitor serum levels of drug and/or clinical status.
[b] Significant interaction causing arrhythmias; avoid combination.

may be erratic because of asymptomatic achlorhydria, which increases with increasing age (38).

Ketoconazole is highly protein bound and distributes poorly into various body compartments. Minimal levels are detected in cerebrospinal fluid, urine, vitreous humor, and peritoneal fluid (39). The drug is metabolized almost totally by the liver, and the serum half-life is very long so that once-daily dosing is adequate (7).

Ketoconazole has several important interactions with other drugs, which have resulted in either drug toxicity or therapeutic failures because of more rapid metabolism of ketoconazole or the concomitantly administered drug (40–44) (Tables 2 and 3). Several of these interactions have important ramifications for elderly patients.

2. *Itraconazole*

Itraconazole is also available only as an oral formulation. It shares with ketoconazole the property of insolubility in water and the requirement for gastric acid to allow absorption (45). Thus, like ketoconazole, there should be some concern that elderly persons with an increased likelihood of achlorhydria may not absorb adequate levels of the drug.

Table 3 Effects of Concomitantly Administered Drugs on Azole Antifungal Drug Levels

Drug affecting azole level	Azole antifungal drug level		
	Ketoconazole	Itraconazole	Fluconazole
Rifampin	↓	↓	↓
Isoniazid	↓	None known	None known
Phenytoin	↓	↓	None known
Carbamazepine	None known	↓	None known

Reductions in azole levels have led to therapeutic failures for some fungal infections.

Itraconazole is highly protein bound and lipophilic (45). It does not distribute well into various body fluids, and serum levels are relatively low (45,46). However, the drug slowly accumulates so that steady state is not reached for several weeks. It accumulates in tissues with high lipid content and has been effective in treating infections, such as meningitis, even though drug cannot be measured in the cerebrospinal fluid (47). Itraconazole is metabolized almost entirely by the liver with no renal excretion (45). The serum half-life is long, so that once or twice daily dosing is appropriate.

There are several important interactions of itraconazole with other drugs, which have led either to toxicity or inadequate drug levels and subsequent therapeutic failure (40,41,48,50) (see Tables 2 and 3). In elderly patients, it is especially important to note the interaction with digoxin, which can result in digoxin toxicity (49,50).

3. *Fluconazole*

Fluconazole differs from ketoconazole and itraconazole in being water soluble; thus, an intravenous as well as an oral preparation are available, and absorption from the gastrointestinal tract is excellent (51). Of the three oral azole preparations, in aging adults there should be the least concern about poor absorption when using fluconazole.

Fluconazole is not highly protein bound and distributes well into all body fluids, including cerebrospinal fluid, vitreous humor, and synovial fluid (52). The drug is excreted almost entirely by the kidneys (51). Thus, in contrast to ketoconazole and itraconazole, the dose should be reduced in renal failure—a 50% reduction for a creatinine clearance of 20–50 ml/min and a 75% reduction for a creatinine clearance <20 ml/min is suggested. With normal renal function, the serum half-life is about 30 h; thus single daily dosing is appropriate.

The interaction of fluconazole with other drugs relates primarily to its inhibition of the P-450–dependent enzyme system (40,41,53–57). Several of these interactions are clinically significant, especially in older patients (see Tables 2 and 3). When treating elderly patients, the most important interactions are those causing an increase in warfarin and phenytoin serum levels.

4. *Miconazole*

Miconazole is available only as an intravenous preparation. It is insoluble in water and must be infused in a polyethoxylated castor oil preparation (Cremaphor EL), which is responsible for many of the side effects of the drug (7,30,31). The drug is highly protein bound, distributes poorly into various body sites, has a short half-life requiring administration every 8 h, and is metabolized by the liver (7,58).

Drug interactions between miconazole and other P-450 metabolized drugs have not been elucidated as have those with the oral azoles, although there is a suggestion that there could be an interaction with warfarin (7).

D. Clinical Indications

1. *Ketoconazole*

In the 1980s, ketoconazole became the drug of choice for treating non–life-threatening histoplasmosis, blastomycosis, and coccidioidomycosis (59,60). However, its use in these endemic mycoses is now challenged by itraconazole, which has been shown to be both less toxic and more effective than ketoconazole in noncomparative clinical trials (61,62).

Ketoconazole has been very effective in treating localized candidiasis, such as denture stomatitis, thrush, vaginitis, and esophagitis (39). Fluconazole, with its good absorption characteristics, perhaps will be a better drug for these infections in elderly patients. However, ketoconazole is much cheaper than fluconazole. Ketoconazole should not be used for disseminated candidiasis and candidemia.

Dermatophyte infections, such as tinea corporis or onychomycosis, continue to be treated with ketoconazole (39). However, in elderly individuals, the physician and patient should discuss whether the infection is severe enough to justify systemic therapy, which in the case of onychomycosis would have to be given for at least 6 months.

2. *Itraconazole*

For most endemic mycoses, itraconazole has supplanted ketoconazole in non–life-threatening clinical situations. It is less toxic, better tolerated, and more efficacious (36,61–65). Thus, the elderly person with chronic cavitary pulmonary or disseminated histoplasmosis, with pulmonary disease or skin lesions due to blastomycosis, and probably with lymphocutaneous sporotrichosis should be treated with itraconazole (36,64,65).

Itraconazole may be an effective alternative to amphotericin B for treating some forms of aspergillosis (35). Studies are currently underway to determine the most efficacious, least toxic drug for this serious infection.

Itraconazole is effective in treating localized candidiasis (63,66) and could supplant ketoconazole for this indication. However, fluconazole will probably continue to be used more commonly. Itraconazole should not be used to treat disseminated candidiasis and candidemia.

3. *Fluconazole*

Fluconazole is approved for use in treating cryptococcal meningitis and candidiasis. Although the approval for cryptococcosis arose from its use in AIDS patients (28,67), the drug has been used in non-AIDS patients with cryptococcal meningitis. However, experience is limited, no prospective study has been reported, and initial therapy for cryptococcal meningitis should remain amphotericin B and flucytosine, with fluconazole used only after the patient's condition has stabilized (14).

Fluconazole is very effective for *Candida* esophagitis (68); given its better absorption characteristics than ketoconazole, it should be used in elderly patients with this problem. *Candida* vaginitis, thrush, and denture stomatitis also respond well to fluconazole (69–71), but creams, lozenges, and suppositories are also effective and cheaper. Fluconazole is currently only a second-line drug for treating disseminated *Candida* infections and candidemia. If and when it is shown to be as effective as amphotericin B in these situations, it may become the drug of choice in elderly patients because of its low toxicity (11,12,72–74).

Although fluconazole is approved for the treatment of *Candida* urinary tract infections, little clinical information is available to show its usefulness. In a patient who does not already have an indwelling catheter in place, fluconazole is preferred over amphotericin B bladder irrigation. Fluconazole should be useful for *Candida* infection of the kidneys, but again data are not available to prove this.

Fluconazole is not approved for treatment of the endemic mycoses, but it has become standard treatment for coccidioidal meningitis in the last few years, obviating the need for intrathecal amphotericin B (75). It may assume a role in treating other endemic mycoses in the future, but only preliminary data are available showing efficacy for these mycoses (76).

4. *Miconazole*

The only indication for the use of intravenous miconazole is treatment of *Pseudallescheria* infections, a very uncommon problem (6,10,31). Because of the toxicity of the vehicle used for infusion and a dearth of information showing efficacy, miconazole is only rarely used to treat disseminated candidiasis (30,31).

E. Administration of Drug

1. Ketoconazole

Ketoconazole is available in 200-mg tablets. The usual daily dose is 200 mg for simple infections, such as tinea or thrush, and 400–800 mg for serious systemic mycotic infections; doses as high as 1200 mg daily may be needed for infections like coccidioidomycosis (60). Ketoconazole is usually given with a meal to ensure adequate gastric acidity, but absorption remains variable, depending on the pH achieved (7,37,41). Once-daily dosing is used unless a large dose cannot be tolerated; then it can be split into two doses. The patient should not take antacids or H_2 blockers, as these decrease absorption. Sucralfate has less effect but may still decrease absorption (P. L. Carver, personal communication). The dose does not have to be decreased with renal failure.

2. Itraconazole

Itraconazole is available in 100-mg capsules. The usual dose is 100 or 200 mg for less serious infections and 400 mg for systemic infections. In treating *Aspergillus* infections, 600 mg has been used (35). Once-daily dosing is used, although larger doses should be given twice daily. All of the caveats regarding gastric absorption noted above for ketoconazole obtain for itraconazole as well. The dose should not be decreased with renal failure.

3. Fluconazole

Fluconazole is available as 50-, 100-, and 200-mg tablets and as an intravenous preparation at a concentration of 2 mg/ml. Unless the patient is vomiting or unable to absorb oral drugs, fluconazole should be given orally. The dose for localized or minor infection is 50–200 mg daily, given as one dose, usually with food. For serious systemic infections, the usual dose is 400–800 mg daily. At higher doses, two daily doses may be better tolerated by the patient. Doses greater than 800 mg have been used in experimental protocols but are not approved at this time. As noted earlier, daily doses should be reduced with severe renal insufficiency.

4. Miconazole

Miconazole is available for intravenous infusion as 200 mg base in 20 ml solution containing 1% Cremophor EL. The daily dose may vary from 600 to 2400 mg. It is infused slowly at a rate of approximately 100 mg/h since rapid infusion has been associated with arrhythmias and cardiac and respiratory arrest (4,31). Because of a short half-life, miconazole must be administered every 8 h (7).

F. Drug Monitoring and Adverse Effects

It is unfortunate that serum levels of the azoles are not readily available. Especially in elderly individuals, who may have asymptomatic achlorhydria, inadequate absorption of ketoconazole and presumably itraconazole may occur with subsequent therapeutic failure. The clinician has no effective way to monitor this.

1. *Ketoconazole*

Ketoconazole has more significant side effects than either itraconazole or fluconazole because of its greater effects on steroid metabolism in mammalian cells (77). These effects are rarely seen at daily doses of 200 or 400 mg, but are common at doses of 800 mg and greater (59,60,77). Both androgenic hormones and glucocorticoid synthesis are suppressed. Decreased libido, azospermia, and gynecomastia are common. These are generally reversible, but this may take months if the patient has been on the drug for a long time. Clinically significant Addison's disease has been described in several patients (78); once-daily dosing rather than twice-daily dosing allows normalization of cortisol levels before the next dose (77).

Hepatitis has been reported with ketoconazole (79). It appears to be idiosyncratic, occurring approximately once in every 15,000 patients, and does not seem to be age-related (79), differing from the situation noted with isoniazid. Although usually reversible, fulminant hepatitis has been described. Other possible side effects include nausea and vomiting (which may require stopping the drug), rash, and fatigue.

Drug interactions occur with concomitant use of ketoconazole and cyclosporine, causing high cyclosporine levels and nephrotoxicity (41,44), and with rifampin and isoniazid, which can lead to failure of both antituberculous and antifungal therapy (42,43). Serious arrhythmias have been noted with concomitant administration of ketoconazole and terfenadine (Seldane) or astemizole (Hismanal). These two antihistamines should never be used with ketoconazole (see Tables 2 and 3).

2. *Itraconazole*

Itraconazole appears to have fewer side effects than ketoconazole in regard to inhibition of steroid metabolism (80). Only at doses of 600 mg or greater have effects on steroid metabolism been noted (81). Nausea, vomiting, edema, and rash occur uncommonly (80). Hepatitis has been reported (82), and the number of cases may increase as more experience accrues with the drug.

Drug interactions with concomitantly administered drugs may cause serious toxicity (Tables 2 and 3). The most important interaction in older adults is a rise in serum digoxin levels in patients taking both drugs. The mechanisms of this interaction and the prevalence are unknown since only a few cases have been reported to date (49,50). Digoxin levels should be carefully monitored in any elderly patient receiving itraconazole. Other drug interactions may also lead to increased serum levels of potentially toxic drugs, such as astemizole (Hismanal) and terfenadine (Seldane) (40,41,48). Serum levels of cyclosporine need to be monitored when patients take this drug with itraconazole. Terfenadine and astemizole should never be given with itraconazole.

3. *Fluconazole*

Fluconazole is relatively nontoxic. It appears to have no effects on mammalian steroid metabolism. Nausea, vomiting, and fatigue can occur. Rash has been described, including Stevens-Johnson syndrome in several AIDS patients (83). Hepatitis has also been described, and can be severe (84). Recently, seizures have been added as a possible effect of fluconazole, but it is not clear if they were actually related to fluconazole.

The interaction of fluconazole with drugs metabolized by the P-450 enzyme system is significant (see Tables 2 and 3). Increased serum drug levels of warfarin, phenytoin, cyclosporine, and carbamazepine have been noticed in patients receiving fluconazole and one of these drugs (40,41,53–57). In elderly patients who might be taking warfarin or phenytoin, this should be a significant concern. The prothrombin time and phenytoin levels should be monitored very carefully in patients treated with fluconazole in addition to warfarin or phenytoin, respectively.

4. *Miconazole*

One of the reasons miconazole has become a second-line drug is the number of significant side effects. Immediate toxicity during the infusion includes anaphylaxis, arrhythmias, chills and fever, nausea, and cardiac and respiratory arrest (4,7,31). Some of these effects can be minimized if the drug is given slowly (31). In addition, hyperlipidemia, pruritus, and phlebitis are common and felt to be related to the diluent used for the drug (4). Unless specifically indicated, such as treatment of *Pseudallescheria* infection, there is no reason to give this drug.

V. POTASSIUM IODIDE

Only brief mention will be made of potassium iodide. For years it has been used to treat lymphocutaneous sporotrichosis with reasonable success, although the exact mode of action is not known. It has rarely been effective in the treatment of systemic sporotrichosis and has no use in treating other fungal infections.

Potassium iodide is usually administered as a saturated solution (SSKI) of 1 mg/ml. Generally, treatment is begun at 10 drops of SSKI three times daily and increased by 1 drop per dose each day reaching a maximum of 60 drops three times daily. Treatment is required for several months and should be continued at least 1 month beyond the time the lesions have disappeared.

Most patients experience some side effects during treatment with SSKI. A metallic taste in the mouth is usually one of the first symptoms. Nasal congestion, skin rash that resembles acne, nausea, and diarrhea are very common. Parotid swelling occurs less commonly. It is likely that itraconazole will supplant SSKI for treatment of lymphocutaneous sporotrichosis (36), and it is unlikely that the drug will have much use in the future.

VI. GRISEOFULVIN

Griseofulvin will be mentioned briefly. It is a systemically administered drug, which has activity only against the dermatophytes and is used only to treat superficial skin and nail infections. Griseofulvin is very insoluble and absorbed poorly, although newer microsize and ultra-microsize formulations have improved its absorption characteristics.

Drug interactions with warfarin are significant, usually requiring an increase in the anticoagulant dose, and demand that careful monitoring of prothrombin time be done in an older individual who is on both drugs. Interactions with phenobarbital and birth control pills also occur with griseofulvin. The side effects of griseofulvin include headache, rash, nausea, vomiting, diarrhea, and peripheral neuropathy, which is uncommon and only occurs after prolonged therapy. Leukopenia and neutropenia have also been described uncommonly.

Griseofulvin should be used for serious tinea infections and onychomycosis (85,86). The usual dose is 500 mg daily, but 1000 mg may be needed for difficult-to-eradicate infections. Therapy is usually given for at least 6–8 weeks for simple tinea infections and for as long as 6 months to a year for nail infections, which may be very recalcitrant to therapy. Although more costly, azoles, such as ketoconazole or itraconazole, could be used for the treatment of dermatophyte infections instead of griseofulvin.

REFERENCES

1. Kauffman CA, Terpenning MS. Deep fungal infections in the elderly. J Am Geriatr Soc 1988; 36:548–57.
2. Fraser DW, Ward JI, Ajello L, et al. Aspergillosis and other systemic mycoses. The growing problem. JAMA 1979; 242:1631–5.
3. Kauffman CA. Fungal infections. Clin Geriatr Med 1992; 8:777–91.
4. Medoff G, Kobayashi GS. Strategies in the treatment of systemic fungal infections. N Engl J Med 1980; 302:145–55.
5. Gallis HW, Drew RH, Pickard WW. Amphotericin B: 30 years of clinical experience. Rev Infect Dis 1990; 12:308–29.
6. Dworzack DL, Clark RB, Borkowski WJ, et al. *Pseudallescheria boydii* brain abscess: association with near-drowning and efficacy of high-dose prolonged miconazole therapy in patients with multiple abscesses. Medicine (Balt.) 1989; 68:218–24.
7. Daneshmend TK, Warnock DW. Clinical pharmacokinetics of systemic antifungal drugs. Clin Pharmacokinet 1983; 8:17–42.
8. Bindschadler DD, Bennett JE. A pharmacologic guide to the clinical use of amphotericin B. J Infect Dis 1969; 120:427–36.
9. Atkinson AJ, Bennett JE. Amphotericin B pharmacokinetics in humans. Antimicrob Agents Chemother 1978; 13:271–8.
10. Terrell CL, Hughes CE. Antifungal agents used for deep-seated mycotic infections. Mayo Clin Proc 1992; 67:69–91.
11. McIlroy MA. Failure of fluconazole to suppress fungemia in a patient with fever, neutropenia, and typhlitis. J Infect Dis 1991; 163:420–1.
12. Kujath P, Lerch K. Secondary mycosis in surgery: treatment with fluconazole. Infection 1989; 17:111–17.
13. Bennett JE, Dismukes WE, Duma RJ, et al. A comparison of amphotericin B alone and combined with flucytosine in the treatment of cryptococcal meningitis. N Engl J Med 1979; 301:126–31.
14. Powderly WG. Treatment of cryptococcal meningitis. Infect Dis Clin Pract 1992; 1:164–68.
15. Fisher JF, Chew WH, Shadomy S, et al. Urinary tract infections due to *Candida albicans*. Rev Infect Dis 1982; 4:1107–17.
16. Wise GJ. Amphotericin B in urological practice. J Urol 1990; 144:215–23.
17. Ellis ME, Al-Hokail AA, Clink HM, et al. Double-blind randomized study of the effect of infusion rates on toxicity of amphotericin B. Antimicrob Agents Chemother 1992; 36:172–9.
18. Sawaya BP, Weihprecht M, Campbell WR, et al. Direct vasoconstriction as a possible cause for amphotericin B-induced nephrotoxicity in rats. J Clin Invest 1991; 87:2097–107.
19. Clements JS, Peacock JE. Amphotericin B revisited: reassessment of toxicity. Am J Med 1990; 88:22N–27N.
20. Branch RA. Prevention of amphotericin B induced renal impairment. Arch Intern Med 1981; 148:2389–94.
21. Butler WT, Bennett JE, Alling DW, et al. Nephrotoxicity of amphotericin B: early and late effects in 81 patients. Ann Intern Med 1964; 61:175–87.
22. Burks LC, Aisner J, Fortner CL, Wiernik PH. Meperidine for the treatment of shaking chills. Ann Intern Med 1980; 140:483–4.
23. Burgess JL, Bircholl R. Nephrotoxicity of amphotericin B, with emphasis on changes in tubular function. Am J Med 1972; 53:77–84.
24. Lin AC, Goldwasser E, Bernard EM, Chapman SW. Amphotericin B blunts erythropoietin response to anemia. J Infect Dis 1990; 161:348–51.
25. Diasio RB, Lakings DE, Bennett JE. Evidence for conversion of 5-fluorocytosine to 5-fluorouracil in humans: possible factor in 5-fluorocytosine clincial toxicity. Antimicrob Agents Chemother 1978; 14:903–8.

26. Schonebeck J, Polak A, Fernax M, Scholer HJ. Pharmacokinetic studies on the oral antimycotic agent 5-fluorocytosine in individuals with normal and impaired renal function. Chemotherapy (Basel) 1973; 18:321–36.
27. Kauffman CA. Flucytosine. In: Peterson PK, Verhoef J, eds. Antimicrobial agents annual 3. Amsterdam: Elsevier Science Publishers, 1988:246–50.
28. Saag MS, Powderly WG, Cloud GA et al. Comparison of amphotericin B with fluconazole in the treatment of acute AIDS-associated cryptococcal meningitis. N Engl J Med 1992; 326:83–9.
29. Kauffman CA, Frame PT. Bone marrow toxicity associated with 5-fluorocytosine therapy. Antimicrob Agents Chemother 1977; 11:244–7.
30. Saag MS, Dismukes WE. Azole antifungal agents: emphasis on new triazoles. Antimicrob Agents Chemother 1988; 32:1–8.
31. Bodey GP. Azole antifungal agents. Clin Infect Dis 1992; 14(suppl 1):S161–9.
32. Fromtling RA. Overview of medically important antifungal azole derivatives. Clin Microbiol Rev 1988; 1:187–217.
33. vandenBossche H, Bellens D, Cooks W, et al. Cytochrome P-450: target for itraconazole. Drug Dev Res 1986; 8:287–98.
34. Uno J, Shigematsu ML, Arai T. Primary site of action of ketoconazole on *Candida albicans.* Antimicrob Agents Chemother 1982; 21:912–18.
35. Denning DW, Tucker RM, Hanson LH, et al. Treatment of invasive aspergillosis with itraconazole. Am J Med 1989; 86:791–800.
36. Sharkey PK, Kauffman CA, Graybill JR, et al. Treatment of sporotrichosis with itraconazole. Am J Med 1993; 95:279–85.
37. Lelawongs P, Barone JA, Colaizzi JL, et al. Effect of food and gastric acidity on absorption of orally administered ketoconazole. Clin Pharm 1988; 7:228–35.
38. Shamburek RD, Farrar JT. Disorders of the digestive system in the elderly. N Engl J Med 1990; 322:438–42.
39. Heel RC, Brogdan RN, Carmine A, et al. Ketoconazole: a review of its therapeutic efficacy in systemic fungal infections. Drugs 1980; 19:7–30.
40. Tucker RM, Denning DW, Hanson LH, et al. Interaction of azoles with rifampin, phenytoin, and carbamazepine: in vitro and clinical observations. Clin Infect Dis 1992; 14:165–74.
41. Carver PL. Clinically relevant drug interactions and adverse effects of antimicrobial agents. Curr Opin Infect Dis 1991; 4:749–56.
42. Doble N, Shaw R, Rowland-Hill C, et al. Pharmacokinetic study of the interaction between rifampin and ketoconazole. J Antimicrob Chemother 1988; 21:633–5.
43. Abadie-Kemmerly S, Pankey GA, Dalvisio JR. Failure of ketoconazole treatment of *Blastomyces dermatitidis* due to interaction of isoniazid and rifampin. Ann Intern Med 1988; 109:844–5.
44. Ferguson RM, Sutherland DER, Simmons RL, Najarian JS. Ketoconazole, cyclosporine metabolism, and renal transplantation. Lancet 1982; 2:882–3.
45. Heykants J, Van Peer A, Van de Velde V, et al. The clinical pharmacokinetics of itraconazole: an overview. Mycoses 1989; 32 (suppl 1):67–87.
46. Perfect J, Durack DT. Penetration of imidazoles and triazoles into cerebrospinal fluid of rabbits. J Antimicrob Chemother 1985; 16:81–6.
47. Tucker RM, Denning DW, Dupont B, et al. Itraconazole therapy for chronic coccidioidal meningitis. Ann Intern Med 1990; 112:108–12.
48. Kramer MR, Marshall SE, Denning DW, et al. Cyclosporine and itraconazole interactions in heart and lung transplant recipients. Ann Intern Med 1990; 113:327–9.
49. Rex J. Itraconazole-digoxin interaction. Ann Intern Med 1992; 116:525.
50. Kauffman CA, Bagnaso FA. Digoxin toxicity associated with itraconazole therapy. Clin Infect Dis 1992; 15:886-7.
51. Brammer KW, Farrow PR, Faulkner JW. Pharmacokinetics and tissue penetration of fluconazole in humans. Rev Infect Dis 1990; 12 (suppl 3):S318–26.

52. Arndt CA, Walsh TJ, McCulley CL, et al. Fluconazole penetration into cerebrospinal fluid: implications for treating fungal infections of the central nervous system. J Infect Dis 1988; 157:178–80.
53. Rowe BR, Thorpe J, Barnett A. Safety of fluconazole in women taking oral hypoglycaemic agents. Lancet 1992; 339:255–6.
54. Lazar JD, Wilner KD. Drug interactions with fluconazole. Rev Infect Dis 1990; 12 (suppl 3):S327–33.
55. Kowalsky SF. Drug interactions with fluconazole. Pharmacotherapy 1990; 10:170S–73S.
56. Blum RA, Wilton JH, Hilligoss DM, et al. Effect of fluconazole on the disposition of phenytoin. Clin Pharmacol Ther 1991; 49:420–5.
57. Sugar AM, Saunders C, Idelson BA, et al. Interaction of fluconazole and cyclosporine. Ann Intern Med 1989; 110:844.
58. Stevens DA, Levine HB, Deresinski SC. Miconazole in coccidioidomycosis. II. Therapeutic and pharmacologic studies in man. Am J Med 1976; 60:191–202.
59. NIAID Mycoses Study Group. Treatment of blastomycosis and histoplasmosis with ketoconazole: Results of a prospective randomized clinical trial. Ann Intern Med 1985; 103:861–72.
60. Ampel NM, Wieden MA, Galgiani JN. Coccidioidomycosis. An update. Rev Infect Dis 1989; 11:897–911.
61. Kauffman CA. Itraconazole, fluconazole, and amphotericin B in antifungal therapy. Curr Opin Infect Dis 1991; 4:764–8.
62. Graybill JR, Stevens DA, Galgiani JN, et al. Itraconazole treatment of coccidioidomycosis. Am J Med 1990; 89:282–90.
63. Cauwenbergh G, deDoncker P, Stoops K, deDier AM, Goyvaerts H, Schuermans V. Itraconazole in the treatment of human mycoses: review of three years of clinical experience. Rev Infect Dis 1987; 9:S146–52.
64. Restrepo A, Robledo J, Gomez I, et al. Itraconazole therapy in lymphangitic and cutaneous sporotrichosis. Arch Dermatol 1986; 122:413–17.
65. Dismukes WE, Bradsher RW, Cloud GA, et al. Itraconazole therapy of blastomycosis and histoplasmosis. Am J Med 1992; 93:489–97.
66. Blatchford NR. Treatment of oral candidiasis with itraconazole. J Am Acad Dermatol 1990; 23:565–7.
67. Powderly WG, Saag MS, Cloud GA, et al. A controlled trial of fluconazole or amphotericin B to prevent relapse of cryptococcal meningitis in patients with the acquired immunodeficiency syndrome. N Engl J Med 1992; 326:793–8.
68. Laine L, Dretler R, Conteas C, et al. Fluconazole composed with ketoconazole for the treatment of Candida esophagitis in AIDS. Ann Intern Med 1992; 117:655–60.
69. Meunier F, Aoun M, Gerard M. Therapy for oropharyngeal candidiasis in the immunocompromised host: a randomized double-blind study of fluconazole vs. ketoconazole. Rev Infect Dis 1990 12(suppl 3):S364–7.
70. Budtz-Jorgensen E, Holmstrup P, Krogh P. Fluconazole in the treatment of *Candida*-associated denture stomatitis. Antimicrob Agents Chemother 1988; 32:1859–63.
71. Lebech PE, Nielsen NC, Lundvall F, et al. Treatment of vaginal candidiasis with a single dose of fluconazole. Eur J Clin Microbiol Infect Dis 1988; 7:364–7.
72. Ikemoto H. A clinical study of fluconazole for the treatment of deep mycoses. Diagn Microbiol Infect Dis 1989; 12:239S–247S.
73. Kauffman CA, Bradley SF, Ross SL, Weber DA. Hepatosplenic candidiasis: successful treatment with fluconazole. Am J Med 1991; 91:137–41.
74. Anaissie E, Bodey, GP, Kantarjian H et al. Fluconazole therapy for chronic disseminated candidiasis in patients with leukemia and prior amphotericin B therapy. Am J Med 1991; 91:142–50.
75. Classen DC, Burke JP, Smith CB. Treatment of coccidioidal meningitis with fluconazole. J Infect Dis 1988; 158:903–4.

76. Diaz M, Negroni R, Montero-Gei F, et al. A Pan-American 5-year study of fluconazole therapy for deep mycoses in the immunocompetent host. Clin Infect Dis 1992; 14(suppl 1): S68–S76.
77. Feldman D. Ketoconazole and other imidazole derivatives as inhibitors of steroidogenesis. Endo Rev 1986; 7:409–20.
78. Khosla S, Wolfson JS, Demerjian Z, Godine JE. Adrenal crisis in the setting of high-dose ketoconazole therapy. Arch Intern Med 1989; 149:802–4.
79. Lewis JH, Zimmerman HJ, Benson GD, et al. Hepatic injury associated with ketoconazole therapy. Gastroenterology 1984; 86:503–13.
80. Tucker RM, Haq Y, Denning DW, et al. Adverse events associated with itraconazole in 189 patients on chronic therapy. J Antimicrob Chemother 1990; 26:561–66.
81. Sharkey PK, Rinaldi MG, Dunn JF, et al. High-dose itraconazole in the treatment of the severe mycoses. Antimicrob Agents Chemother 1991; 35:707–13.
82. Lavrijsen APM, Balmus KJ, Nugteren-Huying WM, et al. Hepatic injury associated with itraconazole. Lancet 1992; 340:251–2.
83. Gussenhoven MJE, Haak A, Peereboom-Wynia JDR, et al. Stevens-Johnson syndrome after fluconazole. Lancet 1991; 338:120.
84. Franklin JH, Elias E, Hirsch C. Fluconazole-induced jaundice. Lancet 1990; 336:565.
85. Jones HE. Therapy of superficial fungal infection. Med Clin North Am 1982; 66:873–93.
86. Roberts MM. Developments in the management of superficial fungal infections. J Antimicrob Chemother 1991; 28:47–57.

25

Antiviral Therapy

Thomas C. Cesario, Shookooh Yousefi Malekpour, Gloria Carandang, and Mary Cesario
University of California–Irvine, Orange, California

Recent discoveries have made the dream of antiviral therapy a reality. While generally producing considerable morbidity, viral infections are not usually associated with increased mortality. In compromised patients, however, including elderly patients, viral infections may be associated with more adverse outcomes. Because of both the morbidity and the mortality, there exists a need for effective treatment. Since aging adults, at least in some cases, are at increased risk from certain viral infections (influenza, herpes zoster), older individuals constitute a possible target group for antiviral treatments. Despite the increasing availability of new antiviral agents and the presence of greater information concerning their pharmacokinetics, relatively little is known about the use of antiviral agents in older patients. In this review we will focus on the pharmacology of antiviral agents, and where it is known, we will discuss the unique features of these agents when used in elderly patients. We will also examine in more depth the treatment of two important viral infections in seniors—influenza and herpes zoster.

I. AMANTADINE

Amantadine is a symmetrically shaped amine with clinically significant activity only against influenza A. This agent is well absorbed from the gastrointestinal tract, is not metabolized, and more than 90% is excreted unchanged by glomerular filtration (1). Blood levels following an oral dose of 2.5 mg/kg approximate 2.0 μmol/L (1), but lung tissue levels may be higher. The half-life of the drug is 24 h (1). In healthy, younger males, amantadine absorption ranged from 55 to 90% (2).

The toxicity of amantadine most often affects the central nervous system. Toxic manifestations include disorientation, confusion, anxiety, and insomnia. Other side effects include nausea, rash, and urinary retention. Elderly persons are particularly predisposed to these side effects, which occur in about 10% of subjects. Reduced renal function and decreased volume of distribution may influence the occurrence of side effects in older patients (3). To avoid such unwanted consequences, the Centers for Disease Control and Prevention (CDC) recommend the use of the lower 100-mg dose at least for nursing home residents (4). Further reductions in dosage, however, lead to suboptimal serum concentrations (5). Even at a dose of 100 mg/day, approximately 22% of older patients residing in nursing homes can be anticipated to experience some evidence of amantadine toxicity (6,7).

The primary use of amantadine is in the treatment and prophylaxis of influenza A (but not influenza B). The drug appears to inhibit an early stage of viral replication, most likely by inhibiting the uncoating of the viral genome (8), and thus is able to influence the ability of the virus to produce disease.

Since influenza is a common cause of severe respiratory illness, particularly in elderly nursing home residents, consideration of the use of amantadine in this setting is warranted. As many as 25% of elderly persons residing in this setting may experience complications of influenza severe enough to lead to hospitalization or even death (9). Thus, the most important consideration is the prevention of influenza. Most would agree that immunization is the first line of defense against the virus. Among the elderly population, however, immunization may have been overlooked or year-to-year variation in viral antigenicity may be so great that immunization may not be effective. Therefore, amantadine is available for older individuals who either were not immunized or are faced with a new influenza strain significantly different in antigenicity than the vaccine strain. Current evidence suggests amantadine at therapeutic doses can prevent 50% of expected infections but will ameliorate 70–100% of illnesses (10).

Amantadine may be given with immunization and will not affect antibody levels (11). The drug can be given in institutional settings where an influenza outbreak is in progress to halt the progression of the epidemic (7). The prophylactic value of amantadine is well established overall (12).

Amantadine also has some therapeutic values for influenza A infections, although specific information on the therapeutic use of amantadine in older adults is limited. Since its antiviral spectrum is limited to influenza A, some laboratory confirmation of the presence of this virus is desirable before the use of the drug. Ideally, this confirmation comes from the individual to be treated, but occasionally other individuals may provide evidence of the presence of the virus in the community. Amantadine when used therapeutically decreases the duration of fever by approximately 50%, but it can also influence other symptoms (13,14).

Amantadine resistance, however, has recently been reported and will have to be monitored in the future (15).

II. RIMANTADINE

Rimantadine is a promising agent not yet licensed in the United States. It appears to resemble amantadine in many respects, including its mechanism of action. It has similar prophylactic (12) and therapeutic value (16) and may be less toxic (12). It differs from amantadine in that it is not as dependent on the kidney for its elimination. Because of its pharmacological profile and seemingly reduced toxicities, it may be more suitable for use in elderly patients.

III. RIBAVIRIN

Ribavirin is a synthetic triazole nucleoside. It is converted by cellular enzymes to the monophosphate, diphosphate, and triphosphate forms and will then inhibit viral or virally induced enzymes (17). It is broadly reactive against a wide range of both RNA and DNA viruses in vitro. It can be given orally, but it is concentrated in red blood cells and can produce a fall in hematocrit. More recently, it has been used in children by the aerosol route to treat infants with severe infections with respiratory syncytial virus (18,19) and intravenously to treat individuals with lassa fever (20). It has as yet no approved indication in the United States for use in geriatric populations; however, since it has activity against influenza (21), it might be considered for use in severe influenza infections in elderly patients. To this end Liss and Bernstein (22) have shown it to be safe when administered by aerosol to older adults.

IV. ACYCLOVIR

Acyclovir is an acyclic analog of guanosine. When phosphorylated by virus-derived thymidine kinase, it can be further phosphorylated to its active state, the triphosphate, by cellular enzymes (23). In this latter form, the drug is an inhibitor of viral DNA polymerase by virtue of its incorporation into DNA with resultant chain termination (23). The virus has in vivo efficacy against herpes simplex virus types I and II and varicella zoster virus (23), but it has reduced efficacy against cytomegalovirus and Epstein-Barr virus.

The drug can be administered orally, intravenously, or topically. With normal renal function, the half-life of the drug is 3 h following an intravenous dose (24). After an intravenous dose of 5 mg/kg body weight, a peak serum level of 30–40 μmol/L is achieved. After oral administration of a 200-mg dose, peak levels range from 1.4 to 4.0 μmol/L (25). Acyclovir is 15% protein bound and has a volume of distribution of 70% of body weight (24).

Excretion of the drug is through both glomeular filtration and tubular secretion. Probenicid will significantly reduce renal clearance (26). Acyclovir is partially removed by dialysis and can be removed slowly by nonrenal routes in the absence of normal renal function (23).

The major deleterious effect of the drug is on renal function. This occurs if the drug is administered too rapidly, the patient is dehydrated, or renal insufficiency is present. This effect is due to crystallization of the drug in the kidneys and is generally reversible (27,28).

Little is known about alterations occurring in the pharmacokinetics of acyclovir with normal aging. Since the drug is excreted largely by the kidney, it might be anticipated that the pharmacokinetics might be altered with age, but future studies must address this in more detail.

Several studies have reported the use of both oral and intravenous acyclovir in immunosuppressed patients as well as older populations (29–32). In these studies no unusual toxic effects were observed. Freris (33), however, reported on serum levels in older patients following an 800-mg oral dose given five times daily. He found several of these patients had blood levels significantly higher than the others, and only two of these had noticeable renal disease. Thus, an occasional older patient may have serum levels of the drug that are higher than anticipated.

Acyclovir is especially useful in the treatment of herpes simplex and varicella zoster infections. While the genital herpes is not a major problem for elderly patients, it should be noted that topical, oral, and intravenous therapy will significantly influence the course of primary genital herpes. Topical therapy decreases symptoms, but oral and intravenous therapy reduce duration of symptoms, virus shedding, and time to healing as reviewed by Whitley et al. (34).

For herpes labialis in individuals of all ages, oral acyclovir has been found to have modest therapeutic benefits (decreased time to crust and extent of lesion area at day 5) (35). When used prophylactically for this condition, oral acyclovir also appears to have modest beneficial effects (36).

Of greater interest to the geriatrician is the effect of acyclovir on herpes simplex infections in the immunocompromised. This is of significance because of the greater numbers of older patients with underlying diseases requiring therapy that will suppress immune function. Topical, oral, and intravenous therapy can reduce morbidity from herpes simplex in this group (34). Additionally, acyclovir is useful at least in younger patients for the treatment of herpes simplex encephalitis (37).

In cases of varicella zoster virus, acyclovir has been reported to be beneficial for the treatment of chicken pox. The oral form of the drug reduced both the height and duration of fever as well as accelerated cutaneous healing in young adults (38). Most critical, however, to older patients is the treatment of herpes zoster or shingles. Early in the acyclovir experience, Balfour et al. (39) demonstrated that intravenous acyclovir reduced complications and accelerated cutaneous clearance of the virus in patients with disseminated disease and some form of immunocompromise.

More recently a number of investigators have addressed the treatment of herpes zoster in settings other than that of the immunocompromised patient. Cobo (40) studied the problem of herpes zoster ophthalmicus. While he did not specify the number of older patients studied, he indicated that he included a group of patients age 60 years and older. Patients were given 600 mg of drug five times daily for 10 days. Cobo found that the duration of viral shedding was significantly reduced. He also indicated that certain complications were significantly decreased, including permanent lid scarring, pseudodendritic keratoapathy, stromal keratitis, and anterior uveitis. Liesegang (41), in reviewing the topic of herpes ophthalmicus, noted that ocular complications occur in 50% of patients with ophthalmic herpes zoster and concluded that patients with herpes zoster ophthalmicus and a presumed normal immune system should receive oral acyclovir.

Dickens et al. (42) and Inamura et al. (31) studied the effects of intravenously administered acyclovir for herpes zoster involving the ear. The two studies included small numbers of patients, and the first was not controlled. Both authors suggested beneficial effects from the drug, and both studies included but were not limited to older patients. It was not clear from these studies if there was a significant effect of the drug on the major complications of this syndrome, mainly facial nerve palsy and deafness.

A number of studies published over the last 10 years have addressed the important question of the use of oral acyclovir for the treatment of herpes zoster in the nonimmunosuppressed patient. This is obviously an important question to practitioners of geriatric medicine.

McKendrick et al. (43) were among the first groups to investigate this problem. The initial study included 41 immunocompetent patients over the age of 50. These patients were given acyclovir 400 mg five times a day for 5 days, in a double-blind, randomized study. Acyclovir was shown to reduce the days of new lesion formation within the effected dermatome. The reduction was from 2 days in the placebo group to 1.2 days in the treated group. No other significant differences were identified. In the same year Peterslund et al. (30) compared intravenous acyclovir to oral acyclovir for the treatment of herpes zoster in 40 patients over the age of 60. The results appeared similar, but no untreated control group was included. In an earlier report using intravenous acyclovir (44), however, these authors detailed a double-blind, randomized, well-controlled study of the intravenous preparation. In that study they found a beneficial effect of acyclovir on the rate of healing and the period of pain. The results were most dramatic in those patients above 67 years old, those with fever, and those with fewer than 4 days of pain before entry.

In 1986, McKendrick et al. (29) compared oral acyclovir at a dose of 800 mg five times daily for 7 days with placebo in a randomized, double-blind trial carried out at three centers in the United Kingdom. Two hundred and five elderly immunocompetent patients were entered within 72 h of the onset of rash. Acyclovir significantly reduced the number of days during which new lesions were discovered (1.7 vs. 2.2 days), the number of days to loss of vesicles (6.4 vs. 8.2 days) and the number of days to full crusting (7.8 vs. 10 days) in those patients whose therapy was initiated less than 48 h after onset of the rash. Furthermore, acyclovir significantly reduced pain (40% vs. 100% at the end of the study). No major adverse effects were appreciated. Wood et al. (45) extended this study 2 years later to include 364 patients. They reached the same conclusions, and their study emphasized the need to begin therapy less than 48 h after the onset of rash. Huff et al. (46) used either a 400- or 800-mg dose of acyclovir five times a day for 10 days in a group of patients of all ages with rash present fewer than 3 days. No beneficial effects were seen in the lower-dosage group, but patients receiving the 800-mg dose experienced a shortened period of viral shedding (2.3 vs. 3.2 days), accelerated time to 50% scabbing (3.3 vs. 4.8 days) and 50% healing (7.1 vs. 9.6 days), and reduced acute pain. Again no major adverse effects were seen.

Morton (47) also demonstrated beneficial effects of acyclovir in a double-blind randomized trial in patients of different ages. He gave 800 mg five times a day for 7 days and found a reduced duration of rash, shortened period of new lesion formation, and reduced pain. However, subsequent studies have supported the contention that acyclovir does *not* influence the course of already established postherpetic neuralgia (48) or the incidence of this complication in those being treated for acute zoster (49).

These studies all suggest that oral acyclovir, if begun early enough, does have a modest beneficial effect on the course acute zoster. The benefit is largely directed at cessation of new lesions and crusting. Because the effects are modest and postherpetic neuralgia is not prevented, the use of acyclovir in this setting is not universally accepted.

Corticosteroid use has been subjected to meta analysis, and these agents have not been found to significantly reduce the incidence or degree of pain in postherpetic neuralgia (50) after 12 weeks of follow-up from the time of onset of the lesions.

A number of reports in the recent literature have now suggested that resistance to acyclovir can develop among members of the herpesvirus family (51,52). However, most cases of resistance have occurred in the setting of severe immune-suppressing disease processes requiring long-term treatment with acyclovir.

V. GANCICLOVIR

Ganciclovir is another acyclic nucleoside analog of guanine. It has similar activity to acyclovir (53) against herpes simplex virus and is approximately 10 times more active against cytomegalovirus and Epstein-Barr virus (15). Ganciclovir is also activated by phosphorylation initiated by viral or cellular kinases. The activated form of the drug causes inhibition of viral DNA polymerase. The drug can only be given intravenously and is generally given at a dose of 5 mg/kg every 12 h. The drug is given for 14–21 days unless the patient is immunosuppressed, in which case maintenance therapy (6 mg/kg 5 days/week) is generally provided. The drug is excreted almost entirely in the urine and is only minimally bound to protein (1–2%). Cerebrospinal fluid (CSF) concentrations approximate 31–67% of concurrent plasma levels (54), and serum levels are similar to those of acyclovir.

The drug is frequently associated with unwanted toxicity, neutropenia and thrombocytopenia being the most common toxicities associated with use of the drug (53). The former is seen in as much as 38% of patients. Fever, rash, and abnormal liver function tests also occur.

Ganciclovir is used primarily for the treatment of cytomegalovirus infections in the immunocompromised. Two areas in particular have lent themselves to treatment with this agent. These include cytomegalovirus retinitis (54), particularly in patients with the acquired immunodeficiency syndrome (AIDS). In this condition, the drug will generally arrest progression of the disease at least for a time. The other condition where the drug has found use is cytomegalovirus pneumonia, especially in the transplant patient (55). The drug may also be useful to treat gastrointestinal (GI) disease induced in AIDS patients by cytomegalovirus.

Other than for those older patients who have been treated for the conditions above, little is known of ganciclovir in the elderly population. No specific pharmacokinetic studies examining age-related differences have been identified.

VI. FOSCARNET

Foscarnet is a recently released pyrophosphate analog which is effective in preventing replication of the herpesviruses and human immunodeficiency virus (HIV) (56). The drug is directly active and does not require phosphorylation by virally derived thymidine kinase to achieve the active state. It is therefore useful in conditions caused by acyclovir-resistant herpesviruses.

The drug is given intravenously 60 mg/kg every 8 h for induction and 90 mg/kg once per day for maintenance. Serum levels of 495 μg/L at the peak and 126 μg/L at the trough have been reported (56). The drug is excreted unchanged in the urine by both glomerular filtration and tubular secretion and is sequestered in bone. The drug achieves a CSF level that is 43% of the mean plasma concentration (57).

The most common adverse effect of foscarnet is an increase in serum creatinine seen in 45% of patients (56). This is usually reversible upon stopping the drug. Additionally hypercalcemia and hyperphosphatemia have been reported during use of the drug.

The primary use of the drug has been for the treatment of acyclovir-resistant herpesvirus infections (56) and cytomegalovirus infections in AIDS patients (56). Again no studies of the unique properties of the drug in the geriatric age group have been identified.

VII. VIDARABINE

Now largely of historical interest, vidarabine was the first parenteral antiviral agent used. It has been successfully employed to treat herpes simplex encephalitis, herpes zoster in the immunosuppressed, varicella in the immunosuppressed, and neonatal herpes. It must be given intravenously except for herpes keratoconjunctivitis, where a topical preparation is available. The drug is not very soluble in water, requires large volumes of fluid to administer, and is rapidly eliminated from blood by metabolism to the hypoxanthine derivative (59).

The drug also produces significant side effects, including GI symptoms, hallucinations, tremors, confusion, and depression of the bone marrow. In most, if not all, cases where vidarabine would be employed in the older patients, other drugs would be preferable.

VIII. INTERFERONS

Three major forms of human interferon are known to exist. These have been designated alpha, beta, and gamma, but only the alpha and gamma types have now been licensed for clinical use. Human alpha interferon has been found to be a family of different proteins consisting of at least 22 different subtypes. Interferons are normally produced in the body under specific circumstances.

Alpha interferon is given subcutaneously or intramuscularly (60). Administration almost invariably causes fever. Other frequent side effects include lassitude, fatigue, leukopenia, thrombocytopenia, and abnormal liver function tests. Doses vary with the diseases. Indications for the administration of alpha interferon include neoplastic diseases, hairy cell leukemia, and Kaposis's sarcoma, but several viral diseases may also be treated with the agent. Intralesional administration of alpha interferon for periods up to 8 weeks has been found beneficial for human papilloma virus infection (61), and systemic administration has been found useful for hepatitis B and C (62). Recently interferon gamma has been licensed for use in chronic granulomatous disease (63).

IX. TRIFLUOROTHYMIDINE

Available only as an ophthalmic preparation, trifluorothymidine is used for herpes simplex keratoconjunctivitis. Specific data on use of this drug in older patients are not available.

X. ZIDOVUDINE

Zidovudine is a thymidine analog that inhibits reverse transcriptase. The drug is phosphorylated by host cell kinases to achieve the active form, which is capable of inhibiting HIV (64).

The drug is well absorbed from the GI tract and reaches peak and trough plasma levels of 7.1 and 0.4 μg/L, respectively. When given 5 mg/kg every 4 h, CSF levels are 50% of corresponding serum levels. The drug is primarily excreted by the kidney as unchanged drug (10–20%) or the glucuronide metabolite (50–80%) (65). The most common side effects include neutropenia and macrocytic anemia.

The drug has been shown effective in the treatment of the AIDS (66) and in asymptomatic individuals with fewer than 500 CD4+ cells/mm^3. The most commonly used dosage is 100 mg five times a day (67). The drug will prolong life, improve CD4 counts, and diminish the risk of opportunistic infections (66).

Most current authors feel that geriatric patient with AIDS should be treated as any other patient (68,69).

XI. DIDANOSINE

Didanosine, or 2′,3′-dideoxyinosine, is a nucleoside compound that is phosphorylated in human cells and metabolized to dideoxyadenosine triphosphate, which inhibits the HIV reverse transcriptase.

Didanosine is well absorbed from the GI tract. It must be protected from gastric acid and therefore is administered with antacid. It has a longer intracellular half-life than either of the other anti-AIDS drugs and can be given twice daily. Didanosine is actively secreted by renal tubules (70). The drug has been shown to decrease levels of the HIV antigen and to increase CD4 counts (71,72).

The major side effect is clinical pancreatitis, which occurs in approximately 1 to 2% of patients. Other side effects include diarrhea, abnormal liver function tests, peripheral neuropathy, headache, and rash.

As of this time, little is known of the effects of didanosine in elderly patients.

XII. ZALCITABINE

Zalcitabine, or 2′,3′-dideoxycytidine, is the most recently licensed anti-AIDS drug. It is phosphorylated by cells to the active triphosphate form.

The drug is well absorbed from the GI tract and has a half-life of 1.2 h. CSF concentrations range from 9 to 37% of plasma levels, and the drug is largely cleared by the kidney (73). Zalcitabine is licensed for use only with zidovudine. The recommended dosage is 0.375 or 0.75 mg three times daily in conjunction with zidovudine (usually 200 mg TID).

The major side effect is painful neuropathy, which is dose related. Thrombocytopenia, neutropenia, oral ulcers, rash, fever, and pancreatitis, can also occur.

The effects of zalcitabine in elderly patients are unknown.

REFERENCES

1. Dolin R. Amantadine and influenza A. Am Fam Pract 1979; 19:127–30.
2. Aoki F, Sitar D. Clinical pharmacokinetics of amantadine hydrochloride. Clin Pharmacokin 1988; 14:35–51.
3. Horadam VW, Sharp J, Smilack J, et al. Pharmacokinetics of amantadine hydrochloride in subjects with normal and impaired renal function. Ann Intern Med 1981; 94:454–8.
4. Centers for Disease Control Immunization Practices Advisory Committee. Prevention control of influenza. MMWR 1988; 37:361–4.
5. Somami S, Degelan J, Cooper S, et al. Comparison of pharmacokinetics and safety profiles of amantadine 50 and 100 mg daily doses in elderly nursing home residents. Pharmacotherapy 1991; 11:460–6.
6. Degelan J, Somami S, Cooper S, et al. Occurrence of adverse effects and high amantadine concentrations with influenza prophylaxis in the nursing home. J Am Geriatric Soc 1990; 38:428–32.
7. Arden NH, Patriarca P, Fasano M, et al. The roles of vaccination and amantadine prophylaxis in controlling an outbreak of influenza A. (H_3 N_2) in a nursing home. Arch Intern Med 1988; 148:865–8.
8. Couch R, Six H. The antiviral spectrum and mechanism of action of amantadine and rimantadine. In: Mills J, Corey L, eds. Antiviral chemotherapy: new directions for clinical application and research. New York: Elsevier, 1986, 50–57.
9. Patriarca PA, Arden N, Koplan J, et al. Prevention and control of type A influenza infections in nursing homes. Ann Intern Med 1987; 107:732–40.
10. Nicholson K, Wiselke M. Amantadine for influenza A. Br Med J 1991; 302:425–6.
11. Douglas R. Prophylaxis and treatment of influenza. N Engl J Med 1990; 322:443–50.
12. Dolin R, Reichman R, Madore HP, et al. A controlled trial of amantadine and rimantadine in the prophylaxis of influenza A infection. N Engl J Med 1982; 307:580–4.
13. Tominack R, Hayden F. Rimantadine hydrochloride and amantadine hydrochloride use in influenza A virus infections. Infect Dis Clin North Am 1987; 1:459–78.

14. Keating M. Antiviral agents. Mayo Clin Proc 1992; 67:160–78.
15. Perelau J, Somani S, Cooper S, et al. Amantadine resistant influenza A in a nursing facility. Arch Intern Med 1992; 152:390–2.
16. Wingfield W, Pollack D, Grunert R. Therapeutic efficacy of amantadine HCL and rimantadine HCL in naturally occurring influenza A_2 respiratory illness in man. N Engl J Med 1969; 281:579–84.
17. Gilbert B. and Knight V. Biochemistry and clinical applications of ribavirin. Antimicrob. Agents Chemother 1986; 30:201–5.
18. Hall C, McBride J, Walsh E, et al. Aerosolized ribavirin treatment of infants with respiratory syncytial viral infection. N Engl J Med 1983; 308:1443–7.
19. Smith D, Frankel L, Mathers L, et al. A controlled trial of aerosolized ribavirin in infants receiving mechanical ventilation for severe respiratory syncytial virus infection. N Engl J Med 1991; 325:24–9.
20. McCormick J, King I, Webb P, et al. Lassa fever: effective therapy with ribavirin. N Engl J Med 1986; 314:20–6.
21. Sidwell R, Huffman J, Khare G, et al. Broad spectrum antiviral activity of virazole 1BD ribofuranosyl 1,24, triazo-3-carboxamide. Science 1972; 177:705–6.
22. Liss H, Bernstein J. Ribavirin aerosol in the elderly. Chest 1988; 93:1235–41.
23. Dorsky D, Crumpacker C. Drugs five years later: acyclovir. Ann Intern Med 1987; 107:859–74.
24. De Miranda P, Whitley R, Blum M. Acyclovir kinetics alter intravenous infusion. Clin Pharmacol Ther 1979; 26:718–28.
25. Van Dyke R, Conner J, Wyborny C, et al. Pharmacokinetics of orally administered acyclovir in patients with herpes progenitalia. Am J Med 1982; 172(1A):5.
26. Laskin O, Longstretta J, Saral R, et al. Pharmacokinetics and tolerance of acyclovir, a new anti-herpes agent in humans. Antimicrob Agents Chemother 1982; 21:393–8.
27. Bridegen D, Rosling A, Woods N. Renal function after acyclovir intravenous infusion. Am J Med 1982; 73(1A):182–5.
28. Bean B, Aeppli D. Adverse effects of high dose intravenous acyclovir in ambulatory patients with acute herpes zoster. J Infect Dis 1985; 151:362–5.
29. McKendrick M, McGill J, White J, et al. Oral acyclovir in acute herpes zoster. Br Med J 1986; 293:1529–32.
30. Peterslund N, Esmann V, Ipsen J, et al. Oral and intravenous acyclovir are equally effective in herpes zoster. J Antimicrob Chemother 1984; 14:185–9.
31. Inamura H, Aoyagi M, Tojima H, et al. Effects of acyclovir in Ramsay Hunt syndrome. Acta Otolaryngol (Stockh) 1988; Suppl 446:111–13.
32. Dickens J, Smith JT, Graham S. Herpes zoster oticus: treatment with intravenous acyclovir. Laryngoscopy 1988; 98:776–9.
33. Freris M. Pharmacokinetic evaluation of oral acyclovir 800 mg, five times/day in elderly patients with herpes zoster. In Wellcome International Antiviral Symposium. Monte Carlo 1987 (abstract).
34. Whitley R, Middlebrooks M, Gnann J. Acyclovir: the past ten years. Adv Exp Med Biol 1990; 278:243–53.
35. Raborn AW, McGaw W, Grace M, et al. Treatment of herpes labialis with acyclovir: review of three clinical trials. Am J Med 1988; 85(2A):39–45.
36. Meyrick R, Dodd H, Yeo J, et al. Oral acyclovir in the suppression of recurrent non-genital herpes simplex infection. Br J Dermatol 1985; 113:731–5.
37. Whitley R, Alford C, Hirsch M, et al. and NIAID Collaborative Study Group. Vidarabine versus acyclovir therapy in herpes simplex encephalitis. N Engl J Med 1986; 314:144–9.
38. Balfour H. Acyclovir for treatment of varicella in immune competent patients. Scand J Infect Suppl 1991; 78:75–81.

39. Balfour H, Bean B, Laskin O, et al. and the Burroughs Wellcome Collaborative Acyclovir Study Group. Acyclovir halts the progression of herpes zoster in immunocompromised patients. N Engl J Med 1983; 308:1448–53.
40. Cobo M. Reduction of the ocular complications of herpes zoster ophthalmicus by oral acyclovir. Am J Med 1988; 85(2A):90–5.
41. Liesegang T. Ophthalmic herpes zoster: diagnosis and antiviral therapy. Geriatrics 1991; 46:64–71.
42. Dickens J, Smith J, Graham S. Herpes zoster oticus: treatment with intravenous acyclovir. Laryngoscope 1988; 98:776–9.
43. McKendrick M, Care C, Burke C, et al. Oral acyclovir in herpes zoster. J Antimicrob Chemother 1984; 14:661–5.
44. Peterslund N, Ipsen J, Schonheyder H, et al. Acyclovir in herpes zoster. Lancet 1981; 2:827–30.
45. Wood M, Ogan P, McKendrick M, et al. Efficacy of oral acyclovir treatment of acute herpes zoster. Am J Med 1988; 85(2A):79–83.
46. Huff JL, Bean B, Balfour H, et al. Therapy of herpes zoster with oral acyclovir. Am J Med 1988; 85(2A):84–9.
47. Morton P. Oral acyclovir in the treatment of herpes zoster in general practice. NZ Med J 1989; 102:93–5.
48. Surman O, Flynn T, Schooley R, et al. A double blind placebo controlled study of oral acyclovir in post herpetic neuralgia. Psychosomatics 1990; 31;287–92.
49. McKendrick M, McGill J, Wood M. Lack of effect of acyclovir on post herpetic neuralgia. Br Med J 1985; 298:66–71.
50. Lycka B. Post herpetic neuralgia and systemic corticosteroid therapy: efficacy and safety. Int J Dermatol 1990; 29:523–7.
51. Burns W, Santos G, Saral R, et al. Isolation and characterization of resistant herpes simplex virus after acyclovir. Lancet 1982; 1:421–3.
52. Jacobson M, Berger T, Fikrig S, et al. Acyclovir-resistant varicella zoster virus infection after chronic oral acyclovir in patients with the acquired immune deficiency syndrome. Ann Intern Med 1990; 112:187–91.
53. Faulds D, Heel R. Ganciclovir: a review of its antiviral activity, pharmacokinetic properties and therapeutic efficacy in cytomegalovirus infection. Drugs 1990; 39:597–638.
54. Buhles W, Mastre B, Tinker A. Ganciclovir treatment of life or sight threatening cytomegalovirus infection: experience in 314 immunocompromised patients. Rev Infect Dis 1988; 10(suppl 3):5495–506.
55. Emanuel D, Cunningham I, Jules-Elypee K, et al. Cytomegalovirus pneumonia after bone marrow transplantation successfully treated with the combination of ganciclovir and high dose intravenous immune globulin. Ann Intern Med 1988; 109:777–88.
56. Chrisp p, Clissold S. Foscarnet: a review of its antiviral activity, pharmacokinetic properties and therapeutic use in immunocompromised patients with cytomegalovirus retinitis. Drugs 1991; 41:104–29.
57. Sjovall J, Bergdahls S, Movin G, et al. Pharmacokinetics of foscarnet and distribution to cerebrospinal fluid after intravenous infusion in patients with human immune deficiency virus infection. Antimicrob Agents Chemother 1989; 33:1023–31.
58. Erlich K, Jacobson M, Koehler J, et al. Foscarnet therapy for severe acyclovir resistant herpes simplex virus type 2 infection in patients with the acquired immune deficiency syndrome. Ann Intern Med 1989; 110:710–13.
59. Nicholson KM. "Vidarabine". In Lambert H. and O'Grady F., eds. Antibiotic and chemotherapy, 6th edition, London: Churchill Livingstone. 1992: page 59 inclusive.
60. Finter NB, Chapman S, David P, et al. The use of interferon alpha in virus infections. Drugs 1991; 42:749–765.
61. Friedman-Kein A, Eron L, Conant M. Natural interferon alpha for treatment of condylomata acuminata. JAMA 1988; 259:533–38.

62. Davis G, Balart L, Schiff E. Treatment of chronic hepatitis C with recombinant interferon alpha. N Engl J Med 1989; 321:1501–05.
63. Todd P, Goa K. Interferon Gamma 1b: A review of its pharmacology and therapeutic potential in chronic granulomatous disease. Drugs 1992; 43:111–122.
64. Klecker R, Collins J, Yarchoan R, et al. Plasma and cerebrospinal fluid pharmacokinetics of 3azido-3deoxythymidine: a novel pyrimidine analogue with potential application for the treatment of AIDS and related diseases. Clin Pharm Ther 1987; 41:407–12.
65. Nicholson KM. Zidovudine. In: Lambert H, O'Grady F, eds. Antibiotic and chemotherapy. 6th ed. London: Churchill Livingstone, 1992:60–1.
66. Fischl M, Richman D, Grieco M, et al. and AZT Collaborative Working Group. The efficacy of azidothymidine (AZT) in the treatment of AIDS and AIDS related complex: a double blind placebo-controlled trial. N Engl J Med 1987; 317:185–91.
67. Volberding P, Lagakos S, Koch M, Peltinelli et al. and AIDS Clinical Trials Group of the National Institute of Allergy and Infectious Disease. Zidovudine in asymptomatic human immune deficiency virus infection: a controlled trial in persons with fewer than 500 CD_4 positive cells per cubic milliliter. N Engl J Med 1990; 322:941–9.
68. Fillit R, Fruchtman S, Sell L, et al. AIDS in the elderly, a case and its implications. Geriatrics 1989; 46:65–70.
69. Boudes P. HIV infection in the elderly. Compr Ther 1991; 17:39–42.
70. Nicholson KM. 2′3′ Dideoxyinosine. In: Lambert H, O'Grady F, eds. Antibiotic and chemotherapy. 6th ed. London: Churchill Livingstone, 1992:69.
71. Cooley T, Kunches L, Saunders C. Once daily administration of 2′3′ dideoxyinosine (DDI) in patients with the acquired immunodeficiency syndrome or AIDS related complex. N Engl J Med 1990; 322:1340–5.
72. Lambert J, Seidlin M, Saunders C. 2′3′ Dideoxyinosine (DDI) in patients with the acquired immunodeficiency syndrome or the AIDS related complex. N Engl J Med 1990; 112:254–61.
73. Nicholson KM. 2′3′Dideoxycytidine. In: Lambert H, O'Grady F, eds. Antibiotic and chemotherapy. 6th ed. London: Churchill Livingstone, 1992:68.

26

Empiric Antimicrobial Therapy

Thomas T. Yoshikawa
George Washington University School of Medicine and United States Department of Veterans Affairs, Washington, D.C.

I. INTRODUCTION

A. Justification

In the first chapter of this book, the high frequency of mortality and morbidity of infections in older patients was discussed. Because of the severe complications of infections, it is imperative that early diagnosis and prompt treatment of an infectious disease be implemented in geriatric patients. However, in many instances or circumstances, a specific etiological diagnosis is not available or readily obtainable in frail elderly patients. Furthermore, in many aging patients, it may not even be certain if an infection is responsible for the symptoms, signs, and/or functional decline—too often clinical manifestations of infections in the elderly person is atypical, nonspecific, or absent (see Chap. 3).

For these reasons, empiric antimicrobial therapy is an important and often necessary approach to managing infectious diseases in aging patients. Reduction in deaths and other complications of infections in older patients will require that treatment—generally empiric treatment—be initiated sooner in clinically diagnosed cases of infections and more often in patients with less well-defined evidence for an underlying infectious process. In some instances, geriatric patients may be "overtreated" for a presumed infection. Nevertheless, such an approach may be justified in order to prevent delays in antimicrobial therapy or to avoid letting infections remain untreated.

B. General Principles

Empiric, according to *Webster's New World Dictionary of the American Language,* is classified as a noun, and *empirical* is considered an adjective meaning "relying or based solely on experiment and observation rather than theory" (1). For purposes of our discussion, empiric, in terms of empiric antimicrobial therapy, will be used as an adjective to mean antimicrobial therapy that is based on previous observations, clinical experiences, and experimental findings that have a scientific basis.

The principles of selecting appropriate empiric antimicrobial therapy include (2):

1. Define the most likely site(s) and microbial cause(s) of the infection.
2. Determine the clinical status of the patient. More seriously ill patients justify more potent and broad-spectrum antibiotics.
3. Know the efficacy of the antibiotics to be selected under similar clinical circumstances.
4. Know the potential adverse effects of the drug(s) and their frequency of occurrence.
5. Evaluate the cost of the drug, i.e., retail price, preparation and administration costs, and costs for monitoring efficacy and/or side effects.

Antibiotic selection should consider all five of these factors before a decision is made to prescribe a particular drug regimen. In the majority of older patients who justify empiric antimicrobial therapy, broad-spectrum β-lactam antibiotics will generally be the drug(s) of choice (e.g., penicillins, cephalosporins, monobactams, β-lactamase inhibitors).

After microbiological data become available that indicate a specific etiology, the empiric regimen should be changed to a more narrow-spectrum antibiotic if deemed appropriate.

The following sections will provide recommendations for empiric antimicrobial therapy for the more common or important infections in older patients.

II. SPECIFIC INFECTIONS

A. Pneumonia

Pneumonia therapy should be classified into three categories: community-acquired, hospital-acquired, and nursing home acquired. (Additional information on nursing home–acquired pneumonia can be found in Chap. 28.)

Community-acquired (C-A) pneumonia in older adults will generally require in-hospital therapy. The most frequently isolated pathogens in older patients with C-A pneumonia are bacteria, i.e., *Streptococcus pneumoniae, Haemophilus influenzae, Staphylococcus aureus,* and gram-negative bacilli (primarily *Klebsiella* spp.) (3,4). Thus, empiric antimicrobial therapy for C-A pneumonia in elderly patients should include a broad-spectrum antibiotic (monotherapy) or a drug-combination regimen that has antimicrobial activity against these pathogens. Recommended parenteral monotherapy could include, but not necessarily be limited to, second-generation cephalosporins (e.g., cefuroxime, cefonicid, cefoxitin, cefotetan), third-generation cephalosporins (e.g., ceftriaxone, cefoperazone), or a β-lactamase inhibitor combined with a β-lactam antibiotic (e.g., ticarcillin-clavulanic acid, ampicillin-sulbactam). Combination regimens could include nafcillin (or oxacillin) or cefazolin plus aztreonam or a quinolone.

More recently, there have been reports of less common pathogens causing C-A pneumonias in older patients. These organisms include *Legionella* spp., *Moraxella catarrhalis,* and *Chlamydia pneumoniae* (5,6). However, until additional data become available, the quantitative role that these organisms have in the etiology of pneumonia in elderly patients remains unclear. Nevertheless, if older patients with C-A pneumonia fail to respond adequately with empiric treatment for the more common respiratory pathogens, the clinician should consider adding or changing therapy that would be effective against these less common organisms. A recommended agent might include erythromycin or one of its new analogs, clarithromycin or azithromycin (7).

Table 1 Empiric Antimicrobial Therapy for Pneumonia

Setting	Organisms	Parenteral antibiotics
Community-acquired	*S. pneumoniae, H. influenzae, S. aureus,* gram-negative bacilli	Second- or third-generation cephalosporins, ticarcillin-clavulanate, nafcillin (or oxacillin) or cefazolin + aztreonam or quinolones
Hospital-acquired	Gram-negative bacilli,[a] *S. aureus, S. pneumoniae,* anaerobes	Third-generation cephalosporins + clindamycin, ampicillin-sulbactam, ticarcillin-clavulanate, piperacillin + quinolones, imipenem
Nursing home–acquired	*S. pneumoniae,* gram-negative bacilli,[a] anaerobes	Second- or third-generation cephalosporins, ampicillin-sulbactam, penicillin (or ampicillin) + quinolones or aztreonam

[a] If *P. aeruginosa* is suspected, an aminoglycoside may be considered as part of the regimen.

Hospital-acquired (H-A) pneumonia, regardless of age, is associated with greater frequency and variety of gram-negative bacilli, as well as increased incidence of *S. aureus* and aspiration (8,9); *S. pneumoniae* remains an important pathogen in H-A pneumonia. However, it appears that in elderly patients in comparison to younger patients with H-A pneumonia, there is a higher incidence of *Pseudomonas aeruginosa, S. aureus,* and aspiration pneumonia (10). With H-A aspiration, not only are gram-negative bacilli deposited in the lung, but large numbers of anaerobic bacteria of the oropharynx also enter the respiratory tract (8,11). It would thus be prudent to include in the empiric therapy of H-A pneumonia in older patients a regimen that is active against aerobic and facultative gram-negative bacilli, anaerobic bacteria, and gram-positive cocci. Suggested regimens include a third-generation cephalosporin such as ceftazidime plus clindamycin, ampicillin-sulbactam, ticarcillin-clavulanic acid, piperacillin plus a quinolone, or imipenem alone. An aminoglycoside may be used if a serious *P. aeruginosa* pneumonia or septic shock was present.

Nursing home–acquired (NH-A) pneumonia is caused by pathogens common to both C-A and H-A pneumonias. *S. pneumoniae* and gram-negative bacilli are the two dominant pathogens with aspiration (presumptively including anaerobes) being an important pathogenic mechanism for NH-A pneumonia. (12,13). Appropriate empiric antibiotic therapy for NH-A pneumonia includes second-generation cephalosporins, third-generation cephalosporins, ticarcillin-clavulanic acid, ampicillin-sulbactam, or penicillin (or ampicillin) plus a quinolone or aztreonam.

Table 1 summarizes recommendations for empiric antimicrobial therapy for pneumonia in older patients.

B. Urinary Tract Infection

Urinary tract infection (UTI) is the most common bacterial infection in elderly persons and is the most frequent cause of bacteremia and sepsis in the community, hospital, or

Table 2 Empiric Antimicrobial Therapy for Urinary Tract Infection

Type of UTI	Organisms	Parenteral antibiotics
Uncomplicated	*E. coli, Proteus* spp., *Klebsiella* spp.	First or second-generation cephalosporins, aztreonam, trimethoprim-sulfamethoxazole
Complicated	As above plus *Enterobacter* spp., *P. aeruginosa, Serratia marcescens*	Third-generation cephalosporins, quinolones, aztreonam, cefoperazone-sulbactam, ticarcillin-clavulanate, aminoglycosides
Chronic catheter	Same as complicated UTI plus *Enterococcus* spp.	As above but add ampicillin (or vancomycin)[a]

[a] For penicillin-allergic patients.

nursing home setting (14–17). The etiology of UTI is dependent on a number of factors including general health and functional status, presence of genitourinary abnormalities, type and severity of underlying illness, presence of a bladder catheter, and use of previous antibiotics (18). From a therapeutic perspective, UTI can be viewed as either *uncomplicated* or *complicated.* Uncomplicated UTI in older persons will be defined in this section as an infection not associated with genitourinary abnormalities, frequent (more than three episodes a year) recurrences, sepsis with hypotension, renal or bladder stones, bladder catheters, fatal underlying diseases (cancer, leukemia), or immunosuppression. *Complicated* UTI would include the above risk factors.

In functionally independent and healthy older adults, UTI generally will be uncomplicated. Common uropathogens are *Escherichia coli, Proteus* spp., and *Klebsiella* spp. The most appropriate empiric parenteral antimicrobial therapies include first- or second-generation cephalosporins, aztreonam, or trimethoprim-sulfamethoxazole. Oral therapy is best begun with amoxicillin-clavulanate, trimethoprim-sulfamethaxozole, or first-generation cephalosporin.

Complicated UTI is frequently caused by uropathogens that are resistant to commonly prescribed antibiotics. In addition to *E. coli, Proteus* spp., and *Klebsiella* spp., such organisms as *Enterobacter* spp., *P. aeruginosa,* and *Serratia marcescens* are isolated in older patients with complicated UTI (19). Moreover, in patients with chronic bladder catheters, polymicrobial bacteriuria including *Enterococcus* spp. (*Enterococcus* is isolated in up to 25–30% of patients) is frequently found (20). Given the potential diverse etiology of complicated UTI, empiric antibiotic therapy should be initiated with drugs with broad-spectrum gram-negative bacillary activity, i.e., third-generation cephalosporins, quinolones, aztreonam, ampicillin-sulbactam, cefoperazone-sulbactam, ticarcillin-clavulanate, aminoglycosides, or imipenem. In patients with chronic catheter-related urosepsis, empiric treatment should include agents effective against *Enterococcus* spp.; a combination of ampicillin (vancomycin for penicillin-allergic patients) plus any of the previously mentioned antibiotics with gram-negative bacillary activity would be appropriate therapy. Older patients with complicated UTI, but who are clinically stable enough to be treated with oral antibiotics, should receive an oral quinolone in most instances as empiric therapy. Table 2 summarizes recommendations for empiric parenteral antimicrobial therapy for UTI in older patients.

C. Skin and Soft Tissue Infections

The three most important skin and soft tissue infections (excluding postsurgical wound infections) in aging adults are simple cellulitis, diabetic lower extremity infections, and infected pressure ulcers (21–23).

Simple cellulitis in healthy or nonimmunocompromised older adults will most often be caused by streptococci, usually group A beta-hemolytic *Streptococcus pyogenes* and *S. aureus*. Severely ill or toxic patients should be treated with a semisynthetic penicillinase-resistant penicillin (e.g., nafcillin, oxacillin) or a first-generation cephalosporin such as cefazolin. Empiric oral therapy may be initiated with cloxacillin, dicloxacillin, amoxicillin-clavulanate, erythromycin, or clindamycin. Immunosuppressed patients, especially those who are leukopenic, are at risk for gram-negative bacillary infections including *P. aeruginosa*. Under these circumstances, a parenteral agent such as ceftazidime, aztreonam, an aminoglycoside, or a quinolone should be part of the empiric regimen.

Diabetic infections of the lower extremities may be seen as cellulitis, ulcers, paronychia, abscess and/or gangrene. Most studies show that these infections are caused by a variety of pathogens, often occurring together as mixed infections that include streptococci, staphylococci, gram-negative bacilli, and anaerobic bacteria (22,24). Older diabetics with such infections and who require parenteral antimicrobial therapy may be empirically begun on cefoxitin, cefotetan, ampicillin-sulbactam, or ticarcillin-clavulanate, as well as a combination regimen that treats anaerobic (e.g., clindamycin, metronidazole) and aerobic (e.g., quinolone, aztreonam, third-generation cephalosporin) organisms (24). Oral empiric therapy could be effectively accomplished with amoxicillin-clavulanate or a combined regimen such as a first-generation cephalosporin or a quinolone plus metronidazole.

Pressure ulcers in their early stages may be infected with aerobic bacteria only (e.g., staphylococci, streptococci, *E. coli*). However, deep ulcers or chronic lesions are invariably infected with a mixture of aerobic and anaerobic bacteria, primarily the fecal flora (23). A superficial, early-infected pressure ulcer may be treated with a second- or third-generation cephalosporin. With more progressive lesions, empiric antimicrobial therapy should be the same as that recommended for diabetic lower extremity infections, i.e., anaerobic and aerobic organisms (25). Table 3 summarizes recommendations for empiric parenteral antimicrobial therapy for skin and soft tissue infections.

D. Bacterial Meningitis

Although bacterial meningitis is a disease primarily of children, the incidence of this infection in adults increases in the elderly population (26). The mortality is exceedingly high with bacterial meningitis in all age groups, but especially in older patients. Thus, early empiric antimicrobial therapy is critical in the management of bacterial meningitis. The most frequently isolated meningopathogens in aging patients are *S. pneumoniae,* gram-negative bacilli, and *Listeria monocytogenes;* at times *Neisseria meningitidis* and *Haemophilus influenzae* may be recovered from the cerebrospinal fluid (CSF).

Antibiotic selection will depend on activity of the drug against the organism, presence of microbicidal properties of the agent, and penetration of the antibiotic into the CSF. Given these restrictions, empiric parenteral antimicrobial therapy for presumed bacterial meningitis in elderly patients should be initiated with a combination of ampicillin (or penicillin) plus a third-generation cephalosporin (except cefoperazone). Aztreonam may be an alternative for the third-generation cephalosporin; aminoglycosides may require intrathecal supplemental doses. Quinolones have not been adequately studied for treatment

Table 3 Empiric Antimicrobial Therapy for Skin and Soft Tissue Infections

Infection	Organism	Parenteral antibiotics
Simple cellulitis		
Nonimmunocompromised	S. *pyogenes, S. aureus*	Nafcillin or oxacillin, first-generation cephalosporin (cefazolin)
Immunocompromised	As above plus gram-negative bacilli, including *P. aeruginosa*	As above plus aztreonam, quinolones, aminoglycosides, ceftazidime (with nafcillin or oxacillin)
Diabetic lesions	Streptococci, staphylococci, gram-negative bacilli, anaerobes	Cefoxitin, cefotetan, ampicillin-sulbactam, ticarcillin- clavulanate, clindamycin (or metronidazole) + third-generation cephalosporins (or quinolones, aztreonam)
Pressure ulcer		
Early, superficial	Streptococci, staphylococci, *E. coli*	Second- or third-generation cephalosporin
Chronic, deep	As above plus other gram-negative bacilli, anaerobes	Same regimen as diabetic lesions

of bacterial meningitis, although ofloxacin appears to have some penetration into the CSF (27).

E. Infective Endocarditis

Infective endocarditis (IE) has become increasingly a disease of older adults during the modern antibiotic era (28). In some series, up to 50% of IE cases occur in persons 60 years and older (29).

The most common pathogens responsible for native valve IE in older patients are streptococci—including viridans group streptococci, *S. bovis,* and *Enterococcus* spp.—and *S. aureus* (30). Empiric antimicrobial therapy should begin with penicillin (or ampicillin), nafcillin (or oxacillin), and streptomycin (or gentamicin) (31). In penicillin-allergic patients, vancomycin plus streptomycin (or gentamicin) are recommended. After culture data become available, if an aminoglycoside is not warranted based on the pathogen isolated, streptomycin (or gentamicin) should be discontinued as soon as possible because of the potential renal and otological toxicities.

Prosthetic valve endocarditis (PVE) is also an infection that occurs in aging adults. The most frequently isolated pathogens are coagulase-negative staphylococci, *S. aureus,* streptococci, and gram-negative bacilli (32). Because of the significant prevalence of

Table 4 Empiric Antimicrobial Therapy for Bacterial Meningitis, Infective Endocarditis, and Intraabdominal Infections

Infection	Organisms	Parentera antibiotics
Bacterial meningitis	*S. pneumoniae, L. monocytogenes,* gram-negative bacilli	Ampicillin (or penicillin) + third-generation cephalosporins[a] (or aztreonam, aminoglycosides)
Infective endocarditis		
Native valve	Streptococci, *S. aureus*	Ampicillin (or penicillin) + nafcillin (or oxacillin) + streptomycin (or gentamicin)
Prosthetic valve	Streptococci, staphylococci, gram-negative bacilli	Vancomycin +gentamicin
Intraabdominal infections		
Cholecystitis	*E. coli Klebsiella* spp., *Enterococcus spp.*	Second- or third- generation cephalosporins, ampicillin + clindamycin (or metronidazole) + quinolones (or aminoglycosides)
Appendicitis, diverticulitis	Anaerobes, gram-negative bacilli	Cefoxitin (or cefotetan), ampicillin + clindamycin (or metronidazole) +quinolones (or aminoglycosides)

[a] Except cefoperazone because of limited cerebrospinal fluid penetration.

methicillin-resistant coagulase-negative staphylococci and methicillin-resistant *S. aureus,* as well as the potential presence of "tolerant" staphylococci (organisms inhibited but not killed by cell-wall active agents such as β-lactams), empiric antimicrobial therapy for PVE is best initiated with a combination of vancomycin and gentamicin; some clinicians recommend adding rifampin. If the offending isolates of PVE are susceptible to β-lactam antibiotics, the regimen should then be changed to one of these agents.

F. Intraabdominal Infections

Acute cholecystitis is a common complication of chronic cholelithiasis. The incidence of gallstones increases to greater than 50% in persons age 70 years and older. The most frequently recovered organisms from bile specimens of elderly patients undergoing either elective or emergency cholecystectomy are *E. coli* and *Klebsiella* spp.; occasionally *Enterococcus* is isolated (33). Anaerobes, such as *Bacteroides fragilis* group, should be suspected in complicated severe biliary tract disease (e.g., due to previous surgery or associated biliary tract carcinoma). In older patients who are clinically stable and not severely ill, empiric antimicrobial therapy for acute cholecystitis should be initiated with a second-generation (cefoxitin, cefotetan) or third-generation cephalosporin (ceftriaxone, cefoperazone, ceftizoxime). In more severely ill patients, a combination of ampicillin, clindamycin (or metronidazole), and quinolone (or aminoglycosides) would be appropriate.

Acute appendicitis is associated with high mortality in aging adults, and acute diverticulitis occurs with high frequency in older persons (34). Both of these intraabdominal infections are caused by the fecal flora, i.e., a mixture of anaerobes and gram-negative bacilli. In community-acquired acute appendicitis or diverticulitis cases in which the patients are not severely ill, empiric therapy may be begun with monotherapy such as cefoxitin (or cefotetan or ampicillin-sulbactam) (35). However, in patients who are severely ill or who develop appendicitis or diverticulitis while in a hospital, it is recommended that treatment be initiated with a combination of ampicillin, clindamycin (or metronidazole), and quinolone (or aminoglycosides) (36).

Table 4 summarizes empiric antimicrobial therapy recommended for bacterial meningitis, infective endocarditis, and intraabdominal infections.

REFERENCES

1. *Webster's New World Dictionary of the American Language.* Second college edition. Cleveland, OH: William Collins Publications, Inc., 1979.
2. Yoshikawa TT. Antimicrobial therapy for the elderly patient. J Am Geriatr Soc 1990; 38:1353–72.
3. Verghese A, Berk SL. Bacterial pneumonia in the elderly. Medicine (Balt.) 1983; 62:271–85.
4. Marrie TJ, Durant H, Yates L. Community-acquired pneumonia requiring hospitalization: 5-year prospective study. Rev Infect Dis 1989; 11:586–99.
5. Fang G-D, Fine M, Orloff J, Arisumi D, Yu VL, Kapoor W, Grayston JT, Wang SP, Kohler R, Muder RR, Yee YC, Rihs JD, Vickses RM. New and emerging etiologies for community-acquired pneumonia with implications for therapy. A prospective multicenter study of 359 cases. Medicine (Balt.) 1990; 69:307–16.
6. Marrie TJ. Pneumonia. Clin Geriatr Med 1992; 8(4):721–34.
7. Neu HC. New macrolide antibiotics: azithromycin and clarithromycin. Ann Intern Med 1992; 116:517–19.
8. Bartlett JG, O'Keefe P, Tally FP, Louie TJ, Gorbach SL. Bacteriology of hospital acquired pneumonia. Arch Intern Med 1986; 146:868–71.
9. Aoun M, Klastersky J. Drug treatment of pneumonia in the hospital. What are the choices? Drugs 1991; 43(6):962–72.
10. Hanson LC, Weber DJ, Rutala WA, Samsa GP. Risk factors for nosocomial pneumonia in the elderly. Am J Med 1992; 92:161–6.
11. Bartlett JG, Gorbach SL. The triple threat of aspiration pneumonia. Chest 1975; 68:560–6.
12. Marrie TJ, Durant H, Kwan C. Nursing-home acquired pneumonia. A case-control study. J Am Geriatr Soc 1986; 34:697–702.
13. Yoshikawa TT. Treatment of nursing home-acquired pneumonia. J Am Geriatr Soc 1991; 39:1040–1.
14. Esposito AL, Gleckman RA, Cram S, Crowley M, McCabe F, Drapkin MS. Community-acquired bacteremia in the elderly: analysis of one hundred consecutive episodes. J Am Geriatr Soc 1980; 28:315–19.
15. Meyers BR, Sherman E, Mendelson MH, Velasquez G, Srulevitch-Chin E, Hubbard M, Hirschman SZ. Bloodstream infections in the elderly. Am J Med 1989; 86:379–84.
16. Setia U, Serventi I, Lorenz D. Bacteremia in a long-term care facility. Spectrum and mortality. Arch Intern Med 1984; 144:1633–5.
17. Emori TG, Banerjee SN, Culver DH, Gaynes RP, Horan TC, Edwards JR, Jarvis WR, Tolson JS, Henderson TS, Martone WJ, Hughes JM. National Nosocomial Infections Surveillance System: nosocomial infections in elderly patients in the United States, 1986–1990. Am J Med 1991; 91(suppl 3B):289S–293S.

18. Yoshikawa TT, Norman DC. In: Aging and clinical practice: Infectious diseases. Diagnosis and treatment. New York: Igaku-Shoin, Inc., 1987:173–84.
19. Yoshikawa TT. Unique aspects of urinary tract infection in the geriatric patient. Gerontology 1984; 30:339–44.
20. Grahn D, Norman DC, White ML, Cantrell M, Yoshikawa TT. Validity of urinary catheter specimen for diagnosis of urinary tract infections in the elderly. Arch Intern Med 1985; 145:1858–60.
21. Yoshikawa TT. Ambulatory management of common infections in elderly patients. Infect Med 1991; 8(12):37–43.
22. Lipsky BA, Pecoraro RE, Larson SA, Hanley ME, Ahroni JH. Outpatient management of uncomplicated lower-extremity infections in diabetic patients. Arch Intern Med 1990; 150:790–7.
23. Galpin JE, Chow AW, Bayer AS, Guze LB. Sepsis associated with decubitus ulcers. Am J Med 1976; 61:346–9.
24. Joseph WS. Treatment of lower extremity infections in diabetics. Drugs 1991; 42(6):984–96.
25. Kurtesz D, Chow AW. Infected pressure and diabetic ulcers. Clin Geriatr Med 1992; 8(4):835–52.
26. Choi C. Bacterial meningitis. Clin Geriatr Med 1992; 8(4):889–902.
27. Bitar N, Claes R, Van der Auwera P. Concentrations of ofloxacin in serum and cerebrospinal fluid of patients without meningitis receiving the drug intravenously and orally. Antimicrob Agents Chemother 1989; 33:1686–90.
28. Cantrell M, Yoshikawa TT. Infective endocarditis in the aging patient. Gerontology 1984; 30:316–26.
29. Garvey FJ, Neu HC. Infective endocarditis—an evolving disease: a review of endocarditis at the Columbian-Presbyterian Medical Center. Medicine (Balt.) 1978; 57:105–27.
30. Terpenning MS, Buggy BP, Kauffman CA. Infective endocarditis: clinical infections in young and elderly patients. Am J Med 1987; 83:626–34.
31. Terpenning MS. Infective endocarditis. Clin Geriatr Med 1992; 8(4):903–12.
32. Tornos P, Sanz E, Permanyer-Miralda G, Almirante B, Planes AM, Soler-Soler J. Late prosthetic valve endocarditis. Immediate and long-term prognosis. Chest 1992; 101:37–41.
33. Margiotta SJ, Horwitz JR, Willis IH, Wallack MK. Cholecystectomy in the elderly. Am J Surg 1988; 156:509–12.
34. Norman DC, Yoshikawa TT. Intraabdominal infections in the elderly. J Am Geriatr Soc 1983; 31:677–84.
35. Wilson SE, Boswick JA Jr, Duma RJ, Echols RM, Jemsek JG, Lerner R, Lewis RT, Najem AZ, Press RA, Rittenburg MS, Stone HH, Ton GT. Cephalosporin therapy in intraabdominal infections. A multicenter randomized comparative study of cefotetan, moxalactam, and cefoxitin. Am J Surg 1988; 155(54):61–6.
36. Yoshikawa TT, Norman DC. Antimicrobial therapy of surgical infection in the elderly. Infect Surg 1984; (Nov.):805–12.

27

Antimicrobial Therapy in the Ambulatory Setting

Thomas T. Yoshikawa
George Washington University School of Medicine and United States Department of Veterans Affairs, Washington, D.C.

Chapter 26 discusses recommendations for antibiotic choices for infections that are often life threatening. The major emphasis is on inpatient, parenteral antimicrobial therapy.

In this chapter, the focus will be on antibiotic recommendations for infections in older patients in an ambulatory setting. Although there will be some overlap with the above-mentioned chapter, the discussion here will be more specific and limited to drug selection, dosages, and duration of treatment. There will not be any discussion of supportive and nonantibiotic aspects of management for these infections. The infectious diseases reviewed will be those most frequently encountered in an ambulatory/office practice setting.

I. PHARYNGITIS

Acute pharyngitis is an inflammation of the pharynx that is most frequently seen in children and young adults. However, older adults do experience this infection. There are seasonal variations in the frequency of pharyngitis, with higher attack rates occurring during winter months.

The microbial causes of pharyngitis are diverse, with the epidemiology of this infection being dependent on season of the year, age of population, severity of illness, and diagnostic methods used for determining the cause of infection (1). When all age groups are considered, the causes of pharyngitis are primarily attributable to the common "cold" viruses (e.g., rhinovirus) and group A beta-hemolytic streptococcus (*Streptococcus pyogenes*).

Pharyngitis associated with the common cold is generally a mild to moderate illness. The pharyngeal complaints are irritation, "scratchy" sensation, and soreness; severe pain in the pharynx and dysphagia are not common. Rhinorrhea, postnasal discharge, and cough are common symptoms. Fever, malaise, pharyngeal exudates, and tender lymph nodes are uncommon. The pharynx is erythematous. In contrast, streptococcal pharyngitis is often associated with marked pharyngeal pain, dysphagia, fever, cervical lymphadenopathy, erythematous and edematous pharynx, which may have an exudate or membrane, and peripheral leukocytosis.

The diagnostic approach is to exclude streptococcal pharyngitis either by throat culture or rapid antigen detection by latex agglutination.

Patients who appear clinically to have viral pharyngitis do not require antibiotics, but they should be tested for presence of *S. pyogenes.* Older patients who appear to have streptococcal pharyngitis on clinical examination or those patients with confirmed *S. pyogenes* infection of the pharynx should be treated with a 10-day course of phenoxymethyl penicillin (250 mg every 6 h). Patients who are allergic to penicillin may be given erythromycin (250 mg every 6 h) or clindamycin (150 mg every 6 h).

II. SINUSITIS

Infection of the paranasal sinuses is very common in elderly persons; acute and chronic sinusitis is reported to occur in 17% of those persons aged 65 years and older (2). However, in many older patients, the infection is unrecognized or is self-limiting (3). Acute sinusitis is a common complication of viral upper respiratory infections, but it is also found in association with maxillary dental infection, nasal foreign bodies or tumors, nasal fractures, and allergic rhinitis. Recurrent sinusitis or chronic sinusitis is also common among elderly persons (2).

In acute sinusitis, *Streptococcus pneumoniae* and *Haemophilus influenzae* account for at least 50% of cases; some patients will be infected with *Moraxella catarrhalis, Staphylococcus aureus,* and facultative or aerobic gram-negative bacilli. Chronic sinusitis is most often caused by anaerobic bacteria commonly found in the normal mouth flora.

The diagnosis of acute sinusitis is made by finding nasal discharge that is yellow or green, especially after a typical upper respiratory infection. Fever, chills, pain over the sinuses, or headache may be found. Chronic sinusitis may not be associated with such acute symptoms, and patients may only complain of nasal obstruction, postnasal drainage (possibly foul-smelling or foul-tasting), hyposmia, sore throat, or cough. Complication of sinusitis should be sought, including orbital cellulitis, meningitis, subdural empyema, brain abscess, or osteomyelitis.

The diagnosis of sinusitis is established by sinus roentgenograms (2). In equivocal or unclear cases by radiology, computed tomographic scans may confirm the diagnosis (2). Most uncomplicated cases of sinusitis will not require microbiological diagnostic procedures (culture of nasal discharge is unreliable because of contamination by indigenous flora). In difficult or refractory management cases, percutaneous puncture of the sinuses may be necessary to determine the microbiology and subsequent appropriate therapy.

The antibiotics most frequently prescribed for acute sinusitis are ampicillin (500 mg every 6 h), amoxicillin (500 mg every 8 h), or amoxicillin (250–500 mg)-clavulanic acid (1 tablet every 8 h). Therapy should last at least 2 weeks. In penicillin-allergic patients, trimethoprim-sulfamethoxazole (TMP-SMX; 160 mg trimethoprim and 800 mg sulfamethoxazole, 1 tablet every 12 h) or erythromycin (500 mg every 6 h) are alternative choices. Oral cephalosporins, e.g., cefuroxime axetil (250–500 mg every 12 h) may also be prescribed. Chronic sinusitis that does not respond to any of the above antibiotic regimens should be treated with the addition of metronidazole (500 mg every 8 h) or with clindamycin alone (300 mg every 8 h). Patients who fail on medical management should be referred to an otolaryngologist for possible surgical intervention.

III. BRONCHITIS

Acute bronchitis is most often initiated by a viral infection (e.g., influenza, rhinovirus). Like chronic bronchitis, acute bronchitis occurs most often in cigarette smokers. Chronic bronchitis—defined as recurrent productive cough that lasts for most days during at least 3 consecutive months for more than 2 consecutive years—has a prevalence as high as 40% in men aged 65 years and older in some parts of the world (4).

Bacterial infection often follows the initial episode of acute viral bronchitis, as well as being an underlying cause of acute exacerbations of chronic bronchitis. The bacteria most frequently isolated in bronchitis patients are *H. influenzae, M. catarrhalis,* and *S. pneumoniae* (5).

Acute bronchitis is diagnosed when there is an acute onset of cough, with or without sputum production. Depending on the presence of underlying lung disease, dyspnea, wheezing, and rhonchi may be present (6); fever is often absent. Acute exacerbations of chronic bronchitis are typically manifested by incessant cough with sputum production in a person who smokes or has a long history of asthma. Physical findings show signs of chronic obstructive lung disease, low-grade or absent fever, and occasional rales or wheezing. Chest roentgenograms show no lung infiltrates in either acute of chronic bronchitis. Sputum examination for bacteria is of limited value because of oropharyngeal contamination (6).

Acute and chronic bronchitis should be treated symptomatically. Antibiotics are indicated if secondary bacterial infection occurs (i.e., first evidence of purulent sputum, fever, or early radiographic changes of pneumonia). Treatment with ampicillin (500 mg every 6 h), amoxicillin (500 mg every 8 h), amoxicillin (500 mg)-clavulanic acid (1 tablet every 8 h), cefuroxime axetil (250–500 mg every 12 h), erythromycin (500 mg every 8 h), or TMP-SMX (160–800 mg, 1 tablet every 12 h) is effective and should be continued for 7 days (6).

IV. URINARY TRACT INFECTION

Urinary tract infection (UTI) occurs in 5–10% of elderly men and 10–30% of elderly women who live in the community (7). However, the majority of older persons with bacteriuria are asymptomatic (8), and thus they will not require antimicrobial therapy in most instances.

The most common uropathogens isolated from older adults with uncomplicated UTI (no genitourinary abnormalities, catheters, sepsis or hypotension, stones, immunosuppressed state, or recurrences) are *Escherichia coli* (50–70%), *Proteus* spp. (10–15%) and *Klebsiella* spp. (10–15%). With complicated UTI (above risk factors), additional organisms such as *Enterobacter* spp., *Pseudomonas aeruginosa, Serratia marcescens* and *Enterococcus* spp. are frequently isolated in the urine.

Clinical manifestations of UTI in elderly patients are similar to those found in younger adults, i.e., frequency, dysuria, urgency, nocturia, fever, lower abdominal pain, or occasionally flank pain. However, older adults may also manifest UTI by acute functional status changes, delirium, urinary incontinence, falls, or loss of appetite.

Diagnosis of bacteriuria or UTI is confirmed by culturing from the urine at least 100,000 colonies/mL urine of a uropathogen. A preliminary presumptive diagnosis of UTI can be made by urinalysis and Gram stain or nitrite test (based on bacteria converting nitrate to nitrite; however, it fails to detect *Streptococcus*) (6). Office screening culture methods using commercially available dip slide culture is able to detect bacteriuria within 24 h.

If treatment is necessary before culture data return, older patients with *uncomplicated* UTI can be begun empirically on amoxicillin (250 mg)-clavulanic acid (1 tablet every 8 h), TMP-SMX (160–800 mg, 1 tablet every 12 h), or cefadroxil (500 mg every 12–24 h). In patients with *complicated* UTI, in whom more drug-resistant organisms are anticipated, TMP-SMX (same dose), cefuroxime (125 mg every 12 h), a quinolone such as norfloxacin (400 mg every 12 h), or cefixime (400 mg every 12–24 h) are potential therapeutic choices. Once culture data become available, the patient should be placed on the least toxic, least expensive, and narrowest-spectrum antibiotic that is active against the pathogens. Duration of therapy is approximately 10 days for older women with uncomplicated UTI. Infected older men and older women with complicated UTI should receive antibiotics for at least 14 days.

V. SKIN AND SOFT TISSUE INFECTION

A. Cellulitis

Cellulitis in older adults most often occurs in the lower extremities, most likely as a result of trauma, peripheral vascular disease, diabetes mellitus, and edema (9). Clinically, the skin is red, tender, warm, and edematous, with no elevation or sharply defined border (as in erysipelas). Systemic complaints (fever, chills, delirium, or weakness) may be present in some patients; these patients and those who have facial and periorbital cellulitis should be hospitalized.

Most cases of uncomplicated cellulitis are caused by beta-hemolytic streptococci and *S. aureus.* Hand infections in older adults may be caused by a mixture of gram-positive and gram-negative bacteria (10). Skin and soft tissue infections related to a human bite are often associated with mixed anaerobic and facultative bacteria (11). Diagnostic microbiological studies are generally not necessary unless purulent drainage or abscess is associated with the cellulitis.

Most cellulitis cases can be treated with dicloxacillin (250 mg every 6 h), cephalexin (500 mg every 6 h), or amoxicillin (500 mg)-clavulanic acid (1 tablet every 8 h). If anaerobic organisms are suspected, clindamycin (150–300 mg every 8 h) is recommended; gram-negative bacilli can be treated with quinolones such as ciprofloxacin (500–750 mg every 12 h). Treatment should be for approximately 10 days.

B. Diabetic Ulcers

Diabetic ulcers occur primarily in the feet and commonly lead to severe consequences such as amputation. Diabetic foot problems may be present in as many as two-thirds of diabetics living in the community (12). Peripheral neuropathy and peripheral vascular disease are the major factors that contribute to diabetic foot ulcers.

The microbiology of diabetic ulcers is polymicrobial with a mixture of anaerobic organisms and facultative and aerobic bacteria (13,14). Common organisms include *Peptococcus* spp., *Bacteroides fragilis, B. melaninogenicus, Proteus* spp., *E. coli, S. aureus,* and *Enterococcus faecalis.*

Diabetic ulcers are easily diagnosed clinically in patients with a history of diabetes mellitus who have peripheral neuropathy and/or peripheral vascular disease. The ulcers may initially be superficial, but they can penetrate deep into soft tissue (muscle, tendons) and bone. Frequently, a foul-smelling odor may be present (due to anaerobes) in the ulcers. Osteomyelitis is a major complication of diabetic foot ulcers and should be evaluated by plain film radiography. The sensitivity, specificity, and cost-effectiveness of various radionuclide and imaging scans have not been determined for chronic contiguous osteomyelitis (12). Surface wound cultures are not diagnostic; bone biopsy to diagnose contiguous osteomyelitis is recommended *except* in diabetic foot ulcers because of potential complications (12).

The antibiotics most appropriate for diabetic foot ulcers would be clindamycin (for anaerobes) (150–300 mg every 8 h [or metronidazole, 500 mg every 8 h]) and a quinolone (for facultative and aerobic bacteria) such as ciprofloxacin (500 mg every 12 h) or ofloxacin (200 mg every 12 h). Alternative agents include amoxillin (500 mg)-clavulanic acid (1 tablet every 8 h), a combination of TMP-SMX (160–800 mg, 1 tablet every 12 h) and metronidazole (500 mg every 8 h), or a combination or cefuroxime (250 mg every 12 h) and metronidazole.

C. Pressure Ulcers

Pressure ulcers are primarily found in hospitalized or chronically institutionalized patients. However, at times older patients may develop pressure ulcers at home, or they will require continuation of pressure ulcer therapy at home postdischarge from a hospital or nursing home.

Early pressure ulcers (e.g., stage 1) may be infected with staphylococci, streptococci, and gram-negative bacilli. These lesions can be treated with local care; however, if cellulitis or acute inflammation appears to be present, systemic antibiotics are recommended. Drugs such as amoxicillin (250–500 mg)-clavulanic acid (1 tablet every 8 h) or cefuroxime axetil (250 mg every 12 h) will be adequate therapy. Infected deeper ulcers are most frequently caused by mixed organisms—as described for diabetic ulcers (see earlier discussion)—which include anaerobic facultative and aerobic bacteria. The same drug regimen prescribed for diabetic ulcers are appropriate for these infected deep pressure ulcers (12).

REFERENCES

1. Gwaltney JM, Jr. Pharyngitis. In: Mandell GL, Douglas RG, Jr, Bennett JE, eds. Principles and practice of infectious diseases. 3rd ed. New York: Churchill Livingstone, 1990:493–8.
2. Slavin RG. Management of sinusitis. J Am Geriatr Soc 1991; 39:212–17.
3. McMahan JT. Paranasal sinusitis: geriatric considerations. Otolaryngol Clin North Am 1990; 23:1169–80.
4. Bulla A, Hitske KL. Acute respiratory infections: a review. Bull WHO 1978; 56:481–98.
5. Nagami P. Respiratory infections. In: Yoshikawa TT, Cobbs EL, Brummel-Smith, eds. Ambulatory geriatric care. St. Louis: Mosby-Year Book Co. 1993:495–503.
6. Yoshikawa TT. Ambulatory management of common infections in elderly patients. Infect Med 1991; 8(12):37–43.
7. Yoshikawa TT. Unique aspects of urinary tract infection in the geriatric patient. Gerontology 1984; 30:339–44.
8. Abrutyn E, Boscia JA, Kaye D. The treatment of asymptomatic bacteriuria in the elderly. J Am Geriatr Soc 1988; 36:473–5.
9. Ginsberg MB. Cellulitis: an analysis of 101 cases and review of the literature. South Med J 1981; 74:530–3.
10. Stromberg BV. Hand infections in the elderly. South Med J 1985; 78:157–8.
11. Goldstein EJC, Citron FM, Wield B, et al. Bacteriology of human and animal bite wounds. J Clin Microbiol 1978; 8:667–72.

12. Kertesz D, Chow AW. Infected pressure and diabetic ulcers. Clin Geriatr Med 1992; 8(4):835–52.
13. Louie TJ, Bartlett JG, Tally FT, et al. Aerobic and anaerobic bacteria in diabetic foot ulcers. Ann Intern Med 1976; 85:461–3.
14. Sapico FL, Witte JL, Canaevati HN, et al. The infected foot of the diabetic patient: quantitative microbiology and analysis of clinical features. Rev Infect Dis 1984; (suppl 6): S171–S176.

28

The Use of Antimicrobials in Nursing Homes

Elizabeth Anne Williams and Steven L. Berk
East Tennessee State University, Johnson City, Tennessee

I. INTRODUCTION

This chapter will concentrate on the prevention and treatment of infection in the patient being cared for in a nursing home (NH) or extended-care facility. These terms will be used interchangeably in the following discussion since the problems encountered are similar. Since the previous chapters discuss in detail the various antimicrobials—spectrum of activity, distribution and pharmacokinetics, toxicity, and synergy and antagonism with other antimicrobials—in the elderly population, this chapter will focus on those aspects of prevention and therapy that are peculiar to the NH setting. In addition, the discussion will address not only the empiric and directed use of antimicrobials, but also the question of using them at all in certain patients, e.g., acutely terminal patients, or the use of less than optimal or "first-line" therapy in patients with "do not hospitalize" orders (1). Finally, the question of cost/benefit in the use of antimicrobials and transfer to hospital will be addressed from the point of view of the NH patient.

The NH patient is almost by definition elderly; 88% were 65 years and older in a nationwide survey in 1985. Even the recent influx of acquired immunodeficiency syndrome (AIDS) patients has not lowered the average age of the NH population. In fact, the trend has been, and will be well into the next century, for NHs to care for an increasing number of elderly persons, especially the oldest old, i.e., those 85 years and over. This is not because a greater percentage of older adults will require institutionalization, but because the demographics of the U.S. population are shifting, resulting in an overall increase in average age of the populace. Thus, while the number of elderly persons will double in 50 years, reaching 50 million, the U.S. population as a whole will increase by only 40%, resulting in there being only four people under the age of 65 for every one person over that age. The number of the oldest old will increase at an even faster rate, tripling in number. And those persons 75 years and older will make up 45% of the elderly population as compared to the 35% that they do now. This demographic shift is due in part to the decrease in average family size, but also to the success of our improved public health and vaccination programs in the twentieth century (2), which have allowed more of our population to live not only to maturity, but to complete the seven ages of man as described by Shakespeare in *As You Like It:*

> The sixth age shifts into the lean and slippered pantaloons, with spectacles on nose and pouch on side. His youthful hose . . . a world too wide for his shrunk shank; and his big manly voice, turning again toward childish treble, pipes and whistles in his sound. Last scene of all . . . is second childishness and mere oblivion, sans teeth, sans eyes, sans taste, sans everything.

Thus, it behooves us to address the problem of infections and the use of antimicrobials in NHs not only because of the >1.5 million patients currently institutionalized, but because of the constantly increasing number of elderly persons who will become institutionalized in these facilities. We must look at the problem as a multifaceted one, viewing it not only from the microbiological perspective but also from an ethical, societal, and financial viewpoint (3), since limited resources may force the medical profession into a triage situation of rationing care to those most likely to benefit from it.

II. THE PATIENT

NH patients are among the most frail and fragile of the elderly population (4), because the largest percentage of them are the oldest old, when one considers those <65 years, those 65–74 years, those 75–84 years, and those 85 years and older. It is this last group that accounted for a 76% increase in elderly residents between 1977 and 1985. These patients bear not only the burden of the usual decrement of physiological function associated with aging, but in addition multiple organ system dysfunction: 96% with diseases of the circulatory system; 63% with cognitive impairment; 31% with disease of the nervous system and sense organs; 27% with diseases of the musculoskeletal system; 12% with diabetes mellitus; and 6% with malignancy (2).

An accumulating body of evidence indicates that as a consequence of the aging process alone, immunological abnormalities develop in addition to the immune dysfunction brought about by underlying diseases or the therapies used to treat them. These immunological abnormalities may contribute to the higher incidence of certain infections and the associated increased morbidity and mortality. Not all older persons have immune deficits, but studies have been limited in the oldest old. Interestingly, cell-mediated immunity, as measured by delayed-type hypersensitivity to a multitest recall panel consisting of tetanus and diphtheria toxoids, candida, tuberculin, streptococcus group C, trichophyton, and *Proteus mirabilis* antigens, showed a reverse correlation with age and with increasing physical dependency. Normal delayed-type hypersensitivity was found in 82.1% of individuals >66 years old living at home, compared to 59% of self-sufficient NH residents, and 40% of dependent NH patients (5). Therefore, it is not surprising that a patient's Karnofsky score (6) and the number of activities of daily living (ADL's) that can be performed correlate with the patient's ability to withstand infection and with their risk of mortality from that infection (7).

The majority of patients enter NHs because of problems related to the circulatory system and/or to mental dysfunction (8); only 0.5% have infection as a primary diagnosis at the time of admission. As time passes these patients become colonized or otherwise exposed to microbial pathogens and subsequently succumb to them (9). Not surprisingly, infections are a primary reason for admission of NH patients to acute-care hospitals, where their length of stay is significantly longer than that of a similarly aged patient with the same problem coming from the community. And the NH patients' mortality is significantly greater in the hospital than community-based elderly patients who are hospitalized. Thus, it behooves the caregivers in NHs and extended care facilities to try to minimize the number of patients who become so severely infected that they require hospitalization. To achieve this goal, increased efforts have been directed at prevention and prophylaxis (an issue addressed later in this chapter). Other approaches require the physician to take a more active role in the NH patient's treatment plans and, if applicable, discharge planning.

When a patient is admitted to a NH, it is imperative that the patient's physician (and the NH physician, if they are separate individuals) explain in a compassionate but detailed manner the choices that a patient and/or family must face in terms of advance directives, living will, and durable power of attorney for health care. This is especially important for the patient who has little if any hope of ever returning to the community. In addition to the familiar (but often misunderstood) "do not resuscitate" (DNR) order, the less familiar, "do not hospitalize" (DNH) decision must be weighed carefully. Such orders would exclude optimal treatment for a serious infection in many circumstances because most NHs are not equipped to deliver intravenous antibiotic therapy and not staffed to provide adequate care for a seriously ill patient, e.g., a patient with a severe multiresistant gram-negative pneumonia who requires intravenous (IV) antibiotics and frequent suctioning (1,10). In addition, decisions about hydration, artificial feedings, blood drawing, oxygen, placement of tubes or catheters, and even the use of antibiotics (11) themselves must be explored. It has recently been demonstrated that elderly people have much more optimistic expectations of the outcome of a "code blue" than is warranted by the actual outcome data. Although it has not been studied, it would not be surprising if this same group of elderly persons were not overly optimistic about the ability of our "wonder drug" antibiotics to effect a cure or at least a substantial improvement in a patient with multiple medical problems, one or more of which will be the ultimate cause of the patient's demise. It is necessary throughout the course of a patient's stay at a NH for the physician to be compassionately realistic with the patient and/or family about ultimate outcomes and determine whether the patient should be hospitalized so that aggressive care, including antimicrobials, can be given (11).

In helping with these decisions, the physician must assess the capabilities of the NH as well as their care for the patient. Can the physician see the patient on a frequent basis if necessary? Is the NH adequately staffed so that patients can be fed, or are feeding tubes (a frequent culprit in lower respiratory infections) routinely placed to save staff time? Can a patient with pneumonia be suctioned, or a patient with a pressure ulcer repositioned every 2 h? Does the NH have a skilled nursing care unit to which the patient can be transferred for more aggressive treatment? Would repeated hospitalization degrade rather than improve a terminal patient's quality of life? And in the unresponsive/chronic vegetative state, does the patient have any quality of life?

III. PREVENTION AND PROPHYLAXIS

A. Influenza (see also Chaps. 25 and 31)

Although the Immunization Practices Committee of the Centers for Disease Control and Prevention (CDC) recommends that >80% of the residents of NHs be immunized each fall against influenza in order to produce "herd" immunity, it is estimated that <20% of this targeted elderly population is actually immunized. This lack of success in carrying out the CDC's recommendations is attributed to (1) poor record keeping due to the number of places at which the institutionalized-elderly person receives care, (2) inability to convince the patient and/or family of the increased importance of the vaccine, and (3) lack of a coordinated protocol by the NH to assure timely administration of the vaccine to both patients and health care personnel. The NH employees are frequently not immunized because the NH does not consider the cost to be worth the benefit and leaves it to the individual employees to arrange and pay for their own immunizations. These same employees often do not have sick leave and thus come to work even when suffering upper respiratory tract infections, including influenza (12–14).

When influenza A does appear in the community, amantadine should be started in those patients who cannot receive the vaccine, e.g., severe allergy to chicken eggs, or have not received the vaccine. The former should receive amantadine for the duration of the outbreak, while the latter can be immunized and amantadine continued until the patient's immune system has been able to develop sufficient antibody to the virus, which is usually about 14 days. (In the immune compromised, amantadine should be given for the duration of the outbreak.) Given as prophylaxis, amantadine is 70–90% effective. It is also effective if administered within 24–48 h after the onset of the illness in reducing the severity and length of the illness, specifically reducing fever and systemic symptoms as well as improving peripheral airway function and cutting in half the amount of viral shedding. For elderly patients the usual adult dose of 200 mg/day is reduced by one-half because of the reduced renal function in this population. If a patient has a creatinine clearance of <40 ml/min/1.73 m^2, then the package insert should be consulted for correct dosing (12–15). NH personnel and frequent visitors who have not received the vaccine should receive the full adult dose of amantadine while simultaneously being given the vaccine. In serious community outbreaks, limiting visitors and curtailing group activities in the NH may be helpful (12–14,16–18).

B. Pneumococcal Disease (see also Chap. 31)

Although the efficacy of the older 14-valent pneumococcal vaccine in high-risk patients, such as those found in NHs, has been questioned (19), the Public Health Service Advisory Committee on Immunization Practices recommends that all persons 65 years of age and older receive a single dose of 23-valent pneumococcal vaccine, which covers 87% of recent bacteremic pneumococcal disease in the United States. This is because pneumococcal pneumonia is still a major killer, especially among elderly persons in whom complications such as respiratory arrest, empyema, bacteremia, and meningitis are most likely to develop. The vaccine is 60–80% effective in healthy older adults and 77% protective in individuals at moderate risk; however, it appears not to be protective in the severely immunocompromised. Unfortunately, only 20% of the high-risk population receive the pneumococcal vaccine. Thus, as with the influenza vaccine, it is necessary to educate both the patient and family as to the importance of receiving the pneumococcal vaccine when the patient is being admitted to a NH. Record keeping is even more essential because Arthus-type reactions have been noted in some patients receiving more than one dose of the vaccine. There is disagreement whether patients who have only been vaccinated with the 14-valent vaccine should receive the 23-valent vaccine. If it is administered, the patient should be closely observed for an Arthus-type allergic reaction (12,16,17).

C. Tetanus (see also Chap. 31)

Clostridium tetani infections occur primarily among older persons, and the mortality is >50% in those over 60. After the age of 60, the incidence doubles with each passing decade. Almost 50% of the infections occur from an indoor wound, such as may be received from a fall from bed or wheelchair; 20% of the cases are found in individuals with chronic wounds, such as pressure sores, which are frequent in NHs. It is estimated that 50–60% of the elderly population lack protective antibodies against tetanus. Upon admission to a NH, those patients with documentation of a complete set of three tetanus toxoid injections should be given a booster if none has been received within the past 10 years. If there is no documentation of immunization, then a complete set of primary immunizations (Td) should be given. All traumatic wounds sustained in NH should be considered dirty; therefore, any patient with more than a minor wound who has not completed the set of three immunizations should be given Td at one site and tetanus immune globulin (TIG) 250 units at another site. While TIG is not 100% effective, it provides protection in most cases. In addition, meticulous wound management is essential, including removal of foreign bodies, drainage of abscesses, irrigation, and debridement (12,17,20,21).

D. Diphtheria

As with tetanus, most older individuals do not have protective antibody levels against diphtheria, thus 25% of the cases of diphtheria occur in persons over 50. There is a risk of nosocomial spread of diphtheria to other patients and health care personnel who lack protective antibody levels. Fortunately, if patients are appropriately immunized against tetanus, they receive diphtheria toxoid simultaneously (12).

E. Tuberculosis (see also Chap. 23)

The threat of an outbreak of *Mycobacterium tuberculosis* among elderly persons in NH environments is well documented by Stead et al. (22–25). However, the appearance of multidrug-resistant strains of *M. tuberculosis* among immigrant populations, especially those from southeast Asia, and human immunodeficiency virus (HIV)–positive individuals has made it more imperative than ever to give all residents as they are admitted to a NH with a relevant clinical history tuberculosis skin testing. As promulgated by the American Geriatrics Society, two-step purified protein derivative (PPD) skin testing with five tuberculin units (intermediate strength PPD) should be applied using the Mantoux method on admission to all residents with a history of negative tuberculin skin tests. If the initial test is negative, then the test is repeated in 1–2 weeks, and only if the second test is negative is the patient regarded as negative (or anergic if dermal control antigens remain negative). If a patient is PPD positive ($\geq$10 mm induration) or anergic, he or she should have a chest radiograph to look for evidence of old or active disease. If the chest radiograph is without evidence of past or recent tuberculosis and the patient is a recent converter without history of exposure to drug-resistant tuberculosis, he or she should be placed on isoniazid (INH 300 mg/day) prophylaxis for 6 months to 1 year. If the chest radiograph is suggestive of past or recent tuberculosis, sputum samples should be collected for smears and cultures. Treatment or prophylaxis will be determined by results of the microbiological studies and whether the patient has risk factors for active tuberculosis. In patients who are anergic and have evidence on chest radiographs of old granulomatous disease, prophylaxis should be considered. Alvarez et al. (26) have shown that INH prophylaxis in elderly patients can be carried out without risk of serious hepatitis as long as the patients are monitored.

All tuberculin skin test–negative patients should be retested every year, or sooner if an active case of tuberculosis is found in the NH. Similarly, all employees should be tested at the beginning of employment, and then at yearly intervals or at the time of possible exposure. Health care workers who are PPD positive should receive prophylaxis if they are recent converters; other PPD-positive employees should receive yearly chest radiographs (12,27).

It is particularly important to have a high index of suspicion for tuberculosis in any patient with unexplained illness, fever, lymphadenopathy, skin lesion (28), or failure to thrive, especially if they have been transferred from a hospital in a large urban area and are immunocompromised individuals, e.g., patients with blood dyscrasias or AIDS, who may be skin-test negative due to anergy (29). Recent studies have shown that multidrug-resistant tuberculosis (MDRTB) is on a precipitous rise and, if not recognized, can result in outbreaks that spread to other patients and health care staff (30). In severely immunocompromised patients, MDRTB often leads to a rapidly fulminant course resulting in death within 4–16 weeks from time of diagnosis. The risk to healthy caretakers is not fully known, but at least eight health care workers have developed active MDRTB, and four have died as a result of occupational exposure (31). In two hospitals the rates of skin test conversion among health care workers were 33 and 50%. Virtually all the isolates from the MDRTB outbreaks were resistant to both isoniazid and rifampin. Health care workers should be thoroughly instructed as to how to avoid nosocomially acquired tuberculosis; they should be made aware of the risk and consequences of acquiring MDRTB. The problem of MDRTB is a rapidly evolving area, and it will be necessary to keep abreast of the latest CDC recommendations for patients and health care workers exposed to MDRTB (28,30–32).

F. Methicillin-Resistant *Staphylococcus aureus* (MRSA)

The problem of MRSA colonization and nosocomial infection in hospitals and NHs has been documented for more than 20 years (33). But it has only been in the past decade that serious attention has been paid to the problem and to the reservoirs that maintain the organism. It is now apparent that both acute-care facilities and long-term-care facilities participate in a vicious cycle of transmission among each other and that individual facilities have internal self-perpetuating cycles as well (34–37). Unfortunately, misunderstanding of these multiple modes of transmission has resulted in patients being denied admission to NHs because they culture positive for MRSA. Similarly, hospitals have denied admission to NH patients for the same reason. There is no question that the presence of a patient with MRSA colonization in a NH requires the implementing of infection control measures (as outlined by the CDC), education of the health care workers about MRSA, and possibly cohorting of patients and staff if there is widespread carriage of MRSA in a NH. Approximately 3–4% of NH patients colonized with MRSA will develop an infection (38).

In terms of chemoprophylaxis for MRSA carriage, mupirocin appears effective (39), especially when combined with chlorhexidine baths, in abolishing nasal carriage and possibly axillary and groin carriage. It is not as clear that it is effective treatment for gastrostomy/jejunostomy feeding tube sites. Rifampin given in doses of 600 mg/day for 7 days has been effective in the past in clearing health care personnel, but not in patients. Unfortunately, MRSA is quick to develop new patterns of resistance to topical as well as oral drug combinations. More recently, MRSA has developed high levels of resistance in many institutions to ciprofloxacin, which was initially successful in treating both carriage and infections (40). It is not uncommon to find MRSA strains that are susceptible only to vancomycin.

At this time, routine chemoprophylaxis against MRSA colonization is not recommended. However, if the number of MRSA infections exceeds the usual prevalence rate in a NH, cultures of patients and employees should be performed. Chemoprophylaxis of MRSA carriers should be considered when an outbreak of MRSA infections occurs. MRSA infections are best treated with vancomycin (38).

G. Pressure Ulcer

Pressure ulcer, also known as "bedsores," "pressure sores," or "decubitus ulcer," is an ever-present problem or potential problem in the NH. Estimates of its prevalence range from 6 to 35%; the wide variation in prevalence is due to the type of patients being served and the quality of the care at the NH or the acute-care facilities from which the NH accepts its patients. Pressure ulcers are particularly serious in frail elderly persons with restriction of mobility and underlying diseases, such as atherosclerotic vascular disease, cerebral hemorrhage, cardiac failure, renal insufficiency, metastatic cancer, and poor nutritional status. Pressure ulcers are access ports for infection especially in those patients who are nonambulatory, fecally incontinent, diabetic, or catheterized (41,42).

Elimination of this source of infection depends on the prevention of its development and on the management of existing pressure ulcers. Prevention is dependent on the ability of NH personnel to determine in advance those patients at high risk (43), as noted above, and to recognize the earliest stage of a pressure ulcer—blanching hyperemia with light finger pressure. At this point the skin damage can be completely reversed by eliminating the causative agent(s), i.e., pressure, shearing forces, friction, and moisture, as well as by correcting host factors such as malnutrition, anemia, circulatory insufficiency, and conditions causing edema, muscle wasting, or locally devitalized tissue. If the causative factors are not eliminated, then the blanching hyperemia progresses to nonblanching hyperemia (stage II), blistering and eschar formation (stage III), and finally sloughing of the devitalized tissue and eschar revealing the underlying ulcer (stage IV). These ulcers can vary in severity from a grade I (partial thickness ulcer, which is still amenable to removal of pressure and local wound care) through grade II (a full-thickness ulcer extending through the dermis to the subcutaneous fat and amenable to removal of pressure and local wound care) to grade III (a deep pressure ulcer, which extends through the subcutaneous tissue to the deep fascia and requires surgical debridement before healing can occur), and finally grade IV (a complicated pressure ulcer with involvement of muscle and bone after breaching of the fascia, which removes the last barrier to extensive spread of infection and may result in osteomyelitis, pyarthrosis, bacteremia, and even meningitis; treatment at this point requires aggressive medical and surgical therapy) (41).

When patients with pressure ulcers become febrile and there are no other obvious sources of infection, it must be assumed that the ulcer is one likely source of the fever, and the patient should be evaluated with a complete blood count including the percent leukocytes, erythrocyte sedimentation rate, blood cultures, and an appropriate specimen from the wound for microbiological studies. If osteomyelitis is suspected, a bone biopsy for culture and histology may be necessary (44). The common practice of swabbing the surface of the ulcer is of little clinical value; aspiration of purulent drainage or tissue biopsy provides more accurate microbiological data.

Most often treatment will be empiric with broad-spectrum antibiotics since organisms that are isolated from wounds and blood are generally mixed anaerobic, facultative, and aerobic organisms, e.g., *Bacteroides fragilis, Peptostreptococcus, Proteus mirabilis,* and *Staphylococcus aureus.* In a study where organisms were obtained by deep aspiration, bone/tissue biopsy, or cotton swab of purulent drainage, aerobic and facultative organisms that were cultured included *P. mirabilis, Enterococcus, Escherichia coli,* staphylococci, and *Pseudomonas* species (45). Thus, in addition to surgical intervention, empirical antibiotic therapy should include coverage for anaerobes, with such antibiotics as clindamycin (45), cefoxitin, metronidazole, or imipenem, as well as for gram-negative bacilli with such agents as a quinolone or a third-generation cephalosporin that is active against *P. aeruginosa.* If MRSA is known to be a problem in the NH or the patient, then therapy with vancomycin should be considered. If osteomyelitis is present then therapy must be prolonged (44).

Any pressure ulcer can result in systemic infection, including bacteremia, osteomyelitis, pyarthrosis, abscess, and meningitis (45,46). In patients who have DNH orders in a NH that is not able to give intravenous antibiotics, a combination of oral ciprofloxacin plus metronidazole or clindamycin along with careful wound management and relief of pressure can result in successful outcomes (47,48).

As to the topical care of pressure sores and ulcers, there are a plethora of management strategies, none of which has been shown superior to standard local wound care. A critical number of bacteria are required for infection to develop (10^5 organisms per gram of tissue appears to be the infective dose for aerobic bacteria). The type of bacteria seem to be less important than the absolute number. Unfortunately, antibiotics alone, either topically or systemically, cannot effectively lower bacterial counts in chronically contaminated pressure ulcers; reduction in contamination depends primarily on careful cleansing and debridement of ulcers, which can best be achieved by frequent changes of wet to dry dressing with fine mesh gauze soaked in normal saline and packed loosely into the wound. To date, none of the enzymatic products that are supposed to act by dissolving denatured collagen and liquefying necrotic debris have been subject to the types of rigorously controlled trials that would allow an assessment of their usefulness (9,42,49,50).

IV. SITES OF INFECTIONS

A. Respiratory Tract

Infections are the leading cause of death in NHs, and pneumonia alone accounts for one-third of all deaths in NHs. Infections of the lower respiratory tract are one of the leading causes, and in some studies the leading cause, of transfer of patients from NHs to acute-care facilities (51). This is not surprising when one considers that the host is frequently compromised by age and multiple medical problems, the treatment of which may make the patient more susceptible to pneumonia, e.g., soporifics, tube feedings (52). Upon entering a NH, a previously healthy adult's oral flora quickly change from a mixture of anaerobic and aerobic organisms to a mixture of aerobic and facultative gram-negative bacilli (53–55). Since the main cause of pneumonias in an elderly population is aspiration of oral contents, it is not surprising that gram-negative organisms are major pathogens in NH-acquired pneumonia (56–58). However, collecting reliable data on this phenomenon is difficult because (1) NH patients often cannot cough up reliable sputum; (2) invasive procedures, such as transtracheal aspiration and bronchoscopy, are not well tolerated by an ill elderly patient; (3) expectorated sputum is likely to be contaminated by oropharyngeal flora; and (4) nasotracheal aspirates are often incorrectly performed and do not get into the trachea and bronchi, so that nasopharyngeal secretions are usually obtained (52,53).

However, with this knowledge, strategies to treat NH-acquired pneumonias (NHAP) in the NH can be devised when the patient and/or family has requested a DNH status for the patient. Moreover, if the NHAP is diagnosed early and the patient is clinically stable, the NH is well equipped and well staffed, and the patient is well known to the NH staff, hospitalization is often not required. The patient may present with only a low-grade fever, but in an elderly person this is a reliable indicator of a serious infection (59,60). Physical findings may be minimal and chest radiography unrewarding if the pneumonia is early in its course or if the patient has lung disease that can obscure a developing pneumonia. If sputum can be obtained, it should be sent for Gram stain and culture, blood cultures should be drawn, and a urinalysis with culture, if needed, obtained, since the same nonspecific signs are found in the elderly patient with urosepsis.

The development of the quinolones, specifically ciprofloxacin and ofloxacin, has substantially filled the need for a potent oral agent that is active against gram-negative bacteria including *P. aeruginosa* (48,61). Initially, MRSA was susceptible to ciprofloxacin, but now many of the organisms are resistant, and *S. pneumonia* has shown itself to be resistant to the usual doses of ciprofloxacin (53,62–64). Therefore, additional coverage such as clindamycin or ampicillin/clavulanic acid should be added to cover potential anaerobes, *S. pneumonia,* and methicillin-sensitive *S. aureus.* If the patient has trouble swallowing or appears to be too ill to tolerate oral therapy, then intramuscular injections of a third-generation cephalosporin (ceftazidime if *P. aeruginosa* is suspected) may be given with or without a penicillin or clindamycin if anaerobes are suspected.

Other more exotic species such as *Neisseria* spp., *Enterococcus,* and *Corynebacterium pseudodiphtheriticum* may occasionally cause pneumonia but may be disregarded by the laboratory as contaminants or normal throat flora. The latter bacterium is particularly important because it can be very resistant to antibiotics (65,66). The development of the more expensive new macrolides, clarithromycin and azithromycin, do not appear to have much advantage over the current therapeutic armamentarium for treating NHAP in elderly patients. However, if Legionnaire's disease is seriously suspected in a DNH patient, clarithromycin may be justified because it causes less gastrointestinal side effects. It is well to remember that one-half of patients pay the direct cost of any prescription they receive in a NH without the coverage of any insurance (67).

For the treatment of tracheobronchitis in NH patients, there are several available oral agents: amoxicillin/clavulanic acid, cefixime, and cefuroxime (68).

B. Urinary Tract

Urinary tract infections (UTIs) are the most common infections in the NH in both males and females. The prevalence of bacteriuria increases sharply after the age of 60 for both, i.e., males become colonized as frequently as females. The prevalence of bacteriuria reaches its peak in institutionalized elderly persons, the majority of whom are female (69). Bacteriuria is largely asymptomatic, and it is not clear whether the presence of this asymptomatic bacteriuria is detrimental to an elderly person's long-term survival (69–72).

Nicolle et al. investigated both elderly institutionalized men and women with asymptomatic bacteriuria and found no differences in genitourinary morbidity and mortality between untreated control subjects and patients who received antibiotic therapy (69,73). These study patients did not have long-term catheters and were functional enough to void when requested. Furthermore, antimicrobial therapy was associated with an increased incidence of reinfection with increasingly resistant organisms, adverse antimicrobial drug effects, as well as increased expense. The treatment group did have a lower prevalence of bacteriuria following therapy, but no short-term benefits (follow-up of one year) were identified.

Dontas et al. did a multifactorial 9-year analysis of survival at the Athens Home for the Aged on 267 ambulatory, nondiabetic, noncatheterized women aged 70–92 years upon admission (72). Bacteriuria emerged as one of five variables related to shortened survival; the other predictors included mildly impaired mobility (74), electrocardiographic abnormalities, smoking, and age itself. The investigators postulate that this increased mortality is not due to the development of urosepsis and shock, but rather to the long-term, low-grade tubular defects from chronic infection that prevent the kidney from maintaining homeostasis during some other life-threatening illness, thus resulting in higher mortality. Alternatively, they speculate that chronic bacteriuria is more common in patients with an underlying fatal illness.

The problem of the long-term catheterized patient is even more complicated (71,75–79) because the bulk of catheterized patients are in NHs where the accepted indications for chronic urinary catheterization are not always followed. Although it is widely recognized that anyone catheterized for >30 days will become colonized with bacteria despite the most meticulous catheter care, it is not widely recognized that catheters differ in their construction and may inflict both medical and chemical damage on the bladder and urethra, which can encourage both colonization and invasive infection (9,80). Most studies analyzing the colonization and UTIs in catheterized subjects differentiated between indwelling and condom catheters, but did not discuss the type(s) of indwelling catheter used or the contribution that a particular type makes in the long-term infectious complications (49,80).

Of the three-quarters of a million nosocomial UTIs that occur in the United States every year, 8 of 10 result from instrumentation, usually related to an indwelling or condom urinary catheter. Autopsies of 75 NH patients revealed that 38% had acute renal but no pyelocalyceal inflammation; only 1 noncatheterized patient had such findings. Therefore, long-term catheterization is resulting in renal damage but a lack of symptomatology, probably because of the lack of pyelitis. It must be stressed that in addition to antimicrobial treatment of serious UTIs in NH patients, management should include the removal of anatomical obstructions and/or foreign bodies (including catheters) if possible. If a patient cannot void without catheterization, intermittent catheterization should be utilized. Unfortunately this takes trained staff time and is insufficiently utilized. Switching to condom catheters from indwelling catheters does not appear to reduce the incidence of UTIs (59,72).

All persons with long-term catheters eventually become colonized, i.e., develop bacteriuria. However, catheter-related bacteriuria should not be treated with antibiotics unless there is evidence of illness (e.g., fever, change in functional status, leukocytosis) (81). Bjork et al. showed that treatment of asymptomatic bacteriuria in catheterized NH patients is followed by a high percentage of cases with bacteriuria with organisms resistant to the antibiotic administered (82).

These resistant organisms are indeed appearing in catheterized NH populations. Many of the most common organisms that produce bacteriuria in patients with catheters, e.g., *Providencia stuartii, Proteus mirabilis, P. aeruginosa,* and *Enterococcus,* are already known to be multidrug resistant. *P. stuartii* has only recently been recognized as a pathogen, and some of its strains are urease-positive, as is the case with the related *P. mirabilis.* They have the ability to alkalinize the urine by metabolizing urea to ammonium hydroxide, resulting in struvite stones and encrustations of the catheter which, when they become large enough, obstruct the catheter. This finally results in pyelonephritis and bacteremia. Epidemiological evidence supports the theory that *P. stuartii* acts as a reservoir for resistant plasmids that then spread to other species. Many strains of *P. stuartii* are resistant to most oral and many parenteral antimicrobials; at present most strains are still susceptible to the quinolones, amikacin, cefotaxime, ceftazidime, aztreonam, and imipenem (83). It has been shown that noncatheterized ambulatory NH patients have significantly greater groin carriage of the tribe Proteeae than their age-matched counterparts in the community. Thus, the NH may be acting as a reservoir from which these organisms can spread to the acute-care setting and the community (82,84,85).

The problem of high-level aminoglycoside-resistant, as well as the rarer vancomycin-resistant, *Enterococcus* has been reported. Fortunately, most of these organisms are still responsive to ampicillin in uncomplicated UTIs. However, in the case of serious bacteremic infections, especially infective endocarditis, a combination of antibiotics is necessary in order to obtain synergistic killing of these organisms, but sometimes even this is ineffective (86). Again, the NH is being pointed to as a reservoir for this organism (87).

In the case of *P. aeruginosa,* the development of the oral fluoroquinolones has allowed much more flexibility in the treating of *P. aeruginosa* UTIs in the NH setting, where previously only intramuscular injections of aminoglycosides were available (88). However, as with all useful drugs, they are being overused and resistance to the fluorquinolones, as well as to the aminoglycosides, is not uncommon.

Another uncommon, often overlooked organism in catheterized patients, especially those with an inflammatory or neoplastic process, is the urease-splitting and struvite-forming *Corynebacterium* Group D2. It is highly resistant to most antimicrobials and should be treated with vancomycin until susceptibility data are available. Even with prolonged treatment and change of catheter, *Corynebacterium* Group D2 frequently recurs because the organism is encrusted at the site of the lesion in the bladder (89,90).

C. Gastrointestinal (GI) Tract

Data on GI infections in the NH is scant. Two definitions of infectious gastroenteritis have been developed by the Consensus Council on Nosocomial Infections in Long-Term Care Facilities: (1) three or more stools in a 24-h period in the absence of a noninfectious cause; or (2) two or more episodes of vomiting in a 24-h period with no evidence of a noninfectious cause after appropriate investigation, *or* diarrhea as defined by an increased number of stools greater than normal for the patient with a >24-h duration and no evidence of a noninfectious cause, *and* abdominal cramps or pain or microbiological findings compatible with a GI pathogen (91).

Although most diarrheas in NHs are a result of noninfectious causes such as medications containing sorbitol, antibiotics, or hyperosmolar tube feedings, an infectious etiology must always be considered, especially when the above causes have been excluded. Most NH-acquired GI infections are sporadic events, but some studies have found many clustered cases associated with increased staff absenteeism, which suggests either a communicable disease or common exposure to a toxin or infectious agent. NHs, even more than acute-care facilities, are potentially at higher risk for harboring GI infections because of a number of factors. Many residents are incontinent of feces (37–82% in several studies), residents are encouraged to take part in group activities and visit each other in their rooms, and the majority of employees who care for the residents often have minimal health care training. Most NHs do not have rooms specifically designed for isolation, and health care workers have to travel long distances to reach sinks for handwashing. Although central kitchens have infrequently been associated with outbreaks of nosocomial gastroenteritis, many outbreaks occur on the ward where meals are often plated out and dishes are often washed by residents or nursing staff who have little if any training in food hygiene (91).

Physiological (increased gastric pH and decreased mucus production) and certain pathological changes associated with aging (e.g., diverticulosis) put the elderly patient at a higher risk for GI infection. Therapeutic interventions can also make the host more susceptible, e.g., antiulcer therapy, which increases gastric pH, and narcotic pain medication, which reduces gut motility and, in conjunction with systemic antibiotics, can lead to bacterial overgrowth (91).

The list of pathogens that can cause gastroenteritis in the NH setting is long, including *Salmonella, Shigella, Entamoeba, Campylobacter, Yersinia, E. coli, Aeromonas, Plesiomonas, Vibrio, Clostridium difficile,* rotavirus, Norwalk agent, and *Strongyloides stercorolis.* Of these, *C. difficile* and rotavirus account for the majority of cases. Almost all of the above pathogens are transferred by the fecal-oral route with the exception of rotavirus, which may also be spread by respiratory transmission (91).

The virus-induced diarrheas can only be treated symptomatically with enteric precautions for the duration of the illness, which is usually short. Diagnosis is usually made on clinical grounds, i.e., a mild illness with vomiting predominating and short-lived diarrhea without pus or blood in the stools. The illness usually occurs during the winter months (91).

Although it is one of the most common causes of NH diarrhea, *C. difficile* has caused considerable confusion among practicing physicians. This gram-positive spore-forming bacillus is probably present in its spore or sporulated form in small amounts in almost everyone. The spore is virtually indestructible and remains dormant until the bowel flora are disturbed by the administration of an antibiotic, most often clindamycin, ampicillin, or a cephalosporin. The spore then reverts to its bacterial toxin-producing or vegetative form, which may produce anything from no symptoms to life-threatening diarrhea. When a patient is found to have *C. difficile* toxin in the stool or a positive culture of the organism, treatment with metronidazole or vancomycin is often started (inappropriately!) without regard to the severity of the illness. In fact, asymptomatic carriers may even be treated. This may be due partially to the fact that many "outbreaks" noted in hospitals and NHs may be artifacts due to overly enthusiastic testing of all patients for the presence of *C. difficile* organisms or toxin when an active case is found (92). The above treatment pattern should be avoided. A recent study shows that treatment of asymptomatic patients for 10 days with metronidazole (500 mg b.i.d.) was not effective. Treatment with vancomycin (125 mg q.i.d.) cleared the stools of *C. difficile* only temporarily, since it returned in approximately 90% of the patients within 20 days. But in the patients who received placebo, only one person was still *C. difficile* culture positive at the end of the study. In each of these groups 50–60% of the asymptomatic subjects were toxin as well as culture positive (93). This is particularly interesting because patients who are not treated for their *C. difficile*–associated diarrhea and colitis never relapse (94). The reason for this may be that in asymptomatic patients no metronidazole reaches the colon, having been absorbed in the small bowel, whereas in the symptomatic patient GI transit time may have increased enough so that not all of the metronidazole is absorbed before it reaches the colon (93). In contrast, vancomycin reaches the gut in high concentration whether the patient has diarrhea or not. Vancomycin can temporarily eliminate enough organisms so that the patients become toxin and culture negative, but apparently a few remaining *C. difficile* spores survive, which lead to relapse. Because 24% of the patients suffered one relapse and 5% had three or more relapses, it may be wise to withhold treatment of *C. difficile* colitis unless a patient has severe and persistent symptoms.

It is the patient with severe *C. difficile* diarrhea and fecal incontinence who is the greatest threat to the spread of the disease (94,95). These patients should be treated with vancomycin 125 mg q.i.d. (a less seriously ill patient may do well on metronidazole, which is substantially less expensive), be isolated in a room with a toilet, and have strict use of enteric precautions that are enforced including room cleansing with a sporicidal agent. If possible, the patient should be withdrawn from the offending systemic antibiotics, or at least have them changed if they consist of clindamycin, ampicillin, and cephalosporins. The patient should improve within 24 h and have reduced bowel symptoms within 4–5 days. If they fail to do so then the diagnosis is suspect and other etiologies for the diarrhea should be sought.

Occasionally other microbes are implicated in antibiotic-associated diarrhea including *Salmonella, Clostridium perfringens,* and possibly *Candida albicans.* However, most cases of antibiotic-associated diarrhea that is *C. difficile* toxin negative have no clear etiology. These diarrheas differ from the *C. difficile*–associated diarrhea/colitis in the following ways: they are rarely associated with systemic signs such as fever and leukocytosis, severe complications are uncommon, and they are dose related in that they resolve when antibiotics are reduced in dosage or discontinued (94,96).

As outlined by Bartlett, when patients relapse with *C. difficile* diarrhea/colitis they should be treated with vancomycin or metronidazole for 10–14 days followed by a 3-week course of one of the following: cholestyramine, one 4-g packet t.i.d.; *Lactobacillus,* 1 g of Lactinex q.i.d.; a combination of the above; pulse doses of vancomycin, 125 mg q.o.d.; or rifampin, 600 mg b.i.d., in addition to the vancomycin (94).

Over a third of *Salmonella* outbreaks are in hospitals and NHs, but of these only 10–40% are foodborne. Person-to-person transmission, either directly or indirectly via the fecal-oral route, account for the rest. Persons over the age of 70 have a very high attack rate, possibly due to a defect in host defenses. The administration of antibiotics may prolong fecal excretion; however, in patients with severe underlying disease, the organism's drug susceptibility pattern should be defined and the patient treated with an appropriate antibiotic. Amoxicillin and ampicillin can no longer be relied upon as effective against *Salmonella* (91,96,97).

Similarly, *Shigella,* usually *S. sonnei,* accounts for most of the epidemics of shigellosis in geriatric hospitals. Again the major mode of transmission of shigellosis is usually person-to-person via the fecal-oral route. However, some cases have been due to contaminated food or water. *Shigella* species have also developed resistance to multiple antibiotics, and susceptibility data must be obtained in order to insure adequate treatment (91,97,98).

Verotoxin-producing *E. coli* serotype 0157 diarrhea has been associated with the serving of contaminated food in a number of NHs. What is usually a mild diarrheal disease can become a syndrome of bloody diarrhea associated with hemorrhagic colitis and hemolytic uremic syndrome, resulting in a high fatality rate. It is not clear whether antibiotic or antidiarrheal treatment decreases the morbidity and mortality. This pathogen should be considered in the differential diagnosis of diarrhea when tests for common pathogens are negative (91,99).

D. Central Nervous System

Many cases of bacterial meningitis in adults occur in individuals >60 years old with mortality rates ranging from 53 to 79%. The exact percentage that occurs in the NH population is unknown because delirium, lethargy, and altered mental status may be attributed to stroke, dementia, hypoxic encephalopathy, or progression of a patient's underlying disease status. Fever and stiff neck are much less common in elderly than in younger individuals (100–102). Thus, delay in diagnosis or overlooking the diagnosis of meningitis leads to high mortality rates in geriatric patients. Patients who have had neurosurgery are particularly prone to such delays or omission of the diagnosis of meningi-

Table 1 Etiology of Bacterial Meningitis in Elderly Patients

Organism	Incidence (%)
Streptococcus pneumoniae	54
Neisseria meningitidis	11
Gram-negative bacilli	8
Listeria monocytogenes	7
Staphylococcus aureus	6
Streptococci (nonpneumococcal)	4
Haemophilus influenzae	2
Unknown	3

Source: Newton JE, et al. Lancet 1979; 2:157; Jonsson M, et al. Scand J Infect Dis 1971;3:141; Quaade F. et al. Geriatrics 1963; 18:860; Massanari RM, et al. Geriatrics 1977; 32:55; Swartz MN, et al. N Engl J Med 1965; 272:725; Weiss W, et al. Arch intern Med 1967; 120:517; Jensen J, et al. Scand J Infect Dis 1969; 1:21.

tis because their symptoms may be attributed to their postoperative course. This is especially true with gram-negative bacillary meningitis because this infection tends to progress more slowly with less symptomatology than meningitis caused by gram-positive cocci. Table 1 lists the common meningopathogens found in older patients. Table 2 summarizes common primary sources of meningopathogens.

Once meningitis is considered in the differential diagnosis, an immediate lumbar puncture to obtain cerebrospinal fluid (CSF) should be done, provided there are no contraindica-

Table 2 Primary Source of Infection in Bacterial Meningitis of Elderly Patients

Etiological agent	Primary source
Streptococcus pneumoniae	Pneumonia
	Otitis media
	Sinusitis
	Skull fracture
Staphylococcus aureus	Acute infective endocarditis
	Pneumonia
	Neurosurgery
Gram-negative bacilli	Neurosurgery
	Head trauma
	Urinary tract
	Pneumonia
	Pressure ulcer
Neisseria meningitidis	Bacteremia
Listeria monocytogenes	Gastrointestinal tract
Haemophilus influenzae	Otitis media
	Pneumonia

Table 3 Antibiotic Therapy for Meningitis in Elderly Patients

Organism	Drugs of choice	Alternate
Streptococcus pneumoniae	Penicillin or ampicillin	Chloramphenicol
Neisseria meningitidis	Penicillin or ampicillin	Chloramphenicol
Listeria monocytogenes	Penicillin or ampicillin	Trimethoprim-sulfamethoxazole
Gram-negative bacilli	Third-generation cephalosporin[a]	Intrathecal aminoglycoside
Staphylococcus aureus	Oxacillin or nafcillin	Vancomycin
Unknown	Ampicillin + third-generation cephalosporin[a]	

[a] Ceftriaxone and ceftazidime are most frequently used. Cefoperazone is not recommended because of limited penetration into the cerebrospinal fluid.

tions such as intracranial hypertension (e.g., due to a space occupying lesion), cellulitis at the puncture site, or a significant coagulopathy. Although no organisms may be seen on Gram or acid-fast stain, evidence of a pleocytosis of 500–10,000 leukocytes with a high percentage of polymorphonuclear neutrophils (PMNs), an elevated protein, and a CSF glucose < 40% of the blood sugar is characteristic of bacterial meningitis. Both *Listeria monocytogenes* and *Mycobacterium tuberculosis* meningitis may lead to a predominance of mononuclear cell in the CSF, but, if diagnosed early, it may also have a predominance of PMNs. Examination and culture of sputum, urine, blood, and other body fluids may also help to determine the meningopathogen as well as the source of infection. Determinations for microbial antigens in CSF by counterimmunoelectrophoresis or latex agglutination or for endotoxin by the limulus lysate test may assist in defining the etiology of the meningitis. These tests are especially helpful when meningitis patients are already receiving antibiotics.

With these findings, rapid, intravenous empiric antimicrobial therapy with a broad-spectrum antibiotic that penetrates the CSF is required unless the CSF Gram stain is characteristic for a particular organism. Antibiotic recommendations for specific menengopathogens are listed in Table 3. For empiric antimicrobial therapy for suspected bacterial meningitis in an elderly patient, a combination of penicillin G (or ampicillin) plus a third-generation cephalosporin (e.g., ceftriaxone or ceftazidime) is recommended (third-generation cephalosporins are ineffective against *L. monocytogenes,* thus, penicillin is necessary). Chloramphenicol or trimethoprim-sulfamethoxazole may be used in penicillin-allergic patients (103). (See also Chap. 26.)

Chemoprophylaxis is indicated for those persons in close contact with a patient who proves to have meningococcal meningitis; this includes frequent visitors, roommates, and health care workers. These individuals should receive rifampin 600 mg every 12 h for 2 days. There are no definitive recommendations for treating those in close contact with a patient with meningitis caused by a *Haemophilus influenzae.* As stated earlier, use of pneumococcal vaccine in elderly persons is likely to reduce the acquisition of a pneumococcal infection or, if acquired, prevent it from progressing to meningitis (101,102)

Brain abscess has not been well studied in elderly persons (103). Although some T-cell abnormalities occur with aging, diseases such as nocardiosis and toxoplasmosis are not problems associated with advanced age. Most elderly patients with brain abscess will have a previous history of sinusitis, dental infection, or pleuropulmonary infection. Brain abscess symptoms of headache, hemiparesis, and visual disturbance may be mistaken for stroke or other space-occupying lesion. Fever is usually low grade and the patient is often not toxic. Focal findings such as papilledema or cranial nerve changes may also be found. Computed tomographic scan with contrast or a magnetic resonance imaging scan will usually provide a definitive diagnosis. Lumbar puncture is contraindicated with space-occupying lesions of brain such as an abscess (104).

Empiric antibiotic therapy is based on the site of the primary infection. Dental infection, sinusitis, and lung infection usually produce anaerobic brain abscess. In patients who have undergone head trauma or neurosurgery, *S. aureus* and gram-negative bacilli are common. Penicillin and metronidazole are commonly used when anaerobes are suspected. In most patients, surgery is required after intravenous antibiotics are initiated (104).

V. CONCLUSION

It is evident that antimicrobial therapy as it is now being administered in NHs could benefit from a true attempt at quality improvement (105–107). It is also obvious that more research needs to be done in NHs, especially in infectious diseases, and that a consensus needs to be reached about common study parameters so that future research is more comparable.

REFERENCES

1. Lipsky MS, Hickey DP, Browning G, et al. The use of do-not-hospitalize orders by family physicians in Ohio. J Fam Pract 1990; 30:61–4.
2. Verghese A, Berk SL. Introduction and epidemiologic considerations. In: Verghese A, Berk SL, eds. Infections in nursing homes and long-term care facilities. Basel: Karger, 1990:1–11.
3. Cowan J, Verghese A. Cost containment and cost effective antibiotic therapy in the nursing home. In: Verghese A, Berk SL, eds. Infections in nursing homes and long-term care facilities. Basel: Karger, 1990:221–30.
4. Garibaldi RA, Brodine S, Matsumiya S. Infections among patients in nursing homes: policies, prevalence, and problems. N Engl J Med 1981; 305:731–5.
5. Smith JK. Immune response and host defense in the nursing home patient. In: Verghese A, Berk SL, eds. Infections in nursing homes and long-term care facilities. Basel: Karger, 1990:12–29.
6. Mor V, Laliberte L, Morris JN, et al. The Karnofsky performance status scale: an examination of its reliability and validity in a research setting. Cancer 1984; 53:2002–7.
7. Mehr DR, Foxman B, Colombo P. Risk factors for mortality from lower respiratory infections in nursing home patients. J Fam Pract 1992; 34:585–91.
8. Scheckler WE, Peterson PJ. Infections and infection control among residents of eight rural Wisconsin nursing homes. Arch Intern Med 1986; 146:1981–4.
9. Franson TR, Duthie EH, Jr, Cooper JE, et al. Prevalence survey of infections and their predisposing factors at a hospital-based nursing home care unit. J Am Geriatr Soc 1986; 34:95–100.
10. Brown NK, Thompson DJ. Nontreatment of fever in extended-care facilities. N Engl J Med 1979; 300(22):1246–50.
11. Wood JS. Nursing home care. Clin Geriatr Med 1986; 2:601–15.

12. Lloyd JC, Lang F, Doane DG. Immunization strategies in the nursing home. In: Verghese A, Berk SL, eds. Infections in nursing homes and long-term care facilities. Basel: Karger, 1990:66–76.
13. Centers for Disease Control. Impact of influenza on a nursing home population—New York. MMWR 1983; 32:32–4.
14. Centers for Disease Control. Outbreaks of influenza among nursing home residents—Connecticut, United States. MMWR 1985; 34:478–82.
15. Centers for Disease Control. Recommendations for prevention and control of influenza: recommendations of the Immunization Practices Advisory Committee. Ann Intern Med 1986; 105:299–404.
16. Berk SL, Alvarez S. Vaccinating the elderly: recommendations and rationale. Geriatrics 1986; 41(1):79–91.
17. LaForce FM. Immunizations, immunoprophylaxis, and chemoprophylaxis to prevent selected infections. JAMA 1987; 257(18):2464–70.
18. Goodman RA, Orenstein WA, Munro TF, et al. Impact of Influenza A in a nursing home. JAMA 1982; 247(10):1451–3.
19. Simberkoff MS, Cross AP, Al-Ibrahim M, et al. Efficacy of pneumococcal vaccine in high-risk patients. N Engl J Med 1986; 315:1318–27.
20. Orenstein WA, Wassilak SGF, Hinman AR. Tetanus. In: Hoeprich PD, Jordan CM, eds. Infectious diseases. 4th ed. Philadelphia: J. B. Lippincott Company, 1989:1173–82.
21. Powers DC, Sears SD. Influenza, pneumonia, tetanus: how effective is vaccination? Geriatrics 1987; 42(10):81–90.
22. Stead WW, To T, Harrison RW, et al. Benefit-risk considerations in preventive treatment for tuberculosis in elderly persons. Ann Intern Med 1987; 107:843–5.
23. Stead WW, To T. The significance of the tuberculin skin test in elderly persons. Ann Intern Med 1987; 107:837–42.
24. Stead WW, Lofgren JP, Warren E, et al. Tuberculosis as an endemic and nosocomial infection among the elderly in nursing homes. N Engl J Med 1985; 312(23):1483–7.
25. Stead WS, Kerby GR, Schlueter DP, et al. The clinical spectrum of primary tuberculosis in adults. Ann Intern Med 1968; 68:731–45.
26. Alvarez S, Kasprzyk DR, Freundl M. Two-stage skin testing for tuberculosis in a domiciliary population. Am Rev Respir Dis 1987; 136:1193–6.
27. Sarubbi FA. Infection control in the nursing home setting. In: Verghese A, Berk SL, eds. Infections in nursing homes and long-term care facilities. Basel: Karger, 1990:55–65.
28. Frampton MW. An outbreak of tuberculosis among hospital personnel caring for a patient with a skin ulcer. Ann Intern Med 1992; 117:312–13.
29. Johnson MP, Coberly JS, Clermont HL, et al. Tuberculin skin test reactivity among adults infected with human immunodeficiency virus. J Infect Dis 1992; 166:194–8.
30. Pearson ML, Jereb JA, Frieden TR, et al. Nosocomial transmission of multidrug-resistant *Mycobacterium tuberculosis:* a risk to patients and health care workers. Ann Intern Med 1992; 117:191–6.
31. Hinman AR, Hughes JM. National action plan to combat multidrug-resistant tuberculosis. MMWR 1992; 41:5–48.
32. Villarino ME, Dooley SW, Jr, Geiter LJ, et al. Management of persons exposed to multidrug-resistant tuberculosis. MMWR 1992; 41:59–71.
33. O'Toole RD, Drew WL, Dahlgren BJ, et al. An outbreak of methicillin-resistant *Staphylococcus aureus* infection: Observations in hospital and nursing home. JAMA 1970; 213:257–63.
34. Hsu CCS, Macaluso CP, Special L, et al. High rate of methicillin resistance of *Staphylococcus aureus* isolated from hospitalized nursing home patients. Arch Intern Med 1988; 148:569–70.
35. Strausbaugh LJ, Jacobson C, Sewell DL, et al. Methicillin-resistant *Staphylococcus aureus* in extended-care facilities: experiences in a Veteran's Affairs nursing home and a review of the literature. Infect Control Hosp Epidemiol 1991; 12:36–45.

36. Storch GA, Radcliff JL, Meyer PL, et al. Methicillin-resistant *Staphylococcus aureus* in a nursing home. Infect Control 1987; 8:24–9.
37. Bradley SF, Terpenning MS, Ramsey MA, et al. Methicillin-resistant *Staphylococcus aureus:* colonization and infection in a long-term care facility. Ann Intern Med 1991; 115:417–22.
38. Bradley SF: Methicillin-resistant *Staphylococcus aureus* infection. Clin Geriatr Med 1992; 8(4):853–68.
39. Abramowicz M. Mupirocin—a new topical antibiotic. Med Lett Drugs Ther 1988; 30:55–6.
40. Schaefler S. Methicillin-resistant strains of *Staphylococcus aureus* resistant to quinolones. J Clin Microbiol 1989; 27:335–6.
41. Burdge DR, Chow AW. The pressure ulcer. In: Verghese A, Berk SL, eds. Infections in nursing homes and long-term care facilities. Basel: Karger, 1990:143–61.
42. Allman RM, Laprade CA, Noel LB, et al. Pressure sores among hospitalized patients. Ann Intern Med 1986; 105:337–42.
43. Moody BL, Fanale JE, Thompson M, et al. Impact of staff education on pressure sore development in elderly hospitalized patients. Arch Intern Med 1988; 148:2241–3.
44. Sugarman B, Hawes S, Musher DM, et al. Osteomyelitis beneath pressure sores. Arch Intern Med 1983; 143:683–8.
45. Chow AW, Galpin JE, Guze LB. Clindamycin for treatment of sepsis caused by decubitus ulcers. J Infect Dis 1977; 135:S65–S68.
46. Galpin JE, Chow AW, Bayer AS, et al. Sepsis associated with decubitus ulcers. Am J Med 1976; 61:346–50.
47. Desplaces N, Acar JF. New quinolones in the treatment of joint and bone infections. Rev Infect Dis 1988; 10(suppl 1):S179–S183.
48. Sanders WE, Jr. Efficacy, safety, and potential economic benefits of oral ciprofloxacin in the treatment of infections. Rev Infect Dis 1988; 10(3):528–43.
49. Woods DR, Bender BS. Long-term urinary tract catheterization. Med Clin North Am 1989; 73:1441–54.
50. Marrie TJ. Bacteremia in the nursing home patient. In: Verghese A, Berk SL, eds. Infections in nursing homes and long-term care facilities. Basel: Karger, 1990:77–94.
51. Stein D. Managing pneumonia acquired in nursing homes: special concerns [published erratum appears in Geriatrics 1990; 45(6):90]. Geriatrics 1990; 45:39–42,47.
52. Nunley D, Verghese A, Berk SL. Pneumonia in the nursing home patient. In: Verghese A, Berk SL, eds. Infections in nursing homes and long-term care facilities. Basel: Karger, 1990:95–113.
53. Yoshikawa TT. Treatment of nursing home-acquired pneumonia [editorial]. J Am Geriatr Soc 1991; 39:1040–1.
54. Marrie TJ, Haldane EV, Faulkner RS, et al. Community-acquired pneumonia requiring hospitalization: is it different in the elderly? J Am Geriatr Soc 1985; 33:671–80.
55. Roth RM, Gleckman RA. Pneumonia in the elderly: a nursing home perspective. Am Fam Physician 1985; 31:131–7.
56. Crossley KB, Thurn JR. Nursing home-acquired pneumonia. Semin Respir Infect 1989; 4:64–72.
57. Marrie TJ, Durant H, Yates L. Community-acquired pneumonia requiring hospitalization: 5-year prospective study. Rev Infect Dis 1989; 11:586–99.
58. Roselle GA. Nosocomial and nursing home-acquired pneumonia. Recent therapeutic advances. Postgrad Med 1987; 81:131–2,135.
59. Mulligan T. Parenteral antibiotic therapy for patients in nursing homes. Rev Infect Dis 1991; 13(suppl 2):S180–S183.
60. Norman DC, Yoshikawa TT. Clinical features of infection and the significance of fever in the elderly nursing home patient. In: Verghese A, Berk SL, eds. Infections in nursing homes and long-term care facilities. Basel: Karger, 1990:30–40.
61. Barriere SL. Economic impact of oral ciprofloxacin. Am J Med 1987; 82(suppl 4A):387–90.

62. Yoshikawa TT. Pneumonia, UTI, and decubiti in the nursing home: optimal management. Geriatrics 1989; 44:32–4,37.
63. Cooper B, Lawlor M. Pneumococcal bacteremia during ciprofloxacin therapy for pneumococcal pneumonia. Am J Med 1989; 87:475.
64. Gordan JJ, Kauffman CA. Superinfection with *Streptococcus pneumoniae* during therapy with ciprofloxacin. Am J Med 1990; 89:383–4.
65. Williams EA, Greene JD, Berk SL. Pneumonia caused by *Corynebacterium pseudodiphtheriticum.* J Tenn Med Assoc 1991; 84:223–4.
66. Morris A, Guild I. Endocarditis due to *Corynebacterium pseudodiphtheriticum:* five case reports, review, and antibiotic susceptibilities of nine strains. Rev Infect Dis 1991; 13:887–92.
67. Abramowicz M. Clarithromycin and azithromycin. Med Lett Drugs Ther 1992; 34:45–8.
68. Berk SL, Verghese A. Antibiotic therapy in the nursing home. In: Verghese A, Berk SL, eds. Infections in nursing homes and long-term care facilities. Basel: Karger, 1990:203–20.
69. Nicolle LE, Mayhew WJ, Bryan L. Prospective randomized comparison of therapy and no therapy for asymptomatic bacteriuria in institutionalized elderly women. Am J Med 1987; 83:27–33.
70. Kunin CM, Douthitt S, Dancing J, et al. The association between the use of urinary catheters and morbidity and mortality among elderly patients in nursing homes. Am J Epidemiol 1992; 135:291–301.
71. Jost PM, Hinthorn DR. Current problems in control of infections. Compr Ther 1991; 17:27–31.
72. Dontas AS. Urinary tract infection in nursing home residents. In: Verghese A, Berk SL, eds. Infections in nursing homes and long-term care facilities. Basel: Karger, 1990:126–42.
73. Nicolle LE, Bjornson J, Harding GKM, et al. Bacteriuria in elderly institutionalized men. N Engl J Med 1983; 309:1420–5.
74. Blocker WP,Jr. Maintaining functional independence by mobilizing the aged. Geriatrics 1992; 47:42–56.
75. Meyers BR. Infectious diseases in the elderly: an overview. Geriatrics 1989; 44 Suppl A:4–6.
76. Kunin CM, Chin QF, Chambers S. Morbidity and mortality associated with indwelling urinary catheters in elderly patients in a nursing home—confounding due to the presence of associated diseases. J Am Geriatr Soc 1987; 35:1001–6.
77. Farber BF, Brennen C, Puntereri AJ, et al. A prospective study of nosocomial infections in a chronic care facility. J Am Geriatr Soc 1984; 32:499–502.
78. Rousseau P, Feuntevilla-Clifton A. Urinary incontinence in the aged, Part 1: patient evaluation. Geriatrics 1992; 47:22–34.
79. Rousseau P, Fuentevilla-Clifton A. Urinary incontinence in the aged, Part 2: management strategies. Geriatrics 1992; 47:37–48.
80. Ruutu M, Alfthan O, Talja M. Cytotoxicity of latex urinary catheters. Br J Urol 1985; 57:82–7.
81. Yoshikawa TT, Norman DC: Aging and clinical practice: infectious diseases, diagnosis and treatment. New York: Igaku-Shoin, 1987:173–84.
82. Bjork DT, Pelletier LL, Tight RR. Urinary tract infections with antibiotic resistant organisms in catheterized nursing home patients. Infect Control 1984; 5:173–6.
83. Warren JW. *Providencia stuartii:* a common cause of antibiotic-resistant bacteriuria in patients with long-term indwelling catheters. Rev Infect Dis 1986; 8:61–7.
84. Ehrenkranz NJ, Eckert DG, Alfonso BC, et al. Proteeae groin skin carriage in ambulatory geriatric outpatients. Infect Control Hosp Epidemiol 1989; 10:150–4.
85. Gaynes RP, Weinstein RA, Chamberlin W, et al. Antibiotic resistant flora in nursing home patients admitted to the hospital. Arch Intern Med 1985; 145:1804–7.
86. Williams EA, Verghese A. Newer pathogens for respiratory infections in the elderly. In: Niederman NS, ed. Respiratory infections in the elderly. New York: Raven Press, 1991:157–87.
87. Zervos MJ, Terpenning MS, Schaberg DR, et al. High-level aminoglycoside-resistant enterococci: colonization of nursing home and acute care hospital patients. Arch Intern Med 1987; 147:1591–4.

88. MacArthur RD, Lehman MH, Currie McCumber CA, et al. The epidemiology of gentamicin-resistant Pseudomonas aeruginosa on an intermediate care unit. Am J Epidemiol 1988; 128:821–7.
89. Soriano F, Aguado JM, Ponte C, et al. Urinary tract infection caused by *Corynebacterium* Group D2: report of 82 cases and review. Rev Infect Dis 1990; 12:1019–34.
90. Brown AE. Other *Corynebacteria.* In: Mandell GL, Douglas RG, Jr., Bennett JE, eds. Principles and practice of infectious disease. 3rd ed. New York: Churchill Livingstone, 1990:1581–7.
91. Huebner J, Daschner F. Gastro-intestinal infections in nursing home patients. In: Verghese A, Berk SL, eds. Infections in nursing homes and long-term care facilities. Basel: Karger, 1990:182–92.
92. Gorbach SL. *Clostridium difficile* settles in a nursing home. Hosp Pract 1989; (Feb. 15):145–60.
93. Johnson S, Homann SR, Bettin KM, et al. Treatment of asymptomatic *Clostridium difficile* carriers (fecal excretors) with vancomycin and metronidazole: a randomized, placebo-controlled trial. Ann Intern Med 1992; 117:297–311.
94. Bartlett JG. The 10 most common questions about *Clostridium difficile* associated diarrhea/colitis. Infect Dis Clin Pract 1992; 1:254–59.
95. Nicolle LE, McIntyre M, Zacharias H, MacDonell JA. Twelve-month surveillance of infections in institutionalized elderly men. J Am Geriatr Soc 1984; 32:513–19.
96. Choi M, Yoshikawa TT, Bridge J, et al. Salmonella outbreak in a nursing home [see comments]. J Am Geriatr Soc 1990; 38:531–4.
97. Abramowicz M. The choice of antibacterial drugs. Med Lett Drugs Ther 1992; 34:49–56.
98. Wiström J, Jertborn M, Ekwall E, et al. Empiric treatment of acute diarrheal disease with norfloxacin: a randomized, placebo-controlled study. Ann Intern Med 1992; 117:202–8.
99. Carter AO, Borczyk AA, Carlson JA, et al. A severe outbreak of *Escherichia coli* 0157:H7–associated hemorrhagic colitis in a nursing home. N Engl J Med 1987; 317:1496–1500.
100. Roos KL. Meningitis as it presents in the elderly. Geriatrics 1990; 45:63–75.
101. Berk SL, Williams EA. Central nervous system infection in the elderly. In: Morley JE, ed. Geriatric care. St. Louis, MO: Mosby & Co., 1994.
102. Berk SL. Bacterial meningitis. In: Gleckman RA, Gantz NM, eds. Infections in the elderly. Boston: Little, Brown and Co., 1983:235–65.
103. Yoshikawa TT, Norman DC. Aging and clinical practice: infectious diseases, diagnosis and treatment. New York: Igaku Shoin, 1987:90–107.
104. Behrman RC, Meyers BR, Mendleson MH, et al. Central nervous system infection in the elderly. Arch Intern Med 1990; 49:1596–9.
105. Leibovici L, Konisberger H, Pitlik SD, et al. Patients at risk for inappropriate antibiotic treatment of bacteraemia. J Intern Med 1992; 231:371–4.
106. Beers MH, Ouslander JG, Rollingher I, et al. Explicit criteria for determining inappropriate medication use in nursing home residents. Arch Intern Med 1991; 151:1825–32.
107. Jones SR, Parker DF, Liebow LS, et al. Appropriateness of antibiotic therapy in long-term care facilities. Am J Med 1987; 83:499–502.
108. Neu HC. The crisis in antibiotic resistance. Science 1992;287:1064–73.

29

Home Intravenous Antibiotic Therapy

Pamela H. Nagami
University of California School of Medicine, Los Angeles, and Kaiser Permanente Hospital, Woodland Hills, California

Stephen A. Landis
Kaiser Permanente Hospital, Woodland Hills, California

I. INTRODUCTION

Only in comparatively recent times has hospital care of patients supplanted home care of the sick. Even as hospitals became larger and more elaborate and nursing services improved, they were, until well into this century, reserved for the care of the indigent and the socially isolated (1). But at the same time that hospitals were losing their stigma and gaining prestige, efforts were being made to return health care to the home.

In 1947, Montefiore Hospital in New York City established the "hospital without walls," the first hospital-based home care program utilizing a team of therapists, nurses, and physicians (2). The first systematic use of home intravenous antibiotic therapy was not in geriatrics, but in pediatrics, in patients with cystic fibrosis. In 1974 Rucker and Harrison (3) reported on the use of home intravenous antibiotic therapy in 62 affected patients who were treated for 1–2 weeks with either gentamicin or colistimethate via gravity drip through a heparin lock. Clinical response was satisfactory in 70% of the antibiotic courses, with many patients maintaining normal activities during therapy.

Subsequent studies demonstrated the feasibility of home intravenous antibiotic therapy in adult patients even when serious intercurrent illness was present. In 1978 Antoniskis et al. (4) published a retrospective pilot study of 13 patients, most with osteomyelitis, who were treated successfully, in most cases, with a variety of antibiotics. In another study, also published in 1978, Stiver and coworkers (5) reported on 23 patients with a variety of infections, including infective endocarditis, who received home intravenous antibiotic therapy after in-hospital training. Patients ranged in age from 12 to 78 years and were visited daily by home care nurses. Antibiotics were infused by gravity drip via a heparin lock. An interesting observation in this study, which has been borne out by subsequent studies of home intravenous antibiotic therapy, was that the phlebitis rate for these patients was lower than that of comparable patients in the hospital. Possible explanations for this observation include more meticulous and unhurried care of intravenous access by the patient, use of family and home care nurse, and less exposure of the patient to nosocomial pathogens.

In 1979, Kind et al. (6) reported on 15 patients treated with intravenous antibiotics at home. Most of their patients were young and were being treated for osteomyelitis and soft tissue infections, but one 61-year-old man was treated successfully for infective endocarditis with penicillin at 6-h intervals. In 1982, Poretz et al. (7) published their experience with 150 patients treated with home intravenous antibiotics over a 2-year period. All of the patients were initially hospitalized at a large community hospital and received training prior to discharge on the administration of antibiotics through a heparin lock via gravity drip. Patients reported to the hospital at regular intervals to replenish their supply of antibiotics. Intravenous catheters were changed through the hospital emergency room or by a visiting nurse. The age distribution of the patients was not described, but the eldest patient enrolled was 86 years old.

Similiar results were obtained in a larger study by Stiver and coworkers (8) published in 1982 and involving 95 patients. Again, antibiotics were infused by gravity through a heparin lock. Interestingly, two patients in this study were not hospitalized prior to the initiation of home intravenous antibiotic therapy but were trained in the outpatient clinic. Patients ranged in age from 4 to 81 years, but further breakdown of patients by age is not given. A wide variety of infections were treated (osteomyelitis, pneumonia, endocarditis, blastomycosis, etc.). No patient required readmission to the hospital because of failure of home intravenous antibiotic therapy.

These and other studies published between 1974 and 1983 show the steady development in the field of home intravenous antibiotic treatment, but in 1983 an event occurred that proved to be a tremendous catalyst for growth within the home health care industry. In that year, Medicare's prospective payment system was passed, by which hospitals receive a flat amount per admission based on diagnosis-related groups regardless of the actual cost of care provided. This new system has created powerful incentives to send Medicare patients home quickly and has contributed to the almost explosive subsequent development of home health care in the United States. Since implementation of these provisions in October 1983, the average hospital stay for Medicare patients has dropped from 13.4 days in 1968 to 7.7 days in June 1985 (9).

At the present time, home health care is the most rapidly growing sector of the health care industry (10). Within home health care the most rapidly growing segment has been outpatient intravenous antibiotic therapy (11). Estimates in the late 1980s projected a 34% expansion before the end of the decade, with estimated expenditure exceeding \$1.3 billion (10). Increased demand for outpatient intravenous antibiotic therapy has led to advances in the techniques of parenteral antibiotic delivery and to the development and marketing of new antibiotics suitable for outpatient parenteral use. These developments in turn have stimulated further expansion within the industry.

The first major advance in the technology of parenteral drug delivery came not from the field of infectious diseases, but from the home care of cancer patients. Programmable infusion pumps were developed to administer patient-controlled analgesia, and the trend has been toward the development of smaller, lighter pumps (12). Thirteen years ago an infusion pump weighed about 40 pounds and was mounted on a pole (13). Modern automated infusion pumps weigh less than a pound, may be worn on a belt or shoulder strap, and are capable of delivering an entire day's supply of intravenous antibiotic accurately and at preset dosing intervals without any intervention by the patient (14,15).

These automated pumps have made home intravenous antibiotic therapy accessible to many elderly patients whose deficits in vision, coordination, and cognition would preclude their participation in antibiotic infusion by conventional gravity drip.

The second area of technological advance has been in the field of intravenous access. Ten years ago home intravenous antibiotics were usually administered via short metal or plastic intravenous catheters, which had to be changed approximately every 3 days, either by a visiting nurse or in the emergency room or clinic. Available sites for peripheral intravenous placement would be exhausted after a few weeks of continuous therapy. Surgical placement of a central venous catheter (e.g., Hickman®, Broviac®) in the operating room was required for treatment courses longer than 2 or 3 weeks, particularly in elderly patients in whom peripheral venous access sites are limited. However, in recent years a variety of peripherally inserted central and midlength catheters have become available, which can be left in place for up to a month (16). In addition, short intravenous catheters made of elastomeric hydrogels (e.g., Aquavene®) are now available, which can remain in place for 2 weeks (17–20). All of these new catheters can be inserted by a nurse trained in the technique.

Finally, the development of new broad-spectrum antibiotics with long half-lives and low toxicity has simplified home intravenous antibiotic therapy, though the parallel developments in automated infusion pumps have made drug half-life less of an issue than it was formerly. Of the new antibiotics, ceftriaxone has received the most attention in the literature and has been widely used in the community.

Despite technological and pharmaceutical advances that have made home intravenous antibiotic therapy more practical for geriatric patients, there is an important financial barrier to its use by patients age 65 years or older. Medicare does not pay for the cost of antibiotics administered to outpatients, even when given by the parenteral route (21). In addition, home health visits for intravenous antibiotic treatment are not reimbursable under Medicare unless the patient is also receiving home health care for one of the reimbursable types of treatment. Most elderly patients, unless they are members of a health maintenance organization, will not have comprehensive insurance coverage for the drugs and services needed to deliver intravenous antibiotic therapy in the home.

II. GENERAL GUIDELINES FOR THE SELECTION OF PATIENTS

The first step in considering elderly patients for home intravenous antibiotic therapy is to determine the type of infection the patient has and what the expected duration of intravenous antibiotic therapy will be (Table 1). This assessment will usually need to be made in consultation with a specialist in infectious diseases. Infections treated with home intravenous antibiotic therapy fall into two categories. The first and most common type are localized infections of soft tissues, bones, or joints that require more than a week a of parenteral antibiotics for cure but do not render the patient medically unstable. The second category comprises infections, such as infective endocarditis, that, though potentially life threatening, require such lengthy courses of therapy that home intravenous antibiotic therapy may be considered.

After the patient is determined to have a condition amenable to parenteral antibiotic therapy at home, an assessment must be made of both the patient's general medical condition and the status of the infection under treatment. For example, patients with diabetic foot infections must have completed necessary surgical debridements and have

Table 1 General Considerations for Patient Selection for Home Intravenous Antibiotic Therapy (HIVAT)

Infection requires intravenous antibiotic therapy for more than a few days
Infection has been stabilized
Other medical conditions permit care at home
Patient and patient's family are motivated to participate in home intravenous antibiotic therapy
No contraindications, such as alcohol or drug abuse, exist
Patient has the necessary insurance coverage

Source: Adapted from Refs. 11, 13, 21.

relatively stable blood sugars before they can be discharged to complete intravenous antibiotics at home. Similarly, patients with infective endocarditis may complete antibiotic therapy in the home, but only after their cardiac infection has come under control in the hospital and only if the patients are hemodynamically stable.

It must be remembered that while hospitalized patients are relatively passive participants in their care, home health patients or their caregivers must be motivated to learn the required techniques (11). Whether they are formally obtained or not, the informed consents of both patients and their families registers their understanding about undertaking home parenteral antibiotic therapy and their commitment to the completion of a course of parenteral antibiotics in the home.

Finally, the home health care team must be alert to any factors that would exclude patients from such care. The most important of these are alcoholism and drug abuse, particularly intravenous drug abuse. Although the home is a bacteriologically less hostile environment than the hospital, patients who are being administered medications by the parenteral route must have a clean and orderly living situation (21).

III. SPECIAL CONSIDERATIONS IN ASSESSING GERIATRIC PATIENTS

In the majority of cases involving elderly patients, home intravenous antibiotic therapy follows inpatient treatment of infectious diseases. Optimally in these patients, evaluation for home intravenous antibiotic therapy occurs as part of the discharge planning process, preferably by a multidisciplinary team. Patients being treated for infections amenable to home parenteral treatment are identified, and their suitability for such treatment is assessed. The levels of functioning of the patients prior to admission to the hospital must be understood as well as the anticipated needs for assistance after discharge.

All of the general conditions for patient selection outlined above must be met (Table 2). In addition, in geriatric patients a comprehensive functional assessment must be made for each patient to assess mobility and physical functioning, cognition, emotional health, and available social supports (22,23). Patients must be sufficiently mobile to be cared for at home (21). The patient or caregiver must have the requisite eyesight, coordination, and cognition to manage the program (11), and everyone involved must have sufficient emotional stability and confidence to follow the patient's clinical course and to recognize adverse drug reactions and signs of failure of treatment.

With the advent of automated infusion pumps and comprehensive home health care, many marginal patients who would not have qualified for home intravenous antibiotic

Table 2 Patient Selection for HIVAT: Geriatric Considerations

Natural history of the infection in a geriatric patient allows HIVAT to be delilvered safely
Patient upon functional assessment has sufficient:
mobility, coordination, and eyesight
cognition
confidence and motivation
social supports
Home environment is sufficiently safe, clean, and uncluttered

Source: Adapted from Refs. 10, 21, 22.

therapy in the past may successfully complete a course of therapy, but these patients must be assessed on a case-by-case basis. There is no substitute for a home visit by a nurse and even an occupational therapist to assess the home environment and the patient's ability to follow the program. It is not unusual to discover that a competent and well-groomed elderly person is living in a condition of squalor, which is ill-adapted to the delivery of antibiotics by the intravenous route (21).

IV. ESTABLISHING INTRAVENOUS ACCESS

In younger patients it is usually possible to give several weeks of intravenous therapy through a succession of plastic or metal intravenous cannulas of short life (3–5 days). In elderly patients, however, the number and strength of suitable veins are diminished, and best use must be made of available veins. For this reason, an extended-life intravenous catheter or periperherally inserted central catheter (PICC) should be inserted early in the acute hospitalization phase of antibiotic treatment while good venous access still exists.

A variety of extended-life peripheral intravenous catheters of varying lengths have become commercially available. For courses of therapy of 7–14 days, a short elastomeric hydrogel (Aquavene®) catheter may be used (19). For antibiotic courses of 3–4 weeks, a longer (152 mm) catheter (e.g., Midline®, Landmark®) may be employed (16,20). These catheters can be inserted at the bedside by a nurse.

Occasional patients are intolerant of the new catheter materials. These patients can be treated by means of conventional peripheral catheters, but if venous access is limited it is best to consult early with a surgeon regarding placement of a peripherally inserted central catheter (21). Central venous catheters (Port-a-cath®, Hickman®, Broviac®) will occasionally have to be used in patients receiving a month or more of therapy in whom all of the above options have failed.

V. CHOOSING THE METHOD OF ANTIBIOTIC ADMINISTRATION

The initial published series on home intravenous antibiotic therapy relied upon the method of gravity drip infusion of antibiotics in minibags (5,7,8). These infusions are delivered through a peripheral steel intravenous catheter (heparin lock) by the patient or a family member trained in the preparation of the site, infusion technique and cleanup, a process that takes 60–90 min (24). This technique is the least expensive, in terms of equipment,

Table 3 Members of the Home Health Team

Physician
Coordinating hospital nurse
Discharge planner or social worker
Home health nurse
Pharmacist

and is best used for antibiotics which are given at 8-h or longer intervals, such as cefazolin or ceftriaxone.

This method presents severe limitations in treating infections, such as infective endocarditis, which require penicillin therapy delivered at 4-h intervals. In addition, many elderly patients and their spouses lack the manual skill or self-confidence required to infuse antibiotics safely via minibags. In some cases daily visits by a home health nurse may be required to set up and infuse antibiotics, and cost considerations usually constrain antibiotic choice to once-daily regimens. For many of these patients ambulatory antibiotic infusion devices have allowed home intravenous antibiotic therapy to be given successfully.

A wide variety of intravenous antibiotic infusion devices are available. Pumps may be battery operated, delivering drug by peristaltic (e.g., CADD-PLUS®) or syringe systems (e.g., Autosyringe®, Bard 400®) or rely simply upon the elasticity of a balloonlike reservoir (e.g., Intermate®) or a spring-loaded pump (I-flow Sidekick®) (12). The elastomeric reservoir systems require the patient to begin each infusion, but the regulation of flow is independent of gravity and the patient can be ambulatory while the antibiotic is infusing. Automated infusion pumps allow the patient to infuse, via cassette or syringe, an entire day's supply of antibiotic at whatever preprogrammed intervals are desired (14,25). The patient must still be trained to recognize the various device alarms (e.g., low battery, high pressure) and to stop and restart the pump if necessary and must still have 24-h-a-day access by phone to a home health nurse or pharmacist. All of these systems are significantly more expensive than minibag systems but may be cost effective if the number of nurse visits to the home are thereby reduced.

VI. PREPARING AND TRAINING THE PATIENT AND FAMILY

The evaluation and training of patients and their families for home intravenous antibiotic therapy and its subsequent administration is best accomplished by a multidisciplinary team (Table 3). Studies on discharge planning of elderly patients have emphasized the importance of active involvement by patients and their families (22,26). When patients are not allowed sufficient time to understand the options available to them in this area, a pattern of defensive avoidance may be established in which patients procrastinate, allowing others to make decisions, or they rush into the most obvious alternative. Since home intravenous antibiotic therapy requires active participation by patients, it is essential that the option be discussed very early in the hospitalization and that patients be introduced, often by their ward nurse, to the techniques used to administer antibiotics (13).

Formal training is usually completed by a registered nurse on the hospital staff or employed by the home health company who gives the patient and family one-on-one

Table 4 Desirable Characteristics of Antibiotics Used in HIVAT

Long serum half-life
High therapeutic index
Appropriate spectrum of activity
Stability
Low incidence of infusion phlebitis
Low cost

Source: Adapted from Refs. 21, 24.

training, shows them appropriate videotapes, and then observes the patient or family member demonstrate all of the necessary techniques (Table 3) (8,27). The patient's treatment course will usually also be followed by a pharmacist who manages delivery of antibiotics and other supplies to the patient's home and interprets the results of serum drug levels (28). The patient's physician oversees all treatment plans and sees the patient in the office as needed and near the end of the planned course of therapy to assess the patient's progress. The physician is also responsible for ordering necessary laboratory tests such as drug levels and serum creatinine concentrations and for reviewing these tests with the home health pharmacist.

Although initiation of therapy is usually hospital based, in areas where free-standing infusion centers exist, patients with mild infections may receive initial treatment and training entirely on an outpatient basis (29–31). Patients with recurrent infections, usually diabetic foot infections or recurrent cellulitis, can reinstitute home intravenous antibiotic therapy easily without hospital admission in many cases.

VII. SELECTION OF ANTIBIOTICS

Desirable characteristics of antibiotics used in home intravenous antibiotic therapy include long serum half-life, high therapeutic index, appropriate spectrum of activity, stability, low incidence of infusion phlebitis, and low cost (Table 4) (21,24). Very specialized agents, such as ticarcillin-clavulanate and aztreonam, are rarely used in home intravenous therapy of elderly patients because of their cost. Other drugs such as nafcillin and potassium penicillin G are usually avoided because they cause phlebitis, especially when given in high concentrations, as through an automated infusion pump. Oxacillin and sodium penicillin are often substituted.

The cephalosporins are a nontoxic class of antibiotics that have found wide use in home health. Cefazolin is an inexpensive, well-tolerated antibiotic, which may be administered by gravity drip or automated pump, 1–2 g at 8-h intervals (32). Cefuroxime, a second-generation cephalosporin, is useful for the outpatient treatment of pneumonias in doses of 750–1.5 g at 8-h intervals. Finally, ceftriaxone, a third-generation cephalosporin, has been widely promoted and extensively used in home intravenous antibiotic therapy because of its broad spectrum of activity and very long half-life allowing once-a-day dose of 1–2 g (24,30,33). Its staphylococcal and streptococcal activities are not as good as cefazolin, however, and it is more expensive than the older compound. Other third-generation cephalosporins (cefotaxime, ceftizoxime, and ceftazidime) are generally safe in elderly patients and may be used in home intravenous antibiotic therapy when required.

The penicillins are less commonly used in home intravenous antibiotic therapy because of their short half-lives, which require 4- to 6-h dosing. Penicillin G is still the best treatment for most cases of viridans streptococcal endocarditis and the sodium salt can be given through an automated infusion pump without difficulty. Ampicillin and ampicillin-sulbactam require 6-h dosing and are not stable in the high concentrations used in automated pumps, so that unless enterococcal coverage is required, alternatives are often selected from among the cephalosporins. Oxacillin will occasionally be required for serious staphylococcal infections, but in most cases cefazolin or vancomycin are selected instead because of their longer serum half-lives.

Of the aminoglycosides, gentamicin is a very inexpensive and active compound whose low cost is offset somewhat by the necessity of twice-weekly visits by the home health nurse to draw serum trough and peak gentamicin levels and serum creatinine concentrations (see also Chap. 13). Age is a risk factor both for nephrotoxicity and ototoxicity due to aminoglycosides, probably because of the normal age-related decline in renal function (34,35). Gentamicin will occasionally have to be used, for example, in the treatment of serious enterococcal infections in combination with penicillin, ampicillin, or vancomycin, and may be undertaken at home provided that close follow-up is maintained.

Vancomycin is frequently used in home intravenous antibiotic therapy because it may be given at 12- to 24-hourly intervals. Unfortunately, the "red man" or "red neck" syndrome is frequent unless care is taken to infuse the drug slowly (over 1 h or more) (see also Chap. 15). In addition, chemical phlebitis is frequent with vancomycin. In one study, elderly patients had higher serum levels of vancomycin than younger subjects given the same dose (36). Although the toxicity of vancomycin is relatively low unless combined with aminoglycosides, drug levels must be monitored carefully in older patients, as hearing loss and nephrotoxicity may occur with vancomycin therapy even when it is given alone (37,38).

Compared to macrolide antibiotics, clindamycin is most often used for home intravenous antibiotic therapy as erythromycin is unstable in solution for periods over 24 h. Diarrhea due to clindamycin is more common in elderly patients (39). It is useful to remember when treating anaerobic infections that metronidazole 500 mg by mouth at 6-h intervals achieves serum levels comparable to those achieved by intravenous administration of the same dose. The drug must be given in combination with antibiotics active against facultative and aerobic bacteria—if these organisms co-exist with the anaerobes—because metronidazole is only effective against bacteria that are strictly anaerobic.

VIII. TREATMENT OF SELECTED INFECTIONS

A. Cellulitis

Cellulitis, particularly of the lower extremity, occurs with increased frequency in elderly persons as a result of trauma, peripheral vascular disease, diabetes mellitus, venous insufficiency, and edema (40,41). Resolution may be slow in elderly patients, particularly where recurrent attacks have damaged lymphatic drainage. At our institution, cellulitis is the most frequent diagnosis on enrollment for home intravenous antibiotic therapy. The usual pathogens in cellulitis are *Staphylococcus aureus* and streptococcal species (42). Most patients may be managed with 7–10 days of cefazolin (32).

B. Diabetic Infections of the Lower Extremity Including Osteomyelitis

Diabetic infections of the lower extremity must be managed primarily by or in close consultation with a podiatrist or orthopedic surgeon because a successful outcome is dependent upon expeditious debridements of devitalized tissue. When possible, the choice of antibiotic therapy should be guided by the results of cultures of material taken at the time of surgery from the interior of the wound or of cultures of infected bone. Intravenous therapy, usually with a cephalosporin (cefazolin or ceftriaxone), may conveniently be supplemented with oral metronidazole when anaerobes are cultured from deep specimens or are suspected on clinical grounds. The length of therapy is determined by clinical response and may have to be continued through several debridements.

C. Other Types of Osteomyelitis

Osteomyelitis of various types was among the first infections to be treated with home intravenous antibiotic therapy (4–6). In many cases, osteomyelitis due to enteric gram-negative bacilli may be treated with oral ciprofloxacin, but the results are variable for staphylococcal osteomyelitis due to the tendency of this organism to acquire resistance to the quinolones. Many patients who come to home intravenous therapy of osteomyelitis have already failed outpatient ciprofloxacin therapy. The importance of accurate cultures for the therapy of osteomyelitis cannot be overemphasized because prolonged therapy (1 month or more) is frequently required. Where possible, cephalosporins (cefazolin, cefonicid, ceftriaxone) are usually chosen because of low toxicity.

D. Pulmonary Infections

The first published series of patients treated with home intravenous antibiotic therapy were those with pulmonary infections and cystic fibrosis (3). However, geriatric patients with pneumonia are more likely to develop bacteremia and other complications of pneumonia, such as empyema and have a higher mortality when compared to younger patients (43–45). For this reason, elderly patients are usually hospitalized until they are clinically stable and become afebrile for 1–2 days by which time it is possible to discharge the patient on oral antibiotics. If home intravenous antibiotic therapy is desired, then cefuroxime 750–1.5 g at 8- or 12-h intervals (depending on renal function) may be used. Severe pneumonia due to enteric gram-negative bacilli (e.g., *Klebsiella*) requires 10–21 days of intravenous therapy; such patients, if clinically stable, could be treated at home, usually with a third-generation cephalosporin (ceftriaxone, cefotaxime, cefoperazone, or ceftizoxime). Finally, patients recovering from drainage procedures for empyema, whether by tube thoracostomy or surgical decortication, frequently require intravenous antibiotic therapy beyond the period of acute hospitalization. Many of these patients will require convalescence in a skilled nursing facility, but some will have the necessary social supports to be cared for at home. The antibiotics selected will depend upon the bacteria isolated at the time of drainage.

E. Infective Endocarditis

Elderly patients with infective endocarditis have a higher mortality rate than do younger patients (46). They are more apt to have nosocomial disease due to resistant organisms (coagulase-negative staphylococci, enterococci) and to suffer from delays in diagnosis

(46). Selected patients with infective endocarditis due to penicillin-sensitive viridans streptococci (minimum inhibitory or bactericidal concentration of 0.1 μ/ml or less) may be treated in the hospital with abbreviated courses of penicillin and gentamicin (47). However, the majority of patients with infective endocarditis will require 4–6 weeks of treatment. Enterococcal endocarditis requires combination therapy with penicillin or ampicillin and gentamicin and carries a high risk in geriatric patients of renal toxicity due to the length of therapy with the aminoglycoside. Home intravenous therapy will require an automated infusion pump for the sodium penicillin or ampicillin. The gentamicin is usually infused by gravity drainage or via a second pump. Gentamicin levels and serum creatinines must be monitored a least twice weekly and more frequently as treatment progresses and the dose quickly adjusted as needed.

IX. ADVERSE EFFECTS AND OUTCOMES IN GERIATRIC PATIENTS

The key to a successful outcome in home intravenous antibiotic therapy is careful patient selection. Outcomes have been very good in well-motivated patients with infections appropriate to home treatment (11,21,48). Adverse effects of treatment experienced by patients on home intravenous antibiotic therapy are similar to those experienced by patients being treated in the hospital and include phlebitis and allergic reactions to antibiotics, especially to β-lactams (4,21). Other adverse effects reported include diarrhea, leukopenia, and abnormal liver tests (24,49).

As discussed earlier, therapeutic outcomes have been favorable in all series reported of home intravenous antibiotic therapy. In general, published studies have not analyzed therapeutic outcome as a function of age. However, in 1990 Chattopadhyay and coworkers (5O) published a comparative study of therapeutic outcomes of elderly and nonelderly patients receiving home intravenous antibiotic therapy. One hundred and fifty consecutive referred patients were accepted into the study. Half of the patients were 62 years and older (mean age 71 years), and half were under 62 (mean age 38 years). Patients with acquired immunodeficiency syndrome (AIDS) or the end stages of terminal diseases were excluded. Osteomyelitis, cellulitis, and wound infections were the most commonly treated infections. There was no significant difference between the therapeutic outcomes in these two groups of carefully selected patients.

X. COST EFFECTIVENESS

Most reported series of patients on home intravenous antibiotic therapy have included some assessment as to their cost effectiveness compared to similar therapy given in the inpatient setting (48). In the early study by Rucker and Harrison (3) on patients with cystic fibrosis, home intravenous antibiotic therapy was thought to have avoided 127 hospitalizations of patients for pulmonary infections. Antoniskis and coworkers (4) estimated the cost of home intravenous antibiotic therapy at $69/day compared with $243/day for inpatient treatment at that time (1978). Similar estimates were published by Stiver and coworkers (5).

Many similar reports followed (6–8), however, most of these studies failed to explicitly address the important distinction between hospital costs and charges. Studies that consider only the charges listed on the hospital bill do not take into account the fact that hospital charges are based on a rate-setting process, which is determined by many factors, of which the economic cost of the particular goods or service provided is only one (51). In addition, most of the above-listed studies did not take into account the nonmedical and indirect costs entailed in inpatient as opposed to outpatient intravenous antibiotic therapy. These include child care costs, hospital housekeeping, physician visits, and lost wages, only some of which are applicable to elderly patients.

An economic analysis of savings from outpatient antibiotic therapy of osteomyelitis published by Eisenberg and Kitz in 1986 (52) attempted to assess costs (as opposed to hospital charges), both direct, indirect, and nonmedical. They reported that early discharge to home intravenous antibiotic therapy was associated with lower medical direct, nonmedical direct, and indirect expenses than conventional inpatient treatment.

While home intravenous antibiotic therapy is a powerful method of allowing early discharge of patients from the hospital, its potential for abuse and overuse is great. The duration of antibiotic therapy for most infections has not been determined in a controlled or prospective way, and, in fact, great variability exists from one medical center to another in the duration of antimicrobial therapy for common infections (53). Length of parenteral treatment for such infections as cellulitis, pyelonephritis, bacteremia, and pneumonia may vary from 5 to 14 days depending on clinical factors and upon the individual practice style of the physician. Even the necessity of intravenous therapy rather than therapy by the oral or intramuscular route is often a matter of individual judgement.

Where a well-organized team (nurse, pharmacist, home health company) is in place, continuation of intravenous antibiotic therapy after hospital discharge and initiation of such therapy in outpatients can be rapidly arranged, often after consultation by telephone between the primary care physician and the infectious diseases consultant. Duration of antibiotic therapy may be somewhat arbitrary (7–10 days) and may be independent of when the patient is to be seen in follow-up in the physician's office. The very efficiency of the agencies in place have led to rapid increases in utilization within this segment of the home health industry. Clearly, careful utilization review procedures will need to be developed to prevent unnecessary or excessive usage of this costly treatment modality.

XI. REIMBURSEMENT CONSIDERATIONS

An important component of patient selection for home intravenous antibiotic therapy involves reimbursement for such treatment by the patient's insurance carrier. Because this is a relatively new modality of treatment, insurance companies vary in their willingness to pay for such treatment. An important member of the home care team is the discharge coordinator or administrator, who is familiar with the insurers' codes for procedural terminology and who is able to contact in advance the insurance company to obtain approval for reimbursement (31). Many third-party payers still provide only 80% coverage for home intravenous antibiotic therapy, and the 20% copayment may be an excessive financial burden on the patient (49).

Unfortunately for the patient age 65 years or older, Medicare does not reimburse for home intravenous antibiotic therapy. Originally this decision was based upon a 1984 report by the Office of Health Technology Assessment that home intravenous antibiotic therapy may not be safe and effective in the geriatric population (50). For these reasons, patients age 65 years or older have been underrepresented in series on home intravenous antibiotic therapy (48). The repealed Medicare Catastrophic Coverage Act of 1988 would have provided reimbursement for home intravenous antibiotic therapy (21), but despite technological advances that render this form of therapy safer and more convenient in elderly patients, the old ruling stands.

Specifically, to qualify for home health care, the elderly patient must be unable to leave the home without assistance. The cost of self-administered antibiotics or those administered by a visiting nurse are not reimburseable under Medicare (54). However, if a home health nurse is visiting the patient for some other reason, such as wound care, Medicare will reimburse the home health company for these visits, and the home health company may absorb or redistribute the cost of the antibiotics themselves.

Medicare will reimburse antibiotics given in the home or office setting if there is a physician present. Therefore, Medicare will reimburse outpatient antibiotic therapy given in the setting of the hospital clinic, physician's office, or infusion center (29).

Elderly patients who are members of health maintenance organizations generally have excellent coverage for home intravenous antibiotic therapy (55). Of 19 such organizations surveyed in 1987, all provided reimbursement for intravenous antibiotic therapy in the home, although half required prior approval for coverage (54). A few Department of Veterans Affairs hospitals also offer home intravenous antibiotic therapy for selected veterans.

XII. LIABILITY ISSUES AND OTHER PROBLEM AREAS

Reviews of home intravenous antibiotic therapy have emphasized the high degree of patient satisfaction with this modality of therapy and the low frequency of lawsuits brought against physicians for any aspect of home care (21,56). Nevertheless, there are important liability issues to be addressed. Frequently, home intravenous antibiotic therapy is administered by a home health company that delivers antibiotics to the patient's home and provides nurse visits to maintain the intravenous line and to draw necessary laboratory tests. When the ordering physician signs lengthy written treatment plans or is informed of the results of laboratory tests by telephone, he or she assumes liability for the patient's care. In one case a patient developed vestibular toxicity on aminoglycoside therapy. The physician was not called because the aminoglycoside levels had been within the recommended range during monitoring by the home health company, but the physician was still liable for the adverse outcome (57).

In addition, the adoption of diagnosis-related groups has resulted in shorter hospital stays. Many patients are angry at being discharged from the hospital early and are increasingly critical of services that they receive at home (2). The legal profession is becoming aware of adverse outcomes of home intravenous antibiotic therapy, and given the rapid growth of these programs and the "deep pockets" of physicians, the number of lawsuits is expected to increase (2,57).

Finally, there are problems with reimbursement of physicians for their involvement in home intravenous antibiotic therapy, especially when it is administered by an independent home health company (9). The current reimbursement system does not provide payment for time spent communicating with home health agencies, devising home treatment plans, or completing certification forms. An insurer that is willing to pay well for hospital visits to the patient by the physician may pay a nurse two or three times as much as a physician to visit the patient at home (57). Efforts by physicians to become more directly involved with the delivery of home health care by ownership in these enterprises may lead to litigation for conflict of interest. However, intravenous therapy provided through a physician's office as an extension of his or her practice appears exempt (57).

XIII. FUTURE DIRECTIONS

Currently, the selection of patients and the types and duration of treatment given them is based on personal experience, with few published guidelines. Research trials involving elderly patients undergoing home intravenous antibiotic therapy are needed so that these decisions may be made on a more scientific basis.

Also needed are more uniform and progressive reimbursement schedules for patients age 65 years or older who undergo this type of therapy. Reimbursement for physicians involved in home intravenous antibiotic therapy should be improved and structured to provide incentives for more direct involvement in case management by physicians. Finally, systems of utilization review must be developed to prevent inappropriate use and overuse of this valuable but costly treatment modality.

ACKNOWLEDGMENTS

The authors wish to thank Elliot Gordon and Marsha Edenburn for invaluable library support.

REFERENCES

1. Fisher RB. Joseph Lister, 1827–1912. New York: Stein and Day, 1977:104–6.
2. Koren MJ. Home care—who cares? N Engl J Med 1986; 314:917–20.
3. Rucker RW, Harrison GW. Outpatient intravenous medications in the management of cystic fibrosis. Pediatrics 1974; 54:358–60.
4. Antoniskis A, Anderson BC, Van Volkinburg EJ, et al. Feasibility of outpatient self-administration of parenteral antibiotics. West J Med 1978; 128:203–6.
5. Stiver HG, Telford GO, Mussey JM, et al. Intravenous antibiotic therapy at home. Ann Intern Med 1978; 89:690–3.
6. Kind AC, Williams DN, Persons G, et al. Intravenous antibiotic therapy at home. Arch Intern Med 1979; 139:413–15.
7. Poretz DM, Eron LJ, Goldenberg RE, et al. Intravenous antibiotic therapy in an outpatient setting. JAMA 1982; 248:336–9.
8. Stiver HG, Trotsky SK, Cote DD, et al. Self-administration of intravenous antibiotics: an efficient, cost-effective home care program. Can Med Assoc J 1982; 127:207–11.
9. Health and Public Policy Committee American College of Physicians. Home health care. Ann Intern Med 1986; 105:454–60.
10. Brown RB. Prescribing antibiotics in home health care. Geriatrics 1988; 43:43–9.
11. Brown RB. Selection and training of patients for outpatient intravenous antibiotic therapy. Rev Infect Dis 1991; 13(suppl 2):S147–S151.
12. Kwan JW. High-technology intravenous infusion devices. Am J Hosp Pharm 1989; 46:320–35.
13. Bernstein LH, Rehm SJ, Faith SRP. When to consider home intravenous antibiotics. Patient Care 1989; 23:161–84.
14. New PB, Swanson GF, Bulich RG, et al. Ambulatory antibiotic infusion devices: extending the spectrum of outpatient therapies. Am J Med 1991; 91:455–61.
15. Williams DN, Gibson JA, Busch D. Home intravenous antibiotic therapy using a programmable infusion pump. Arch Intern Med 1989; 149:1157–60.
16. Smeed C. Use of a midline catheter in PWAs. Aids Patient Care 1990; 4:34–7.
17. Hickey RF, Cason BA, Charles R. Lower incidence of intravenous catheter complications with an elastomeric hydrogel catheter. Anesth Analges 1989; 68(2S):S121.
18. Cooke JE, Loftus J, Michelson S. Thrombophlebitis following insertion of two types of intravenous catheters. Anesth 1989; 71(3A):A436.

19. Crocker KS, Devereaux GB, Ashmore DL, et al. Clinical evaluation of elastomeric hydrogel peripheral catheters during home infusion therapy. JIN 1990; 13:89–97.
20. Fontaine PJ. Performance of a new softening expanding midline catheter in home intravenous therapy patients. JIN 1991; 14:91–9.
21. Bernstein LH. An update on home intravenous antibiotic therapy. Geriatrics 1991; 46:47–54.
22. Sharp JWI. Social work in a home intravenous antibiotic program. Soc Work Health Care 1986; 12:93–101.
23. Fretwell MD. Comprehensive functional assessment in everyday practice. In: Hazzard WR, Andres R, Bierman EL, et al, eds. Principles of geriatric medicine and gerontology. New York: McGraw-Hill Information Services Company, 1990:218–24.
24. Grizzard MB. Home intravenous antibiotic therapy. Postgrad Med 1985; 78:187–95.
25. Kamen BA, Gunther N. Administration of a 24-hour supply of antibiotics with a programmable automated syringe pump. Am J Hosp Pharm 1985; 42:2715–16.
26. Coulton CJ, Dunkle RE, Goode RA, et al. Discharge planning and decision making. Health Social Work 1982; 7:253–61.
27. Rehm SJ, Weinstein AJ. Home intravenous antibiotic therapy: a team approach. Ann Intern Med 1983; 99:388–92.
28. Ackerman BH, Wolfe JJ. Monitoring chronic outpatient infections: providing comprehensive home healthcare pharmacy services. DICP Ann Pharmacother 1991; 25:840–8.
29. Poretz DM. The infusion center: a model for outpatient antibiotic therapy. Rev Infect Dis 1991; 13(suppl 2):S142–S146.
30. Tice AD. An office model of outpatient parenteral antibiotic therapy. Rev Infect Dis 1991; 13(suppl 2):S184–S188.
31. Green SL. Practical guidelines for developing an office-based program for outpatient intravenous therapy. Rev Infect Dis 1991; 13(suppl 2):S189–S192.
32. Quintiliani R, Nightengale CH. Cefazolin. Ann Intern Med 1978; 89:650–6.
33. Poretz DM, Woolard D, Eron LT, et al. Outpatient use of ceftriaxone: a cost-benefit analysis. Am J Med 1984; 77(suppl 4C):77–83.
34. Bauer LA, Blouin RA. Gentamicin pharmacokinetics: effect of aging in patients with normal renal function. J Am Geriatr Soc 1982; 30:309–11.
35. Moore RD, Smith CR, Lipsky JJ, et al. Risk factors for nephrotoxicity in patients treated with aminoglycosides. Ann Intern Med 1984; 100:352–7.
36. Cutler NR, Narang PK, Lesko LJ, et al. Vancomycin disposition: the importance of age. Clin Pharm Ther 1984; 36:803–10.
37. Downs NJ, Neihart RE, Dolezal JM, et al. Mild nephrotoxicity associated with vancomycin use. Arch Intern Med 1989; 149:1777–81.
38. Yoshikawa TT. Antimicrobial therapy for the elderly patient. J Am Geriatr Soc 1990; 38:1353–72.
39. Neu HC, Prince A, Ortiz Neu C, et al. Incidence of diarrhea and colitis associated with clindamycin therapy. J Infect Dis 1977; 135:S120–S125.
40. Ginsberg MB. Cellulitis: an analysis of 101 cases and review of the literature. S Med J 1981; 74:530–3.
41. Yoshikawa TT, Norman DC. Skin and soft tissue infection. In: Aging and clinical practice: infectious diseases. Diagnosis and treatment New York: Igaku-shoin, 1987:185–92.
42. Hook EWIII, Hooten TM, Horton CA, et al. Microbiologic evaluation of cutaneous cellulitis in adults. Arch Intern Med 1986; 146:295–7.
43. Verghese A, Berk SL. Bacterial pneumonia in the elderly. Medicine 1983; 62:271–85.
44. Marrie TJ, Haldane EV, Faulkner RS, et al. Community-acquired pneumonia requiring hospitalization. Is it different in the elderly? J Am Geriatr Soc 1985; 33:671–80.
45. Sims RV. Bacterial pneumonia in the elderly. Emerg Clin North Am 1990; 8:207–20.
46. Terpenning MS, Buggy BP, Kauffman CA. Infective endocarditis. Clinical features in young and elderly patients. Am J Med 1987; 83:626–34.

47. Wilson WR, Geraci JE. Treatment of streptococcal infective endocarditis. Am J Med 1985; 78(suppl 6B):128–37.
48. Balinsky W, Nesbitt S. Cost-effectiveness of outpatient parenteral antibiotics: a review of the literature. Am J Med 1989; 87:301–5.
49. Poretz DM. Home management of intravenous antibiotic therapy. Bull NY Acad Med 1988; 64:570–6.
50. Chattopadyay T, Catania PN, Mergener MA. Therapeutic outcome of elderly and nonelderly patients receiving home intravenous antimicrobial therapy. Am J Pharm 1990; 47:335–9.
51. Finkler SA. The distinction between cost and charges. Ann Intern Med 1982; 96:102–9.
52. Eisenberg JM, Kitz DS. Savings from outpatient antibiotic therapy for osteomyelitis. JAMA 1986; 255:1584–8.
53. Turck M, Smith J. Prospective pricing system and its effect on the principles and practice of infectious disease. Am J Med 1985; 78(suppl 6B):23–8.
54. Balinsky W. Reimbursement for outpatient parenteral antibiotic therapy: update. Rev Infect Dis 1991; 13(suppl 2): S193–S195.
55. Grizzard MB, Harris G, Karns H. Use of outpatient parenteral antibiotic therapy in a health maintenance organization. Rev Infect Dis 1991; 13(suppl 2):S174–S179.
56. Health and Public Policy Committee American College of Physicians. Long-term care of the elderly. Ann Intern Med 1984; 100:760–3.
57. Tice AD. Growing pains in outpatient intravenous antibiotic therapy. Infect Dis Clin Pract 1992; 1:74–6.

30

Antimicrobial Prophylaxis

Chester Choi
UCLA School of Medicine, Los Angeles, and St. Mary Medical Center, Long Beach, California

The prevention of infectious complications in surgical and nonsurgical situations has direct importance for the geriatric population. A large and increasing number of complex surgical procedures are carried out in this population, and the prevention of infective endocarditis, late prosthetic joint infections, and other "medical" problems is important to the well-being of many older adults. This chapter will attempt to summarize the available data and recommendations regarding prophylaxis in elderly patients and will delineate those situations where additional studies appear to be necessary to aid in clinical decision making.

I. PREOPERATIVE SURGICAL PROPHYLAXIS

A. General Comments

One of the most important impacts of antimicrobial technology on our society may be its influence on the evolution of modern surgery (1). In helping to control the rates and severity of postoperative infection, antibiotics have made possible both routine and technically advanced procedures to the benefit of many patients. Yet, Wenzel has stated that postoperative wound infections complicate the recovery of at least 920,000 of the 23 million patients who undergo surgery each year in the United States (2). The rates vary from 3 per 100 clean procedures to 9 or more per 100 for grossly contaminated procedures, and for inpatients, postoperative stay is often doubled and costs may be more than \$1.5 billion annually. Disability may last more than 6 months in some 18% of those with postoperative wound infections. Thus, despite advances in understanding and implementation, postoperative infections remain a significant problem (2).

Historically, antibiotic use in the perioperative period was relatively poorly understood or studied (3,4) until the salient investigations of Burke demonstrated the crucial relationship between the timing of administration of antibiotics and the prophylactic efficacy (5).

Table 1 Most Likely Pathogens in Postoperative Wound Infections

Category of surgery	Most likely pathogen(s)
Clean	
Cardiac/Vascular	*Staphylococcus epidermidis* *Staphylococcus aureus* Gram-negative bacilli (GNB)
Breast	*S. aureus*
Orthopedic	*S. aureus, S. epidermidis,* GNB
Dialysis access	*S. epidermidis, S. aureus*
Neurological	*S. epidermidis, S. aureus,* GNB
Clean contaminated	
Burns	*S. aureus, Pseudomonas aeruginosa*
Head and neck	Streptococci, *S. aureus,* anaerobes
Gastrointestinal tract	GNB, anaerobes
Urogenital tract	GNB, group D streptococci
Dirty	
Ruptured viscera	GNB, anaerobes
Traumatic wound	*S. aureus,* group A streptococci, Clostridia

Source: Ref. 15.

These studies showed that proper timing of administration of systemic penicillin, i.e., shortly before or at the time of intradermal inoculation of a sensitive *Staphylococcus aureus,* resulted in a marked reduction in the size of the erythema resulting from this experimental infection in guinea pigs. Delaying the antibiotic administration resulted in lesions that were similar in size and histology to those in animals who had not received antibiotics. Thus, the study convincingly showed that a key to the effectiveness of prophylaxis was the presence of antibiotic in sufficient amounts in tissues at the time of bacterial contamination (5).

These and other studies established important prophylactic principles (6–8). These principles include the use of effective antibiotics, achieving inhibitory levels in the tissues at the time of contamination from the procedure, the lack of benefit of antibiotics given too early, and the lack of utility of continuation of antibiotics beyond the risk period. Thus, it was noted that the earlier practice of administration of antibiotics to patients "on call" to the operating room often led to insufficient levels of antibiotic in the tissues at the time of the actual surgical procedure (4). In a large study examining the effect of timing of administration of prophylactic antibiotics in clean or clean-contaminated surgical procedures at a community hospital, Classen and his colleagues showed that administration of antibiotics in the 2 h before surgery significantly reduces the risk of wound infection (9). The most current *Medical Letter* advises that drug administration take place approximately 30 min before the actual procedure.

Most earlier studies have divided the types of surgical procedures into clean, clean-contaminated, contaminated, or dirty (10,11). Earlier opinions doubted the efficacy of antibiotic prophylaxis in clean surgeries (12); however, recent investigations have shown that these procedures often result in bacterial contamination of the surgical wound and have variable rates of subsequent postoperative infection. More recent studies have now shown that antibiotic prophylaxis in even these "clean" surgeries is of benefit and may

Table 2 Criteria for Designing or Assessing Studies of Antimicrobial Prophylaxis of Surgical Wound Infection

The study is prospective, randomized, and double blind
Written definitions of surgical wound infection are established
Comparability of host risk factors is present in all arms of the study
The various operative procedures are well defined and equally distributed in all arms of the study
The choice of antimicrobial agent is appropriate for the expected pathogens and their antimicrobial susceptibilities
The doses of antimicrobial agents, as well as the initiation, route, frequency and duration of their administration are chosen to provide adequate tissue levels throughout the operative procedure
Concomitant use of nonstudy perioperative antibiotics and antiseptics is controlled or eliminated
The antimicrobials used carry a minimum risk of toxic or allergic reactions
The costs of the various approaches, including the cost of any infections, are compared
Sufficient numbers of patients are included to demonstrate whether significant differences do or do not exist between antibiotic regimens

Source: Ref. 4.

be cost effective (13). The largest of these studies was performed for breast surgery and herniorrhaphy. The authors concluded that a single dose of cefonicid prior to the procedures decreased the rate of postoperative infection overall and also appeared to be cost effective (14). Whether the same conclusions would be valid for each procedure analyzed separately is not entirely clear, since the study was not designed with sufficient power to discern the effects in the separate procedures, but it seems likely that the conclusions would hold for mastectomy (14). Similar conclusions with smaller studies have been reached in the clean surgeries of vascular and neurosurgical variety.

Waldvogel and colleagues (15) reviewed the microbial factors affecting prophylactic efficacy. They review the importance of adherence mechanisms, staphylococcal carriage, the production of glycocalyx, which may influence bacterial adherence and resistance, and the need for additional studies in patients and animal models. The most likely pathogens in postoperative wound infections are shown in Table 1.

Several comprehensive reviews of antibiotic prophylaxis, including specific recommendations for a number of procedures, have recently been published (4,16–22). These studies also set forth key criteria for the evaluation of prophylaxis trials (Table 2) and methodology for assessing cost effectiveness (23). The following equations may be used to determine 1) whether or not to give prophylaxis:

$$\frac{C}{B} = \frac{(NP)\ (C)}{(NP)\ (RO)\ (B)}$$

and 2) Which drug or regimen to give:

$$\frac{C}{B} = \frac{(NP)\ (\Delta C)}{(NP)\ (B)\ (\Delta O)}$$

where:

NP = number of procedures
C = costs associated with prophylaxis administration
RO = reduction in occurrence of postoperative infection
B = benefits associated with occurrence of postoperative infection
ΔC = differences in costs for new drug/regimen compared with current standard
ΔO = difference in occurrence of postoperative infection when new drug/regimen is given, compared with current standard antimicrobial agent or regimen

A summary of antibiotic recommendations for procedures commonly encountered in the treatment of a geriatric population is presented in Table 3, with the following additional comments.

B. Abdominal Operations

Most cases of elective operation for colorectal processes should be adequately prophylaxed with an oral regimen, which usually includes erythromycin and neomycin or metronidazole and neomycin (16,18). Bowel cleansing with agents such as "GoLYTELY" is often prescribed as well, but does not appear to be effective without the additional use of the oral antibiotic regimen. Whether the use of parenteral cephalosporins with the oral regimen provides additional effect is unclear, although Lau and colleagues (24) obtained a better outcome with parenteral agents than with these oral drugs alone, and Weaver and his associates (25) noted a difference of 41% postoperative infections with the oral agents compared to 10% with intravenous metronidazole plus ceftriaxone.

In more emergent cases where the oral regimen cannot be instituted in a timely manner, parenteral antibiotics should be utilized. Most experts would recommend a second-generation cephalosporin (cefoxitin or cefotetan) in such an event, in order to provide antimicrobial activity against intestinal anaerobes including *Bacteroides fragilis.* Gorbach has also recommended the addition of cefoxitin or cefotetan in situations where the onset of surgery is delayed (probably more than 10–12 h), where the procedure is prolonged for more than 3.5 h or when rectal resection is required (18).

Gastroduodenal procedures are often complicated by intestinal dismotility, bowel obstruction, or alteration of gastric pH (12). These factors may provide a setting for bacterial replication and give added importance to antibiotic prophylaxis. The *Medical Letter* additionally recommends cefazolin prophylaxis for gastric bypass or percutaneous endoscopic gastrostomy procedures (16).

Elective cholecystectomy generally is associated with sufficiently low infection rates that perioperative antibiotics are not needed; however, in elderly patients (>70 years of age), patients with previous biliary surgery, or patients with a history of acute symptoms or jaundice, antibiotic prophylaxis has been shown to be beneficial (4,12,26,27).

C. Orthopedic Procedures

Total joint replacement is a procedure being carried out with increasing frequency in the geriatric population (28–30). The rates of postoperative infection have been decreased with operating room techniques including ultraclean air systems. Perioperative antibiotics also seem to decrease the infection rates; however, whether the combination of ultraclean air systems and perioperative antibiotics is additive or synergistic has not been established. Persson and colleagues (31) concluded that from a cost-benefit perspective, departments

Table 3 Antimicrobial Prophylaxis in Surgery

Surgical procedure	Antibiotic regmens
Intraabdominal	
Colorectal	oral ERY,[a] NEO[a] (elect): iv CFX 1 g q6h ×4 or CTN 1 g q12h ×2 (emerg)
Appendectomy	oral ERY,[a] NEO[a] (elect); iv CFX 1 g q6h ×4 or CTN 1 g q12h ×2(emerg)
Cholecystectomy	iv CFZ 1 g q8h ×3 (>70y, acute cholecystitis, obstructive jaundice, common duct stones)
Gastroduodenal	iv CFZ 1 g q8h ×3
Genitourinary	
Hysterectomy	iv CFZ 1 g q8h ×3 (vaginal, abdominal or radical abdominal)
TURP	iv CFZ 1 g q8h ×3 no prophylaxis may be necessary if urine sterile preoperatively
Orthopedic	
Total joint replacement	iv CFZ 1 g q8h × 4 +/-ultraclean air
Other	iv CFZ 1 g q8h × 4 or CFM (closed hip fracture, use of fixation devices, procedures of >2h)
Cardiac	
Coronary bypass	iv CFZ 1 g q8h ×6
Valvular surgery	iv CFZ 1 g q8h ×6
Thoracic	
Elective, noncardiac	iv CFZ 1 g q8h ×3
Chest tube placement	no prophylaxis
ENT	
Clean contaminated	iv CLINDA 600 mg q6h ×4 or AMOX/CLAV
Oncological surgery	same
Neurosurgery	
Clean or clean contaminated	VANCO 1 g iv + GENT 80 mg (repeat doses if procedure longer than 6h) or CFZ 1 g+ GENT 80 mg (repeat at 6 h)
Peripheral vascular	
Lower extremity deep surgery with graft implant	iv CFZ 1 g q8h ×3
Other clean surgery	
Mastectomy and herniorrhaphy	iv CEFONICID 1 g

CFZ = cefazolin; CLINDA = clindamycin; AMOX/CLAV = amoxicillin + clavulanic acid; VANCO = vancomycin; CFM = cefamandole; CFX = cefoxitin; CTN = cefotetan; ERY = erythromycin; NEO = neomycin; GENT = gentamicin; TURP = transurethral resection of prostate; elect = elective; emerg = emergency.

[a]1 g each at 1, 2, and 11 p.m. on day before surgery, after appropriate diet and catharsis.

Source: Refs. 4, 16, 17, 18–22.

performing more than 100 total joint replacements per year should use the ultraclean air system in combination with parenteral antibiotics, while those performing fewer such operations should utilize parenteral and perhaps local (antibiotic-impregnated cement) antibiotics (32) without the costly air systems.

Norden (20) has also summarized the use of antibiotics in other orthopedic procedures. For operative management of closed hip fractures, either nafcillin or a first-generation cephalosporin appeared effective when administered for 48 or 72 h. For those procedures involving internal fixation devices, superficial wound infections were decreased by the use of a cephalosporin. Additionally, Henley and colleagues (33) showed that perioperative antibiotics reduced the incidence of infections in those patients undergoing general orthopedic procedures for operations lasting more than 2 h.

D. Genitourinary Procedures

Hemsell (19) has recently summarized the use of prophylactic antibiotics in gynecologic-obstetric surgery. For vaginal, abdominal, and radical abdominal hysterectomies, Hemsell recommends the use of 1 or 2 g of intravenous cefazolin; doxycycline is recommended for those patients allergic to cephalosporins or those with a type I allergic reaction to penicillin.

The issue of perioperative antibiotics for transurethral prostate resection (TURP) is not entirely clear. Several studies demonstrating efficacy of antibiotic regimens included patients with preoperatively infected urine; thus, for some, the antibiotics were doubtless therapeutic and not preventative or prophylactic (17,34–39). For the majority of individuals undergoing this procedure, no perioperative antibiotics seem necessary; however, a recent study by Slavis and associates (40) purports to show that a single intramuscular dose of cefonicid lowers the postoperative infection rate from 37% in the placebo treated group to 12% in the antibiotic group. Urine cultures were performed to exclude those with preoperative bacteriuria; however, the clinical endpoint chosen for this study was $>10^4$ cfu/cc urine. Thus, pyuria and clinical symptoms were not described, nor were the organisms cultured postoperatively identified. It is possible that a subset of those undergoing TURP might benefit from antibiotics, but additional data would seem to be needed. Conte (17) summarized a large number of studies of prophylaxis in urological surgery and recommended short-term intravenous cefazolin usage (1g q8h $\times$ 3) in those with sterile preoperative urine. The data presented, however, were largely for drugs other than cefazolin and were of various types (some were not placebo-controlled trials or double-blinded and some were studies of single-dose therapy). The *Medical Letter* (16) states that patients with positive preoperative urine cultures should be treated with appropriate antibiotics, but that those with sterile preoperative urine do not require prophylaxis. Similarly, Kaiser recommends against the use of prophylactic antibiotics in patients with abacteriuria undergoing prostatectomy.(4)

E. Peripheral Vascular Surgery

Some increasingly common forms of surgical procedures for older persons are those to improve peripheral vascular blood flow. Hopkins (13) and Conte (17) have both summarized the available literature in this field and have concluded that perioperative antibiotics, particularly directed against staphylococci and especially used when implantation of grafts is involved, are useful. In a double-blind, prospective, randomized comparison of cefazolin versus placebo, the wound infection rate was 0.9% versus 6.8%, respectively (41).

F. Head and Neck Surgery

Velanovich (42) has published a meta analysis of prophylactic antibiotics for head and neck surgery and concluded that a one-day course of clindamycin may be the best regimen. Shapiro (22) reviewed the literature, concluding that (1) in clean otological and oncological operations of the head and neck, prophylaxis is not indicated; (2) in clean contaminated oncological operations, either clindamycin or amoxicillin/clavulanic acid is appropriate; (3) in clean and clean-contaminated neurosurgery, prophylaxis is indicated, probably with vancomycin plus gentamicin or cloxacillin alone (other possibilities include gentamicin and cefazolin and vancomycin alone); and (4) the evidence suggests the need for prophylaxis in shunt operations, but further studies are needed to determine the proper drug and assess an appropriate endpoint and stopping rule (43).

G. Controversies

Some of the current controversies regarding surgical prophylaxis include the following issues.

1. Choice of Parenteral Agent

In order to demonstrate a difference between two agents, particularly in a situation of relatively low risk, a very large number of patients would need to be entered into the study. Additionally, to demonstrate that there is no difference between two regimens may require an even larger study. Thus, most available studies are unable to show a difference due to lack of statistical power.

2. Use of Antibiotics in Other Clean Surgeries

Again, large studies would be necessary to demonstrate efficacy, since the probable rates of postoperative infection would be low. The data would be meaningful, however, since large numbers of these procedures are often performed and small differences between prophylaxis and no prophylaxis may add up to a significant difference overall (2,9,13).

3. Topical Antibiotics

The probable cost savings and presumably lower incidence of side effects with topical agents would be advantageous in many procedures. Their effectiveness in preventing bacterial contamination of deeper tissues of surgical wounds remains to be proven (4). Some studies have shown significant serum levels with topically applied antibiotics, suggesting that some of the putative advantages may be unclear and that some of these topical agents may have efficacy in part due to their systemic and tissue absorption (44).

4. Duration of Therapy

Most recent studies have utilized single-dose prophylaxis, but some have utilized agents of longer duration in an attempt to ensure adequate serum and tissue levels in the perioperative period. In surgical procedures of longer duration, the antibiotic levels may not be sufficient to provide effective prophylaxis during the entire period of risk. Repeat dosing has been employed for some agents of shorter duration, and clearly, knowledge of the pharmacokinetics of these drugs is essential (2,45).

5. Risk Stratification

More recently, investigators in this field have attempted to better classify the risk of postoperative infection and have formulated stratification criteria that include such factors

Table 4 Prevention of Infective Endocarditis: Selected Cardiac Conditions

Prophylaxis Recommended
Prosthetic cardiac valves (bioprosthetic and homograft)
Previous bacterial endocarditis
Most congenital cardiac malformations
Rheumatic and other acquired valvular dysfunction (even after valvular surgery)
Hypertrophic cardiomyopathy
Mitral valve prolapse with valvular regurgitation (thickening or redundancy of valve leaflets, esp. men > 45)
Prophylaxis Not Recommended
Isolated secundum atrial septal defect
Surgical repair without residua beyond 6 months of isolated secundum atrial septal defect, ventricular septal defect, patent ductus arteriosus
Previous coronary artery bypass graft surgery
Mitral valve prolapse without valvular regurgitation
Physiological, functional, or innocent heart murmurs
Previous Kawasaki disease without valvular dysfunction
Previous rheumatic fever without valvular dysfunction
Cardiac pacemakers and implanted defibrillators

Source: Ref. 53.

as age, underlying illness, etc. (46). This may result in improved selection of groups or subgroups in whom prophylactic antibiotics may be beneficial.

II. PROPHYLAXIS TO PREVENT LATE COMPLICATIONS

A. Infective Endocarditis

Infective endocarditis in elderly patients is increasing in incidence (47,48). Kaye cited data from three series of endocarditis patients observed from 1967 to 1977 in which the mean ages were 44, 55, and 57 (49). In the study by Terpenning and colleagues (50), 7.4% of cases in patients over age 60 were due to mitral valve prolapse. In this age group overall, most patients were not known to have a predisposing cardiac lesion and often had a more occult presentation. Additionally, the inciting causes were nosocomial in nature in many instances (23%) and the organsims were often *Streptococcus bovis,* enterococci, and coagulase-negative staphylococci.

A comparison of a community cohort of endocarditis patients with a group at a tertiary referral center revealed that the community group was much more frequently elderly (≥65 years) and had worse outcomes with increased age (51). Friedlander and Yoshikawa reported a 50% mortality from infective endocarditis or its complications in the elderly population (52).

The American Heart Association updated its recommendations for antibiotic prophylaxis for infective endocarditis in December 1990 (Tables 4–9) (53). The major features of the update include a simplification of the antibiotic protocols, emphasizing the use of oral amoxicillin, and a reassessment of the relative risks of various invasive procedures. In regard to the latter, physicians are given the option of administering prophylactic antibiotics to patients with high-risk cardiac lesions (prior infective endocarditis, prosthetic

Table 5 Prevention of Infective Endocarditis: Procedures

Prophylaxis Recommended
Dental procedures known to induce gingival or mucosal bleeding, including professional cleaning
Tonsillectomy and/or adenoidectomy
Surgical operations involving intestinal or respiratory mucosa
Bronchoscopy with rigid bronchoscope
Sclerotherapy for esophageal varices
Esophageal dilatation
Gallbladder surgery
Cystoscopy
Urethral dilatation
Urethral catheterization if urinary tract infection present
Urinary tract surgery if urinary tract infection is present
Prostatic surgery
Incision and drainage of infected tissue
Vaginal hysterectomy
Vaginal delivery in presence of infection
Prophylaxis Not Recommended
Dental procedures unlikely to induce gingival bleeding
Injection of local intraoral anesthetic (except intraligamentary injections)
Shedding of primary teeth
Tympanostomy tube insertion
Endotracheal intubation
Bronchoscopy (flexible bronchoscope, with or without biopsy)
Cardiac catheterization
Endoscopy with or without gastrointestinal biopsy
Cesarean delivery
In the absence of infection: urethral catheterization, dilatation and curettage, uncomplicated vaginal delivery, therapeutic abortion, sterilization procedure, insertion or removal of intrauterine devices

Source: Ref. 53.

Table 6 Infective Endocarditis Prophylaxis: Standard Regimen for Oral or Upper Respiratory Tract Procedures in Patients at Risk

Amoxicillin 3 g orally 1 h before procedure, then 1.5 g 6 h after initial dose
For amoxicillin/penicillin-allergic patients:
Erythromycin ethylsuccinate 800 mg or erythromycin stearate 1 g orally 2 h before a procedure; then one half the dose 6 h after initial administration
or
Clindamycin 300 mg orally 1 h before a procedure and 150 mg 6 h after initial dose

Source: Ref. 53.

Table 7 Infective Endocarditis Prophylaxis: Alternative Regimens for Genital, Oral, or Upper Respiratory Tract Procedures in Patients at Risk

For patients unable to take oral medication
  Ampicillin 2 g iv (or im) 30 min before procedure; then ampicillin 1 g iv (or im) or amoxicillin 1.5 g orally 6 h after initial dose
 For ampicillin/amoxicillin/penicillin-allergic patients unable to take oral medications:
  Clindamycin 300 mg iv 30 min before a procedure and 150 mg iv (or orally) 6 h after initial dose
For patients considered to be at very high risk
  Ampicillin 2 g iv (or im) plus gentamicin 1.5 mg/kg iv (or im) (not to exceed 80 mg) 30 min before procedure, followed by amoxicillin 1.5 g orally 6 h after the initial dose; alternatively, parenteral regimen may be repeated 8 h after initial dose
 Amoxicillin/ampicillin/penicillin-allergic patients considered to be at very high risk:
  Vancomycin 1 g iv administered over 1 h, starting 1 h before the procedure. No repeat dose is necessary.

Source: Ref. 53.

Table 8 Infective Endocarditis Prophylaxis: Regimens for Genitourinary and Gastrointestinal Procedures

Standard regimen
  Ampicillin 2 g iv (or im) plus gentamicin 1.5 mg/kg iv (or im) (not to exceed 80 mg) 30 min before procedure, followed by amoxicillin 1.5 g orally 6 h after the initial dose; alternatively, parenteral regimen may be repeated once 8 h after initial dose
 For amoxicillin/ampicillin/penicillin-allergic patients:
  Vancomycin 1 g iv administered over 1 h plus gentamicin 1.5 mg/kg iv (or im) (not to exceed 80 mg) 1 h before procedure. May be repeated once 8 h after initial dose
Alternate oral regimen for low-risk patients
 Amoxicillin 3 g orally 1 h before procedure, then 1.5 g 6 h after initial dose

Source: Ref. 53.

Table 9 Infective Endocarditis Prophylaxis: Prophylactic Regimens for Cardiac Surgery with Placement of Foreign Material

Cefazolin 2 g iv immediately preoperatively and every 6 h for 24–48 h plus gentamicin 1.7 mg/kg iv immediately preoperatively and every 8 h for 24 h
In institutions with a high incidence of methicillin-resistant staphylococci:
 Vancomycin 15 mg/kg iv over 1 h immediately preoperatively, followed by 10 mg/kg iv immediately after cardiopulmonary bypass surgery plus gentamicin as above

heart valves, or surgically constructed systemic-pulmonary shunts or conduits) even with low-risk invasive procedures.

Kaye and Abrutyn (54) reviewed the AHA recommendations and raised several important points. The risk of infective endocarditis associated with individual cardiac lesions and specific procedures is unknown and may never be known with precision. Only a fraction of all infective endocarditis cases could be prevented even if the prophylaxis was entirely effective. Only about half the patients found to have infective endocarditis have a recognized or recognizable predisposing cardiac condition that would qualify them for prophylaxis, and fewer than 25% of patients with infective endocarditis caused by streptococci of oral origin and about 40% of those with enterococcal endocarditis develop valve infection in association with a procedure for which prophylaxis could be given. Enterococci and streptococci together account for only about 65% of all infective endocarditis cases; thus, fewer than 10% of cases overall are preventable even with the best compliance with these recommendations.

Several other controversial issues remain. The use of such prophylaxis for patients with mitral valve prolapse (the cardiac lesion most often associated with infective endocarditis) remains to be clarified (55–59). Many cardiologists choose to utilize such prophylaxis only in those patients with mitral valve prolapse associated with a holosystolic or late systolic murmur that is detectable with or without physical examination adjuncts such as the Valsalva maneuver (55,56,60). Others rely on echocardiographic findings of "classic" mitral valve prolapse such as valvular leaflet thickening and redundancy before initiating prophylaxis (61). It would be useful to stratify the risk with this valvular abnormality, since the administration of antibiotic prophylaxis to all with echocardiographic or clinical mitral valve prolapse may not be cost effective or beneficial. The AHA recommendations cite mitral valve prolapse with valvular "regurgitation" for infective endocarditis prophylaxis and state that "individuals who have a mitral valve prolapse associated with thickening and/or redundancy of the valve leaflets may be at increased risk for bacterial endocarditis, particularly men who are 45 years of age or older." In a study of mitral valve prolapse and recommendations for infective endocarditis prophylaxis by practicing physicians (62), neither physical examination findings nor echocardiographic findings were associated with antibiotic recommendation. Prophylaxis was recommended more frequently in persons under 40 years of age than in those more than 60 years old. For every 10-year upward increment in age, there was a 30% independent reduction in recommendations for infective endocarditis prophylaxis. Thus, practitioners in this study seem to discount the risk of infective endocarditis in older adults with mitral valve prolapse and do not seem to utilize any stratification other than age.

Adherence to the AHA recommendations by physicians and dentists has been suboptimal in past surveys. The questionnaire by Nelson and Van Blaricum (63) during the time when the prophylaxis was slightly more complex than currently resulted in appropriate prophylactic prescription rates of 58.9% for dentists and 36.1% for physicians when presented with patients with valvular heart disease and no drug allergies. Compliance rates diminished to approximately 25% when prosthetic heart valves were considered.

An assessment of failures of infective endocarditis prophylaxis revealed that only 6 of 52 patients received regimens recommended by the AHA at the time, but that the etiological organisms were often (63%) sensitive to the antibiotics used (usually oral penicillin) (64). Thus, failures can occur even when the organism is sensitive to the antibiotics used. In addition, the regimens used in these patients did not conform to the current recommendations at that time. At least two studies attempting to quantify the efficacy of antibiotic prophylaxis in preventing postdental infective endocarditis have been published (65,66). Both are case-control studies with reliance on patient interviewing and record review to determine details and outcome. Both studies are hampered by the low rates of infective endocarditis and the relatively low usage of antibiotic prophylaxis. Imperiale and Horwitz (65) concluded that antibiotic prophylaxis is 91% protective, while van der Meer et al. (66) arrived at a maximal protective effect of 49%. However, in the latter case-control study, the authors admitted that to detect a statistically significant protective effect of antibiotic prophylaxis of 49% would require well over 100 cases of medical or dental procedure–related infective endocarditis and several hundred controls who underwent similar procedures without developing infective endocarditis. Their data included only 18 such cases of infective endocarditis after surveying all microbiology departments in The Netherlands for 2 years.

The simplified antibiotic regimens should, however, improve both the administration and compliance by practitioners and patients (54). Patients with prosthetic valves and other high-risk cardiac conditions can now be given the oral regimen of amoxicillin or its oral alternatives, eliminating the logistical problems of the prior parenteral regimens. This recommendation seems to have been effective in Great Britain with better compliance and few failures. Physicians and dentists are provided the option of the parenteral regimens per their preference (53).

The elimination of some low-risk procedures from the list of those requiring prophylaxis has been controversial in some subspecialties. A survey of fellows in training for colorectal surgery and colorectal surgery program directors (67) revealed that the majority would give prophylactic antibiotics to patients undergoing colonoscopy (even without biopsy) if the patients had valvular hear disease, mitral valve prolapse with murmur, prosthetic heart valves or a previous history of endocarditis. A somewhat similar response resulted from a survey of directors of infectious disease training programs about the use of prophylactic antibiotics in colonoscopy (68). In responding to the controversy, the American Society of Gastroenterology and the American Society of Colon and Rectal Surgeons recommended that prophylactic antibiotics be used only in patients with a prosthetic heart valve, a surgically constructed systemic-pulmonary shunt, or a history of infective endocarditis if they are to have gastrointestinal endoscopy (69,70). In dissent, Meyer as well as Steinberg pointed out that complications, particularly allergic reactions, from the antibiotics may outweigh the theoretical advantages of prophylaxis (71,72). Some endoscopists have raised concern that other procedures, including esophageal dilatation, injection sclerotherapy for esophageal varices, and endoscopy for debulking malignancy, might have a higher risk of causing bacteremia and subsequent infective endocarditis. However, the data seem insufficient to make specific recommendations for these procedures (73,74).

B. Prophylaxis for Late Prosthetic Joint Infection (LPJI)

It is estimated that prosthetic joint infections occur in about 1–4% of the more than 200,000 such procedures performed each year. One estimate is that more than half of these infections occur more than 12 weeks after the surgery (75–78). The possibility of preventing some fraction of these late infections with the use of prophylactic antibiotics has generated considerable controversy. Most studies of this problem have focused on the postdental procedure aspect, extrapolating from the problem in preventing infective endocarditis. In reviews of these infections, however, the major pathogens appear to be *Staphylococcus aureus* or *Staphylococcus epidermidis* (78). Therefore, prevention of such infections may require prophylaxis for a variety of conditions that are likely to lead to sufficient bacteremia and would "seed" the prosthetic device; the antibiotic administered would need to be directed at the likely pathogen(s). In addition, most such late infections may be caused by hematogenous seeding of the prosthesis, but persistence of organisms from the original surgical procedure could also account for late infections (79).

The majority of analyses of this problem have reached the conclusion that routine prophylaxis for those patients with prosthetic joints is not advisable (67,79–82). Statements from the American Dental Association, the Working Party for the British Society for Antimicrobial Chemotherapy, and the American Society of Colon and Rectal Surgeons have recommended against the administration of prophylactic antibiotics for dental and endoscopic procedures except when obvious infection is present.

A dissenting opinion is expressed by Blackburn and Alarcon (83). In their cost-benefit analysis, if one makes small changes in the presumed rate of protective effect of antibiotic prophylaxis for LPJIs, the number of LPJIs related to dental procedures, and the yearly risk of late infection, one could reach a conclusion favoring the use of antibiotic prophylaxis for prevention of LPJIs. These authors recommend the use of prophylaxis for patients likely to have a poor outcome and those who may be at higher risk for LPJI, i.e., patients with rheumatoid arthritis or other chronic debilitiating disease or those taking immunomodulatory drugs. The antibiotic used would depend upon the type of procedure and the patient's history of drug allergies. For those with less risk, individualization based upon analysis of cost-benefit ratios in the local community is recommended (83).

Tsevat and associates (84) developed a decision tree model to assess whether patients with artificial joints should take penicillin, erythromycin, or no antibiotics before dental procedures. Erythromycin prophylaxis was felt to be the most effective, albeit the most expensive, strategy, and sensitivity analysis demonstrated that the risk of developing a joint infection is the key parameter in the analysis.

A more complex decision-utility analysis model for this problem was developed by Jacobson and colleagues (85). The model included such factors as quality-of-life adjustments, costs, adverse outcomes, anaphylaxis, and different antibiotic regimens. No definite conclusion could be reached based upon the available data, but the most cost-effective strategy was no prophylaxis. This hypothesis, however, yielded greater calculated numbers of deaths and amputations (1.93 and 2.93 per million dental visits) as opposed to a 1-day oral cephalexin strategy (0.75 deaths and 0.46 amputations per million dental visits). Sensitivity analysis indicated that the key, additional research to determine better estimates of the risk of late prosthetic joint infections should focus on quantifying the risk of LPJIs after dental therapy.

From the available studies, it appears difficult to recommend routine antibiotic prophylaxis for dental or most invasive procedures in patients with prosthetic joints without the benefit of additional data. Certainly, these patients should be monitored and aggressively treated for infections likely to result in bacteremia and subsequent joint seeding. Additionally, foci of infection such as dental abscesses, skin infections, and urinary tract infections should be sought and treated prior to placement of the prosthetic device. It seems reasonable to target prophylaxis to those with higher risk of bad outcomes, such as patients with rheumatoid arthritis or those on immunosuppresive drugs, but precise data to defend this practice are limited.

C. Prevention of Other Late Infections in Indwelling Prostheses

There appear to be insufficient data to evaluate the risk or recommend appropriate prevention strategies for other prosthetic devices. Some have recommended prophylaxis for patients with vascular grafts for the first year after implantation on primarily theoretical grounds. No data are available to evaluate this practice. Similarly, others have been concerned about intraocular lens implants and cardiac pacemakers and defibrillators. In regard to the latter, the AHA recommends against the use of routine prophylaxis for these devices (53). No firm recommendations can be made about the intraocular lens implants.

III. FUTURE DIRECTIONS

With continued increases in the geriatric population, issues of appropriate prophylaxis for surgical procedures, infective endocarditis, and late prosthetic joint infections have become more prominent. The widespread publication of rational prevention strategies are of help to the practitioner in dealing with these common patient care issues. Cost-effective regimens for surgical prophylaxis are now better established, but the role of prevention with antibiotics requires better definition in clean procedures. The possibility of utilizing less expensive oral therapies needs to be addressed. In the prevention of infective endocarditis, assessing and improving efficacy and compliance seem to be needed. In addition, identification of additional risk groups and more standardized means of prevention in those with mitral valve prolapse could be undertaken. Late prosthetic joint infections will be an increasing problem as the procedures become more widespread. Basic data regarding the risks of invasive and routine procedures would immensely aid in our understanding of the problem.

REFERENCES

1. McDermott W, Rogers DE. Social ramifications of control of microbiologic disease. Johns Hopkins Med J 1982; 151:301–12.
2. Wenzel RP. Preoperative antibiotic prophylaxis. N Engl J Med 1992; 326:337–8.
3. Nichols RL. Surgical wound infection. Am J Med 1991; 91(suppl 3B):54S–64S.
4. Kaizer AB. Antimicrobial prophylaxis in surgery. N Engl J Med 1986; 315:1129–38.
5. Burke JF. The effective period of preventative antibiotic action in experimental incision and dermal lesions. Surgery 1961; 50:161–8.
6. Platt R. Antibiotic prophylaxis in surgery. Rev Infect Dis 1984; 6(S4):S880–86.
7. Crossley K, Gardner LC, Task Force on Prophylactic Antibiotics in Surgery. Antimicrobial prophylaxis in surgical patients. JAMA 1981; 245:722–6.
8. Redington J, Ebert SC, Craig WA. Role of antimicrobial pharmacokinetics and pharmacodynamics in surgical prophylaxis. Rev Infect Dis 1991; 13(suppl 10):S790–9.
9. Classen DC, Evans RS, Pestotnik SI, et al. The timing of prophylactic administration of antibiotics and the risk of surgical wound infection. N Engl J Med 1992; 326:281–6.
10. Sandusky WR. Use of prophylactic antibiotics in surgical patients. Surg Clin North Am 1980; 60:83–92.
11. Culver DH, Horan TC, Gaynes RP, et al., the National Nosocomial Infections Surveillance System. Surgical wound infection rates by wound class, operative procedure, and patient risk index. Am J Med 1991; 91(suppl 3B):152S–157S.
12. Hirschmann JV, Inui TS. Antimicrobial prophylaxis: a critique of recent trials. Rev Infect Dis 1980; 2:1–23.

13. Hopkins CC. Antibiotic prophylaxis in clean surgery: peripheral vascular surgery, noncardiovascular thoracic surgery, herniorrhaphy, and mastectomy. Rev Infect Dis 1991; 13(suppl 10):S869–73.
14. Platt R, Zaleznik DF, Hopkins CC, et al. Perioperative antibiotic prophylaxis for herniorrhaphy and breast surgery. N Engl J Med 1990; 322:153–60.
15. Waldvogel FA, Vaudaux PE, Pittet D, et al. Perioperative antibiotic prophylaxis of wound and foreign body infections: microbial factors affecting efficacy. Rev Infect Dis 1991; 13(suppl 10):S782–9.
16. Antimicrobial prophylaxis in surgery. Med Letter Drugs Ther 1992; 34:5–8.
17. Conte JE. Antibiotic prophylaxis: non-abdominal surgery. In: Remington JS, Swartz MN, eds. Current clinical topics in infectious diseases 10. Boston: Blackwell Scientific Publications, 1989:254–305.
18. Gorbach SL. Antimicrobial prophylaxis for appendectomy and colorectal surgery. Rev Infect Dis 1991; 13(suppl 10):S815–20.
19. Hemsell DL. Prophylactic antibiotics in gynecologic and obstetric surgery. Rev Infect Dis 1991; 13(suppl 10):S821–41.
20. Norden CW. Antibiotic prophylaxis in orthopedic surgery. Rev Infect Dis 1991; 13(suppl 10):S842–6.
21. Dellinger EP. Antibiotic prophylaxis in trauma: penetrating abdominal injuries and open fractures. Rev Infect Dis 1991; 13(suppl 10):S847–57.
22. Shapiro M. Prophylaxis in otolaryngologic surgery and neurosurgery: a critical review. Rev Infect Dis 1991; 13(suppl 10):S858–68.
23. McGowan JE. Cost and benefit of perioperative antimicrobial prophylaxis: methods for economic analysis. Rev Infect Dis 1991; 13(suppl 10):S879–89.
24. Lau WY, Chu KW, Poon GP, et al. Prophylactic antibiotics in elective colorectal surgery. Br J Surg 1988; 75:782–5.
25. Weaver M, Burdon DW, Youngs DJ, et al. Oral neomycin and erythromycin compared with single-dose systemic metronidazole and ceftriaxone propylaxis in elective colorectal surgery. Am J Surg 1986; 151:437–42.
26. Kaufman Z, Engelberg M, Eliashiv A, et al. Systemic prophylactic antibiotics in elective biliary surgery. Arch Surg 1984; 119:1002–4.
27. Lykkegaard NM, Moesgaard F, Justesen T, et al. Wound sepsis after elective cholecystectomy: restriction of prophylactic antibiotics to risk groups. Scand J Gastroenterol 1981; 16:937–40.
28. Nasser S. Prevention and treatment of sepsis in total hip replacement surgery. Orthoped Clin North Am 1992; 23:265–77.
29. Nelson CL. The prevention of infection in total joint replacement surgery. Rev Infect Dis 1987; 9:613–18.
30. Friedman RJ, Friedrich LV, White RL, et al. Antibiotic prophylaxis and tourniquet inflation in total knee arthroplasty. Clin Orthoped 1990; 260:17–23.
31. Persson U, Montgomery F, Carlsson A, et al. How far does prophylaxis against infection in total joint replacement offset its cost? Br Med J 1988; 250:99–102.
32. Josefsson G, Gudmundsson G, Kolmert L, et al. Prophylaxis with systemic antibiotics versus gentamicin bone cement in total hip arthroplasty. A five-year survey of 1688 hips. Clin Orthoped 1990; 253:173–8.
33. Henley MB, Jones RE, Wyatt RWB, et al. Prophylaxis with cefamandole nafate in elective orthopedic surgery. Clin Orthop 1986; 209:249–54.
34. Houle AM, Mokhless I, Sarto N, et al. Perioperative antibiotic prophylaxis for transurethral resection of the prostate: is it justifiable? J Urol 1989; 142:317–9.
35. Taylor EW, Lindsay G, West of Scotland Surgical Infection Study Group. Antibiotic prophylaxis in transurethral resection of the prostate with reference to the influence of preoperative catheterization. J Hosp Infect 1988; 12:75–83.

36. Prescott S, Hadi MA, Elton RA, et al. Antibiotic compared with antiseptic prophylaxis for prostatic surgery. Br J Urol 1990; 66:509–14.
37. Crawford ED, Berger NS, Davis MA, et al. Prevention of urinary tract infection and bacteremia following transurethral surgery: oral lomefloxacin compared to parenteral cefotaxime. J Urol 1992; 147:1053–5.
38. Cox CE. Comparison of intravenous ciprofloxacin and intravenous cefotaxime for antimicrobial prophylaxis in transurethral surgery. Am J Med 1989; 87(suppl 5A):252S–257S.
39. Marshall A. Prophylactic antimicrobial therapy in retropubic prostatectomy. Br J Urol 1959; 31:431–8.
40. Slavis SA, Miller JB, Golji H, et al. Comparison of single-dose antibiotic prophylaxis in uncomplicated transurethral resection of the prostate. J Urol 1992; 147:1303–6.
41. Kaiser AB, Clayson KR, Mulherin JL Jr, et al. Antibiotic prophylaxis in vascular surgery. Ann Surg 1978; 188:283–9.
42. Velanovich V. A meta-analysis of prophylactic antibiotics in head and neck surgery. Plastic Reconstr Surg 1991; 87:429–35.
43. Djindjian M, Lepresle E, Homs J. Antibiotic prophylaxis during prolonged clean neurosurgery. J Neurosurg 1990; 73:383–86.
44. Duff P, Gibbs RS, Jorgensen JH, et al. The pharmacokinetics of prophylactic antibiotics administered by intraoperative irrigation at the time of cesarean section. Obstet Gynecol 1982; 60:409–12.
45. Redington J, Ebert SC, Craig WA. Role of antimicrobial pharmacokinetics and pharmacodynamics in surgical prophylaxis. Rev Infect Dis 1991; 13(suppl 10):S790–9.
46. Wilson APR, Treasure T, Sturridge MF, et al. A scoring method (asepsis) for postoperative wound infections for use in clinical trials of antibiotic prophylaxis. Lancet 1986; 1:311–12.
47. Korzeniowski ON, Kaye D. Infective endocarditis. In: Braunwald E, ed. Heart disease. A textbook of cardiovascular medicine. 4th ed. Vol 2. Philadelphia: W.B. Saunders Company, 1992:1078–105.
48. Gantz NM. Geriatric endocarditis: avoiding the trend toward mismanagement. Geriatrics 1991; 46:66–8.
49. Kaye D. Changing pattern of infective endocarditis. Am J Med 1985; 78(suppl 6B):157–62.
50. Terpenning MS, Buggy BP, Kauffman CA. Infective endocarditis: clinical features in young and elderly patients. Am J Med 1987; 83:626–34.
51. Steckelberg JM, Melton LJ 3rd, Ilstrup DM, et al. Influence of referral bias on apparent clinical spectrum of infective endocarditis. Am J Med 1990; 88:582–8.
52. Friedlander AH, Yoshikawa TT. Pathogenesis, management and prevention of infective endocarditis in the elderly dental patient. Oral Surg Oral Med Oral Pathol 1990; 69:177–81.
53. Dajani AS, Bisno AL, Chung KJ, et al. Prevention of bacterial endocarditis. Recommendations by the American Heart Association. JAMA 1990; 264:2919–22.
54. Kaye D, Abrutyn E. Prevention of bacterial endocarditis: 1991. Ann Intern Med 1991; 114:803–4.
55. MacMahon SW, Hickey AJ, Wilcken DEL, et al. Risk of infective endocarditis in mitral valve prolapse with and without precordial systolic murmurs. Am J Cardiol 1986; 58:105–8.
56. Rahko PS. Prevalence of regurgitant murmurs in patients with valvular regurgitation detected by doppler echocardiography. Ann Intern Med 1989; 111:466–72.
57. Corrigall D, Smolen J, Hancock WE, et al. Mitral valve prolapse and infective endocarditis. Am J Med 1977; 63:215–22.
58. Devereux RB, Kramer-Fox R, Kligfield P. Mitral valve prolapse: causes, clinical manifestations, and management. Ann Intern Med 1989; 111:305–17.
59. Baddour LM, Bisno AL. Infective endocarditis complicating mitral valve prolapse: epidemiologic, clinical, and microbiologic aspects. Rev Infect Dis 1986; 8:117–37.
60. Cheng TO. Should antibiotic prophylaxis be recommended for all patients with mitral valve prolapse? Am J Cardiol 1991; 68:564.

61. Marks AR, Choong CY, Sanfilippo AJ, et al. Identification of high-risk and low-risk subgroups of patients with mitral-valve prolapse. N Engl J Med 1989; 320:1031–6.
62. Lavie CJ, Khandheria K, Seward JB, et al. Factors associated with the recommendation for endocarditis prophylaxis in mitral valve prolapse. JAMA 1989; 262:3308–12.
63. Nelson CL, Van Blaricum CS. Physician and dentist compliance with American Heart Association guidelines for prevention of bacterial endocarditis. JADA 1989; 118:169–73.
64. Durack DT, Kaplan EL, Bisno AL. Apparent failures of endocarditis prophylaxis. Analysis of 52 cases submitted to a national registry. JAMA 1983; 250:2318–22.
65. Imperiale TF, Horwitz RI. Does prophylaxis prevent postdental infective endocarditis? A controlled evaluation of protective efficacy. Am J Med 1990; 88:131–6.
66. van der Meer JTM, van Wijk W, Thompson J, et al. Efficacy of antibiotic prophylaxis for prevention of native-valve endocarditis. Lancet 1992; 339:135–9.
67. Rosen L, Abel ME, Gordon PH, et al. Practice parameters for antibiotic prophylaxis—supporting documentation. Dis Colon Rectum 1992; 35:278–85.
68. Meyer GW. Prophylaxis of infective endocarditis during colonoscopy. Report of a survey. Gastrointest Endosc 1981; 27:58–9.
69. Infection control during gastrointestinal endoscopy: guidelines for clinical application. Gastrointest Endosc 1988; 34:37S–40S
70. The American Society of Colon and Rectal Surgeons. Practice parameters for antibiotic prophylaxis to prevent infective endocarditis or infected prosthesis during colon and rectal endoscopy. Dis Colon Rectum 1992; 35:277.
71. Meyer GW. Endocarditis prophylaxis and gastrointestinal procedures. Am J Gastroenterol 1989; 84:1492–3.
72. Steinberg W. Antibiotic prophylaxis for gastrointestinal procedures: the case against antibiotics. Am J Gastroenterol 1990; 85:1043.
73. Neu HC, Fleischer D. Recommendations for antibiotic prophylaxis before endoscopy. Am J Gastroenterol 1989; 84:1488–91.
74. Baskin G. Prosthetic endocarditis after endoscopic variceal sclerotherapy: a failure of antibiotic prophylaxis. Am J Gastroenterol 1989; 84:311–12.
75. Davenport J. Late prosthetic joint infections: a problem for family physicians. Am Fam Physician 1989; 40:115–19.
76. Ainscow DA, Denham RA. The risk of haematogenous infection in total joint replacements. J bone Joint Surg (Br). 1984; 66:580–2.
77. Gristina AG, Kolkin J. Total joint replacement and sepsis. J Bone Joint Surg (Am) 1983; 65:128–34
78. Powers KA, Terpenning MS, Voice RA, et al. Prosthetic joint infections in the elderly. Am J Med 1990; 88:5-9N–5-13N.
79. Segreti J, Levin S. The role of prophylactic antibiotics in the prevention of prosthetic device infections. Infect Dis Clin North Am 1989; 3:357–70.
80. Council on Dental Therapeutics. Management of dental patients with prosthetic joints. JADA 1990; 121:537–8.
81. Simmons NA, Ball AP, Cawson RA, et al. Case against antibiotic prophylaxis for dental treatment of patients with joint prostheses. Lancet 1992; 339:301.
82. Thyne GM, Ferguson JW. Antibiotic prophylaxis during dental treatment in patients with prosthetic joints. J Bone Joint Surg (Br) 1991; 73-B:191–4.
83. Blackburn WD Jr, Alarcon GS. Prosthetic joint infections. A role for prophylaxis. Arth Rheum 1991; 34:110–17.
84. Tsevat J, Durand-Zaleski I, Pauker SG. Cost-effectiveness of antibiotic prophylaxis for dental procedures in patients with artificial joints. Am J Public Health 1989; 79:789–43.
85. Jacobson JJ, Schweitzer SO, Kowalski CJ. Chemoprophylaxis of prosthetic joint patients during dental treatment: a decision-utility analysis. Oral Surg Oral Med Oral Pathol 1991; 72:167–77.

31

Immunoprophylaxis

Stefan Gravenstein
University of Wisconsin, Madison, Wisconsin

Barbara A. Miller
Institute on Aging, Madison, Wisconsin

Paul J. Drinka
University of Wisconsin, Madison, and Wisconsin Veterans Home, King, Wisconsin

I. INTRODUCTION

Infection is the fourth leading cause of death in persons aged 65 and older. In addition to antimicrobial chemophrophylaxis, prevention of infectious diseases includes hygiene and isolation techniques. The spread of many infections, however, cannot be prevented with these simple measures because of drug costs, potential adverse drug reactions, development of antibiotic resistance, pathogen prevalence, and ease of transmission of the pathogen.

Immunoprophylaxis has been repeatedly demonstrated to be effective in preventing or limiting disease caused by a variety of pathogens including influenza viruses, *Streptococcus pneumoniae,* and *Clostridium tetani.* However, physicians in the United States and Canada frequently fail to administer recommended vaccinations.

For vaccine-preventable diseases, rapid humoral immunity has been an important determinant of protective efficacy and reduced pathogenicity. Because of lifelong experiences, it would be expected that acquired immunity increases with time. However, T-cell–dependent humoral immunity declines with age (immune senescence) (see Chap. 2). Hence the impact of many infectious diseases changes with age. Tetanus, pneumococcal, and influenza mortalities are dramatically influenced by age. For example, despite lifelong exposure to a variety of influenza viruses, influenza and pneumonia comprise the leading infectious cause of death in elderly persons. Also, tetanus occurs at the greatest rate among people aged 65 years and older. Living in long-term care facilities enhances the likelihood of infection such as influenza and pneumonia. Co-morbidity with cardiovascular or pulmonary disease increases susceptibility to infectious diseases, especially of the lower respiratory tract. Thus, factors affecting immune senescence and acquired immunity need to be considered when planning and preparing vaccine programs.

Pathogenic organisms that are spread by aerosol (e.g., tuberculosis and influenza) are of the greatest concern for person-to-person transmission and have caused outbreaks in closed settings such as long-term care facilities. Once such contagious organisms are in an institution, it is difficult to control the spread to susceptible persons. Under these circumstances, immunoprophylaxis is highly desirable as a means for primary prevention of institutional outbreaks.

Only influenza, pneumococcal, and tetanus-diphtheria vaccines are specifically recommended for routine use for persons 65 years and older by the Immunization Practices and Advisory Committee (1) and the American College of Physicians Task Force on Adult Immunization (2), although no vaccine is specifically contraindicated in this population. Although these vaccines are efficacious, immune senescence may impair vaccine-induced antibody response and cellular immunity. This impairment has led to considerable research to improve vaccine effectiveness, and this topic is reviewed elsewhere (3). This chapter will discuss primarily vaccination programs, the vaccines currently recommended for elderly people, and vaccine effectiveness.

A. Importance and Implementation of Organized Vaccination Programs

Control of vaccine-preventable infections depends on the delivery of effective vaccines. A suboptimal proportion of people aged 65 and older are immunized with the vaccines recommended by the Centers for Disease Control. Less than 30% of the aged target group received an annual influenza vaccine, less than 10% received the pneumococcal vaccine (4), and less than 20% are up to date with their tetanus-diphtheria toxoid booster vaccination. The low vaccination rates stem in part from difficulty in educating health practitioners and the public, both of whom have been described as uninformed (4). Immunization programs demonstrating substantially larger vaccination rates have been those in which formal vaccination programs are in place (5).

The types of vaccination programs that are successful differ depending on the setting, but the key factors seem to be education of the target population and health care providers as well as efficient use of personnel (6). If the vaccine is administered by a nurse, the medical consultation cost would be reduced. Nichol and coworkers (personal communication) have found that informational mailings with reminder postcards to patients receiving VA outpatient care was associated with high influenza vaccination rates. Their 60% vaccination acceptance rate may also have been attributed to inservices for clinic nurses and establishment of vaccination clinics. Whether such success would be achievable for other types of vaccines or in other clinical settings is unknown.

Policies in long-term care facilities could require that, upon admission, residents or guardians of incapacitated residents give consent for annual influenza vaccination (7). This saves time needed for annual consents. Generally, a physician's order must be written for this intervention. Having this order preprinted as a routine medication renewal will decrease the potential for a missed vaccination opportunity if the physician forgets to write this specific order. A tetanus-diphtheria (Td) toxoid booster is to be given every 10 years after completion of the primary series. One study found only a few nursing homes that responded to a survey had a policy to immunize residents with Td (8). Such a policy could be established to focus on Td boosters during decadal years, e.g., 1990, 2000, 2010. However, the cost effectiveness of this practice is unsubstantiated (see next section).

B. Cost Effectiveness of Vaccination Programs

Persons aged 65 and older currently comprise approximately 13% of the U.S. population, yet consume over half of the health care dollars. Much of the cost benefit from vaccination is derived by preventing expensive hospitalization and care required for such diseases as pneumonia. However, cost effectiveness depends upon vaccine efficacy, which differs between vaccines. Influenza (9,10) and pneumococcal (11–13) vaccines are each estimated to be 60–70% protective against pneumonia and hospitalization. It has been estimated from a prospective population-based study of 40,000 people conducted in Finland during 1981–82 (C. Jokinen, doctoral thesis, Kuopio University), that the baseline incidence of pneumonia for people aged 65 years and older was 30 cases/1000 persons/year. Consistent with this data was the 2% incidence of pneumonia among elderly persons in an enrolle-based study of Group Health care patients over a 3-month period from January to March of 1990 in the Minneapolis area (K. L. Nichol, personal communication). Both organisms may be responsible for 30–50% of all pneumonias in older persons (14). Thus, of the approximately 15 cases of influenza/1000 elderly individuals, 9 cases could be prevented with vaccination (14). The rate for pneumonia is 15–19 cases of pneumococcal pneumonia/1000 elderly persons, many of whom will have a concurrent or antecedent viral infection. Since approximately 90% of the pneumococcal pneumonias are caused by strains represented in the current pneumococcal vaccine, 7–12 cases of pneumococcal pneumonia/1000 elderly individuals could be prevented each year with vaccination (14). With a conservative estimated cost of care for pneumonia as $2500/case based on in-hospital costs only, a vaccinated United States elderly population of more than 30 million should save over $1 billion annually for the cases of influenza and pneumonia prevented. The annual cost of vaccination is approximately $11/person ($10/year influenza and $10 every 10 years for pneumococcal vaccine). Costs for vaccinating all elderly persons ($11 × 30 million) would net an annual savings of $0.7 billion in hospitalization costs alone.

Tetanus and diphtheria vaccines are highly effective in preventing disease and, thus, can potentially prevent several hundred cases of tetanus and diphtheria annually. The reported incidence of tetanus and diphtheria infection is low, but it is likely underestimated (see below). The net savings from vaccine-prevented disease are more difficult to calculate. The cost to prevent both tetanus and diphtheria is only $1/person/year ($10 for one vaccination every 10 years), or ~$30 million each year in the United States.

Medicare has covered the cost of pneumococcal vaccination since 1981, but the cost of influenza vaccination has not been covered except for persons residing in states participating in the Medicare Influenza Vaccine Demonstration program (1988–1992). Even if not covered by Medicare, insurers could save significant capital by underwriting at least the expense of influenza and pneumococcal vaccinations (15). As indicated above, assuming each vaccine costs $10, an annual net savings of $20/person in hospitalization costs could be anticipated. The cost effectiveness of tetanus vaccination in uncertain, but the cost per case prevented has been estimated over $1 million for a mail-reminder program targeting elderly Canadians (16). Thus, the benefit of tetanus vaccination to the population at large may be debatable, but it could be more cost effective if only high-risk older individuals were targeted for routine vaccination. [Editor's note: Beginning in 1993, Medicare will pay for cost of influenza vaccination.]

II. INFLUENZA

Influenza-related illness costs more health care dollars and lives lost than any other virus-caused disease in the United States. The influenza virus genome is segmented so that different combinations of segments yield a phenotypically different virus. The process of recombination of the genetic segments is referred to as antigenic shift. Antigenic drift or point mutations of the genome also occurs. These phenomena enable the influenza virus to escape immune recognition and allow annual epidemics (as with antigenic drift) or pandemics (as with antigenic shift). (See also Chap. 25.)

Typically, influenza infection causes abrupt fever and sore throat. Elderly persons are at increased risk for complications related to secondary bacterial infection, and they are more likely to require hospitalization and experience a higher mortality rate. Over 80% of the influenza-related deaths occur in persons 65 or more years old (17). Influenza and pneumonia rank fifth among the leading causes of death in persons aged 65 years and older and fourth in persons aged 75 years and older (18). In nursing homes, up to 70% of the residents may contract influenza-like illnesses during an outbreak; during nonepidemic years an attack rate of 10–20% is the norm. The case fatality ratio during an outbreak may be as high as 30% (19). Because individuals over 80 years of age are the fastest growing segment of the United States population (20), the impact of influenza will continue to intensify unless we attain better control of the disease.

A. Vaccine Effectiveness

The cornerstone to influenza prevention remains vaccination. Vaccination is far more cost effective than the alternative intervention, i.e., amantadine prophylaxis (10). A well-matched vaccine is effective in reducing the incidence and severity of influenza illnesses. Vaccination can reduce the number of influenza-related hospitalizations, radiologically diagnosed cases of pneumonia, and deaths (9,10,21).

Amantadine and rimantidine can complement vaccination, but their use to prevent influenza A infections is not cost effective if given for the duration of influenza A presence in the community. When amantadine is used to treat influenza A symptoms, it is therapeutic if given within the first 48 h of onset of illness; its efficacy in elderly recipients who are treated later in their illness remains unproved. (See also Chap. 25.)

Despite these preventive measures, outbreaks of influenza occur annually. The influenza vaccine can fail to provide the intended protection because of several factors including immune senescence, weak vaccine immunogenicity, lack of herd immunity, antigenic drift, or antigenic shift. Because of advanced age and underlying disease, only about one half of nursing home residents develop "protective" vaccine-induced antibody titers compared with 70–90% of young healthy adults. Supplemental vaccination and vaccines with higher concentrations of antigen have not consistently demonstrated increased antibody response in elderly persons, but they have demonstrated more side effects (22). Nevertheless, elderly persons may benefit from vaccination despite low antibody titers; the influenza illness may be less severe and the risk of complications, hospitalization, and death may be reduced.

Retrospective studies of vaccine efficacy following influenza outbreaks have found that vaccine efficacy varies from about 30 to 80% (21). However, one prospective study suggested that the Centers for Disease Control and Prevention case definition for influenza may only be 51% sensitive and 63% specific for detecting laboratory-confirmed H3N2 influenza (23). The low sensitivity and specificity of this case definition (oral temperature $\geq$ 100°F accompanied by either sore throat, cough, or coryza) may occur because the clinical features of an influenza illness are largely indistinguishable from other viral illnesses that occur primarily during the influenza season. The sensitivity of the case definition for influenza may also be reduced because elderly persons are less likely to have a fever in response to infection and therefore do not meet the temperature requirement of the case definition (24). Clinical influenza may also be attenuated in previously vaccinated individuals, further compromising the case definition's sensitivity. Thus, retrospective studies reporting vaccine efficacy relying on clinical symptoms for case detection may underestimate the ability of the vaccine to prevent infection. Nevertheless, when infection occurs in vaccinated individuals, the vaccine is quite effective in preventing serious morbidity and death. Reduction of influenza-associated hospitalization and death has been reported in both community and nursing home settings (9,10).

B. Indications

Annual influenza vaccination is recommended for high-risk individuals and their caregivers, including physicians. High-risk individuals include residents of nursing homes and other long-term care facilities, persons ≥65 years of age, those with chronic disorders of the pulmonary or cardiovascular system, and those requiring regular medical follow-up or hospitalization during the preceding year because of chronic metabolic disorders, renal dysfunction, hemoglobinopathies, or immunosuppression (17).

Annual influenza vaccination rates in nursing homes across the United States range from 0 to 100% (10,21,25). The proportion of vaccinated nursing home staff is frequently less than 30% (21). The rate of vaccination of nursing home residents and staff depends on the energy and enthusiasm of the medical director, director of nursing, and/or infection control practitioner, as well as implementation of nursing home education programs and vaccination policies.

One purpose of influenza immunization programs in long-term care facilities is to induce herd immunity, thereby reducing the probability of virus transmission within a population (26). The ambitious vaccination rate of 80% for residents and staff is calculated to generate herd immunity, and it is a goal that nursing homes should set.

C. Administration and Revaccination

An intramuscular injection of 0.5 ml of the trivalent influenza vaccine is recommended in the United States. Although subcutaneous and intradermal routes have been used, their efficacy has not been adequately compared. Annual vaccination is necessary as the protective response to current influenza vaccines is short-lived and the virus's rapid antigenic change renders the previous year's vaccine ineffective.

The question of optimum timing of the influenza vaccine is important and not easily answered. If vaccination takes place too early, protective antibody titers may no longer be present when the virus circulates, while late vaccination permits viral exposure before protective antibody develops. Because it may take 4–6 weeks for elderly individuals to develop optimum antibody titers (27), it is advisable to vaccinate 4–6 weeks before the influenza season is expected. In most states, vaccination during November is reasonable, while vaccination during August and September is probably premature. Influenza typically circulates from December to March, making vaccination of new staff and residents in January or later justifiable. When an influenza outbreak is identified, unvaccinated staff and residents should be reoffered the vaccine. Those accepting the vaccine during an influenza A outbreak should also be offered amantadine for the 2-week interim following vaccination to allow time to develop vaccine-induced immunity. Unvaccinated persons with acceptably low risks for amantadine-associated side effects should be offered amantadine for the duration of the influenza A outbreak.

D. Adverse Reactions

The unfounded concern that the influenza vaccine causes an influenza illness constitutes a major obstacle to vaccination (28). Because the current vaccine contains only noninfectious virus particles, preservatives, and trace amounts of egg protein, it *cannot* cause an influenza infection. Occasional cases of respiratory disease following vaccination represent coincidental illnesses unrelated to the vaccine (17). Less than one-third of influenza vaccine recipients complain of injection site tenderness for 1–2 days following vaccination. Fever, malaise, or myalgia occur in less than 10% of vaccine recipients and most often in persons naive to the influenza vaccine. The rate of these systemic reactions in elderly people is similar to that in saline placebo recipients (29). The potential for an allergic-type response exists, although it is rare. These reactions likely result from hypersensitivity to vaccine components like residual egg proteins or vaccine preservatives. Only the 1976 influenza vaccine was associated with the Guillain-Barré syndrome (six cases), and this relationship is not expected to recur. The influenza vaccine is contraindicated in persons with anaphylactic hypersensitivity to eggs. Persons with an acute febrile illness (temperature $> 100°F$) may be vaccinated when the fever abates. Pregnancy (in care providers) is not a contraindication for vaccination (17).

The dose of amantadine treatment and prophylaxis should be adjusted for creatinine clearance because the drug is principally cleared by the kidneys. The usual dosage for older adults who do not have significant renal impairment is 100 mg a day (standard dosage for younger adults is 100 mg twice daily). The benefits of symptom amelioration and protection against influenza A infection must outweigh the side effects. Amantadine can cause confusion, dizziness, and insomnia, and increases the risk for falls in elderly people. The risks for amantadine side effects are greater in persons with a history of confusion, agitation, or balance disturbance. Persons with seizure disorders should not receive amantadine.

III. TETANUS AND DIPHTHERIA

Although tetanus and diphtheria are completely preventable, partially or nonimmunized individuals acquire these diseases each year. Tetanus has become a disease of older adults. Although tetanus is a rare disease in the United States, 60% of tetanus cases occur in people over 60 years of age, and the case fatality ratio is approximately 50% in this population (30). In the United States, 560 cases of tetanus were reported in 1947, but fewer than 330 cases were reported in the last 5 years combined (31). Similarly, 11 cases of diphtheria occurred in the United States between 1985 and 1989 (31). About a third of diphtheria cases occurred in persons aged over 60 years. The morbidity and mortality of these diseases is expected to grow in the future as America's aging population increases over the next 40 years, since this age group has low levels of immunity (32).

A. Tetanus (see also Chap. 28)

Tetanus is an acute illness caused by the neurotoxin produced by *Clostridium tetani,* an ubiquitous anaerobic, spore-forming bacillus. Its typical clinical presentation is tonic rigidity and painful spasms of the masseter and cervical muscles; less frequently, trunk and other muscles are involved. The case fatality ratio remains near 50%, which is virtually unchanged in the last several decades (33); some believe the mortality data may be underreported (34). The risk for tetanus and its associated mortality increases with age. Elderly persons are more prone to this disease principally because (1) the proportion of individuals with protective antitoxin levels declines with age; (2) vascular ulcers and surgical wounds are more common in older people; and (3) hospitalized or institutionalized elderly persons may develop pressure ulcers. An estimated 10% of people are fecal carriers of *C. tetani,* which makes pressure ulcers high-risk lesions for potential contamination. Twenty percent of tetanus cases have been associated with chronic wounds or abscesses, and 55% of these cases occurred in individuals age 60 and over. Clinical tetanus might be unrecognized and underreported in debilitated elderly patients who die with malnutrition and necrotic skin lesions. The overall decline in the occurrence of tetanus has been secured by widespread use of the tetanus toxoid vaccine and improved wound care. Wound cleaning, debridement, and proper immunization are important. If a contaminated wound is found in a person who has not completed a primary series, tetanus immune globulin should be given if no contraindication exists. A booster alone is appropriate if the patient completed a primary series but has not received tetanus toxoid within the preceding 5 years. A thorough attempt should be made to determine whether a person has completed primary immunization. Patients with unknown or uncertain previous immunization histories should be considered to have no previous tetanus toxoid doses. Persons who had military service since 1941 can be considered to have received at least one dose, although most may have completed a primary series. However, this cannot be assumed for all persons. The number of people at risk for tetanus will increase unless elderly persons are more conscientiously given tetanus toxoid vaccines.

A study of 69 nursing home residents with an average age of 80 years found 51% with protective antitetanus antibodies (35). Another study of 111 institutionalized elderly persons in Los Angeles with an average age of 82 years reported 29% with protective antitetanus titers (32). Protective antibody titers decline with age, especially in elderly women, while elderly men with previous military service show better immunity to tetanus (36).

B. Diphtheria (see also Chap. 28)

The incidence of diphtheria has gradually declined to only a few cases each year (37). As with tetanus, such cases are limited to partially or nonimmunized individuals, the majority of whom are elderly persons. Diphtheria results from a toxin elaborated by a noninvasive organism, *Corynebacterium diphtheriae,* which replicates in wounds such as surgical sites, abrasions, and injured mucous membranes. The toxin typically induces symptoms of moderate fever, malaise, and sore throat with a local exudative necrosis and characteristic pseudomembrane in the respiratory tract or on the skin that rapidly spreads (within hours) and is associated with systemic toxemia. Major complications include thrombocytopenia, myocarditis, and cranial or peripheral nerve involvement.

Widespread use of diphtheria toxoid in United States has limited the annual occurrence of the disease to five cases, and a case fatality rate less than 10%. More than 90% of diphtheria cases occur in adults, virtually all of whom are unprotected. About half (41–84%) of adults aged 60 years or older have protective titers of circulating antitoxin. Adult susceptibility to diphtheria reflects reduced lifetime exposure (to *C. diphtheriae*) and failure to administer the primary series of the vaccine and decadal boosters throughout life.

C. Vaccine Effectiveness

Tetanus-diphtheria toxoids (Td) are among the most immunogenic of vaccines indicated for older adults, and they are virtually 100% effective in immunocompetent adults who have kept their vaccination status up to date. Naturally acquired immunity to tetanus toxin does not occur. Evidence indicates that complete primary immunization with tetanus toxoid provides 10 or more years of protection. Appropriately timed boosters are needed to maintain antitoxin titers.

Recent outbreaks of diphtheria in countries where the disease had been considered eliminated highlights the risk for outbreaks of diphtheria even in populations with high rates of immunization (38,39). Following a 23-year period without reported cases of diphtheria, the disease reemerged in Sweden. Although 95–99% of the children were vaccinated and 81% of the population under 20 years of age had protective immunity, only 19% of women and 44% of men over 60 years of age had protective immunity (40). All those individuals who died or had neurological complications had low levels of antibodies, while 33 of 36 symptom-free carriers of the same strain had protective antibody titers. In the United States, the number of older adults with protective antibody to both tetanus and diphtheria is similarly low (36,41), making an experience similar to the one in Sweden likely if we are unable to better vaccinate our population.

D. Indications

All elderly persons should be actively immunized against both tetanus and diphtheria through the initial primary series and then revaccinated every 10 years. Anyone who has not received the complete primary series should complete it with the combined Td vaccine, although earlier doses need not be repeated if the schedule is delayed. A booster dose even 30 years after primary vaccination results in rapid protection for both tetanus and diphtheria. Getting the series up to date is especially relevant if travel to developing countries is anticipated.

Td prophylaxis is recommended with clean, minor wounds if the primary series is incomplete or the last booster vaccination was more than 10 years ago. More serious wounds require both active and passive immunization.

The Canadian experience of few adult cases of tetanus was reviewed, and the need for booster immunization programs for adults was questioned (42). Tetanus is rare enough such that the cost for each case prevented and for each year of life gained is large, resulting in a recommendation to target only high-risk adults, such as those with vascular ulcers or those seen at time of injury, for revaccination (16). Benefits may actually be greater than previously thought if tetanus is underdiagnosed in debilitated malnourished nursing home residents who die with chronic skin ulcers.

E. Administration and Revaccination

The primary series used for adults consists of two 0.5-ml doses of Td given intramuscularly at least 4 weeks apart, followed by a third 0.5-ml dose 6 or more months later. The Td vaccine contains only 10% of the diphtheria toxoid contained in the pediatric DTP, making it much less reactogenic.

F. Adverse Reactions

Present vaccines have been well tolerated with minimal reactions. The high reactogenicity of childhood DTP vaccines has been largely attributed to the pertussis component. The only contraindication to tetanus and diphtheria toxoid is a history of a neurological or severe hypersensitivity reaction after a previous dose, or sensitivity to the preservative.

In previously immunized adults, the local reactions rate is 40–50%. Less than 10% of vaccinees develop an area of redness or swelling larger than 5 cm (43). Potential side effects include local reactions, fever, chills, hypersensitivity, arthralgia, rash, and encephalopathy. Reactions may be related to high antitoxin titers or mediated by hypersensitivity to the mercury preservative.

Td vaccination occurred without major sequelae following a vaccination program for 161 institutionalized veterans. Nine percent of the participants had local reactions generally considered insignificant. One person fell. The single fall, with the associated risk for fracture, was attributable to a sore deltoid muscle. A sore arm may be only a minor inconvenience in a healthy adult, however, an individual who depends on arm support for environmental stability and transfers may be placed at risk for falls and fractures.

IV. PNEUMOCOCCAL DISEASE

Pneumococcal disease remains a significant cause of morbidity and mortality in all populations (44). Pneumococcal pneumonia ranks as one of the 10 leading causes of death. In the United Kingdom, over a third of pneumonias resulting in hospitalization are pneumococcal infections. An estimated 45–95 cases of pneumococcal pneumonia occur annually per 100,000 persons in the United States. This figure increases to 150–250 cases per 100,000 persons aged 65 years and older (1). An estimated 40,000 deaths occur annually in the United States from all pneumococcal disease (1).

Streptococcus pneumoniae is a facultative gram-positive organism closely related to other streptococci. It usually occurs in pairs or short chains when viewed by microscopy. Virulent organisms are encapsulated and usually spread by respiratory secretions. Asymptomatic colonization of the nasopharynx averages between 25 and 50% in children and 5% in adults. The organism can give rise to systemic manifestations such as septicemia and meningitis. Pneumococcal otitis media, which is common among children, is unusual in elderly individuals. Besides extremes of age, associated risk factors for developing pneumococcal infections and their complications are immune deficiency, metabolic abnormality, and chronic cardiovascular or pulmonary disease.

A. Vaccine Effectiveness

There are currently 83 known serotypes of *S. pneumoniae* based on differences in the polysaccharide capsule. Many of these serotypes are closely related to each other and to other encapsulated organisms. Although the protective antibody titer has not been determined, protective immunity to pneumococcal pneumonia is directly related to an individual's titer of type-specific anticapsular polysaccharide antibody (45,46). Vaccine efficacy against pneumococcal pneumonia varies among studies and ranges between 0 and to 77% (47,48). Variations or biases in study design and populations may account for this wide range. Despite the variance in reported efficacy, there is evidence that vaccination is worthwhile, especially in elderly persons.

In most cases of pneumococcal pneumonia, antibiotics can be used to treat the disease; however, the emergence of multiple antibiotic–resistant strains of *S. pneumoniae* and development of irreversible physiologic lung damage with invasive disease emphasize the importance of immunoprophylaxis. The current 23-valent vaccine that was licensed in 1983 contains 88% of the most frequently reported capsular types of *S. pneumoniae.* Vaccines composed of purified pneumococcal capsular polysaccharide have been shown in adults to be effective in preventing infections against serotypes included in the vaccine, but the duration of protective antibody levels appears to be age-dependent. A case-controlled study showed that invasive pneumococcal infection was a measure for vaccine efficacy (48). Pneumococcal vaccine was 93% effective in those aged under 55 years, but only 46% effective in those aged over 84 years in individuals vaccinated during the previous 3 years. Overall efficacy was 61%.

B. Indications

Healthy adults aged 65 years and older and those with increased risk for infection or complications from infection should be vaccinated. Those with chronic cardiac and pulmonary disease, functional or anatomical asplenia, chronic liver disease, alcoholism, and diabetes mellitus are especially at risk. Reduced vaccine responses can be expected in those with anatomical asplenia, functional asplenia (lymphomas), hematological malignancies, chronic renal failure (whether or not receiving dialysis), or those receiving immunosuppressive therapy (transplant recipients, chest or bone radiotherapy, and chemotherapy). Ideally, individuals should receive their primary vaccination 2 weeks or more before splenectomy or immunosuppressive therapy.

C. Administration and Revaccination

The duration of vaccine-induced protection is not known but believed to last several years (45). Antibody titers fall over the years in elderly persons, and revaccination 6 years after the initial vaccination is recommended for those persons with reduced vaccine responses, such as individuals with asplenia, nephrotic syndrome, renal failure, or organ transplants. Recommendation to revaccinate other elderly individuals cannot yet be made. Early reports suggest an increased risk for side effects with revaccination, but these data were not acquired from elderly subjects (49,50). Serious side effects may be uncommon with revaccination among elderly vaccinees (51). Total antibody response in revaccinated individuals may be somewhat less than that following primary vaccination.

D. Adverse Reactions

As expected, some injection site tenderness, erythema, or induration may occur. Fever, myalgia, and severe local reactions have been reported in <1% of those vaccinated. Severe systemic reactions are rare. Simultaneous vaccination with the influenza vaccine will not increase the risk for side effects and will provide antibody responses to both vaccines. The injections should be given at different sites. Serious adverse reactions have not been reported among persons recommended to be revaccinated. Arthuslike reactions are infrequent in persons revaccination with the 23-valent formulation after initial vaccination with the older 14-valent formulation.

ACKNOWLEDGMENTS

Supported by NIH Grants (KO8-AG00548-01 and RO1-AG09632-01A1) and the University of Wisconsin Graduate and Medical Schools. This is publication number 53 Madison VA GRECC.

REFERENCES

1. Centers for Disease Control. Update on adult immunization. Recommendations of the Immunization Practices Advisory Committee (ACIP). MMWR 1991; 40:1–94.
2. American College of Physicians. Guide for adult immunization. 2nd ed. Philadelphia: American College of Physicians, 1990:15–17
3. Powers DC. Immunological principles and emerging strategies of vaccination for the elderly. J Am Geriatr Soc 1992; 40:81–94.

4. Williams WW, Hickson MA, Kane MA, et al. Immunization policies and vaccine coverage among adults. Ann Intern Med 1988; 108:616–25.
5. Siewert M, Drinka PJ, Langer E. A successful nursing home vaccination program. Am J Infect Control 1988; 16:228–30.
6. Nichol KL, Korn JE, Baum P. Estimation of outpatient risk characteristics and influenza vaccination status: validation of a self-administered questionnaire. Am J Prev Med 1991; 7:199–203.
7. Gravenstein S, Miller BA, Drinka P. Prevention and control of influenza A outbreaks in long-term care facilities. Infect Control Hosp Epidemiol 1992; 13:49–54.
8. Richardson JP, Knight AL, Stafford DT. Beliefs and policies of Maryland nursing home medical directors regarding tetanus immunization. J Am Geriatr Soc 1990; 38:1316–20.
9. Barker WH, Mullooly JP. Influenza vaccination of elderly persons. Reduction in pneumonia and influenza hospitalizations and deaths. JAMA 1980; 244:2547–49.
10. Patriarca PA, Weber JA, Meissner MA, et al. Use of influenza vaccine in nursing homes. J Am Geriatr Soc 1985; 33:463–6.
11. Bolan G, Broome CV, Facklam RR, et al. Pneumococcal vaccine efficacy in selected populations in the United States. Ann Intern Med 1986; 104:1–6.
12. Shapiro ED, Berg AT, Austrian R, et al. The protective efficacy of polyvalent pneumococcal polysaccharide vaccine. N Engl J Med 1991; 325:1453–60.
13. Sims RV, Steinmann WC, McConville JH, et al. The clinical effectiveness of pneumococcal vaccine in the elderly. Ann Intern Med 1988; 108:653–7.
14. Mäkelä PH, Jokinen C, Pyhälä R, et al. Use of vaccines for respiratory infections; strategies for influenza and pneumococcal vaccines. Scand J Infect Dis 1990; 70(suppl):141–8.
15. Fedson DS. Clinical practice and public policy for influenza and pneumococcal vaccination of the elderly. Clin Geriatr Med 1992; 8:183–99.
16. Hutchison BG, Stoddart GL. Cost-effectiveness of primary tetanus vaccination among elderly Canadians. Can Med Assoc J 1988; 139:1143–51.
17. ACIP. Prevention and control of influenza. Recommendations of the Immunization Practices Advisory Committee. MMWR 1992; 41:1–17.
18. Silverberg E, Lubera Ja. Cancer statistics 1989. Cancer 1989; 39:3–20.
19. Patriarca PA, Weber JA, Parker RA, et al. Efficacy of influenza vaccine in nursing homes. JAMA 1985; 253:1136–9.
20. Schneider EL, Guralnik JM. The aging of America. Impact of health care costs. JAMA 1990; 263:2335–40.
21. Kendal AP, Patriarca PA, Arden NH. Policies and outcomes for control of influenza among the elderly in the USA. Vaccine 1985; 3(suppl):274–6.
22. Peters NL, Meiklejohn G, Jahnigen DW. Antibody response of an elderly population to a supplemental dose of influenza B vaccine. J Am Geriatr Soc 1988; 36:593–9.
23. Gravenstein S, Miller BA, Ershler WB, et al. Low sensitivity of CDC case definition for H3N2 influenza in elderly nursing home subjects. Clin Res 1990; 38:547A.
24. Yoshikawa T. Approach to the diagnosis and treatment of the infected older adult. In: Hazzard WR, Andres R, Bierman EL, Blass JP, eds. Principles of geriatric medicine and gerontology. New York: McGraw-Hill, 1990:1055–61.
25. Arden NH, Patriarca PA, Kendal AP. Experiences in the use and efficacy of inactivated influenza vaccine in nursing homes. In: Kendal AP, Patriarca PA, eds. Options for the control of influenza. New York: Alan R. Liss, 1986:155–68.
26. Fox JP, Elveback L, Scott W, et al. Herd immunity: basic concept and relevance to public health immunization practices. Am J Epidemiol 1971; 94:179–89.
27. Gravenstein S, Duthie EH, Miller BA, et al. Augmentation of influenza antibody response in elderly men by thymosin alpha one. A double-blind placebo-controlled clinical study. J Am Geriatr Soc 1989; 37:1–8.

28. Centers for Disease Control. Adult immunization: knowledge, attitudes and practices-DeKalb and Fulton Counties, Georgia, 1988. MMWR 1988; 37:657–64.
29. Margolis KL, Nichol KL, Poland GA, et al. Frequency of adverse reactions to influenza vaccine in the elderly. A randomized, placebo-controlled trial. JAMA 1990; 264:1139–41.
30. Centers for Disease Control. Tetanus—United States, 1987 and 1988. JAMA 1990; 263:1192, 1195.
31. Centers for Disease Control. Diphtheria, tetanus, and pertussis: recommendations for vaccine use and other preventive measures. Recommendations of the Immunization Practices Advisory Committee (ACIP). MMWR 1991; 40:1–28.
32. Weiss BP, Strassburg MA, Feeley JC. Tetanus and diphtheria immunity in an elderly population in Los Angeles County. Am J Public Health 1983; 73:802–4.
33. Faust RA, Vickers OR, Cohn I. Tetanus: 2449 cases in 68 years at a charity hospital. J Trauma 1976; 16:704–12.
34. Sutter RW, Cochi SL, Brink EW, et al. Assessment of vital statistics and surveillance data for monitoring tetanus mortality, United States, 1979–1984. Am J Epidemiol 1990; 131:132–42.
35. Ruben F, Nagel J, Fireman P. Antitoxin response in the elderly to tetanus-diphtheria (TD) immunization. Am J Epidemiol 1978; 108:145–49.
36. Gareau AB, Eby RJ, McLellan BA, et al. Tetanus immunization status and immunologic response to a booster in an emergency department geriatric population. Ann Emerg Med 1990; 19:1377–82.
37. Mumford RS, Ory HW, Brooks GF, et al. Diphtheria deaths in the United States, 1959–1970. JAMA 1974; 229:1890–3.
38. Rappuoli R, Perugini M, Falsen E. Molecular epidemiology of the 1984–1986 outbreak of diphtheria in Sweden. N Engl J Med 1988; 318:12–14.
39. Karzon DT, Edwards KM. Diphtheria outbreaks in immunized populations. N Engl J Med 1988; 318:41–3.
40. Christenson B, Böttiger M. Serological immunity to diphtheria in Sweden in 1978 and 1984. Scand J Infect Dis 1986; 18:227–33.
41. Crossley K, Irvine P, Warren JB, et al. Tetanus and diphtheria immunity in urban Minnesota adults. JAMA 1979; 242:2298–300.
42. Mathias RG, Schechter MT. Booster immunisation for diphtheria and tetanus: no evidence of need in adults. Lancet 1985; 1:1089–91.
43. Björkholm B, Granström M, Wahl M, et al. Adverse reactions and immunogenicity in adults to regular and increased dosage of diphtheria vaccine. Eur J Clin Microbiol 1987; 6:637–40.
44. Mufson MA, Krause HE, Schiffman G, et al. Pneumococcal antibody levels one decade after immunization of healthy adults. Am J Med Sci 1987; 293:279–84.
45. Koskela M. Serum antibodies to pneumococcal C polysaccharide in children: response to acute pneumococcal otitis media or to vaccination. Pediatr Infect Dis J 1987; 6:519–26.
46. Lee CJ. Bacterial capsular polysaccharide-biochemistry, immunity, and vaccine. Mol Immunol 1987; 24:1005–19.
47. Simberkoff MS, Cross AP, Al-Ibrahim M, et al. Efficacy of pneumococcal vaccine in high-risk patients. Results of a Veterans Administration Cooperative Study. N Engl J Med 1986; 315:1318–27.
48. Shapiro ED, Berg AT, Austrian R, et al. The protective efficacy of polyvalent pneumococcal polysaccharide vaccine. N Engl J Med 1991; 325:1453–60.
49. Borgono JM, McLean AA, Vella PP, et al. Vaccination and revaccination with polyvalent pneumococcal polysaccharide vaccines in adults and infants. Proc Soc Exp Biol Med 1978; 157:148–54.
50. Schwartz JS. Pneumococcal vaccine: clinical efficacy and effectiveness. Ann Intern Med 1982; 96:208–20.
51. Mufson MA, Hughey DF, Turner CE, et al. Revaccination with pneumococcal vaccine of elderly persons 6 years after primary vaccination. Vaccine 1991; 9:403–7.

Index

About the Editors

THOMAS T. YOSHIKAWA is Assistant Chief Medical Director for Geriatrics and Extended Care at the United States Department of Veterans Affairs Central Office, and Adjunct Professor of Health Care Sciences at George Washington University School of Medicine, Washington, D.C. The coauthor or coeditor of several books that examine geriatric care and infectious diseases, he is a Fellow of the Infectious Diseases Society of America, the Gerontological Society of America, and the American College of Physicians, and a member of the American Geriatrics Society, the American Federation for Clinical Research, and the American Society for Microbiology. Dr. Yoshikawa received the M.D. degree (1966) from the University of Michigan, Ann Arbor.

DEAN C. NORMAN is Chief of Staff at the West Los Angeles Veterans Affairs Medical Center, California, and Associate Professor of Medicine at the University of California School of Medicine, Los Angeles. He is a member of the Gerontological Society of America, the Infectious Diseases Society of America, the American Geriatrics Society, and the American Federation for Clinical Research, among other organizations, and the coauthor of one book and the author or coauthor of over 120 professional papers, book chapters, and abstracts. Dr. Norman received the M.D. degree (1976) from the University of California Medical School, Los Angeles.